# Communicating About Health

# Communicating About Health

*Current Issues and Perspectives*

THIRD EDITION

## Athena du Pré
*University of West Florida*

New York   Oxford
OXFORD UNIVERSITY PRESS
2010

Oxford University Press, Inc., publishes works that further Oxford University's
objective of excellence in research, scholarship, and education.

Oxford    New York
Auckland    Cape Town    Dar es Salaam    Hong Kong    Karachi
Kuala Lumpur    Madrid    Melbourne    Mexico City    Nairobi
New Delhi    Shanghai    Taipei    Toronto

With offices in
Argentina    Austria    Brazil    Chile    Czech Republic    France    Greece
Guatemala    Hungary    Italy    Japan    Poland    Portugal    Singapore
South Korea    Switzerland    Thailand    Turkey    Ukraine    Vietnam

Copyright © 2010 by Oxford University Press, Inc.

Published by Oxford University Press, Inc.
198 Madison Avenue, New York, New York 10016
http://www.oup.com

Oxford is a registered trademark of Oxford University Press

**Library of Congress Cataloging-in-Publication Data**
Du Pré, Athena.
    Communicating about health : current issues and perspectives / Athena du Pré.—3rd ed.
       p. ; cm.
    Includes bibliographical references and index.
    ISBN 978-0-19-538033-0 (pbk. : alk. paper)    1. Communication in medicine.    2. Medical personnel and patient.    3. Health
education.    4. Health promotion.    I. Title.
    [DNLM:    1. Communication.    2. Delivery of Health Care.    3. Health Promotion.    4. Interprofessional Relations.
5.  Professional-Patient Relations. W 84.1 D942c 2010]
    R118.D87 2010
    613—dc22
                                                                                                        2009001737

9  8  7  6  5  4  3  2  1

Printed in the United States of America
on acid-free paper

# CONTENTS

**Part II. The Roles of Patients
and Caregivers**

*Chapter 3*
**PATIENT–CAREGIVER
COMMUNICATION**  47

## *Chapter 4*
## CAREGIVER PERSPECTIVE 75

### BOXES

## *Chapter 5*
## PATIENT PERSPECTIVE 109

### Chapter 6
## DIVERSITY AMONG PATIENTS 131

My fascination with health communication began with individuals who were generous enough to share their stories:

- the woman who allowed me to be present when the bandages were removed from her eyes and she saw her children for the first time in 20 years
- the 34-year-old police officer I met in his parents' front room, occupying the left side of a hospital bed, the right side reserved for his faithful canine companion, Shep, who, along with hospice, provided warmth and comfort during the final joyful and sad months of the man's life
- the doctor who ushered everyone from the room when the patient (myself) seemed scared and nervous. "She's shaking," exclaimed Dr. Williamson. Then she sent everyone away and sat on the edge of my bed, holding my hands in hers to warm them, telling me that, in Japan, long fingers like mine are revered as a sign of beauty.

Stories such as these occur every day in health settings. I've been privileged to witness them as a news reporter, a public relations director, a researcher, and sometimes a participant. Such stories are the reason we do what we do—whether that be designing health campaigns, caring directly for patients, helping manage and guide health care organizations, researching and teaching health communication, or studying the issues so that we and our loved ones will be better prepared when we are the patients.

In this edition of *Communicating About Health: Current Issues and Perspectives* my objective is twofold: (1) to update coverage of the latest issues and research (and there is a lot of exciting news to cover) and (2) to give voice to the stories of people who live and embody the issues we study. If I have been successful, you will find this to be an insightful, rich, and thorough overview of health communication. My wish is that readers come away with sophisticated knowledge about current issues and research, a real-life appreciation of the human side of health care and advocacy, and practical strategies for communicating more effectively and ethically about health.

## MY APPROACH

Because health care is so dynamic and complex, it's difficult to keep up with everything. We feel we're doing well to stay up to date in any one sector. That's understandable. But it's also the greatest weakness in the system, and it can be a fatal flaw. As specialists, we miss opportunities for innovative teamwork. Our efforts are often duplicative and contradictory. And we often don't see the larger patterns at work. As the great systems theorist Peter Senge (2006) observes, "*Structures of which we are unaware hold us prisoner*" (p. 93).

In health care, this often equates to mistakes and duplications, expensive care that might have been avoided, well-intentioned campaigns that don't work, and administrative oversight that is cumbersome and distracting rather than smooth, supportive, and integrated. Effective communication isn't a nicety. It's good medicine, and it's good business. The stakes are high. The system will go broke if we don't fix it. At the current rate, Medicare will be insolvent by 2019 (Barkley, 2008), and 47 million Americans are already unable to afford health insurance (U.S. Census Bureau, 2007). There is hope. In almost every case the solution lies in better communication, not just within our own spheres of experience, but across boundaries. Solutions require systems-level awareness and problem solving. I have written this book with that goal in mind.

If I have done my job well, the book is readable enough to serve as an introduction to the field. But as feedback from experienced health professionals bears out, this is not a skim-the-surface book. It offers sophisticated insight that is helpful even for experienced practitioners and researchers. By the book's end, readers should be able to speak knowledgeably, not just about one aspect of health care, but about how the many pieces fit together and influence each other.

## INTENDED AUDIENCE

This book is designed primarily for people pursuing careers in the health industry and those with a research interest in health communication. This includes caregivers, public relations professionals, media planners and producers, public health promoters, marketing professionals, educators, human resources personnel, health care administrators, researchers, educators, and others.

It may seem that such a diverse audience could not be served by the same text, and that is true to some extent. By all means, read other works well. Explore specialized texts. But my advice is to read this book first or alongside the others. It provides something that specific-interest books cannot— a revealing overview of how various professions, cultures, and current concerns converge in health care. I believe that, where health is concerned, understanding the big picture is as important as mastering a particular skill set. Your success will be enhanced if you are able to speak knowledgeably about current issues in the health care field overall. (And truth be told, I'm counting on you to help solve some of the problems.)

## MY BACKGROUND

I have a professional and a theoretical interest in health communication. In recent years, I have devoted myself to teaching health communication, studying health transactions, consulting with health care organizations, and writing books and articles on the subject. Earlier in my career, I covered health news for newspaper and television audiences and served as public relations director for a large medical center. In these capacities, I wrote news stories, directed public health campaigns, designed advertising, produced a monthly television program about health issues, assisted in strategic planning and marketing efforts, and worked alongside health caregivers and administrators.

As a former journalist, I understand the difficulties in keeping the public informed, and I am uncomfortably aware that unethical practices sometimes degrade the value of what the media has to say. My experience in a health care organization reminds me of how challenging it is to maintain morale, encourage open communication, and adjust to market pressures. As a scholar and researcher, I appreciate more than ever how important (and difficult) it is to manage the multiple goals and diverse influences on health communication.

Together, these experiences make me especially sensitive to the weaknesses and strengths of health communication. It is impossible to observe (and be part of) health communication efforts and believe they are all good or all bad. You will notice throughout the book that issues are described in terms of their potential advantages and drawbacks. For instance, public health promotion is an immensely valuable way to inform and motivate people. However, promoters must be careful to avoid stigmatizing ill persons and making people unnecessarily anxious. I believe communicators are most effective when they have given careful thought and ethical consideration to the communication strategies available to them.

Another result of studying and working in the health industry is my immense respect for the diverse people who comprise it. I am frustrated by scholars who criticize the actions of health professionals and patients without also acknowledging what they are up against—time limits, stress, overwhelming emotional demands, and so on. I believe health communication can be improved in many respects, but it is naive to call for reform or expect it to happen without understanding and modifying the factors that influence it. This book provides insight about many of those factors.

## FEATURES IN THE NEW EDITION

I have preserved features that were popular in the previous editions. For example, while updating information in every chapter, I have continued to integrate research evidence, real-life examples, suggestions for practical application, and current issues. Among the features I have preserved are the following.

- A *Theoretical Foundations* box in each chapter showcases an important theory relevant to health communication.
- *Resources* boxes suggest articles, books, websites, organizations, and other means to continue exploring communication issues.
- *Perspectives* boxes describe actual episodes of health communication as described by patients, professionals, family members, health care leaders, and others.
- *Communication Skill Builders* feature practical strategies for communicating with patients and caregivers, avoiding burnout, talking to children about illness, listening, facilitating social support, talking about death, developing cultural competence,

stimulating teamwork, designing public health campaigns, and more.
- *Communication Technology* features describe the impact of virtual communities, telemedicine, tailored health messages, and the Internet, to name just a few.
- *Ethical Considerations* boxes present the pros and cons of issues such as paternalism, privacy, media responsibility, the politics of prevention, health care rationing, affirmative action in medical school, and more.
- *Key Terms* and *Discussion Questions* are provided at the end of each chapter to stimulate dialogue.

The following features are new to the third edition.

- *Career Opportunities* boxes throughout the book showcase more than 100 careers related to health communication, along with links to more information and job listings.
- *Can You Guess?* boxes challenge readers to consider questions such as "Which state has the highest percentage of uninsured residents?" and "In which country do people have the longest life expectancy on earth?"
- A new *Instructor's Manual*, available both in print and online at www.oup.com/us/dupre, features sample syllabi, test questions, class activities, and more.

As mentioned, this edition includes substantially more real-life examples and brief case studies. It builds on the previous coverage of diversity to include even more information about cultures and health systems around the world and in the United States. I have also included more discussion-starter questions.

As you will see in the following descriptions, this edition features a new chapter (Chapter 12), devoted to coverage of public health issues, risk and crisis communication, and health care reform.

### Part One: Establishing a Context for Health Communication

The first two chapters provide an introduction to health communication. Chapter 1 establishes the nature and definition of health communication, current issues, and important reasons to study health communication. It also provides tips for making the most of features such as *Ethical Considerations, Theoretical Foundations,* and *Career Opportunities* boxes that appear throughout the book.

Chapter 2 provides an account of how health has been shaped by centuries of philosophy and scientific discovery. Understanding these issues allows for deeper appreciation of topics described in the rest of the book. The chapter culminates with a description of current issues in health care. The section on managed care is updated to describe the array of new options available, such as point of service (POS) plans, health savings accounts, and high-deductible health plans.

## Part Two: The Roles of Patients and Caregivers

Part Two focuses on interpersonal communication between patients and caregivers. Chapter 3 describes patient–caregiver communication in terms of who talks, who listens, and how medical decisions are made. It includes a discussion of power differences and a feature on health communication as a collaborative interpretation. This edition contains updated coverage of telemedicine, the link between poor communication and malpractice lawsuits, and the value of communication in reducing pain. It includes a new feature on motivational interviewing, an extensive list of journals relevant to health communication, and career opportunities for people with expertise in health communication research.

In Chapter 4, readers view health from the perspective of professional caregivers. The chapter describes the rewards of caregiving as well as the stress, competition, time limits, and self-doubt that often influence how caregivers communicate. The chapter describes recent research about the ways physicians are socialized to think and act "like doctors," outlines the controversy surrounding privacy regulations, and reveals patients' (mostly favorable) reactions to knowledge coupling, whereby physicians use computers to help with diagnosis and

treatment recommendations. New to the chapter are tips for communicating with difficult patients, communicating when time is limited, and disclosing medical mistakes. Information is provided about careers in medicine, dentistry, and medical executive positions.

Chapter 5 looks at health communication through patients' eyes, considering what motivates patients, what they like and do not like about health care, and how they express themselves in health encounters. The chapter looks closely at how communication is influenced by the nature of an illness, patient disposition, and threats to personal identity. It includes information about communication skills training for patients and additional information about patient narratives, self-advocacy, and individuals' willingness to communicate about health. The chapter also includes new resources and career information for people who wish to serve as patient advocates.

Chapter 6, Diversity Among Patients, presents information and tips on communicating effectively with patients who differ in terms of social status, gender, sexual orientation, race, language, ability, or age. This chapter includes a new section on genetic profiling, outlining the promise of dramatic medical breakthroughs as well as concerns about ethics, privacy, and discrimination. The section on health literacy is substantially updated and is followed by tips for serving marginalized populations. Case studies describe the experiences of a Spanish-speaking woman in an English-speaking hospital and a college student coping with a physical disability. The chapter features career information for diversity officers, interpreters, and Equal Employment Opportunity personnel.

## Part Three: Social and Cultural Issues

Part Three focuses on the ways that cultural and social issues influence health. Chapter 7 illustrates the importance of social support and provides tips for supportive communication. This edition features expanded coverage of lay caregiving, end-of-life experiences, and virtual communities. It also includes new sections on transformative health care experiences and organ donation decisions. A *Career Opportunities* box showcases careers in social services and mental health.

Chapter 8 describes social conceptions of health and healing. It describes the increasing importance of focusing on global health and creating intercultural teams. The chapter includes a new section about the health beliefs of Asians and Pacific Islanders as well as Hispanic and Arab cultures and a new sidebar contrasting Eastern and Western ideas about health. This chapter highlights the importance of cultural competence, examines culturally diverse ways of defining health, and describes the different roles patients and caregivers may be expected to play. It includes a feature about the theory of health as expanded consciousness and suggestions for communicating more effectively across cultural lines.

## Part Four: Communication in Health Care Organizations

Part Four investigates communication in health organizations. This unit emphasizes the impact that organizations have on caregiver attitudes, patient satisfaction, who receives medical care, and service excellence.

Chapter 9 focuses on communication as a medium for creating and reflecting organizational cultures. The chapter presents the latest figures on gender and racial equity in medicine, the role of communication in addressing the current nursing shortage, and emerging issues about alternative/complementary care. It also includes new coverage of retail clinics and the pros and cons of hospitalists. The chapter includes a description of conflict in health organizations and suggestions for using communication to manage conflict and diversity effectively. The *Career Opportunities* box presents an extensive list of jobs and resources in allied health.

Chapter 10, Leadership and Teamwork, is filled with many new examples of innovation and service excellence. It presents new information on Six Sigma, boutique hospitals, service excellence strategies, and careers in health care administration. The chapter describes how people in some health care organizations are using communication to become more patient-centered, more adaptive and competitive, and more pleasant places to work. Experts share advice on training new leaders, managing by collaboration, promoting a shared vision, working in teams, and rewriting the rules by which health care organizations operate. (The previous unit on careers relevant to health communication has been expanded into coverage throughout the book.)

## Part Five: Public Health: Media, Crisis, Policy, and Health Promotion

Chapter 11 provides the latest information about health images in advertising, news, and entertainment. It features expanded discussions of direct-to-consumer drug advertising, race and media, health narratives, and media literacy. The chapter also includes a new unit on the international impact of entertainment-education and information about careers in health journalism. It includes tips for reporting health news, using interactive media to present health information, and developing media literacy.

Chapter 12 is a new chapter. It focuses on public health, crisis, and health care reform. The chapter opens with a series of mini-case studies about mad cow disease, AIDS, SARS, anthrax, and avian flu, presenting lessons about risk and crisis communication from each of these experiences. The chapter includes a discussion of public health and an up-to-date exploration of health care reform options, drawing from health care models around the globe. Readers will learn more about universal coverage, multi- and single-payer systems, play-or-pay provisions, individual mandates, and more. A *Career Opportunities* box features information about careers in public health.

Chapters 13 and 14 guide readers through the creation and evaluation of public health campaigns. Both chapters include new campaign exemplars and sample PSAs as well as expanded coverage of campaign design resources and message framing. A new section discusses the lessons of the critical-cultural approach as we contemplate the ethics of persuading people in diverse cultures to change health-related behaviors. These chapters showcase careers in health promotion and health campaign design.

## STRENGTHS OF THE BOOK

*Communicating About Health* has several advantages. For one, it offers up-to-date coverage of issues and research. It describes how managed care, telemedicine, health care reform, the Internet, and other factors are changing the nature of health communication. More than most health communication texts, this one goes beyond research data to explain the larger social issues and policies that influence health care and health advocacy.

Second, this book provides extensive coverage of diversity in health care. It describes culturally diverse ways of thinking about health and healing and reveals how such factors as gender, age, and race influence health communication. Readers are able to look at health care through the eyes of caregivers, patients, administrators, health promoters, and others who contribute to the process.

Third, *Communicating About Health* is a useful guide for people interested in improving their health-related communication skills. It includes suggestions for encouraging patient participation, providing social support, listening, developing cultural competence, working in teams, designing health promotion campaigns, and more.

Fourth, this text situates health communication within the contexts of history, culture, and philosophy. This gives a depth of understanding and allows readers to grasp better the significance of health communication phenomena. For instance, evidence that doctors tend to dominate medical transactions takes on added importance when readers understand the influence of science and technology on medicine. By the same token, managed care comes into focus in light of the way health care has evolved in the United States.

Fifth, this book is designed to promote critical thinking and discussion. It poses ethical considerations and discussion questions and is supported by an instructor's manual that presents a wide range of class activities and discussion-starters to encourage active involvement with the material. Additionally, case studies and interviews with health professionals bring health communication to life.

In summary, *Communicating About Health* is much more than a literature review. It explores the diverse perspectives of people involved in health communication and shows how they blend and negotiate their ideas to create communication episodes. The book integrates research, theories, current issues, and real-life examples. This blend of information enables students to understand the implications of various communication phenomena. At the same time, readers learn how they can contribute to health communication in a positive way as professionals, patients, and researchers.

## ACKNOWLEDGMENTS

A great number of people have contributed to the creation of this text. My first thanks go to Peter Labella, Josh Hawkins, Courtney Roy, Preeti Parasharami, Lisa Grzan, Elliot Simon, Paula Schlosser, Ari Hill, and their colleagues at Oxford University Press for their remarkable guidance, enthusiasm, and good humor. I am also grateful to the following reviewers who suggested ideas for the third edition: Mariaelena Bartesaghi, University of South Florida; Ellen Cohn, University of Pittsburgh; Michael Dennis, University of Kansas; Stephen Haas, University of Cincinnati; Amy Hedman, Minnesota State University, Mankato; Haywood Joiner, Louisiana State University at Alexandria; JJ McIntyre, University of Central Arkansas; Jill O'Brien, DePaul University; Jim Query, James Madison University; Pam Secklin, Saint Cloud State University; Jiunn-Jye Sheu, University of Florida; Juliann C. Scholl, Texas Tech University; Sharlene Thompson, James Madison University; Kandi Walker, University of Louisville; Catherine Woells, Bellevue University; Kevin Wright, University of Oklahoma.

I continue to be grateful, as well, to those who have edited and reviewed previous editions, including Nanette Giles, Holly Allen, Mary L. Brown, Rebecca Cline, June Flora, Stephen Hines, Katherine Miller, Donna Pawlowski, Rajiv N. Rimal, Claire F. Sullivan, Teresa Thompson, Monique Mitchell Turner, and Gust A. Yep.

I would also like to thank colleagues and students who have contributed ideas, narratives, and feedback, most notably Jennifer Terry, Susanne Fillmore, Dawn Murray, Praewa Tanuthep, Beverly Davis Willi, Jennifer Seneca, Lori Juneau, Stefanie Howell, Melanie Barnes, Amy Jenkins, Bridget King, Micah Nickens, Samantha Olivier, and Gwynné Williams. I owe heartfelt thanks to Grant Brown, who inspired me throughout the process, and to Ken Brown, M.D., who served as my advisor on medical details, managed care, and many aspects of health care administration.

As always, I am indebted to mentors Sandy Ragan, Sonia Crandall, Jon Nussbaum, and the late Larry Wieder and Jung-Sook Lee. Heartfelt thanks also to Betty Adams and Cris Berard, who will always be the kind editors in my head. Finally, to Ron and my family (Jordan, Hannah, Ginger, Ed, Dale, Sarah, Andrew), who accommodated the many hours devoted to this project and provided endless support, I am deeply grateful.

# ESTABLISHING A CONTEXT FOR HEALTH COMMUNICATION

# CHAPTER
## I

# Introduction

*When my 9-year-old daughter came home from her grandparents with a rash from poison ivy, I wasn't alarmed. She'd had it before. I smeared her with sticky white ointment from a tube promising to "soothe minor rashes and skin irritations." A few days later, however, Hannah awoke with one eye nearly swollen shut. The inflamed rash had spread to her face. I felt I had failed miserably as Dr. Mom.*

*I called the HMO and learned our regular doctor was out, but another doctor could see us at 11 a.m. In the meantime, I called Hannah's school to explain and brought her to the university with me. In the hallway, a colleague stopped to ask in horror, "Is that poison ivy!? You better get her to a doctor. It can cause blindness around the eyes like that." I felt even more frightened and guilty. The only comfort was that Hannah said it didn't itch much.*

*In the car, I mentally rehearsed what I would say to this doctor I didn't know: "The ointment worked last time.... She wasn't this bad last night.... Maybe I should have brought her in sooner.... I'm a good mom!" My guilt escalated when I realized these statements sounded more like a courtroom defense than an explanation of my daughter's symptoms. I wondered if my little girl was going to be all right and why I was feeling such a mixture of emotions.*

How many instances of health-related communication can you identify in this real-life example? You might have counted five or more, including the ointment label, the call to the doctor's office, my call to school, the colleague's frightened warning, and my daughter's comments. All of these fall within the domain of health communication.

In addition, the story hints at several factors that influence health communication—emotions, expectations about good parenting, effects of health maintenance organization (HMO) membership, cultural ideas about parenting, and so on. All this before we even reached the doctor's office!

Episodes like the one described illustrate that health communication is a part of everyday life. Everyone is involved in some way. Our ideas about health are influenced by health care professionals, friends, family members, coworkers, educators, advertisers, entertainers, public health promoters, and many others. Television medical dramas may influence what people expect from actual health care encounters. At the same time, we influence the people around us with our own actions and thoughts about health.

One reason health communication is so dynamic and interdependent is that health itself is dynamic and interdependent. The World Health Organization (WHO) defines **health** as "a state of complete physical, mental and social well-being and not merely the absence of disease or infirmity" (WHO, 1948). This definition, unchanged for more than 60 years, reminds us that *healthy* is not the opposite of *sick*. Being healthy means more than that. It is a state of harmony and equilibrium between many aspects of life. Health involves inner feelings, physical abilities, and relationships with others. Throughout the book, we will discuss diverse theories about the nature of health and its relation to communication.

A central theme of this book is that one aspect of health communication affects others. To be effective in any arena, you must understand how various components of the system rely on and influence each other. For example, a well-meaning campaign director unfamiliar with cultural ideas about health may create messages that are unappealing or offensive to the audience he or she is trying to reach. A marketing/public relations director who does not understand the dynamics of patient–caregiver communication is unable to help shape and promote services that meet the needs of internal and external shareholders. A caregiver ignorant about health care administration misses out on leadership opportunities and has relatively little chance to influence how organizations are run. Moreover, caregivers who do not communicate well among themselves can confuse patients with contradictory information.

Knowledge gaps are understandable, even among people who have been in health-related careers for some time. Ideas about health, health care, and prevention are changing rapidly. Whereas specialization was once encouraged, now effective health care scholars and practitioners are attuned to broader contexts. They consider situations from many perspectives. They understand the historical, cultural, and market pressures that influence health. They are skillful at encouraging feedback, listening, analyzing, experimenting with new communication techniques, and selling their ideas to others.

In Chapter 2 we learn more about current issues in health care by going back in time. Following the evolution of medicine from ancient Egypt to twenty-first century managed care reveals a lot about where we are today. When we understand the philosophy and events that have shaped the modern system, we're in a better position to decide what has worked well, where we went wrong, and where we should go from here.

Perhaps the most rewarding aspect of studying health communication is putting what we learn to good use. Throughout the book, *Communication Skill Builders* sections present practical tips for communicating more effectively about health. Based on research evidence, we'll develop communication strategies for communicating with diverse patients, presenting our concerns as patients, avoiding burnout, engaging in leadership and teamwork, listening, managing conflict, attaining service excellence, designing health campaigns, and more.

It's an exciting and challenging time to be involved with health. Perhaps more than ever before, health care leaders are open to innovative ideas. They are also facing critical challenges—to control costs, attract clients, earn employees' loyalty, and more. The changes are both destabilizing and exciting. In Richard T. Pascale's (1999) terms, it can sometimes feel like "surfing the edge of chaos" (p. 198). The good news is that disequilibrium opens the field to new ways of thinking and behaving. People involved with health care today have the potential to reshape and improve the system. In Chapters 9 and 10 we'll discuss innovative ways health care organizations are pursuing these goals.

The remainder of Chapter 1 is divided into four sections. The first defines health communication. The second introduces two approaches to health care—the biomedical and the biopsychosocial models. The third outlines the importance of studying how (and why) people communicate as they do about health. The chapter concludes with a look at current issues that underline the importance of understanding health communication.

## Profile of More Than 100 Health-Related Jobs

Career boxes throughout the book showcase opportunities in health promotion, allied health, medicine, nursing, dentistry, health journalism, public relations, health care administration, diversity, patient advocacy, social services and mental health, and more. Each box provides links where you can find more information and job listings.

## WHAT IS HEALTH COMMUNICATION?

Health communication is shaped by many influences, including personal goals, skills, cultural orientation, situational factors, and consideration of other people's feelings. The definitions presented in this section emphasize the interdependence of these factors. As you will see here and throughout the book, communicators influence—and are simultaneously influenced by—the people and circumstances around them. They rely on others to help them meet goals, develop a satisfying awareness of self and others, and make sense of life events.

### Defining Communication

To attempt a conversation with someone who does not understand you is usually neither satisfying nor productive. There is more to effective communication than putting thoughts into words. Understanding other people's perceptions and clearly expressing your own are important aspects of communication. The definition of **communication** offered by Judy Pearson and Paul Nelson (1991) underscores these concerns: "Communication is the process of understanding and sharing meaning" (p. 6). The significance of this definition becomes clear when we examine communication in terms of process, personal goals, interdependence, sensitivity, and shared meaning.

*Process* Defining communication as a process recognizes that people are involved in an ongoing effort to understand each other and the world around them. Meaning is interpreted in light of past, present, and future expectations.

Some factors that influence communication are set in motion before a word is ever spoken. Consider the scenario at the beginning of this chapter. As I chatted with my daughter on the way to the doctor's office I was already wondering what would be said during the visit. The physician also approached the transaction with assumptions and expectations. In many ways, the groundwork for communication episodes begins to take form long before the participants even meet.

Just as communication has no set beginning, it has no definite ending either. People may reevaluate the meaning of a conversation long after it has ended. For instance, you might say to a friend: "When I began physical therapy, I thought my therapist was mean. But now I realize he was doing me a favor by making me work so hard."

As a process, communication is influenced by its placement in the ongoing stream of life and events. Good communicators realize that it is often helpful to know what people expect going into a communication episode and how they feel about it later. In health care situations this may mean collecting information about events leading up to an illness or health care visit and making follow-up phone calls or visits to answer any questions or concerns that arise later. In Chapters 3 through 5 we will explore the nature of patient–caregiver communication and look at health through the eyes of professional caregivers and patients.

*Personal Goals* Researchers have found that participants approach health encounters with a range of goals and expectations. The main goal of caregivers is presumably to maintain or restore patients' health, but caregivers may have other goals as well, such as

# True Stories About Health Communication Experiences

In *Perspectives* boxes you'll read about the real-life experiences of people involved with health communication. These true accounts represent the viewpoints of patients, loved ones, caregivers, executives, social activists, health campaign managers, and others. They provide insight about how people of different races, cultures, ages, languages, abilities, sexual orientations, and educational levels experience health communication. See Box 1.5 for the first in a series of *Perspectives* boxes that appear throughout the book.

---

saving time, preventing burnout, displaying their knowledge, and so on. Likewise, patients may have many goals, including the need to vent emotions, be forgiven, be reassured, or simply to be healed.

As I drove my daughter to the doctor, my confidence as a parent was shaken. I craved reassurance that I had not made her condition worse. Although I didn't take my colleague's warning about blindness too seriously, it did escalate my anxiety. These concerns influenced my goals for the encounter. Emotions and identity are tied to how people behave in medical settings.

One measure of effective communication is how well participants feel their goals have been met. Knowing what people expect from a health encounter is a useful way to increase participants' satisfaction.

*Interdependence* Although it is important to consider personal goals, communication ultimately relies on how well people work together to coordinate their goals and establish common understanding. Defining communication as "understanding and sharing" emphasizes that no one communicates alone. Communicators are **interdependent**; that is, they rely on each other and exert mutual influence on communication episodes.

Communication is a process of acting, reacting, and negotiation. For example, if the waiting room receptionist seems curt and unfriendly, patients are likely to feel defensive. This may affect their willingness to be open about embarrassing or frightening concerns in the exam room. By contrast, pleasing communication can alter a health care encounter for the better. In the poison ivy episode the receptionist who greeted us was friendly and sympathetic. She showed my daughter a rash on her own arm, caused by poison ivy in her garden. The waiting room was quiet and pleasantly decorated, and it was not long before a nurse called Hannah's name. The nurse smiled and joked with us, greatly easing the anxiety we felt. By the time the doctor entered the examination room, my daughter and I were much less anxious than before.

Being friendly and receptive in health care encounters will encourage others to be friendly and open in return. It is unrealistic to expect people to be honest, trusting, and friendly when they feel discouraged by the behavior of people around them. Interdependence also serves to emphasize that everyone involved in the communication has some influence on it. Patients, family members, receptionists, and others often affect health communication as much as doctors do.

*Sensitivity* Many theorists consider that the best communicators are sensitive to other people's feelings and expectations. Sensitivity enhances health communication on many levels. Research shows that public health campaigns are most effective when they are designed with the audience's concerns and resources in mind (Murray-Johnson & Witte, 2003). By the same token, people are usually most satisfied with physicians who listen attentively and seem to understand what they are feeling (Grant, Cissna, & Rosenfeld, 2000; Tarrant, Windridge, Boulton, Baker, & Freeman, 2003).

Being sensitive means looking and listening carefully. It also means interpreting the cues offered by other communicators. Whether Hannah and I realized it or not, we were probably presenting a number of cues that we were anxious about the visit. My arm around her shoulders, her hesitant smile, our tone of voice—all of these might have cued the staff that we were apprehensive. They were sensitive to the cues and responded in a way that was culturally appropriate and pleasing to us personally.

Sensitivity is more difficult when communicators do not share the same cultural expectations. In a different culture, a well-intended joke might seem offensive rather than kind. Interpreting subtle cues and responding to them in a sensitive way requires an awareness of **cultural display rules** (ways of showing emotions in different cultures) and an understanding of personal preferences and cultural expectations. To be effective, health communicators must be concerned enough to pay close attention to people's behavior and knowledgeable enough to recognize cultural and personal preferences that make people different.

In Chapter 8 we go around the world, exploring the diverse ways that culture influences health and healing. For example, we'll contrast the Western concept of *fighting for one's life* with the Eastern belief that health isn't a battle, but *harmony*. In this way and many others, culture provides a rich context for understanding others and expanding our own ideas. The more we know, the more likely we are to be culturally competent communicators. On the other hand, people who do not understand and respect cultural differences often do harm even when they are trying to help (Dutta & de Souza, 2008). We'll explore the idea of health disparities, social capital, and the health/power relationship in Chapters 6, 13, and 14.

*Shared Meaning* What an action means depends largely on the people and the circumstances involved. For instance, trading teasing put-downs with a friend means you like each other, but the same put-downs from someone you barely know might make you angry. Meaning exists in the participants' mutual interpretation of it.

So how do people know if they are sharing the same meaning? Usually, they can tell by the way

other people respond. A nod of the head, a smile, an angry look, or a question may signal how a conversational partner is interpreting the conversation. People send and receive messages constantly, although they may not be aware of it. Hannah and I were not trying to look anxious, but we probably showed that we were in multiple ways. Likewise, we displayed our willingness to engage in humor and light conversation when the receptionist held out her arm and we both looked at her, laughed, and relaxed our rigid posture. We got along easily. But imagine that Hannah and I had exhibited behaviors more in keeping with a Native American or Asian culture, politely (from our perspective) avoiding direct eye contact. A receptionist unaware of the cultural difference might assume we were unfriendly or dismissive. Even from such a simple example, it's easy to see how people get different types of care based on the cultural assumptions of the people involved. Consequently, we may be more or less inclined to trust the caregivers and to return for future visits.

Because communication is a cooperative process, it's inappropriate to blame one partner or the other when communication between them is unsatisfactory. In the past, scholars often blamed doctors for being insensitive to patients' wishes. However, theorists such as Teresa Thompson (1984) and Gary Kreps (1990) caution that patients should not be considered the underdogs in health situations. Patients are active agents who can influence the way health communication is conducted. For example, doctors are sometimes criticized for doing most of the talking in medical encounters. At the same time, however, patients are known to be particularly submissive around doctors. Whether patients realize it or not, they may contribute to the very dynamic they dislike.

## Defining Health Communication

Kreps and Barbara Thornton (1992) define **health communication** as "the way we seek, process, and share health information" (p. 2). People are actively involved in health communication. They are not passive recipients of information. Instead, people seek

## BOX 1.3 RESOURCES

# Health Communication Organizations and Resources

This book is designed to give you a rich and current overview of health communication. We'll visit a number of locations (social settings, doctors' offices, board rooms, movie theatres, and more) and look at health through different people's eyes. My hope is that, as you explore each perspective, your appreciation of the nuances that influence health and health communication will increase. Along the way you will probably want to know more than I could fit into the book, so *Resources* boxes in each chapter provide information about relevant websites, organizations, publications, and more.

To get you started, here is a list of organizations and websites you might wish to investigate for more about health communication:

American Academy of Communication in Healthcare: www.aachonline.org

American Communication Association: www.americancomm.org

American Public Health Association: www.apha.org

Association for Education in Journalism & Mass Communication: www.aejmc.org

Centers for Disease Control and Prevention: www.cdc/gov

Central States Communication Association: www.csca-net.org

Coalition for Health Communication: www.healthcommunication.net

Eastern Communication Association: www.ecasite.org

Exchange: A Networking and Learning Programme on Health Communication for Development: www.healthcomms.org/index.html

European Association for Communication in Health Care: www.each.nl

European Public Health Association: www.eupha.org

Graduate programs in health communication: www.gradschools.com/Subject/Health Communication/74.html and www.gradschools.com/Subject/Health-Communication International/74.html

Health Care Public Relations Association: www.hcpra.org/home.aspx

Health Communication Partnership: www.hcpartnership.org

Health Communication Research: blog.healthcommunicationresearch.com

Health e Communication Forum, sponsored by the Communication Initiative: forums.comminit.com/index.php?style=1

International Communication Association (Health Communication Division): www.icahdq.org

International Union for Health Promotion and Education: www.iuhpe.org

National Cancer Institute: www.cancer.gov/aboutnci/office-of-communications

National Center for Health Marketing: www.cdc.gov/healthmarketing

National Center for Health Statistics: www.cdc.gov/nchs

National Center for Public Health Informatics: www.cdc.gov/ncphi

National Communication Association (Health Communication Division): www.natcom.org

National Institute of Health: www.nih.gov

National Prevention Information Network: www.cdcnpin.org/scripts/campaign/strategy.asp

Pan American Health Organization: devserver.paho.org

Partnership for Clear Health Communication: www.npsf.org.pchc

Public Relations Society of America, Health Academy: healthacademy.prsa.org/index.html

South Asia Public Health Forum: www.saphf.org

Southern States Communication Association: ssca.net

U.S. Department of Human Services Health Communication Activities: www.health.gov/communication

Western States Communication Association: www.westcomm.org

World Federation of Public Health Associations: www.wfpha.org

World Health Organization: www.who.int/en

## BOX 1.4  THEORETICAL FOUNDATIONS

# The Basis for Health Communication

*He who loves practice without theory is like the sailor who boards the ship without a rudder and compass and never knows where he may cast.*
                    —LEONARDO DA VINCI

As we explore the field of health communication, theories connect the dots, just as constellations reveal patterns in the stars. Good theories make sense of diverse information and help us to get our bearings. They help us know, in advance, where we are headed and what paths are available to us. A *Theoretical Foundations* box in each chapter showcases a theory relevant to health communication. These theories address such issues as:

- What is health?
- How do we make sense of health crises?

- What behaviors enhance and compromise coping efforts?
- How do interpersonal relationships influence health?
- How does multiculturalism influence health and health care?
- How can health care organizations stimulate teamwork and innovation?
- In what ways do media messages influence our health?
- How do people respond to public health campaigns?
- What factors influence people to become more knowledgeable and proactive about their own health?

Each *Theoretical Foundations* box poses questions that invite you to analyze the theory as it applies to your experiences and beliefs.

---

and share messages and mingle what they hear and see with their own ideas and experiences. A great deal of health communication involves professional caregivers, such as doctors, nurses, aides, therapists, counselors, and technicians. But we serve as caregivers for friends and loved ones as well. Chapter 7 demonstrates the value of social support when we are ill, healthy, and even (perhaps especially) when we cope with death and dying.

## History of Health Communication

Health communication emerged as a defined area of study in the late 1960s. Interest was spurred most notably by researchers and practitioners in psychology, medicine, sociology, and persuasion who were attentive to the idea that communication is central to the process of health and healing (Kreps, Query, & Bonaguro, 2008, p. 5). They realized that, in many cases, particularly in counseling situations, communication *is* the means of treatment. And even when the goal is physical care, communication is the vehicle

by which people (both professionals and patients) learn about health and reach agreement about what is wrong and what should be done. Communication was, and still is, a priority for people interested in psychology and medicine. At the same time, persuasion scholars offer insight about how and why people behave as they do (T. Thompson, Robinson, Anderson, & Federowicz, 2008). As you know, our personal health is shaped in part by the choices we make as individuals. Communication—be it through news stories, PSAs, entertainment programming, or conversations with health professionals, neighbors, friends, or family members—often has an impact on whether we smoke, exercise, drink and drive, get enough sleep, take part in health screenings, and so on. Consequently, persuasion theories (Chapter 14) are of paramount interest to people interested in public health, health education, and health promotion. Persuasion is also important at community and societal levels as we negotiate issues of social equity, justice, community resources, and the environment. As you will see, these issues are sometimes more important than individual choices at determining people's health status.

Today, health communication research thrives within a wide variety of disciplines. One of the most interdisciplinary and organized communities comprises communication scholars devoted to the study of interpersonal, social and cultural, organizational, and mass-mediated communication relevant to health (T. Thompson, 2006). From this group has emerged the journal *Health Communication*, first published in 1989 and still led by founding editor Teresa Thompson at the University of Dayton, as well as *Qualitative Health Research* (launched in 1991), the *Journal of Health Communication* (first published in 1996), *Communication & Medicine* (first released in 2004), the *Handbook of Health Communication* (T. Thompson, Dorsey, Miller, & Parrott, 2003), and many other publications. (See Chapter 3 for a more comprehensive list of journals).

As you are probably beginning to appreciate, health communication is quite diverse. It unites practitioners and scholars and covers a gamut of issues ranging from patient–caregiver interaction, to cultural ideas about health, media images, public health efforts, health campaigns, health care administration, and much more. It also involves the work of scholars around the world—from Europe, to Australia and New Zealand, to Asia, Canada, the United Kingdom, and the Americas (T. Thompson et al., 2008). (For opportunities to become involved in the health communication dialogue, see Box 1.3.)

The following section introduces two approaches to health care that are fundamental to considering how and why people communicate as they do about health.

## MEDICAL MODELS

What causes ill health? If your answer is germs, you've probably been influenced by the biomedical model, which is not surprising, considering that it has been the basic premise of Western medicine for the last 100 years. But if you believe illness is caused by a variety of factors, including a person's frame of mind, your views more closely reflect the biopsychosocial model, which is gaining favor in today's health care system. Following is a description of each model and its impact on health communication. By way of illustration we will return for a final time to the poison ivy episode to see what the doctor said.

## Biomedical Model

The **biomedical model** is based on the premise that ill health is a physical phenomenon that can be explained, identified, and treated through physical means. Biomedicine is well suited to a culture familiar with engines and computers. "Repairing a body, in this view, is analogous to fixing a machine," writes Charles Longino (1997, p. 14). Physicians are like scientists or mechanics. They collect information about a problem, try to identify the source of it, and fix it. For instance, while the doctor was examining my daughter's poison ivy rash, he asked these questions: "When were you exposed to the poison ivy?" "When did you first notice the rash?" "Does it itch?" "Is it spreading?"

Health communication influenced by the biomedical model is typically focused and specific. Doctors' questions require only brief answers (e.g., "Last weekend." "Sunday." "No." "Yes."). Patients may have little input, and talk is largely restricted to physical signs of illness (Roter, Stewart, et al., 1997).

At its best, the biomedical approach is efficient and definitive. Medical tests and observations may yield evidence that can be logically analyzed and treated with well-established methods. One criticism of the biomedical model, however, is that it marginalizes patients' feelings and social experiences, sometimes to the extent of treating people as impersonal collections of parts or symptoms. As you will see in Chapter 5, people are often dissatisfied when caregivers do not listen to their concerns surrounding an illness, and they may not trust diagnoses if they feel the doctor did not fully understand the problem.

# A Memorable Hospital Experience

In my short 27 years I have visited hospitals in four states, and only one stands out in my memory, St. Jude Children's Research Hospital in Memphis, Tennessee. My family spent nearly 2 years of our lives walking in and out of the doors of St. Jude while my sister was being treated for leukemia.

Walking into the administrative office the first day we arrived was like being in grandma's house seated by a warm, open fireplace. During those first hours of our shock and fear over my sister's diagnosis, the hospital staff worked quickly on her paperwork without making us feel the least bit rushed. The warmth and tone of their voices was like that of a family member. We were assured we could always reach them, if not at work, at home! They were our new family.

The doctors at St. Jude stopped and spoke with families and patients and answered any questions they were asked. The doctors were not the only gems in the hospital, though. I remember two very special nurses, Jackie and Mary. One night my parents and I went to eat and were late getting back (it was shrimp night!). We found Mary, who had gotten off work 1½ hours earlier, reading to my sister. Jackie assisted my sister with manicuring her nails, even though it was not part of her technical duties. The nurses at St. Jude stepped out of their textbook roles to accommodate the needs of their patients.

Members of the housekeeping and dietary staff were always helpful too. When my sister thought she had an appetite for a hamburger or macaroni and cheese, they always did their best to get some up to her before she realized she did not want anything at all.

The last person I recall from the support staff was Mrs. Fran, our social worker. She was a dream, not just a friend you could talk to but one you could count on to take care of the little things you naturally forget in situations such as ours. When my sister died, Mrs. Fran was there for my family and made all the arrangements to get us back home to Louisiana.

There were many difficulties in dealing with the death of a loved one, and my sister was only 15. However, my parents and I feel an incredible debt to St. Jude. We have founded a fundraising chapter for St. Jude in Baton Rouge and I hope to pursue a career to help caregivers, families, and the public understand the importance of interpersonal communication skills in hospitals and other health care centers.

—Gwynné Williams

---

## Biopsychosocial Model

The **biopsychosocial model** takes into account patients' physical conditions (biology), their thoughts and beliefs (psychology), and their social expectations. From this perspective illness is not solely a physical phenomenon but is also influenced by people's feelings, their ideas about health, and the events of their lives.

Caregivers influenced by the biopsychosocial model are likely to be concerned with patients' thoughts and emotions as well as the physical conditions of their illnesses. For example, consider this dialogue.

*Doctor:* That must really itch. Is it driving you crazy?

*Child:* (giggling) Not really.

*Parent:* I thought the ointment would help, but the rash seems to be getting worse.

*Doctor:* That was a reasonable treatment. I'm not sure why it didn't help. At any rate, I can put your mind at ease....

With his comments the doctor addressed Hannah's (itchy) feelings and my concern. His reassurance that the ointment was "a reasonable treatment" did not take long but was immensely comforting to

## BOX 1.6

# Can You Guess?

1. Does the United States spend more on national defense or on health care?
2. Order the following countries, from who spends the least on health care per capita (total dollars divided by the number of citizens) to who spends the most: Australia _____, Iceland _____, the United Kingdom _____, China _____, USA _____, France _____
3. Which, if any, of the following countries outranks the United States on the World Health Organization's ranking of national health systems? France, Japan, Cyprus, Saudi Arabia, Morocco, Chile, Costa Rica, Cuba, Colombia, Malta

*Answers appear at the end of the chapter.*

me. Hannah and I left feeling that the doctor had respectfully addressed the situation *and* our feelings. Plus, we had a prescription for medicine that cured the rash overnight. The biopsychosocial approach is supported by evidence that people's thoughts and emotions have an influence on their overall health. Researchers have long known that emotional stress tends to elevate people's heart rates and blood pressure. They are now finding that excessive stress reduces the body's resistance to disease (e.g., Gouin, Hantsoo, & Kiecolt-Glaser, 2008). On the bright side, health is enhanced by good humor, a positive attitude, and social support (e.g., Gallagher, Phillips, Ferraro, Drayson, & Carroll, 2008).

The biopsychosocial approach is appealing for its thoroughness and personal concern. The case study in Box 1.5 points out how grateful people can be to caregivers who go beyond strictly physical concerns. However, implementing a biopsychosocial approach is no easy task. At a time when health professionals are conscientiously conserving resources, broadening the scope of medicine may

seem unrealistic. Some health professionals feel it is too time consuming to evaluate all aspects of a patient's well-being. You will read more about caregivers' concerns in Chapter 4.

Although it is a useful shorthand to speak of medical models, it's important to remember that models are only prototypes. As such, they are open to interpretation and blending. Few patients or caregivers operate solely within one model, nor would most people wish the entire health care system to adopt a single model. Ultimately, the best option may be the awareness that health can be approached in different ways and the versatility to use different aspects of these models appropriately.

## IMPORTANCE OF HEALTH COMMUNICATION

Health communication is important to individuals, organizations, and society overall. It's crucial to meeting medical goals, enhancing personal well-being, saving time and money, and making the most of health information. Following are six reasons to study health communication. Each of these is addressed more fully in the chapters that follow.

### Six Important Issues

First, *communication is crucial to the success of health care encounters*. Without it, caregivers cannot hear patients' concerns, make diagnoses, share their recommendations, or follow up on treatment outcomes. "Health communication is the singularly most important tool health professionals have to provide health care to their clients," write Kreps & Thornton (1992, p. 2). Patients who take an active role in medical encounters are more likely than others to be satisfied with their doctors, trust diagnoses, and carry out treatment regimens (e.g., Jadad & Rizo, 2003; Tarrant, Windridge, Boulton, Baker, & Freeman, 2003).

Interpersonal communication is crucial, considering that about 90 million people in the United States (roughly 1 in 2 adults) are unable to read more than a simple children's storybook. Added to that figure are people who, although they can read, have language differences and physical challenges that make it difficult to understand and use health information ("Health Literacy Overview," 2003). All of these fall within the category of healthy literacy. People with health literacy challenges are usually less knowledgeable about health issues than others, and they may miss appointments, avoid medical care because they are embarrassed or frustrated, prepare incorrectly for surgery and other procedures, misinterpret the instructions on medicine bottles, and more. Experts estimate that health literacy challenges result in avoidable medical costs totaling more than $106 billion a year in the United States (Vernon, Trujillo, Rosenbaum, & DeBuono, 2007), and the loss in productivity and quality of life is immeasurable. Effective interpersonal communication can offset these tragic and costly consequences of low literacy. We'll focus on health literacy and relevant communication strategies in Chapter 6.

Second, *wise use of mass media can help people learn about health and minimize the influence of unhealthy and unrealistic media portrayals.* Health promoters use communication skills to assess public needs, inform people about health issues, and encourage them to behave in healthy ways. Media consumers—especially those who rely on newspapers, magazines, and computers—are likely to be well informed about health issues and to take an active role in maintaining their own health (Rowe & Toner, 2003; van der Pal-de Bruin et al., 2003). However, the media is also filled with glamorous images of people engaging in unhealthy behaviors, making media literacy especially important. Researchers have found that media-literate individuals are less likely than others to believe unrealistic images of eating, drinking, using drugs, and being unnaturally thin (Singer & Singer, 1998). In Chapters 11 through 14 we'll explore health images in the media, media literacy, and how to create effective health campaigns.

Third, *communication is an important source of personal confidence and coping ability.* Health professionals are less likely to experience burnout and less likely to leave the profession if they are confident and satisfied (Landon, Reschovsky, Pham, & Blumenthal, 2006). Likewise, patients cope best when they feel comfortable talking about delicate subjects like pain and death. And people involved in support groups often cope better and even live longer than similar persons who are not members. In short, good communication is conducive to good health.

Fourth, *effective communication saves time and money.* Caregivers who listen attentively and communicate a sense of caring and warmth are less likely than others to be sued for malpractice (Nichols, 2003). Likewise, patients who communicate clearly with their caregivers have the best chance of having their concerns immediately addressed (Cegala & Broz, 2003), which is likely to improve their health and save time and money.

Fifth, *communication helps health care organizations operate effectively.* Communication skills are useful in recruiting employees, establishing innovative teams, creating efficient systems, and sustaining service excellence (Vestal, Fralicx, & Spreier, 1997). Survey results show that supervisors' communication skills are one of the most important determinants of nurses' job satisfaction and their intention to stay on the job (Thorpe & Loo, 2003). Organizational leaders can also use communication to assess market needs and respond to patient preferences. In Chapter 10 we explore techniques for accomplishing these objectives.

Sixth, *health communication may be important to you because the health industry is rich with career opportunities.* A background in health communication is an asset in a range of careers, including clinical care, public relations, marketing, health care administration, human resources, education, community outreach, crisis management, patient advocacy, and more. In fact, health care is a rare source of optimism in today's tense economic climate. Analyst Charles Lauer (2008a) reports that the United States lost 310,000 manufacturing jobs between mid-2007 and mid-2008—but it *added* 363,000 jobs in the health industry. As Lauer puts it, health care is "an economic lifeboat in many communities" (p. 25).

To get an idea of how large and dynamic the health industry is, consider these statistics.

In the United States, health care accounts for $2,400,000,000,000 in domestic spending per year. That's $2.4 trillion (National Coalition on Health Care, 2008). The U.S. Bureau of Labor Statistics (2008) reports that more than 14 million people are employed in the U.S. health care system, and 3 million new jobs are expected between 2006 and 2016. That means that 7 of the 20 fastest-growing occupations are health related. Reasons for the increase are twofold: Baby Boomers are retiring, and health needs are simultaneously escalating as the average age of the population increases. Experts predict particularly high demand for nurses, allied health professionals, and people qualified to educate the public about health issues. Communication skills are a valuable asset no matter what aspect of health care interests you.

## CURRENT ISSUES IN HEALTH COMMUNICATION

The chapter concludes with a brief overview of current issues in health care. We'll discuss the influence of these issues on health communication throughout the book.

### Emphasis on Efficiency

As demand for health services increases there is more concern than ever that they be affordable. Although the United States spends more on health, per capita, than any other nation, it lags behind most industrialized nations in terms of equitable care for all citizens. More than 47 million Americans are uninsured (U.S. Census Bureau, 2007) because they cannot afford rising premiums. Medicare covers many health costs for people age 65 and older; but without significant changes, analysts predict, it will be insolvent by 2019 (Barkley, 2008). The culprit, say many, is unwise use of resources. When researchers at the Commonwealth Fund issued their 2008 scorecard on U.S. health system performance, they gave the nation an F (53%) on efficient use of health resources, citing uncoordinated patient care, avoidable

hospitalizations, too-high administrative costs, and slow adoption of time-saving communication technology (Commonwealth Fund, 2008c). Improving these is mostly a matter of communicating more effectively.

Managed care, begun in the late 1980s, is one effort to monitor and reduce health expenses. However, some people worry that managed care has gone overboard, skimping on care in the zeal to cut costs. We'll discuss these issues in Chapter 2.

As we look ahead, it's important to be well informed about the options for health care reform. Terms such as *universal coverage, individual mandates,* and *single-payer vs. multipayer models* are likely to become familiar in the lexicon. In Chapter 12 we'll explain these terms, survey health systems around the world, and lay out options for health care reform in the United States.

### Prevention

Prevention has become a health priority for two main reasons: It increases people's quality of life, and it costs less than medical treatment. Although the first reason has always been true, the second has become an important concern in recent years. S. Renée Gillespie (2001) observes that the dual pressures of competition and cost-containment have created "a new conceptualization of the patient as both valued customer and dangerous consumer of health care resources" (p. 99). Within this framework, recruiting the "right" patients (those who do not require expensive care) may keep a health care organization in business. However, patients with expensive health needs can drain the organization's resources. It's in everyone's best interest to keep people healthy.

Prevention is cost-efficient because it is usually less expensive to prevent diseases and injuries than to treat them. For example, it costs less to provide cardiovascular exercise programs than to perform open-heart surgeries. Prevention efforts are often led by diverse teams of physicians, nurse practitioners, physician assistants, dietitians, therapists, and others. The rewards are great, for both patients and caregivers. The challenge is to become skillful at interdisciplinary

## BOX 1.7 ETHICAL CONSIDERATIONS

# An Essential Component of Health Communication

*Our customers routinely bare their bodies, as well as their souls, within our organizations. I can think of no other enterprise in our society where so much is placed in the hands of others.*
—*LARRY SANDERS, CHAIR OF THE AMERICAN COLLEGE OF HEALTH CARE EXECUTIVES*

Sanders (2003) advises those who provide and study health care: "One of the most significant ways we can demonstrate how much we care about those we serve is to visibly display our personal commitment to operating with extraordinary integrity, ethics and morality each and every day" (p. 46).

It is imperative that people involved with health care understand the ethical implications of their actions and conduct themselves with honor and integrity. They must also be aware of others' perceptions. If people perceive—rightly or wrongly—that health-related professionals are not ethical, they may experience stress, avoid medical care, lie to health care providers, or withhold information to protect themselves.

I once studied a hospital unit in which several of the patients had AIDS but were afraid to tell their caregivers about their diagnosis. The caregivers were justifiably angry that they might become infected because they were not aware which patients were contagious. However, the patients had a good point as well. They felt their diagnosis would not be kept confidential, and they were probably right. Patient records were often left open on the counter of the nurses' unit, posted outside patients' rooms, and handled by more than a dozen employees, including clerks, secretaries, pages, and more. There was no reasonable assurance of confidentiality. Consequently the caregivers distrusted the patients, and the patients distrusted everyone in the organization.

Many of the ethical dilemmas that people in health care face are essentially matters of communication. Issues frequently arise concerning honesty, privacy, power, conflicts of interest, social stigmas, media images, advertising, and persuasive messages about health. In most cases, there is more than one option but no simple solution. What seems right in one situation may be wrong in another. Personal preference and culture, among other factors, shape what people want and expect. Even so, there is value in thinking through the implications and exploring diverse reactions with others.

An *Ethical Considerations* box in each chapter presents an ethical dilemma and a list of discussion questions and additional resources. I encourage you to discuss and debate these issues, eliciting diverse viewpoints. Do not be afraid to change your mind or to argue both sides of an issue. It is usually easier to behave ethically if you have thought the issues through *before* you find yourself in a real-life dilemma. Following are some questions you might ask yourself as you consider your options concerning ethical challenges posed in this book and elsewhere.

- Is this option legal?
- Is it honest? Is deception or omission of the truth involved?
- Who will be hurt? Who will be helped?
- Will the decision benefit me personally but hurt others?
- Are the results worth the hardship involved?
- Is it culturally acceptable?
- Will my decision compromise people's privacy or trust?
- Will my decision be demeaning or degrading to anyone?
- Is it fair? Will my action unfairly discriminate against anyone?
- Is the action appropriate for the situation?
- Have I considered all the options?
- How would I wish to be treated in the same situation?
- How would I feel if my decision or action were published in tomorrow's newspaper?

teamwork and collaborative problem solving, factors we'll discuss more in Chapter 10.

Holistic medicine is also becoming popular. Four in 10 Americans now use alternative therapies such as chiropractic, acupuncture, and relaxation therapy (Barrett, 2003). These are relatively inexpensive and are geared toward prevention and long-term health maintenance. As you will see in Chapter 9, holistic therapists often spend a good deal of time talking with patients about lifestyle choices and emotional well-being.

Communicating well is at the heart of prevention efforts. Conversations, brochures, news stories, and mass media campaigns influence what we know and how we act. To be successful, information must be useful, accurate, culturally sensitive, interesting, and motivational.

### Patient Empowerment

It's easier than ever to be knowledgeable about health. It's the subject of cable television channels, magazines, best-selling books, news programs, advertisements, and extensive computer databases. News media in the United States release more than 3,500 health-related stories in a typical 18-month period (Kaiser Family Foundation, 2008). It is said that knowledge is power, and that may be the case in health care. The current Information Age coincides with a move toward **patient empowerment** (Hardey, 2008). Empowerment means patients have considerable influence in medical matters. Their ideas count. They ask questions and state preferences, and they may visit doctors or other caregivers, not because they are ill, but because they would like information or feedback on a health issue.

Patient empowerment is also encouraged by increased competition in the health industry. People are now courted by health plans and medical centers vying for their business. Advertising appeals make it plain that health care agencies are not simply a source of assistance but are part of an industry that relies on consumers.

Increased knowledge and the awareness that health agencies need patients' business may reduce the status difference between patients and their caregivers. As Tom Ferguson (1997) puts it:

> As we move farther into the Information Age, health professionals will do more than just treat their patients' ills—they will increasingly serve as their coaches, teachers, and colleagues, working side-by-side with empowered consumers in a high-quality system of computer-supported, low-cost, self-managed care. (paragraph 34)

It will be interesting to see if (and how) patients and caregivers adapt to the idea that they are well-informed partners working toward common goals. On the one hand, patient empowerment relieves some of the pressure on caregivers to "fix" people who do very little to maintain their own health (R. Kaplan, 1997). On the other hand, patient empowerment dispels the notion that people should simply follow doctors' orders. It is no longer enough (if ever it was) simply to tell patients what to do. Empowered patients want information and the right to make their own decisions. Changing expectations require new communication skills and different styles of interaction on the part of patients and caregivers.

### Global Health Needs and Intercultural Competence

In today's world environment, travel, immigration, and the international exchange of food and products mean that diseases are continually carried across national borders. The outbreak of severe acute respiratory syndrome (SARS) in 2003 provided a striking example of how quickly a communicable disease can spread around the globe. Within 100 days, the disease that began in southern China had killed more than 100 people in 20 countries. Remarkably, the world health community was able to contain the outbreak of SARS within a few months.

The AIDS epidemic has been far more difficult to keep in check. The number of new HIV/AIDS cases has leveled off since 2000, partly because of aggressive health promotion efforts. UNAIDS (2008) reports that HIV-prevention efforts around the world have tripled since 2005. Slower spread of the virus is an intermediate victory for health educators, but the situation remains critical. Some 33 million people (down from 42 million in 2003) are infected, and the spread is still rapid in some parts of the world, particularly sub-Saharan Africa and India.

In Chapter 12 we'll focus on international teamwork and the intercultural competence necessary to deal effectively with SARS, AIDS, mad cow disease, avian flu, and more.

## Changing Populations

Population shifts are also changing health care needs in the United States. One shift is toward an older society. In 2011, about 20,000 baby boomers a day will reach age 65. By 2020, about 1 in 5 Americans will be 65 or older (U.S. Census Bureau News, 2008). Although many older adults are healthy, they are more likely than others to have chronic diseases, which will increase the need for medical care, assisted living facilities, social services, and home care.

The racial and cultural mix of American society is also changing. By 2042, people from current minority racial and ethnic groups will comprise the majority of the U.S. population (U.S. Census Bureau News, 2008). This presents an unprecedented richness of diversity. Unfortunately, it is still anticipated that people from minority groups will have fewer educational and professional opportunities than others, meaning that the number of underprivileged individuals in the United Sates will probably rise. People with limited education and income are typically most in need of health care but are least likely to be informed about health issues and to utilize health services (Bochner, 1983; M. Williams et al., 1995). The challenge is to provide affordable care to the people who need it and to use prevention efforts to keep people as healthy as possible.

Furthermore, diversity among health care workers is not expected to keep pace with the overall population. Currently, minorities comprise less than 15% of physicians and less than 11% of nurses in the United States, which is about half their representation (29%) in the overall population (American Association of Medical Colleges, 2007). As a result, the odds are that patients will be treated by caregivers who differ markedly from them in terms of knowledge, need, and cultural beliefs. Communication is a valuable tool for meeting this challenge. It is important to understand and appreciate culturally diverse views of health and illness and to become skillful at intercultural communication, topics we'll cover in Chapters 6, 8, and 9.

## Technology

Technology may address many of the issues just described. The ability to communicate with health care clients across great distances may avail people of medical care, information, and social support they would not otherwise receive. Using technology, health messages can be broadcast around the world or tailored (*narrowcast*) to meet the needs the needs of specific individuals. At another level, electronic medical records can save time, prevent mistakes, and help coordinate patient care. Some analysts predict that we will eventually have medical ATM-type cards or microchips inserted under our skin so that our medical profiles will be accessible anywhere we are, even if we are unable to answer questions. In yet another application of medical technology, scientists have used computers to map nearly all the genes in the human body. This has the potential to unlock the mystery of many diseases, maybe even cancer. But for genetic testing and all the forms of technology just listed, many questions about privacy, quality, cost, and access remain to be resolved. In *Communication Technology* sections throughout the book we'll learn more about these issues and more.

In closing, although it may seem that the average person is not affected by changes in the health industry, that is far from the case. Changes influence the type of caregivers people are apt to see, what services are available, and what role individuals play in maintaining their own health. People who work in the health industry are likely to experience the stress and promise of change, the pressure to save money, the imperative to use new technology, and the need to communicate effectively with a variety of people and to include them as partners in their own care and disease prevention efforts. We are all influenced by health issues, not only in the United States, but around the world.

## SUMMARY

Effective health communication involves an extensive number of people. Physicians often seem to call the shots, but they are affected by a range of factors themselves, including budget limitations and public expectations. And doctors do not work alone. Nurses, therapists, technicians, counselors, public health experts, friends, and others also shape our health attitudes and behaviors. In the larger scope of things, health care administrators, media professionals, and public health promoters play important roles. Furthermore, everyday citizens affect the process more than they may realize.

In a context of rapid change, the most effective people are those who keep the larger picture in sight, are open to new ideas, and work with others to identify and implement options that serve multiple goals at the same time. The emphasis is on communicating as leaders and team members. In this climate of change and consolidation, communication specialists can help assess community needs, market new services, keep people informed about changes, and facilitate team efforts to design high-quality, affordable care systems. Caregivers, administrators, and researchers who wish to influence the transformation of health care will need to draw on a range of communication skills.

Communication about health issues is achieved within a complex array of influences. It is partly the result of individual action and partly the result of social contexts and expectations. Participants in health care must strive not only to attain their personal objectives but also to maintain the good faith of those around them, without whom they cannot achieve long-term success. Social equity and opportunities are profoundly important in determining who is healthy and who is not.

With this philosophy it seems important to emphasize that if health communication is good

(or bad), then we have a host of people to thank (or blame). Almost always we are among those people. We influence the process throughout our lives, as patients, caregivers (professional or otherwise), citizens, policy-makers, and friends. We all have something to gain by understanding the process and, hopefully, something to contribute as well.

There are different ways of looking at health. Two of the most popular perspectives are the biomedical model, which assumes that disease is best understood and treated in physical terms, and the biopsychosocial model, which treats health as a broad concept that includes social, personal, and physical factors.

Health communication is important for several reasons. It allows patients and caregivers to share concerns and establish trust. Effective communication also helps people cope and builds their self-confidence. Communicating well saves time and money and helps health care organizations solicit, organize, and implement new ideas. Finally, media messages have the potential to improve or discourage healthy habits. Part of effective communication is discerning between helpful and harmful information.

Health communication is especially important now as the industry and the public work toward a more affordable health system, disease prevention, patient empowerment, and treatment for a diverse population. The current health care system is quickly evolving amid diverse global pressures, making the nature of medicine and the importance of health communication a dynamic and important consideration in the twenty-first century.

## KEY TERMS

health
communication
interdependent
cultural display rules
health communication
biomedical model
biopsychosocial model
patient empowerment

## DISCUSSION QUESTIONS

1. Why is it important for people in one aspect of health (e.g., campaign management, public relations, clinical care) to be knowledgeable about broader issues relevant to health?
2. What is the significance of defining communication as a process?
3. How do personal goals, interdependence, and sensitivity affect the communication process?
4. How do communication partners establish shared meaning?
5. What are the implications of describing health communication in terms of seeking, processing, and sharing information?
6. Have you ever felt like the underdog in a health care encounter? What contributed to this feeling? Is there anything you or other people might have done differently?
7. Why is it important to study theories in conjunction with research about health communication?
8. How are the biomedical and biopsychosocial models different? How are they alike?
9. Do you believe health is affected by moods and communication with others? Why or why not?
10. Have your health care experiences been characterized more by the biomedical approach or the biopsychosocial approach? How? Which do you prefer and why?
11. What do you think of the case study about St. Jude Hospital (Box 1.5)? How have your experiences with hospitals been similar or different?
12. What are six reasons to study health communication?
13. Why is it especially important that people involved in health care maintain high ethical standards?
14. What questions might you ask as you evaluate the options presented by an ethical dilemma?
15. What role can communication specialists play as health agencies strive to cut costs?
16. How is the emphasis on disease prevention likely to affect health communication?
17. How does patient empowerment affect health communication?
18. What shifts are expected in the U.S. population over the next 50 years? How will these changes affect health care and health communication?
19. Why should we be concerned about health crises around the world? What role does communication play in striving for global health?

## ANSWERS TO *CAN YOU GUESS?*

1. The United States spends 4.3 times more on health care than on national defense (National Coalition on Health Care, 2008).
2. China ($81), UK ($3,064), Australia ($3,181), France ($3,819), Iceland ($5,154), United States ($6,350) (WHO, 2008b)
3. The only country on the list that doesn't outrank the United States is Cuba (WHO World Health Report, 2000). We'll examine the reasons why in Chapter 12.

# CHAPTER
# 2

# History and Current Issues

---

*On one of my trips, I received an urgent call that my mother had been in a terrible accident, in which she had fallen asleep at the wheel and hit a tree. In the accident my father was killed and my mother had broken her neck, her sternum, one leg in three places, and the other leg just above the knee.... I took the first plane I could get to be by her side. I wondered if the nurses in ICU would be strict about how long I could spend with my mother. I pictured them telling me that I could spend only 10 minutes out of the hours with her. The more I thought about being chased out of ICU, the more I decided I was going to be belligerent about my rights to be with my mother as long as she wanted me there.... I finally arrived at the ICU waiting room.... As I walked into the unit, I was a time-bomb ready to go off if anybody tried to limit my time with my mother. When I entered her room, it was a shock to see her on the ventilator. Her head was in a steel halo with rods running from the rim into her skull. Her face was swollen beyond recognition. Her bandages made her seem twice as big.... Off to one side of her bed was a nurse facing a bank of electronic equipment with blinking lights. She was writing my on mother's chart. I hoped she didn't notice me enter the room as I went over to other side of the bed and took my mother's hand. Not knowing if she was awake or not, I said softly, "Mother, this is Fred and I am here now to be with you." I felt a gentle squeeze and knew she heard and understood me.... As if on cue, the nurse turned around and looked at me. I thought, Here it comes. Give it your best shot, lady. But instead, the nurse smiled and said, "My, my, my, you should see what your touch just did to your mother's vital signs. It's amazing. We need you here all of the time!" (F. Lee, 2004, pp. 61–62)*

This story, told by Fred Lee in his book *If Disney Ran Your Hospital*, illustrates many of the facets in modern-day medicine. Health care today is a mix of life-saving technology, institutional rules and guidelines, and, at its best, a deep appreciation for the role that compassion, love, and touch play as well. The example also points to the powerful role of communication. Lee reflects: "Could she have come up with a more perfectly timed thing to say? It was as if she had read my mind and in one gracious comment had made me feel needed and welcome, an essential part of the healing team" (p. 62).

Unfortunately, the opposite is also true. Lee's trepidation about being turned out from his mother's room reflects the reality that health care professionals and patients are sometimes at odds about what constitutes good care. To understand how and why health communication has evolved as it has, we take a journey through history in this chapter. You will see how ideas (some ancient, some modern) influence the way people think and talk about health today. You may be surprised to find that your assumptions about health care have roots in the philosophies of ancient Egypt, medieval Europe, or colonial America. By chapter's end, we will explore current issues, including the evolution of managed care.

## MEDICINE IN ANCIENT TIMES

Many Westerners date medicine to ancient Greece and think of Hippocrates as the first physician. This would make medicine about 2,000 years old, a period during which tremendous change has taken place. However, the first doctor in history was actually Imhotep of ancient Egypt, who lived about 2,000 years before Hippocrates was born.

### Imhotep

As the first known physician, **Imhotep** was part of an ancient medical community that is still admired for its vast knowledge. Translations of early texts suggest Egyptians were aware of blood circulation and the functions of bodily organs thousands of years before the Western world attained that knowledge. A learned observer of archeology once remarked that the accomplishments of ancient Egypt would make citizens of the modern world "blush for shame" (Thorwald, 1962, p. 15).

Imhotep was not only a healer but a priest, a sculptor, and an architect as well. He designed the first stone pyramid, which was built for King Zoser about 2600 B.C. In the centuries after his death, Imhotep attained godlike status. Some legends portrayed him as the son of Ptah, the Egyptian god of architecture. Others revered Imhotep as a medicine god and evoked his name in healing ceremonies.

The ancient Egyptians took a **religio-empirical approach** to medicine, combining spiritualism and physical study. Healers were holy men such as Imhotep, but the ancients also recognized a physical component of illness (Thorwald, 1962). They developed an impressive variety of instruments, including surgical appliances, sutures, drugs, and immobilizing casts. Mummies show that the ancient Egyptians were prone to many disorders that plague people today, including dental ailments, cancer, and arteriosclerosis (hardening of the arteries).

It is believed that Imhotep was the basis for the Greek god Aesculapius, whose name is mentioned in the famous Hippocratic oath (Garrison, 1929). In fact, historians believe Hippocrates was strongly influenced by the writings of ancient Egypt.

### Hippocrates

**Hippocrates** (460–370 B.C.) is often considered the founder of scientific medicine and Western medical ethics. Perhaps his most enduring legacy is the oath that bears his name.

The **Hippocratic oath** (Box 2.1) established a code of conduct for physicians that has influenced the Western world until the current day. In a collection of succinct sentences, the oath says a great deal about medical ethics then and now. For centuries medical students took the Hippocratic oath when they received their degrees. The tradition has largely been abandoned, but most doctors are familiar with the oath and continue to be influenced by the ethical framework it presents.

Parts of the Hippocratic oath—particularly the appeal to medicine gods Apollo and Aesculapius—seem archaic today. More remarkable, however, are the issues that remain current. The oath's edict to "give no deadly medicine" is relevant to modern debates over physician-assisted suicide. Likewise, the mention of abortion and sexual misconduct could be straight from modern headlines, as could issues of patient confidentiality.

The oath's pledge not to "cut persons laboring under the stone," but to leave such work to specific practitioners, reflects the distinction in Hippocrates' day between medicine and surgery. It is believed that this passage refers to bladder and kidney stones, which were then extracted by surgeons but not by physicians (Edelstein, 1967).

Hippocrates' views on the nature of disease are as important as the oath that bears his name. At the

## BOX 2.1  THE HIPPOCRATIC OATH

I swear by Apollo the physician, and Aesculapius and Hygeia, and Panacea, and all the gods and goddesses, that according to my ability and judgment, I will keep this oath and its stipulations—to reckon him who taught me this art equally dear to me as my parents, to share my substances with him, and to relieve his necessities if required; to look upon his offspring in the same footing as my own brothers; and to teach them this art if they shall wish to learn it, without fee or stipulation, and that by precept, lecture, and other mode of instruction, I will impart a knowledge of the art to my own sons, and those of my teachers, and to disciples bound by a stipulation and oath according to the law of medicine, but to none other.

I will follow that system of regimen which, according to my ability and judgment, I consider for the benefit of my patients, and abstain from whatever is deleterious and mischievous. I will give no deadly medicine to anyone if asked, nor suggest any such counsel; and in like manner I will not give to a woman a pessary to produce abortion. With purity and holiness I will pass my life and practice my art. I will not cut persons laboring under the stone, but will leave this to be done by men who are practitioners of this work. Into whatever houses I enter, I will go into them for the benefit of the sick, and will abstain from every voluntary act of mischief and corruption; and, further, from the seduction of females or males, of freemen and slaves. Whatever, in connection with my professional practice, or not in connection with it, I see or hear, in the life of men, which ought not to be spoken of abroad, I will not divulge, as reckoning that such ought to be kept secret.

While I continue to keep this oath unviolated, may it be granted to me to enjoy life and the practice of this art, respected by all men, in all time. But should I trespass and violate this Oath, may the reverse be my lot.

—This version of the Hippocratic oath was published in 1910 by P. F. Collier and Son in *Harvard Classics* (Vol. 38). It was placed in the public domain in June 1993.

---

time Hippocrates lived, many people believed disease was God's punishment, and they were shamed by it (Amundsen & Ferngren, 1983). Hippocrates' ideas helped dispel this notion. In place of spiritual explanations, he presented a rational/empirical model of medicine. From a **rational/empirical approach**, disease is best understood by careful observation and logical analysis.

Hippocrates promoted the idea of health as a harmonious balance between many factors, including diet, contact with nature, relationships, and physical strength. He also advocated a balance between different body fluids, which he called body *humors*—blood, phlegm, yellow bile, and black bile (J. R. Moore, Van Arsdale, Glittenberg, & Aldrich, 1987). Thus, although Hippocrates strengthened the notion that physical factors are a significant part of disease, he acknowledged social and personal influences as well. In this way Hippocrates' philosophy was an early forerunner to the biopsychosocial approach.

The treatment of body humors had a substantial impact on the practice of medicine, forming the basis for bloodletting and other purging practices. Bloodletting involved lancing a vein or applying leeches to allow a portion of the patient's blood to drain from the body. It was believed this would purge impure blood or balance blood levels with other humors. Other purging practices include vomiting, sweating, and the use of laxatives.

Bloodletting may seem archaic today (in fact, it is still used in some rare cases), but Hippocrates' influence on health communication has endured through the centuries. By establishing medicine as rational and empirical, Hippocrates helped shape the role of physicians as scientists and intellectuals rather than spiritualists. As a result, medical talk began to focus on physical, social, and personal factors. If the rational/empirical perspective had never taken root, you might now visit a minister rather than a doctor when you become ill. By the same token, treatment and diagnosis might involve spiritual exploration more than physical remedies.

Hippocrates' ideas were not always well received, however. His views on medicine were overshadowed for a time when early Christianity brought about a resurgence of spiritualism in western Europe.

## MEDIEVAL RELIGION AND HEALTH CARE

Christianity dominated the course of Western medicine for hundreds of years during the Middle Ages, also known as the medieval period (A.D. 500–1450). Medical spiritualism, which waned but never fully died under Hippocrates' influence, was renewed with vigor.

### Medical Spiritualism

As Donald Bille (1981) defines it, **medical spiritualism** is the belief that illness is governed by supernatural forces such as gods, spirits, or ghosts. Medical spiritualism was supported by the belief that Jesus performed healing miracles. Healing was so closely tied to Christianity that monks were the principle physicians during much of the Middle Ages (White, 1896/1925).

As the only recognized religion in medieval Europe, the Catholic church was involved in making laws, allocating land and resources, and caring for the sick and homeless. As such, it had immense influence over people's well-being and way of life. The church's ideology affected the nature of health communication. From a spiritualist perspective, disease was treated through prayer and faith and, sometimes, through application of natural (God-given) substances such as plants. People generally believed that illness was manifested differently in each person (T. L. Thompson, 1990). As a result, patients' thoughts and feelings, faith, and behaviors were directly relevant to the subject of healing.

During a portion of the Middle Ages, the church banned the practice of secular medicine, particularly surgery. Surgeons were often regarded as sorcerers, butchers, and atheists (White, 1896/1925). Because the soul was believed to inhabit a persons'

entire body, to cut into the body (before or after death) was to interfere with God's work.

### Barber Surgeons

During the Middle Ages, health care was provided mostly by monks and by a limited number of secular practitioners, most of whom did not perform surgery. Barbers began offering surgical procedures in addition to hairstyling because they had the sharp instruments and public facilities necessary. **Barber surgeons** were called on to perform simple surgeries, bloodletting, and tooth extractions (C. Douglas, 1994). It is believed that the modern barber pole was derived from the image of white and bloodstained bandages swirling in the wind as they dried outside barbershops. If these images sound harrowing by today's standards, consider that during the time of barber surgeons people were still unaware of germs and had no effective anesthesia!

Although it is easy to regard the church as antiprogressive for discouraging secular medicine, it is perhaps understandable considering how dreadful surgery seemed at that time. As medical historian John Duffy (1979) describes it, prior to the 1860s surgery was "a grim and bloody business" requiring the surgeon "to be a strong, fast, forceful operator, ruthlessly immune to the screams and struggles of the patient" (p. 130).

### Science and Magic

Monastic medicine varied from the scholarly to the superstitious. It was, in turn, praised and condemned. In cathedral schools such as Salerno in southern Italy, the clergy studied medical theory. These institutions became models for European medical schools to follow. The church founded the first hospitals as we know them and staffed them with its own learned practitioners, forming what Darrel Amundsen and Gary Ferngren (1983) laud as a "vast charitable institution" (p. 15).

In contrast to this academic atmosphere, however, was the exercise of **Christian magic,** the use of bizarre ceremonies and exorcisms condoned by the church (Amundsen & Ferngren, 1983). In an effort to disgust evil spirits into leaving a person's body, for instance, the patient might be instructed to eat toad livers or drink rat's blood (White, 1896/1925). (In fairy tales to come, of course, these ingredients made up the imaginary contents of witch's brew.)

The church also became involved in selling fetishes and hosting miracles, some of which were later exposed as hoaxes. **Fetishes** were holy relics said to protect those who purchased them from calamities such as shipwreck, fire, lightning, and difficult childbirth (White, 1896/1925). Those who could afford to buy fetishes or visit holy sites made lavish offerings to the church in exchange for divine intervention.

### End of an Era

Ironically, as medicine advanced with the monks' practice of it, their work began to seem disturbingly secular and altogether overwhelming. The very technology and pharmacology they developed were at odds with the church's position on healing by faith and were diverting the monks from other spiritual pursuits (Ackerknecht, 1968). In 1311 the church forbade monks to practice medicine any longer.

As with any enterprise of such vast duration and involvement, the church's role during the Middle Ages had both positive and negative aspects. The church has been criticized for profiting from its caregiving role and for suppressing the development of secular medicine. At the same time, it is lauded for helping establish a compassionate perspective toward the ill and founding institutions of care and learning that served as a model of Western medicine. Today, even in the context of high-tech biomedical care, this influence is reflected in the existence of church-funded and other nonprofit medical centers devoted to public service and in the presence of clergy and chapels in many hospitals.

## RENAISSANCE PHILOSOPHY AND HEALTH CARE

From one extreme to another, the religion-oriented thought of the Middle Ages was followed by the intellectual skepticism of the European Renaissance.

The Renaissance began in the 1300s (overlapping with the Middle Ages) and continued into the 1600s.

Confronted with the age-old question "What is real?", artists and philosophers of the Renaissance looked to mathematics and matter for answers. Their theories changed the Western worldview, including the nature of medicine.

Partly in reaction to the religious dominance of the Middle Ages, Renaissance thinkers tended to be skeptical about anything they could not prove. **René Descartes** (1596–1650), an influential philosopher and mathematician of the time, introduced his method of doubt, prescribing that the thinker systematically doubt the existence of all things until that existence could be verified. (Such a method eventually led him to doubt his *own* existence until, realizing he had to *exist* to be *doing* the doubting, he reached the famous conclusion "I think, therefore I am.")

### Principle of Verification

The **principle of verification**—do not believe it if you cannot prove it—changed the nature of health care. No longer were people considered ill based solely on their feelings. Instead, physicians and others began to look for verifiable signs of illness (a perspective consistent with today's biomedical approach).

Surgery and autopsies became acceptable. In fact, not only physicians but artists became interested in human dissection (Dowling, 1997). Renaissance artists, including Michelangelo and Leonardo da Vinci, studied the human body inside and out to make their representations of it more precise. Mathematical precision and a knowledge of anatomy became mainstream in both science and art.

The principle of verification affected health communication. If illness is physically verifiable, it follows that people may believe they are ill even though they really are not. This idea is still pervasive in Western medicine. You know this if you have ever gone to the doctor feeling ill and been told that tests confirm you are "just fine." In fact, some people avoid going to the doctor because it

BOX 2.2 **PERSPECTIVES**

# Sick in the Head?

After two months with a 101-degree temperature but no real discomfort, a 21-year-old woman presented her concerns to a doctor. "From the beginning, I got the feeling he really didn't want to see me," she remembers. "I waited 4 hours in the waiting room."

During a brief consultation, the doctor scolded the woman for smoking and prescribed two medications. "Those were to relieve the congestion in my chest (which I didn't have) and strep throat (which I also didn't have). We paid and left. I knew I didn't have strep throat, and I wasn't sick from smoking, but I took the medicine because it might help, and he was a doctor," says the woman.

The medicine made her feel worse, and the woman eventually went to a physician assistant who diagnosed a urinary tract infection and prescribed medication that provided immediate relief. Looking back, the woman muses: "I wondered why the first doctor was so incompetent. He came highly recommended. I guess he figured I was a young hypochondriac. I didn't really spend that much more time with the physician assis-

tant, but she believed I was sick, where the other doctor obviously didn't."

This true story brings up an interesting question. What makes an illness real? Is it symptoms, lab tests, a certain look or demeanor? A by-product of organic medicine is the belief that an illness is not real unless it is physically verifiable, and society frowns on those who complain of "imaginary" conditions.

The phrase "sick in the head" is typically a put-down, an insult that suggests one is crazy or out of touch with reality. Yet in reality there is strong evidence that what people think does affect how they feel, germs or no germs.

## What Do You Think?

1. How do you feel if a doctor tells you there is nothing wrong, but you feel sick?
2. If you feel sick but the doctor can find nothing wrong with you, are you sick?
3. How would you feel if you were told your illness was "all in your head"?
4. What would you do if you thought the doctor's diagnosis was incorrect?

---

seems a sign of weakness to complain about something that (medically speaking) is trivial or does not exist. (See Box 2.2.) My experience producing health campaigns bears this out. I once directed a campaign to encourage people to go to an emergency room if they experienced chest pains. The campaign was spurred by evidence that people were dying of heart attacks because they were afraid to go to the emergency room and find out, to their embarrassment, that they had nothing more than indigestion.

## Cartesian Dualism

Renaissance thinkers were challenged to explain the relationship between body and soul. As mentioned, during much of the Middle Ages the soul was believed to inhabit the entire body. Descartes

proposed an alternative in the form of a mind–body dualism.

**Cartesian dualism** (named for Descartes) contends that every person has both a soul and a body but that the two are not the same. Descartes believed that the soul dwells only temporarily in the human body, a belief based on the conviction that the soul lives after the body dies (Cottingham, 1992). Furthermore, Descartes theorized that the soul was seated in the human brain (other animals being presumably soulless). Thus, in Descartes' view, the soul is most closely associated with the mind, not spread throughout the body.

The medical implications of Cartesian dualism are profound, including the separation of medicine into two branches, one for the mind and one for the body. From this perspective, disease (a physical condition) is distinguishable from illness (the condition as it is experienced). Of course, this distinction goes only so far. Few people would argue that the mind and the body have no influence on each other. Nevertheless, dualism was (and still is) accepted as a general principle. For the most part, medical doctors (e.g., internists, cardiologists, neurologists) consider it their primary function to treat physical ailments. Mental health is more the domain of psychiatrists, psychologists, social workers, and the like.

## HEALTH CARE IN THE NEW WORLD

Near the end of the Renaissance, European settlers began inhabiting North America. Despite our romantic notions of it, the New World was not a healthy place, physically or emotionally.

### Health Conditions

The relatively good health enjoyed by Native Americans before 1600 was replaced by widespread epidemics after European settlers began arriving, and the early settlers fared little better. James Cassedy (1991) reports that 80% of the settlers in Virginia died between 1607 and 1625, and contact with settlers resulted in the death of 90% of the Native American population. The settlers suffered from exhaustion, malnutrition, and, very often, severe depression. In addition, both settlers and Native Americans were threatened by exposure to diseases uncommon in their homelands. Without the immunity that might have resulted from previous exposure, many died of conditions such as measles, dysentery, malaria, and the flu.

Health care consisted mainly of family efforts and home remedies. Caregivers were diverse, including physicians as well as folk therapists specializing in herbs, hypnosis, acupuncture, phrenology (based on the size and shape of the skull), and other forms of treatment. Many of these folk remedies remained quite popular until the late 1800s (Cassedy, 1991).

### Hippocrates' Influence

People nostalgic for the age of humble country doctors may not wish to turn time back quite so far as the 1700s. Physicians in colonial America adhered largely to Hippocrates' idea of body humors, bloodletting, and purging. Early accounts describe patients who died after being induced to vomit 100 times or enduring days of sweating and bleeding (Cassedy, 1991). Cotton Mather, a Boston minister and healer, spoke out against such aggressive treatments. He once wrote:

> Before we go any farther, let this Advice to the Sick be principally attended to: *Don't kill 'em!*...If we stopt here, and said no more, this were enough to save more *Lives* than our *Wars* have destroyed. (as cited in Duffy, 1979, p. 35)

It's no wonder that people preferred more gentle folk remedies and often summoned doctors only as a last resort.

### Women's Role

In early America women played an important but unofficial role in health care. Most care was provided in the home, and women were expected to nurse ill family members. Schools of nursing had yet to be established. During the Civil War, female nurses and a small number of unlicensed female physicians were accepted as military medics, but the prevailing assumption was that most women were too delicate and uneducated to be doctors (Bonner, 1992). We will explore the role of women and ethnically diverse people more in Chapters 6 and 9.

## THE RISE OF ORTHODOX MEDICINE

The Industrial Revolution was made possible by mass production and diverse power sources available in the United Sates by the late 1800s. The revolution brought people to urban centers to work in factories and made health care a booming business. This dramatically widened the schism between what Cassedy (1991) calls **orthodox practitioners**, who were educated in medical schools, and **sectarians**, who practiced folk medicine taught to them by friends and family members.

Folk medicine had long been popular as a safer and less painful alternative to orthodox medicine (also referred to as *conventional medicine*). However, these advantages were diminished by the introduction of anesthesia and sterilization in conventional medical centers, medical research and technology, medical school reform, and a campaign to wipe out disease through orthodox medicine. Together these factors contributed to the decline of sectarian medicine.

## Population Shifts

Industrialization increased the demand for medical care. The number of crippling injuries rose with the introduction of heavy machinery in factories and on farms (Cassedy, 1991). Contagion was also a threat in dense population centers, a factor aggravated by inadequate drainage and waste disposal.

Medicine became more lucrative, but also more demanding. Larger patient-to-physician ratios made house calls impractical and required physicians to develop more intricate methods of keeping records. Hospitals and clinics were opened to bring patients and doctors together. The image of the solitary traveling country doctor gave way to that of the physician situated at the hub of an overwhelming number of patients, professionals, and technical facilities.

## Germ Theory

At about the same time, a scientific breakthrough helped hospitals and medical centers become safer and more appealing than in the past. That breakthrough was germ theory, which became widely accepted in the late 1800s through the work of Louis Pasteur.

Simply put, **germ theory** states that disease is caused by microscopic organisms (Twaddle & Hessler, 1987). The ramifications of such a simple notion are astounding. An awareness of microscopic agents has allowed communities to remove the threat of many contagious diseases, reduce the incidence of infection, and develop inoculations

against smallpox, measles, polio, and other diseases. Based on germ theory, Joseph Lister revolutionized surgery by sterilizing medical instruments and environments (Raffel & Raffel, 1989). Hospital personnel began cleansing their instruments and separating people with contagious diseases from other patients.

## Research and Technology

Medical centers made it possible to collect patient data systematically and to acquire expensive technology. As research and technology advanced, so did the demands on health professionals to expand their knowledge, increase their patient loads, and track the health of a diverse population (Raffel & Raffel, 1989). With so many demands, it was necessary for physicians to limit the time they spent with each patient, promoting the idea that medical communication should be brief and to the point.

Medical developments also made it important for doctors to be well trained. Physicians increasingly gained legitimacy through attendance at medical schools, membership in medical societies, contributions to professional journals and research, and eventually through laws requiring doctors to be state licensed. The American Medical Association (AMA) was organized in 1846 to unite doctors across the continent and to speak on their behalf.

## Campaign of Orthodox Medicine

In his book *The Silent World of Doctor and Patient*, Jay Katz (1984) makes a case that conventional practitioners in the early 1900s sought to distinguish themselves as the legitimate guardians of people's health. In Katz's view, this campaign was not entirely self-serving. Many people believed scientific knowledge and technology could be used to eradicate disease. Whether conventional medicine was more concerned with this goal or with attaining professional dominance, the effect was the same. Folk medicine was largely discredited as quackery, and "orthodox" medicine gained a virtual monopoly over health care. As Katz describes it, this monopoly seemed to eliminate the need for physicians to explain or justify their actions:

Since they no longer had to defend themselves against the criticism of rival groups, doctors asserted more adamantly, and now without fear of contradiction, that laymen could not judge medical practices and had to comply with medical orders. (p. 39)

Physicians' authority was considered unquestionable. Doctors were not expected to express doubts or uncertainties, and they were not to be influenced by the opinions of people (including patients) less educated than themselves.

The image of physicians as all-knowing authorities inspired public trust. But defining medical professionalism in terms of certainty and scientific expertise discouraged doctors from showing emotions or admitting doubts or mistakes (Katz, 1984). At the same time, patients and their loved ones were effectively silenced into submission. Soon, many patients were too trusting or intimidated to speak freely to their doctors (Katz, 1984).

### Flexner Report

One part of the campaign to promote scientific medicine took the form of medical school reform. Prior to 1900, most medical schools in the United States were run as private businesses, oriented more toward profit than toward rigorous education (Cassedy, 1991). Such schools produced thousands of physicians with little knowledge of biology or physiology.

Disturbed by the low scientific standards in these schools, the AMA commissioned Abraham Flexner of the Carnegie Foundation to evaluate U.S. medical schools and make recommendations. The **Flexner Report**, published in 1910, was a stinging indictment. It charged that all but a few medical schools in the country—the notable exceptions were Harvard, Johns Hopkins, and Western Reserve—were lax in their coverage of biology and other sciences. The report also criticized medical schools for not offering more supervised, hands-on experience with patients.

Of the 155 medical schools he evaluated, Flexner recommended that all but 31 cease operation (Raffel & Raffel, 1989). In fact, nearly two-thirds of U.S. medical schools did close, unable to meet the reform standards (Twaddle & Hessler, 1987). Most of the schools that remained open were incorporated within universities.

The chief model for reform was Johns Hopkins Medical School, with its alliance to Johns Hopkins Hospital (both located in Baltimore, Maryland). The staff at Johns Hopkins incorporated the most up-to-date knowledge of healthy ventilation, efficiency, and infection control. They emphasized science, laboratory and research experience, and clinical experience with actual patients (Raffel & Raffel, 1989). Following this example, medical schools across the country became more demanding and began to focus intensely on organic aspects of disease as well as clinical and laboratory experience.

### Decline of Sectarian Medicine

For the most part sectarian healers were not prepared to fight the emerging dominance of conventional medicine. Americans were enamored with science and technology—both of which were firmly rooted in the camp of conventional medicine by the early 1900s. Moreover, there was little to unite diverse healers, and because their treatments promised gradual and long-term effects, outcomes were hard to isolate and measure (Cassedy, 1991).

Osteopathy and chiropractic were among the only sects to maintain popularity. Other forms of therapy, such as acupuncture and herbal remedies, faded from significance for several decades, at least in the United States. Interestingly, the very reasons that led to their decline—long-term results, low-tech methods—are now contributing to a resurgence of popularity as people seek to reduce costs and to prevent ill health. You will read more about that in Chapter 9.

### TWENTIETH CENTURY HEALTH CARE

Medicine began to depend ever more on technology, and by 1900 physicians were using x-rays to see inside the body. High-powered microscopes identified a long list of diseases, including malaria, influenza, pneumonia, tuberculosis, and more (Reiser, 1978). With the new technology, a small vial of blood could be the basis for dozens of diagnostic procedures. The phrase "a battery of tests" became common. The efficiency of technology, combined with Americans' confidence in it, made technology an appealing option in medical care.

People's confidence in medicine grew, but as health care became high tech it lost some of the intimacy to which people were accustomed. Emotional concerns can seem out of place in the sterile, scientific atmosphere of clinics and hospitals, and caregivers trained in the sciences were not necessarily prepared to deal with psychosocial aspects of illness. Added to this, doctors were so greatly outnumbered by their patients that it became difficult to establish close relationships with them all.

Social conditions affected medicine as well. Racial segregation continued well into the twentieth century. African American patients and caregivers were not allowed into most hospitals in the United States until the 1960s (a topic to be covered more thoroughly in Chapter 9). Even as the United States was building one of the most respected medical systems in the world, its benefits were not available to all citizens.

## Specialization

The immense growth in medical knowledge and technology spawned an era of **specialization**, in which doctors focused on particular aspects of health. Neurologists, allergists, radiologists, cardiovascular surgeons, and oncologists—to name a few—began limiting their practices to specific concerns. A patient with an ailment in any of these categories could see an expert rather than a generalist, a prospect that was appealing but expensive. Before long it became more prestigious and profitable to be a specialist than to be a general practitioner. As you will see, this trend eventually led to a critical shortage of general practitioners that continues today. It also changed the nature of health communication. Talk about broader concerns often seems out of place when seeing an expert who focuses on a specific body part or system.

## Medicine and Free Enterprise

As health care evolved over the course of U.S. history, it came to be treated largely as a free market commodity. That is, consumers, commanding what buying power they could, were soon able to choose between a range of caregivers who charged fees for the care they provided.

Insurance became particularly important in the United States as health care costs rose to cover the expenses of medical technology, education, specialization, staffing, and facilities. The premise of insurance is to pool resources so that expenses are spread over a great number of people, saving any one subscriber from overwhelming debt. This assumes that most people will not require more than they contribute and that enough people will subscribe to establish an adequate treasury. These premises were about to topple.

## PUTTING THE BRAKES ON HEALTH CARE COSTS

The strength of the United States after World War II made it a model for rebuilding countries, many of which received medical aid from the United States. However, a crisis was building. In this section, we discuss the financial dilemma surrounding health care that has given rise to managed care.

## Health and Wealth

By the mid-1900s, Americans who could afford health insurance had access to specialists and facilities as superb as any in the world. It seemed for a while that no expense was too great, especially when the government or insurance companies were footing the bill.

The emphasis on individuality and the value of human life in the United States fostered the expectation of equal treatment for all and immense expenditures for the sake of single individuals (Balint & Shelton, 1996). In practice, of course, the system fell far short of that ideal. Discrimination has never been fully abolished, and the poor have always been underserved. Nevertheless, the ideology of individualism justified using every resource available for any patient deemed to be in need of it.

## Problems

Eventually, the rising cost of health care became more than Americans could afford. The population increased as life expectancy lengthened. Today, U.S. residents live an average of 77.8 years—32 years longer than most settlers in colonial America (National Center for Health Statistics, 2007a; D. Taylor, 1999). That is partly because of better living conditions and better medical care. Diseases once fatal have become treatable, allowing us to extend our lives, albeit sometimes with expensive long-term treatment.

It became clear by the 1960s that health care was too expensive. Health insurance rates began to climb out of the reach of many Americans. In 1965 the government stepped in with the creation of Medicare and Medicaid, publicly funded health insurance programs for impoverished children and pregnant women, people with disabilities, and people 65 and older. Even so, tens of millions of U.S. residents were still uninsured (McDermott, 1995).

A tragic spiral developed. As Americans were forced to drop their insurance coverage, insurance treasuries decreased, leading to steep rate hikes for those who continued to subscribe, forcing more people to drop their coverage, and so on.

Government-sponsored health programs forecast bankruptcies, unable to keep up with rising medical costs and the growing number of uninsured and needy people.

The United States also began to experience a shortage of primary care doctors, especially in rural and low-income areas. This was particularly lamentable because primary care physicians are valuable in tracking and monitoring people's overall care. Without primary care, the uncoordinated efforts of various specialists may lead to treatment duplications and unforeseen drug interactions. Moreover, systemic illnesses are more apt to go undetected by doctors with a very specific focus. Finally, many patients became discontent because specialists were not focused on them as whole persons.

## Reform Efforts

Beginning in the late 1970s, several measures were taken to curb costs and improve medical care. One was increased surveillance. Utilization review boards began to review patient records to identify treatment duplications and to see if costs were justified. Second, funding agencies (government and private insurers) began to require that patients see specialists only with referrals from primary care physicians.

Finally, funding agencies established specific reimbursement rates for health services. For example, **diagnosis-related groups (DRGs)** establish in advance what the funding agency will pay hospitals for certain procedures or the treatment of specific ailments. One effect of set reimbursement rates is that funding agencies largely control the market value of health services. A major player in this process is the government. The U.S. health system is ostensibly private rather than state run, but the government has substantial influence because it pays for about 39% of the nation's health care expenses through Medicaid and Medicare (Cowan & Hartman, 2005).

Reimbursement rates limit the care health agencies are willing or able to provide. If reimbursement rates are too low, health organizations may discontinue services or stop treating certain patients. Especially worrisome is funding for diagnostic tests, AIDS treatment, care for dying individuals, and long-term care. For example, in 2008 the U.S. legislature considered cutting nursing home reimbursements by two-tenths of a percent. That sounds small, but the measure would take $5 billion out of nursing home budgets in just five years ("Nursing Homes," 2008).

Reimbursement restrictions have had several effects besides influencing what services are marketable. First, health care organizations are under pressure to keep their costs under reimbursement rates. If their expenses fall below those rates, they get to keep the difference. However, if their expenses exceed reimbursement rates, they take a loss. Furthermore, paperwork to justify expenses has increased, and health professionals accustomed to professional autonomy sometimes chafe under the scrutiny of third parties who second-guess their judgments.

## MANAGED CARE

Another response to cost containment was the creation of managed care. About 97% of U.S. residents with employer-sponsored health plans and about 88.5% of U.S. physicians now participate in managed care plans (Henry J. Kaiser, 2007; O'Malley & Reschovsky, 2006). **Managed care organizations** essentially coordinate the costs and delivery of health services. Whereas health decisions used to be made almost entirely by caregivers and patients, managed care organizations now recruit patients, match them up with caregivers and facilities, and monitor expenses. As such, managed care represents the influence of people (or entities) other than patients and caregivers. By "managing" resources such as money, labor, technology, and facilities, managed care organizations seek to make health care more efficient and affordable.

It is easiest to understand managed care (and how it compares to traditional health insurance) if we look at it from the consumer's perspective. Imagine that Sam is trying to decide between traditional health insurance and managed care.

**Percent Insured U.S. Workers in Each Plan**

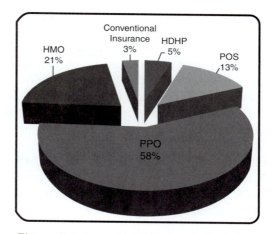

**Figure 2-1** Insured U.S. Workers in Each Plan
Source: Henry J. Kaiser Family Foundation Employer Health Benefits Study, 2007

### Conventional Insurance

At one point, nearly everyone who had health insurance in the United States had conventional (also known as *indemnity*) insurance. Now that managed care has become the standard, this type of insurance is rare. Particularly if Sam is counting on health insurance offered through his employer, conventional insurance is probably not an option. Only 3% of employee-sponsored plans meet this description (Henry J. Kaiser, 2007). (See Figure 2.1.)

However, let's assume Sam can pay for insurance on his own, so he meets with an agent. The agent explains that Sam will pay a set monthly amount (his **insurance premium**) and will pay for the first $500 (his **insurance deductible**) of medical expenses he incurs every year. If Sam's expenses exceed his deductible, his insurance will pay 80% of the remaining medical bill and Sam will pay 20%. To prevent Sam from going into overwhelming debt, there is an upper limit, called a **catastrophic cap**, on the amount of out-of-pocket money he will be required to pay each year. Beyond that limit, insurance pays 100%. Amounts vary, but let's say that Sam's cap is $1,500 a year for covered services.

Conventional insurance is classified as **fee-for-service** because providers are paid (reimbursed) for specific care they provide. In other words, doctors, hospitals, physical therapists, and so on, only make money if patients use their services. Traditional insurance is also known as a **third-party payer** system because, as you can see, there are three parties involved—the provider, the patient, and the payer (insurance company). Practically speaking, this means that if Sam has knee surgery this year, he will pay the first $500 and 20% of the remaining medical bills in addition to his monthly premiums. The insurance company will pay the rest.

As mentioned, this is how almost all insurance used to work, meaning that it's quite possible care providers overprescribed tests and treatment at times. For one thing, more treatment means more pay in a fee-for-services system. But also keep in mind that diagnostics is detective work. It's hard to know which medical tests will help solve the puzzle until the results are in. Furthermore, providers wary of being sued were (and still are) reluctant to overlook or undertreat patients, for fear they will be considered negligent if things don't go well.

With traditional insurance, there isn't much financial incentive to keep people well. Most policies don't cover routine checkups. That means Sam would pay for those visits entirely from his own pocket. This is a significant difference between conventional insurance and managed care.

Here are two final considerations for Sam. Conventional insurance premiums are usually more expensive than other forms of health insurance. However, the advantage is freedom of choice. Under this type of plan, Sam may choose his own caregivers.

Next Sam considers managed care. The most obvious benefit—if Sam is fortunate enough to work for an organization that offers health insurance benefits—is that his employer probably *does* offer some type of manage care plan, perhaps

several types. This means the employer will help pay for Sam's monthly premium, usually about 85% of it (Henry J. Kaiser, 2007). (Larger firms typically cover more than smaller firms.) The confusing part may be deciding which managed care plan to choose. So let's walk through the typical options. The averages presented here are based on the Henry J. Kaiser Family Foundation's 2007 study of employee-sponsored health plans.

### Health Maintenance Organization

A **health maintenance organization (HMO)** is designed to be, more or less, a one-stop shop for members' health needs. An HMO hires physicians and other care providers, who work directly for the HMO. Their salaries are covered by the premiums that members (like Sam) pay each month.

If Sam chooses an HMO through his employer, his portion of the monthly premium will probably be about $59 a month (for one-person coverage) and he will be charged a **copay** (usually $15, $20, or $25) every time he visits a doctor[1]. This includes checkups and preventive care visits. (See Figure 2.2 for a comparison of premium costs.)

Let's pause for a moment to look back in time. In the beginning, premiums and copays were usually the only costs associated with HMO membership. All other medical costs were absorbed by the HMO. Knowing that he would never pay more than $25 a visit, Sam would probably be more willing than with conventional insurance to have annual checkups and to see a doctor about minor health concerns. This incentive to seek well-care is meant to save money in the long run, both for members and for HMOs, because, where health care is concerned, a pound of prevention is often less expensive than an ounce of cure.

Things have changed a bit, and now most HMOs charge a deductible (usually $400 or so a

---

[1] For now, let's leave prescription drugs, outpatient surgery, and hospital care out of the mix. With managed care, separate copays and deductibles usually apply to those services.

## Average Worker Contribution to Annual Premiums

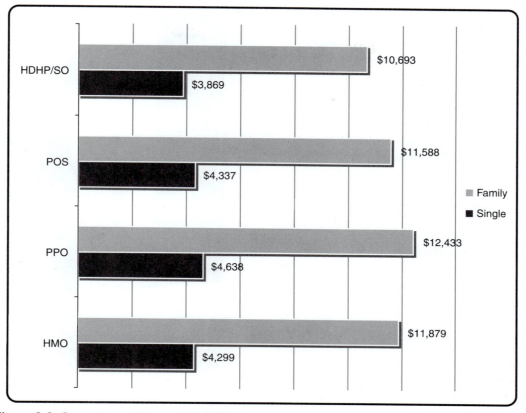

**Figure 2-2** Comparison of Managed Care Premiums
Source: Henry J. Kaiser Family Foundation Employer Health Benefits, 2007

year). Thus, the incentive to seek preventive and minor care is not quite as great as before. But if Sam needs a lot of medical care, HMO membership might still save him money. He can feel confident that he won't have exorbitant medical bills no matter what. (With traditional insurance, even 20% of a surgery bill is pretty high!) The trade-off is that Sam cannot choose any doctor he wants. He is limited to providers who work for the HMO, and he cannot see specialists (even if they are part of the HMO) unless such care is recommended by his primary care physician in the HMO. This is designed to avoid unnecessary visits and costs, but the approval process and limitations can be frustrating.

You guessed it: HMOs are not third-party payer systems. In their case, it's as if the insurance company and the medical center merged into one. And they are not based on fee-for-service. Instead, HMOs are **capitated systems**. They receive a set (capitated) amount, in the form of premiums (plus minor copays), no matter what care they provide. HMOs' job is to manage both the budget and the care.

Some people (including many physicians) worry that combining the insurance company and the medical center into one presents a conflict of interest. We'll talk more about that shortly. But first, let's continue the tour of managed care options.

### Preferred Provider Organization

A **preferred provider organization (PPO)**, also in the managed care family, works a little differently. If Sam joins a PPO, he will pay a monthly premium roughly equivalent to HMO membership. He might also have a deductible. (About 48% of PPOs have deductibles, compared to 71% of HMOs. See Figure 2.3 for more details.) The difference is that, as a PPO member, Sam's copay is not a prescribed amount. Instead, he pays a percentage of the medical bill.

Here's how it works. Rather than hiring care providers outright, as HMOs do, PPOs contract with independent care providers. The PPO agrees to put the provider on a "preferred" list if the provider offers services at agreed-on discount rates to the PPO's members.

Sam's copay is a percentage of this discounted fee. This means he will pay different amounts for different services. It also means he can choose any health care providers he wishes, with one caveat. As the name implies, providers on the "preferred" list cost less than those who are not. There are often higher copays and/or separate deductibles for providers not on the list. But unlike HMO members, Sam will receive *some* financial coverage no matter which caregivers he chooses. (As with conventional insurance, there is usually an annual catastrophic cap for PPO members.)

If Sam requires a lot of care or sees nonpreferred providers, he is likely to pay more as a PPO member than as an HMO member. But he has more freedom of choice. He may also encounter less conflict of interest because (1) PPO providers do not work directly for the managed care organization, so they may be spared some of the pressure to cut costs and speed up patient visits, and (2) they operate on a fee-for-service basis that gives them more incentive to prescribe (rather

### Percentage of Plans that Have Deductibles

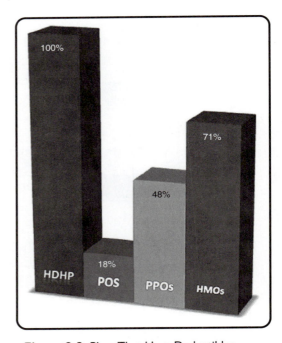

**Figure 2-3** Plans That Have Deductibles
Source: Henry J. Kaiser Family Foundation Employer Health Benefits, 2007

than avoid) tests and treatment. These advantages may be why the majority of people with employee health plans choose PPOs (58% compared to 21% in HMOs).

HMOs and PPOs used to be the only two options in managed care. But a few others have emerged.

### Point of Service

**Point of service (POS)** plans combine features of HMOs and PPOs. If Sam chooses to see only preferred providers, the POS plans feels like an HMO. He pays a set, minimal copay every time he seeks care, and his primary care provider oversees his care and determines if he should see specialists or not.

However, Sam also has the option to see providers outside the network. At that point, the POS plan functions like a PPO. That is, Sam pays a portion of the medical bills, and he may have to meet a deductible. In sum, although Sam has greater choice than with HMO membership, there are still financial incentives to see preferred providers.

POS plans are relatively new. So far, about 13% of people with employee health plans subscribe to them. On average, monthly premiums are slightly less expensive than HMOs and PPOs. (Employees' portion is usually about $52 per month.) Only 18% of POS plans have deductibles, and although these deductibles are usually higher than with other managed care plans (about $621 per year compared to $400–$460 in HMOs and PPOs), they often apply only to out-of-network providers.

### High-Deductible Health Plan

Imagine that Sam is in excellent health and almost never seeks medical care. He may wonder, "Why should I pay such high premiums when I never meet the deductible anyway? My money goes in, but it doesn't come out—at least it doesn't come to me." And if he is really thinking long-term, he might also wonder, "Rather than paying high premiums, why can't I save that money for the future, when my medical bills are likely to be higher?"

These are the basic concepts behind **high-deductible health plans (HDHPs)**. Members pay relatively low monthly premiums (about $43.50 per month in employer-sponsored plans). In exchange, their deductibles are three to four times more than for other plans (about $1,729 per year), and the catastrophic cap is several thousand dollars higher. HDHPs are typically coupled with other managed care plans. Thus, members enroll in either an HMO, a PPO, or a POS. The difference is in the out-of-pocket expenses they absorb.

Furthermore, membership in an HDHP qualifies one to invest in a tax-deferred **health savings account (HSA)**. This is why you often see the abbreviations HDHP/SO (HDHP with a savings option) or HDHP/HSA. Sam and his employer can contribute to his HSA over time, creating a fund he can use to pay for future medical expenses. As long as they invest the money while Sam is an HDHP member and he uses the money only for medical bills, Sam doesn't pay taxes on it.

The U.S. government approved tax breaks for HSAs in 2003 to give people an incentive to control their own health costs. After all, if you have a high deductible or are paying the medical bills from your own savings account, you might think twice before seeing a doctor.

Unfortunately, this is also the downside of HDHPs. Some people buy into them because they can afford the lower premiums but then find out that they can't afford the out-of-pocket costs that lie ahead. Reports abound of people who are insured but still cannot afford to buy prescription drugs or see a doctor. Even if Sam hasn't needed much medical care in years past, one accident or appendicitis attack can wreck his finances if he is not adequately insured.

Critics of HDHPs point out that premiums, once quite low, continue to rise and that the true audience for HDHP/HSAs have been the wealthy, who use them as tax shelters. The numbers bear this out. The average taxpayer in the United States makes $51,000 per year. The average income among people claiming HSA tax benefits is $133,000 (Woodbury, 2007). Another criticism is that enticing people to pay lower premiums further depletes the money available to pay for health costs across the nation. In Sam's case, maybe he hasn't needed insurance payouts so far, but the day may come when his benefits outpace his contributions. This only works if people at every need level are invested in the system.

As you can see, managed care has given rise to its own vocabulary, and the system and terms continue to evolve. For a handy synopsis of relevant terms see Box 2.4.

### Organizations' Perspective

Managed care also affects hospitals, medical centers, treatment and diagnostic centers, and other

## Managed Care at a Glance

**managed care:** A health care system in which income, resources, and health services are supervised by a managing body such as a health maintenance organization or preferred provider organization. Patients pay the organization a set fee each month to receive health services.

**health maintenance organization (HMO):** A managed care organization that offers enrollees a variety of health services for a set monthly fee and copays. Caregivers are usually employed directly by the HMO and provide services only to HMO members.

**preferred provider organization (PPO):** A managed care organization that pays caregivers a discounted fee for each service they provide to PPO members. Patients may visit providers not on the preferred list, but they pay higher fees to do so.

**point of service (POS):** A hybrid between an HMO and a PPO. Members may pay an established copay to see providers affiliated with the plan. But they are also covered (at a higher cost) if they see providers not on the list.

**high-deductible health plan (HDHP):** A managed care plan with lower-than-normal premiums but higher deductibles and out-of-pocket spending caps. Most HDHPs qualify members to establish tax-exempt health savings accounts.

**health savings account (HSA):** A tax-exempt savings plan (a lot like an IRA) in which people can set aside money to pay future medical bills. United States taxpayers qualify for HSAs if they are part of high-deductible health plans. Money saved can be used over many years' time.

**health reimbursement account (HRA):** Not to be confused with an HSA, a health reimbursement account (HRA) is a temporary fund in which an employee can set aside tax-exempt money for health care costs incurred within the plan year. For example, you might have $100 set aside from each paycheck before taxes. Your employer will use this money to reimburse you for up to $1,200 of medical expenses during the year. Typically, if you do not use the money in a HRA by year's end, you forfeit the balance.

**premium:** A membership fee paid by subscribers in a conventional insurance or managed care plan. Usually deducted from one's paycheck.

**capitation:** A set fee paid to cover a person's health needs, regardless of the care actually required.

**catastrophic cap:** An upper limit on the amount of out-of-pocket expense a subscriber is required to pay each year.

**copay:** The portion of a health care bill the patient is required to pay when services are rendered.

**deductible:** The amount of out-of-pocket medical expense an insured individual is required to pay before receiving financial assistance from the insurer. For example, you might pay the first $500 of your emergency room bill, and insurance will pay 80% of the remaining cost.

**fee-for-service:** The practice of being paid for specific care provided.

organizations in the health care industry. These organizations may contract with managed care agencies to provide care for their members, or they may offer their own managed care plans. Either way, their income is largely governed by the terms of managed care, with its reliance on discounts and capitated fees.

I was public relations director at a large medical center in the early 1990s, when managed care tipped the scales in our market. Prior to that point, we received daily census reports detailing how many patients were in the hospital. The higher the census, the greater was our revenue. But I remember a pivotal meeting at which the CEO said to us:

We now rely on DRGs and capitation to such an extent that "beds filled" doesn't mean much. We could just as easily lose money on a patient as make money. And sometimes we make more money when the beds are empty!

What he meant, of course, was that capitation agreements provided us money even when patients didn't need care. But, on the flip side, reimbursements rates below previous market value meant we had to cut costs or we would quickly find ourselves in a hole.

Capitation, discounted fees, DRGs, and other cost-curtailment efforts may be especially hard on not-for-profit medical organizations. These organizations are granted tax exemptions because they provide care for needy persons and they reinvest the money they earn in the organization rather than paying owners or stockholders (Bruck, 1996). However, even with tax breaks, making less money on insured patients means these organizations have less surplus to cover the care of people who cannot afford to pay. And nonprofit organizations are typically not at liberty to discontinue services that yield low reimbursements.

Overall, there are upsides and downsides to managed care. Following are a few considerations both ways. One note before we begin. In the parlance of health care, *insurers* includes both conventional insurance companies and managed care organizations. However, as you have seen, as much as 97% of insurance policies are now managed care memberships. So when people talk about "insurers" these days, they mostly mean managed care.

## Advantages

Imagine yourself around the table at a health care center in the early days of managed care. You are at a historical turning point. Rather than earning income after the fact for specific services you perform, the health center will now have an annual budget paid by member fees. It's not a huge budget. It's actually less than you made before. But it's predictable, so you can plan ahead. The beauty of capitation is the freedom to be proactive, to accomplish some things you could never do before. You have the opportunity—in fact,

the obligation—to redesign how medical care is provided.

Physicians Joseph Dorsey and Donald Berwick were around that table. They were on staff at Harvard Pilgrim Health Care when managed care began. "Capitation gave us the flexibility to use our budget with creativity limited only by our imaginations and habits," they recall (Dorsey & Berwick, 2008, p. A9). The Harvard Pilgrim team invested in innovative and patient-friendly services such as reminder calls, after-hour phone access, extended clinic hours, time-saving technology, and more. They devoted themselves to providing better, more patient-centered care for less money than before. As a result, their patient members made half as many visits to emergency rooms as the state average. "The innovations that managed care and capitation made possible were good for almost everyone" (Dorsey & Berwick, p. A9).

***Incentive to Collaborate and Conserve*** That is one advantage of managed care in its purest form— it gives health care professionals a means and an incentive to work together to provide innovative care in a cost-effective way. With managed care, there is a strong incentive to streamline processes and eliminate wasteful practices.

***Affordability Goal*** A related benefit is that managed care is designed to make health care more affordable. In a global sense, it is oriented to making the most of every health care dollar. At an individual level, membership in a managed care organization, particularly an HMO, curbs financial risk because subscribers pay set (or reduced) fees even if they need a lot of care. This can be especially valuable to people with chronic illnesses, who benefit from regular treatment (Nussbaum, Ragan, & Whaley, 2003).

***Wellness*** Third, managed care presents an incentive to keep patients well. In the long run, organizations make more money if people do not require costly treatments. And everyone stands to benefit if managed care invests in disease prevention and public education. (As you will soon see, this potential has not been well fulfilled so far.)

So far we have talked mostly about the advantages for patients. But providers may also benefit from managed care.

### Administrative Assistance

*Administrative Assistance* Working for an HMO has the potential to ease the administrative demands of running a private medical practice. The HMO handles facilities, maintenance, administrative and support staff (receptionists, nurses, and so on), billing procedures, marketing, and more. This can mean more stability, fewer headaches, and better working hours because providers can share the patient load with others in the organization.

A physician I know says that managed care gave him his life back. He doesn't make as much money as before, but he is only on call one day a week, and he can schedule days off—luxuries he didn't have as a physician entrepreneur.

*Patient Load* For health professionals who are just getting started and those worried about attracting new patients, managed care organizations can offer a ready-made caseload. Signing on as an HMO employee or a preferred provider means built-in advertising among hundreds or thousands of available patients.

### Disadvantages

Unfortunately, as the system has evolved, the disadvantages of managed care have become numerous. Public opinion about managed care has not been favorable since 1995. In 2006, *Modern Healthcare* magazine proclaimed: "Over the past 20 years, managed care has gone from industry hero to industry villain and then to health care has-been" ("Managed Care," 2006, p. 20). Similarly, the staff of Deloitte's highly respected Center for Health Solutions quips on their website: "If the U.S. health care system is in crisis—and just try to find someone who says it isn't..." (Deloitte Center, 2008, paragraph 1). All in all, it's no stretch to say that managed care is unpopular. Nearly everyone agrees that the system is badly flawed. It may help as you read the following list of drawbacks to keep in mind that *something* had to

be done. It is conceivable that we would be in even worse shape without the managed care revolution. But clearly, we still have a long way to go!

*Costs Still Prohibitive* One disappointment is that the goal of cutting overall costs, thus insuring a greater proportion of the population, has not been met. Managed care may have slowed spiraling costs to some extent, but premiums have climbed steadily, as has the percentage of uninsured Americans.

Let's look back. Managed care organizations originated in the mid-1980s and doubled in number during the 1990s. But, during the 1990s, health insurance premiums rose by 53%, far outpacing inflation and wage increases. And health care costs rose even more—up 57% in the same timeframe (Economic Research Initiative, 2005). By the decade's end, the number of uninsured Americans didn't shrink. It grew by 23%, from 34.7 million to 42.6 million (Economic Research Initiative). And it hasn't gotten much better since.

In 2005 the number of uninsured in the United States jumped from 44.8 million to 47 million in one year—the largest leap since 1992 (U.S. Census Bureau, 2007). To put that into perspective, consider that 47 million is more than the combined populations of Alabama, Alaska, Colorado, Delaware, Connecticut, Idaho, Hawaii, Iowa, Kansas, Maine, Montana, Oregon, Vermont, West Virginia, North Dakota, Oklahoma, Arizona, South Carolina, and Wyoming!

Some people assume that the uninsured are covered by programs such as Medicaid and Medicare. Actually, people in those programs count as *insured*. The 47 million have no insurance of any type—not even government-sponsored assistance. (We'll talk more about these issues in Chapter 12.)

Spokespersons for managed care say premium hikes are necessary because health expenses are rising and the population is getting older. However, critics charge that managed care organizations are making profits while patients and providers lose money. Some hospitals in California have even begun what is known as **balance billing**, charging customers for the amount their insurance companies don't reimburse. One hospital chain in

## BOX 2.5 ETHICAL CONSIDERATIONS

### Classroom Debate on Managed Care

Managed care is currently the most controversial issue in health care. You have already been exposed to several viewpoints about it. Some people fear managed care will lessen the quality of medical decisions by limiting what doctors can say and do. Others favor the managed care emphasis on wellness and applaud the effort to cut health care costs. There are other issues, both pro and con. Read up on the managed care debate (a few sources are listed at the end of this box) and develop your own viewpoints.

Hold a classroom debate. Divide the class into four groups: (a) those in favor of HMOs, (b) those who support PPOs, (c) those who propose specific alternatives, and (d) those who support HDHPs. Appoint team captains or have the instructor moderate. One group at a time should present its arguments, with time after each argument for questions and challenges.

(Make sure talking time is divided fairly among the participants.)

As the debate progresses, people may change their minds. If so, they should get up and move to the group that best represents their viewpoint.

### Suggested Sources

Anderlink, M. R. (2001). *The ethics of managed care: A pragmatic approach.* Bloomington, IN: Indiana University Press.

Shapiro, R. S., Tym, K. A., Eastwood, D., Derse, A. R., & Klein, J. P. (2003). Managed care, doctors, and patients: Focusing on relationships, not rights. *Cambridge Quarterly of Healthcare Ethics, 12*(3), 300–307.

Ulrich, C. M., Soeken, K. L., & Miller, N. (2003). Ethical conflict associated with managed care: Views of nurse practitioners. *Nursing Research, 52*(3), 168–175.

*Also see resources in Box 2.6.*

---

California sent thousands of patients bills for up to $50,000 each (Costello, 2008). Imagine receiving such a bill even though you are fully insured and have paid your copays and deductibles. Courts are reviewing the lawfulness of balance billing, which puts patients in the middle of pricing disputes between insurers and providers.

*Prevention Expectations Unrealized* It is sometimes said that the United States doesn't have a health care system, it has an illness care system. Managed care was supposed to change that by shifting the focus to cost-saving prevention. That hasn't happened on the scale many people had hoped. This is mostly because prevention efforts cost in the short run but save in the long run. "I think that [the rising cost of premiums] is primarily due to the short-sighted nature of many of the for-profit companies," said a managed care executive on an anonymous survey. "The managed care plans don't think

it's worthwhile to invest in prevention programs when people change their plans frequently, trying to get lower costs" ("Health Economics," 2003, p. 56). In other words, predictably enough, managed care organizations are often reluctant to invest in the long-term health of short-term members.

*Undertreatment* Critics are also troubled that managed care organizations sometimes pressure providers to limit care and speed up patient visits. Journalists have coined the phrase "death by HMO" to refer to instances in which people's health was hurt or destroyed when their managed care organizations refused to authorize expensive treatments or delayed approval until it was too late.

Some people worry that these incentives will interfere with caregivers' professional judgment. It is common for HMOs to withhold a portion of physicians' pay, to be awarded only if the treatment they prescribe comes in under budget and only if they see a specified (usually large) number of patients per day. Equally as worrisome are so-called **gag rules** that prohibit physicians from telling patients about costly treatment options. For example, if the doctor believes a cancer patient might benefit from a certain treatment but the treatment is expensive or not covered by the health plan, the doctor would be disciplined for even mentioning it to the patient. Although the AMA and the federal government have banned the use of gag rules, many say they are at least implicitly enforced. About 31% of managed care physicians surveyed said they had avoided mentioning useful medical procedures to patients because those procedures were not covered by the health plan (Wynia, VanGeest, Cummins, & Wilson, 2003). Physicians worry that patients' mistrust is damaging their professional reputations and diminishing how much patients trust their doctors (Gorawara-Bhat, Gallagher, & Levinson, 2003). (To debate the managed care issue yourself, see Box 2.5.)

*Restricted Options*   Fourth, patients in managed care lose some of the ability to choose or switch caregivers. Even with PPOs and POS plans, there is a strong financial incentive to see providers on the short list. To receive full benefits, members are limited to providers who participate in their care plans, and they may be forced to switch providers if they change employers or if their employers change managed care affiliations. Such disruptions may compromise the quality of patient–caregiver relationships. Some people are more worried than others. Of older adults surveyed, only 44% said they would willingly give up their choice of doctors if it meant lower medical bills (Tu, 2005). However, among people ages 18 to 34, 70% were willing to sacrifice choice for lower costs (Tu).

*Confidentiality at Risk*   Fifth, medical information becomes less confidential when patient records and caregiving decisions are scrutinized by members of a managed care organization. Of the 51 hospital patients Maria Brann and Marifran Mattson

(2004) interviewed, 81% were concerned that their confidential medical information would be inappropriately shared by people within the health care organization. In an earlier study (Eastman, Eastman, & Tolson, 1997), 80% of physicians surveyed said they might divulge sensitive information (such as drug abuse) to other members of a health maintenance organization, even if patients asked them not to tell.

*Bureaucratic Hassles*   Sixth, a great deal of energy in managed care is diverted to paperwork, authorizations, and procedures. Many caregivers say it is nearly impossible to do their jobs well and meet the increased demand for paperwork. When Locum Tenens, a physician staffing agency, surveyed 2,400 physicians across the United States, only 3% were satisfied with the current health system. The most common complaint was frustration about the hassles and delays of managed care organizations ("Physicians Report," 2008).

Of a similar mind, Bhpinder Singh, a New York general practitioner, told the *New York Times:*

> Thirty percent of my hospital admissions are being denied. There's a 45-day limit on the appeal. You don't bill in time, you lose everything. You're discussing this with a managed care rep on the phone and you think: "You're sitting there, I'm sitting here. How do you know anything about this patient?" (quoted by Jauhar, 2008a, p. 5)

Likewise, Texas physicians surveyed about managed care gave the system a resounding thumbs-down (J. Greene, 2008). Here's a brief summary of what they said.

- 83% of the physicians have had to hire extra staff to help with the paperwork required by managed care organizations,
- 65% of doctors felt insurers make it needlessly cumbersome and time-consuming to get treatment options approved,
- 64% indicated that managed care payments to doctors are often late and less than promised, and

## BOX 2.6 **RESOURCES**

# Before You Select a Managed Care Plan

Here are some questions to ask when reviewing health insurance plans.

1. What are my monthly premiums, and, if applicable, what portion of the premium will my employer pay?
2. Will I have copays? If so, how much are they?
3. Is there an annual deductible? If so, how much is it? *(If you are considering a family plan, ask if this amount applies to each person's care or to the family overall.)*
4. Does the deductible apply to preventive care visits?
5. Do separate deductibles or copays apply to preventive care, prescription drugs, outpatient surgery, hospital stays, or visits to nonpreferred providers?
6. Is there an annual catastrophic cap (a limit on my out-of-pocket) on expenses? If so, what is it? What expenses count toward this amount?
7. How many (and which) physicians and specialists are on the plan or the preferred provider list? *(It's a good idea to call a few of these before you sign on, to see if they are accepting new patients and to gauge how long patients typically wait to get an appointment. Just because a provider appears on the list doesn't mean he or she has time for more patients.)*
8. Are there conditions or treatments not covered by this plan? *(Managed care has not been particularly good about funding care for mental health and some*

*other concerns. Ask in advance what is covered and what isn't.)*
9. Does this plan include care for preexisting conditions?
10. Is it required that I establish a primary care physician? If so, who are my options? If an HMO, will I be able to see the same physician every time, or will I be required to see whoever is available?
11. To what extent will the plan restrict the prescription drugs I am able to buy with benefits? *(Every plan has formularies, which are lists of approved drugs the plan covers. Some plans have long lists, and some have short ones. Particularly if you know which drugs you prefer or need to take, it's wise to ask in advance if they are covered.)*
12. Which hospitals are covered by this plan? If more than one, can I choose from among them?

*For more, see the following:*

The U.S. Department of Health and Human Service's Guide to Choosing a Health Plan: ahrq.gov/consumer/qnt/qnthplan.htm#rate
Center for Studying Health System Change: hschange.com
Henry J. Kaiser Family Foundation: kff.org
Deloitte Center for Health Solutions: deloitte.com/dtt/section_node/0,1042,sid%253D80772,00.html
National Center for Health Statistics: cdc.gov/nchs
American Association of Health Plans: aahp.org
*American Journal of Managed Care:* ajmc.com
Managed Care Information Center: themcic.com

---

- 58% charged that insurers do not educate patients well about their coverage, copayments, and deductibles.

The discontent begins even before many physicians enter practice. Of more than 2,000 medical students surveyed, 35% strongly agreed (and only 5% disagreed) with the statement that "physicians have a responsibility to take care of patients

regardless of their ability to pay" (Frank, Modi, Elon, & Coughlin, 2008, p. 140). But only 1 in 10 agreed that managed care, as it is currently implemented, does a good job at providing that care.

The extra paperwork translates to less time with patients. An extensive study of hospital nurses revealed that the nurses spent less than one-fifth of their time (just shy of 2 hours per 10-hour shift) providing direct patient care (Hendrich, Chow, Skierczynski, & Lu, 2008). The nurses spent the most time (nearly 4 hours per shift) doing required paperwork. (The rest was spent communicating with other care team members, getting supplies, moving between rooms, and so on.)

Patients are frustrated by the red tape as well. Says one managed care Medicaid patient:

> It's hard to get a doctor who takes Medicaid. They send out a list of doctors who'll see us, but they don't tell you that only a few'll take new patients. Nobody wants Medicaid patients. The doctors hate dealing with us, the insurance is such a pain in the butt. (Gillespie, 2001, p. 109)

All in all, the managed care landscape is pretty unsatisfying and even downright frightening. It has changed significantly from the early days when, as physicians Dorsey and Berwick (2008) recall, "neither of us can recall a single instance of being told by management to withhold from a patient any care that we thought, based on evidence, could help" (p. A9). Now, they charge, managed care has been "hijacked by insurance companies" such that physicians are "handcuffed" to procedures and limitations meant to save money today rather than provide high-quality care that will pay off in the long run (p. A9).

For some questions to ask as you consider various managed care plans and for online reviews, see Box 2.6.

## Managed Care Around the World

The United States is not the only country grappling with issues of health care costs and access. People in India, China, and Russia rank affordable health plans as the most important benefit an employee can offer (Korkki, 2008). The Japanese health care system, one of the best in the world, has traditionally offered care to every citizen without out-of-pocket expense. But the demands of a disproportionately elderly population threaten the solvency of the national system (Kakizoe, 2008). Similarly, leaders of the Singapore health system, which is ranked sixth in the world by the World Health Organization,

are debating tough choices such as the need to improve patient–caregiver ratios versus investing in expensive cutting-edge medicines. An address by the Singaporean Minister of Health, Khaw Boon Wan, echoes the concerns of people throughout the world: "Our doctors and health care professionals are overworked, and at some point they need a life too," he says, adding, "But the patients keep coming" ("World-Class," 2008, np).

## SUMMARY

A historical perspective suggests why patients and caregivers communicate as they do and why they devote themselves to certain topics but not to others. The ancient Egyptians established a basis for considering health in both spiritual and physical terms. About 2,000 years later, influenced partly by Egyptian ideals, Hippocrates of ancient Greece proposed a rational/empirical model for medicine. Within that model, illness was believed to reflect people's physical well-being as well as their harmony with nature and other people. Parts of the Hippocratic oath continue to influence Western medical ethics.

During the Middle Ages, illness was assumed to be a spiritual matter, to be treated with prayer and holy redemption. Patients' spirituality and behaviors were central to talk between patients and caregivers. In the centuries that followed, fervor for accuracy and physical proof characterized the European Renaissance. Talk of faith or emotions was treated as inappropriate, even misleading, to scientific analysis. Cartesian dualism strengthened the separation of mental and physical factors. The basic assumption (which continues to influence medicine) is that patients' thoughts and feelings are largely separate from their physical conditions.

Today, the United States is renowned for its scientific, high-tech medical system. However, spiraling costs and overutilization have made it necessary to allocate health resources with care. Managed care, which developed from the need to rein in medical costs, has spawned new concerns about the quality of care Americans will receive from organizations that have a vested interest in saving money. Few are satisfied that managed care has lived up to its potential to cut costs, promote wellness, stimulate teamwork, and trim waste. Instead, managed care is often criticized for creating hassles and roadblocks, increasing paperwork, second-guessing doctors' judgments, and restricting patients' options.

The challenge to provide citizens of the world with excellent, affordable health care is a challenge worthy of our best efforts. Throughout the rest of the book, we will examine health care from multiple perspectives—both personal and global—to better understand the needs and opportunities that lie before us.

## KEY TERMS

Imhotep
religio-empirical approach
Hippocrates
Hippocratic oath
rational/empirical approach
medical spiritualism
barber surgeons
Christian magic
fetishes
René Descartes
principle of verification
Cartesian dualism
orthodox practitioners
sectarians
germ theory
Flexner Report
specialization
diagnosis-related groups (DRGs)
managed care organizations
insurance premium
insurance deductible
catastrophic cap
fee-for-service
third-party payer
health maintenance organization (HMO)
copay
capitated system
preferred provider organization (PPO)

point of service (POS)
high-deductible health plan (HDHP)
health savings account (HAS)
health reimbursement account (HRA)
balance billing
gag rules

## DISCUSSION QUESTIONS

1. Why was medicine in Imhotep's time referred to as religio-empirical?
2. How did Hippocrates' ideas about medicine affect the role of physicians and the nature of health communication?
3. How did the medical spiritualism of the Middle Ages affect health communication?
4. For what reasons (spiritual and practical) did the church ban surgery during the Middle Ages?
5. From your experience, what role does religion play in modern health care?
6. Based on the principle of verification, how do you know if you are ill? Who is better able to know the state of your health, you or a doctor?
7. Do you mostly agree or disagree with Cartesian dualism, that the mind and body are separate? If what ways are they separate? In what ways intertwined? What effect has dualism had on health care and health communication?
8. Have you ever known anyone who imagined himself or herself to be ill or caused the illness to occur when there was no physical basis for it? Have you ever felt this way yourself?
9. How did Hippocrates' ideas influence health care in colonial America?
10. What was women's role in health care in colonial America?
11. The Flexner Report led medical schools to focus intensely on science. In your opinion, what is lost and gained by this?
12. What factors led to the rise of conventional ("orthodox") medicine in the United States?
13. How have reimbursement restrictions affected the health care industry?
14. Have you or anyone you know ever gone without health insurance? Why? In your experience,

what are the effects of risks of being uninsured?

15. How do fee-for-service and capitated systems differ from a consumer's perspective? From a care provider's perspective?

16. Which type of health insurance do you prefer as a consumer? Why? What type do or would you prefer as a health professional? Which do you think is best for the country overall?

17. If you could open a tax-exempt health savings account, would you? Why or why not?

18. Statistics show that less than half of Americans understand their health insurance plan. Do you feel confident that you understand yours? Why or why not?

19. How is it possible that a doctor's office, hospital, or other health care agency could make money when no patients visit? How can they lose money when they have a full patient load?

20. Do you worry that your doctor might not prescribe tests or treatments because he or she is being pressured to cut costs? Why or why not?

21. Which is more important to you, to save money or to choose your own caregivers? Why?

22. What are potential advantages and disadvantages of managed care?

23. If you were able to change managed care for the better, what might you do?

## ANSWERS TO *CAN YOU GUESS?*

1. Only 1% of the uninsured in America are past retirement age (U.S. Department of Health and Human Services, 2005). This is largely because about 90% of older adults in the United States qualify for Medicare benefits. Keep in mind, however, that unregistered immigrants, homeless individuals, and some other populations do not show up much on the statistical radar. And being insured does not mean older adults have it easy. Many still pay large amounts for prescription drugs and long-term care.

2. All of these states, plus much more. The number of uninsured people in the United States is equal to the total combined populations of Maine, Alabama, Oklahoma, Alaska, Colorado, Delaware, Connecticut, Idaho, Hawaii, Iowa, Kansas, Maine, Montana, Oregon, Vermont, West Virginia, North Dakota, Arizona, South Carolina, and Wyoming.

# PART II

# THE ROLES OF PATIENTS AND CAREGIVERS

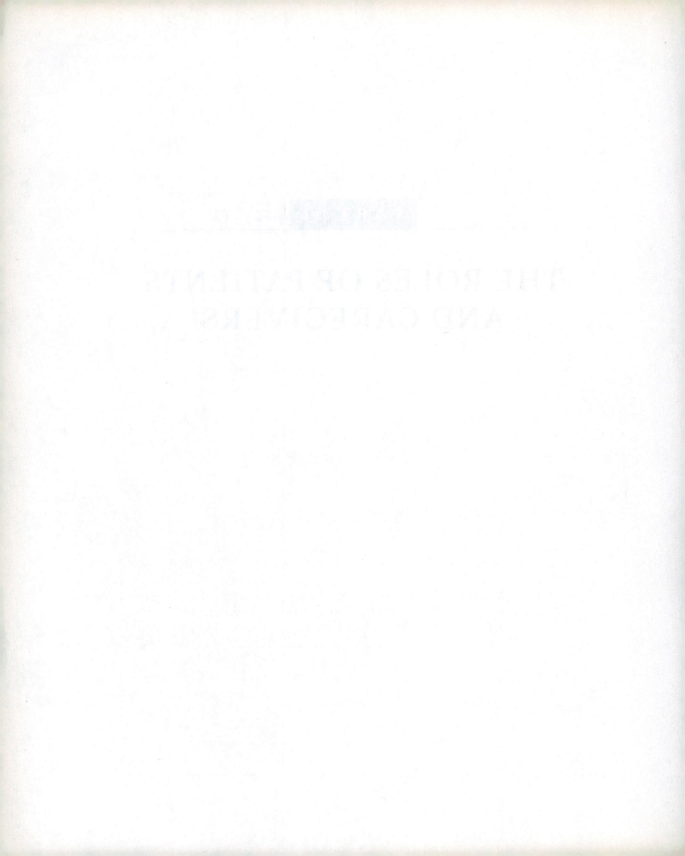

# CHAPTER 3

# Patient–Caregiver Communication

*Ben noticed a lump in his breast just after his 58th birthday. Embarrassed about the problem, he avoided mentioning it to his wife for several months, thinking it would probably go away on its own. When she learned about it, his wife encouraged, then begged, Ben to see a doctor. In the next few months other family members joined her entreaties. Finally, Ben made a doctor's appointment. On the day of the appointment the family was anxious to hear what the doctor said. Imagine their surprise when Ben returned and said the visit went "just fine," but he did not tell the doctor about the lump. When the shocked family asked why, Ben shrugged and said, "He didn't ask."*

This story illustrates some of the complex factors that affect patient–caregiver communication. Although it may sound foolish not to tell a physician about your health concerns, research suggests that episodes like Ben's occur quite frequently. In a classic study of 800 visits to a pediatric emergency clinic, 26% of the parents said they did *not* tell the doctor what concerned them most (Korsch & Negrete, 1972). Their explanations were similar to Ben's. Most said the doctor did not encourage them or even give them a chance to share the information. Health professionals may see the matter differently, wondering why patients seem to play guessing games with them rather than coming straight to the point. Recent evidence suggests that many patients and caregivers continue to experience this impasse.

This chapter examines what happens during medical transactions—who talks, who listens, and how people behave. As you will see, communicating well is important for a number of reasons. Patient–caregiver communication has an impact on how well patients recover, how they tolerate pan, how much stress they experience, and whether people follow medical advice.

Moreover, doctors are less likely to be sued for malpractice if they communicate effectively with patients. Physicians and dentists who have never been sued are observed to spend more time with patients, use more humor, and solicit patients' participation more often than doctors who have been sued (Dym, 2008; Levinson, Roter, Mullooly, Dull, & Frankel, 1997). We'll talk more about this in Chapter 4.

Because patient–caregiver communication is so important, researchers and others tend to judge it by high standards. As you read about (and experience) patient–caregiver communication, you may be tempted to blame one party or another if the communication seems insensitive or ineffective. One of my students, when asked to sum up health communication literature, declared quite candidly, "What I get is that doctors are mean and patients are dumb." Few people might be so blunt, but experts and students alike are often guilty of similar assumptions.

Resist the urge to draw simplistic conclusions. Keep in mind that patients and caregivers work together to shape their communication patterns. Communication is a transactional process. No one communicates alone, and participants are not completely at liberty to behave as they might wish (Rawlins, 1989, 1992; Watzlawick, Beavin, & Jackson, 1967). Relational communication, or **transactional communication,** means that communicators exert mutual influence on each other such that the approach one participant takes suggests how the other might respond. For instance, if a physician acts like a parent, the patient is encouraged to behave in the complementary role of a child (and the other way around). Patients sometimes become frustrated with their caregivers' parentlike behavior, unmindful that they have encouraged it by adopting meek and submissive roles themselves (Pendleton, Schofield, Tate, & Havelock, 1984). Stephen Bochner (1983) urges people not to consider patients and caregivers as adversaries but as "reasonable people of good will, trying to exchange views with other reasonable people of equally good will" (p. 128) in circumstances that are sometimes very challenging.

The chapter is divided into five sections. The first two describe physician-centered and collaborative communication, respectively, including communication skill builders for caregivers. The next two describe, respectively, environmental restructuring and the impact of telemedicine on patient–caregiver communication. The chapter concludes with communication tips for patients who wish to take an active role in medical encounters.

## PHYSICIAN-CENTERED COMMUNICATION

Medical transactions in the United States have traditionally utilized **physician-centered communi-**cation, in which health professionals do most of the talking, choose conversational topics, and begin and end communication episodes. The disproportionate power granted to clinicians, particularly physicians, is partly a result of cultural expectations. Westerners tend to regard doctors as scientific experts with the unique ability to understand and treat disease. Consequently, patients may feel unqualified to take an active role in medical encounters.

Medical tradition and medical education also contribute to clinician-centered talk. Katz (1984) describes the long-standing belief that physicians should act on their own authority "without consulting their patients about the decisions that need to be made" (p. 2). He observes that, traditionally, doctors felt it was wrong to "confuse" patients with medical details or "burden" them with making medical decisions.

Added to the conviction that clinicians know best is the conventional belief that patients will waste time describing irrelevant details unless others keep a tight rein on medical interviews. Medical schools have traditionally taught doctors to keep interviews brief and to the point. Doctors tend to assert themselves verbally and nonverbally, ask focused questions, and block discussion of highly emotional topics. In extreme cases, clinicians may treat patients as if they are ignorant or childlike.

### Assertive Behavior

Physicians often communicate more assertively than patients. In patient interactions Richard Street Jr. and Bradford Millay (2001) studied, physicians devoted only about 2% of their talking time to partnership-building and supportive communication. Patients supported the dynamic by devoting only 7% of their talking time asking questions and assertively conveying their concerns. Patients rarely asserted themselves as active participants unless their doctors actively encouraged them to do so.

Similarly, in her study of online birthing stories, Carma Bylund (2005) found that only 57% of the narratives indicated that the women had participated in medical decision making (usually about pain medication). However, women who *were* active participants described their experiences using more positive emotional terms than other women.

Doctors' interruptions also display their control over medical encounters. Physicians typically ask some version of "What seems to be the problem?" at the beginning of medical exams. That may seem like an easy question, but try answering it in a third of a minute! In a famous study, Howard Beckman and Richard Frankel (1984) studied 74 doctor's office visits and found that most patients talked for no longer than 18 seconds before the physician interrupted them and began asking specific questions. None of the patients who were allowed to keep talking took more than 2½ minutes. And notably, only 1 patient of the 52 who were interrupted returned to the original subject.

More recent research has revealed similar results. In a study published in 2005, researchers found that internal medicine residents interrupted patients 59% of the time after asking about their concerns. The interruptions occurred after patients had talked for an average of 16.5 seconds (Dyche & Swiderski, 2005). In the same study, residents began 37% of medical exams *without* asking patients about their concerns. Presumably, in those instances the residents felt they already knew what was on the patients' minds. But when researchers talked to patients afterwards, they found that doctors who neglected to ask for input were 24% less likely than others to identify correctly and address the patients' main concerns.

We should note that interruptions are not always assertive or intrusive. They can be used to encourage further talk, as in "I understand," "Tell me more," or "Say that again." And doctors are not the only ones who interrupt. Patients do so as well. But when physicians interrupt patients, they tend to claim the floor or change topics (Li, Krysko, Desroches, & Deagle, 2004). By contrast, patients (especially female patients) typically interrupt their doctors to show cooperation. Female patients that Li and colleagues studied were 11 times more likely to offer cooperative interruptions than were male patients. But male and female patients were similar in that they all tended to yield the floor (94% of the

time) when physicians began talking. By contrast, physicians yielded to patients' attempted interruptions only 68% of the time (Li et al.) The researchers concluded that, much of the time, "physicians are firmly in charge of the process and/or content of the conversation" (p. 152).

When patients don't speak up, doctors may have inadequate information with which to make diagnoses and suggest acceptable options, and patients may feel frustrated and belittled, lamenting that they have wasted time and money addressing concerns that are not chief on their minds. One implication is that it's important to enlist patients' involvement in setting the medical agenda. That means not just asking, but asking in ways that encourage honest input.

John Heritage and Jeffrey Robinson (2006) found that patients' responses to their doctors' question are shaped partly by the doctors' word choices. In their analysis of 302 patient visits, Heritage and Robinson identified five types of opening questions. The most prevalent (accounting for 89%)[1] were openers in which the physician posed a general inquiry such as "What can I do for you today?," "So you're sick, huh?," or "You're having body aches" (treated as an implied query) (pp. 92–95). Of these examples, the first is the most general and resulted in the most detailed patient responses. But let's review the other two, which campaign for confirmation of something the doctor displays as "already known." With these, the physicians may be signaling that they remember the patient or have reviewed what he or she told the nurse or receptionist. This may be gratifying in a sense, and it may seem efficient in terms of getting right to the point. But as Heritage and Robinson point out, since the rules of polite conversation discourage people from repeating information that is (ostensibly) already known, respondents may be dissuaded from saying very much (Heritage & Robinson, p. 93). Patients' answers to these types of questions were indeed markedly briefer and less detailed than to open-ended questions. With the

---

[1] Other, less common opening questions involved "How are you?" greetings (5%) and history-taking questions (6%).

## BOX 3.1  DOORKNOB DISCLOSURES

The instant intimacy demanded in medical situations is tricky to manage. The physician may wish to get right to the point, but the patient may consider it extremely risky (or even rude) to disclose information in the first few seconds of the conversation. However, delaying disclosures or beating around the bush can waste valuable time, often at the expense of other people.

While studying interactions in a family practice office a few years ago, I noticed that patients often began with small concerns, not their main worries. One woman said initially that she was suffering from a sore throat. Only halfway through the medical visit did she admit that depression was her biggest problem. In fact, she eventually told the doctor she had tried to commit suicide several days earlier. Many other patients blurted out their main concerns just as the physician was leaving the room. These so-called **doorknob disclosures** occur at what seems to be the last instant of the medical visit. The physician in such a situation can postpone the main concern until another time or, as more often happens, launch what is in effect *another* medical interview with the patient. Remember this the next time you are frustrated with a physician for keeping you waiting!

---

more leading questions, the implication (true or not) is that the doctor has reviewed the patient's concerns and identified the most important or salient of them (e.g., body aches) or has already concluded that the patient is sick. (Don't we often go to the doctor wondering *if* we are sick? To begin a question with that assumption may seem logical to the doctor but may suggest a more definitive assessment than he or she intended.) With this study in mind, it is easy to see that the *way* a doctor asks a question can have a powerful influence on what is said and what agenda emerges. These considerations are especially important in light of evidence that patients often build up to their most important concerns, and they may not share them at all unless encouraged to do so. (See Box 3.1 for more on this.)

As suggested by the tenets of transactional communication, physician-centered communication is a collaborative enterprise. Physicians are often quite assertive, but for their part, patients are typically quick to acquiesce. In a study of 72 patient visits with a family physician, Kandi Walker and colleagues (2002) noted that the patients displayed a general willingness to let the physician guide the encounter, and in various ways the physician conveyed that her understanding of health conditions was superior to the patients' (Walker, Arnold, Miller-Day, & Webb, 2002). For example, when a patient who had had kidney infections before said she recognized the symptoms of a current infection, the physician responded, "Let me take a look. Since I am the doctor here . . ." (Walker et al., p. 52). The patient briefly objected that she was sure of the diagnosis, but then she relinquished the argument and was relatively submissive during the remainder of the medical visit.

### Questions and Directives

Caregivers use their talking time mostly to ask questions and issue **directives** (instructions or commands). For example, during physical therapy visits, therapists talk about twice as much as their patients, mostly asking about health history and giving instructions (Roberts & Bucksey, 2007). A Canadian study showed that medical residents, although assertive, were less so than physicians. Residents asked 80% of the questions during medical exams (compared to physicians' 89%) and spent twice as long (about 19.7 minutes) with patients as did most physicians (Pahal, 2006). Pahal speculates that the residents were more comfortable extending exams and entertaining patients' questions because they were not under the same time constraints as doctors and because unlike doctors, the residents were not paid based on the number patients they saw.

Doctors may keep medical conversations focused to save time and prevent patients from rambling. Researchers suggest that patients tend to stammer and stutter, especially when they are afraid the doctor will disapprove of their behavior (du Pré & Beck, 1997). Ironically, these stutters and stammers, which may sound like wasted time, are often signals that the patient is working up to an especially important disclosure. The doctor who too quickly diverts the conversation may lose an important opportunity to learn what's on the patient's mind.

### Blocking

Research on patient–caregiver communication refers to **blocking**, a process by which caregivers steer talk away from certain subjects. Through topic shifts or questions, nurses are sometimes observed to block complaints or avoid patients' emotional disclosures (Jarrett & Payne, 1995), as are physicians. For example, in one conversation a patient asked, "You know how you get sorta scared?" and the physician responded, "How long were you on the estrogen?" (Suchman, Markakis, Beckman, & Frankel, 1997). In a different episode, when an 80-year-old patient told a doctor that she was "very nervous, very nervous" and said she had recently suffered the sudden death of two friends and watched her husband committed to an intensive care unit, the physician simply asked, "Do you smoke?" (M. G. Greene, Adelman, & Majerovitz, 1996, p. 270).

On the other hand, some caregivers are quite responsive and patient-centered. Greene and coauthors (1996) describe an encounter during which an 84-year-old patient told the doctor she was being pressured to provide care for a mentally ill family member. "They've been putting a lot of pressure on me and it's made me very nervous," the patient said. The physician responded, "Maybe there's a way I can help. Well, I can see [by] what you said that you have a lot of things on your mind. An awful lot of pressure and tension" (p. 273). The doctor wrote a letter that resolved the dilemma, and he received

effusive thanks from the patient. The researchers point out that the doctor in this episode acknowledged the woman's feelings, offered specific assistance, and reassured her that he was concerned.

### Patronizing Behavior

Because of physicians' high social status and their extraordinary ability to influence people's lives, if patients are not happy with the care they receive they may be reluctant to criticize or protest. It follows that patients of relatively low social status will feel this effect most strongly. The powerlessness of women and minorities in medical situations is sometimes quite shocking.

Critical theorists such as Alexandra Todd point out ways in which some doctors **patronize** patients (treat them as if they are inferior) by withholding information, speaking down to them, and shrugging off their feelings as childish or inconsequential. Many of these episodes involve **transgressions**, which are episodes in which a doctor or patient acts inappropriately (Farber, Novack, & O'Brien, 1997). For example, Todd (1984) describes an examination she witnessed during which the gynecologist exclaimed, "This is all girl" while examining a patient's breast for lumps. When the patient did not respond, he repeated, "I *said*, this is all girl." After the exam, the physician told the women to "get dressed like a good girl" and he would give her some "happy pills" (birth control pills) (p. 182). (See Box 3.2 for tips on handling transgressions.)

Even experts find health situations challenging. Health communication scholar Christina Beck describes her panic and frustration when a doctor refused to take her seriously (Beck, Ragan, & du Pré, 1997). Previously diagnosed with a hormone deficiency that had already caused one miscarriage, Beck pleaded with her new doctor to begin hormone replacement therapy at the beginning of her next pregnancy. Calling her "honey" and telling her "don't worry," the doctor declined do so. Within weeks Beck suffered another miscarriage. Writing of the experience, she expresses regret that she, "a normally assertive, intelligent, and well-educated woman," did not take a firmer stand or switch doctors.

## BOX 3.2 STEPPING OVER THE LINE

It is sometimes difficult to establish what behaviors are appropriate between a patient and a caregiver. Touch, personal disclosures, and body exposure usually reserved for intimate relationships are often required in medical settings.

Usually both parties recognize the boundary between intimacy (a unique sense of closeness, interdependence, and trust) and detached concern (the effort to understand another person, but with restricted emotional involvement). However, patients and caregivers sometimes cross the line. Farber et al. (1997) call actions that cross the line between intimacy and professionalism *transgressions* (from the Latin phrase meaning "to step across").

Transgressions frequently have painful and confusing results. Feelings of heartache, disappointment, guilt, and loss of reputation may result. Patients, typically in positions of lesser power, may feel violated or forced into behaving against their wishes. Professionals may feel harassed or embarrassed and may face legal action and loss of professional privileges.

Sexual contact is an obvious transgression, but other behavior can be inappropriate as well. Doctors say patients sometimes transgress by demanding more time than the caregiver can afford, asking for money or favors, being overly flirtatious or seductive, giving frequent or expensive gifts, and even being verbally abusive (Farber et al., 1997). Nurses are sometimes harassed by patients who grab them and make suggestive comments (R. Zook, 1997). Caregivers may transgress by making sexual advances, asking unnecessary personal questions, insulting patients, or sharing confidential information with others.

Researchers propose that transgressions may result from patients' vulnerability, their need for assurance, and the trust they place in their caregivers. Caregivers, too, may experience strong feelings (either positive or negative) in relation to patients, feelings that may be heightened by a sense of isolation from family and friends.

Farber et al. (1997) and R. Zook (1997) suggest these steps for avoiding or terminating transgressions:

- Take stock of personal needs and social expectations that may motivate a transgression (loneliness, need for approval, etc.).
- Establish clear boundaries for touch and talk.
- Be careful not to send ambiguous or mixed messages.
- Seek the counsel of support groups, friends, and colleagues.
- Have others present during transactions.
- Acknowledge transgression attempts and discuss them in a calm way with the other person.
- If inappropriate behavior does not stop, let the other person know you intend to take formal action. If it still does not stop, contact the health care management or the local medical society.

Episodes such as these point to the pitfalls of a power inequity between patients and caregivers. Although most professionals do not abuse the power difference, when they do, patients may perceive that they have little recourse. This situation is particularly unfortunate for patients of low socioeconomic status, who may feel the effects of discrimination more than others but may not be at liberty to choose or switch doctors.

### Power Difference

It is true that patients do not have to do what the doctor says. But because people have traditionally sought medical care when they are ill or hurt, they may not be in much of a position to argue. Throughout history, patients (who are quite literally weak) have relied on their caregivers to be strong. In the current political climate in which doctors are criticized for being domineering, it is easy to forget that for many generations society expected them to be dominant.

It is also important to remind ourselves that power is granted to physicians by others. Doctors do not have license to treat patients without their consent. Nor can they require them to follow medical advice. They cannot even require patients to show up for exams. However, patients may not perceive that they have much choice in these matters, based on the alternatives.

A powerful example is emergency room care. Across the country, emergency departments are often overcrowded and understaffed. This is partly because of laws that require emergency personnel to treat anyone who arrives, even if they are not able to pay. An unintended consequence of these laws is that people who do not have insurance, and thus who may be turned away from doctors' offices, often rely on ER care instead. For most hospitals ER isn't a money maker, it's a financial drain, hence the understaffing. The hectic, high-anxiety atmosphere affects patients and professionals. While studying an urban emergency department for 6 months, Eisenberg, Baglia, and Pynes (2006) noted the enforced passivity of patients and their families, who were often required to wait for hours and watch people with more serious concerns (or more political clout) "jump the line" to be seen ahead of them. The researchers observe: "Patients are expected to play a 'sick role' in which they passively and cooperatively submit to the expert opinion of the professionals" (p. 205). In one case they witnessed, a father brought his daughter in for evaluation after she fell and bloodied her nose.

> After waiting for 20 mins, the man approached the window and asked when his daughter would be seen. "We have more serious cases, sir," replied the triage nurse. "This is serious," said the father. "But I saw her walk in," returned the nurse. "Yeah, but now she's complaining about a headache." "Well, if she fell on her nose, she's going to have a headache." (Eisenberg et al., p. 201)

The incident illustrates the powerlessness of the father to get immediate care for his daughter and

the subtext—an environment in which caregivers are often too harried to feel compassion and patience. In these situations, cultural expectations, combined with the desire to stay in caregivers' good graces, may be enough to silence patients into submission, whether they follow doctors' advice when they leave or not.

## Criticism of Clinician–Centeredness

Not everyone is satisfied with clinician-centered communication. For one thing, as people become more educated about health matters, many are no longer content answering closed-ended questions and following doctors' orders. They wish to discuss options and participate in medical decision making. "It's the rare physician who doesn't acknowledge that now, more than ever, physicians learn from their patients," says Weiss (2008, paragraph 3). It must be said, however, that not all doctors agree. Some long for the days when patients mostly listened and learned from them directly. They resent having to "de-educate" patients about erroneous information they pick up online, and they may perceive that well-informed patients are challenging their authority. Says a patient in Broom's (2008) study:

> We extensively searched the Internet [and] at one urologist's office I was asking about certain information and this went on for some time. I went back to his secretary and we are paying the bill. He [the doctor] was talking into a Dictaphone and he was making the referral to somebody else and he said, "[patient's name] is somewhat difficult and overinformed." . . . They definitely don't really like well-informed people. (p. 101)

A second criticism of physician-centered communication (as mentioned) is that if patients don't speak up, it's difficult to know what they want and need. Physicians trying to guess may have a difficult time considering that patient expectations typically differ according to anxiety level, age, education, and familiarity with the caregiver (Street, 1990).

A third criticism is that, although physician-dominated communication seems efficient in the

## BOX 3.3 ETHICAL CONSIDERATIONS

### Therapeutic Privilege

Although Anna (age 68) is seriously ill, she feels relatively well and her spirits seem high. She often remarks to those around her that she is feeling much better and she is eager to talk of future plans. However, it is obvious to her caregivers and to her family that she will not live more than a few months. The family has asked Anna's physician not to tell her she is dying. They argue that she probably knows she is dying but that her behavior implies a request that people not bring up the issue. They feel that Anna's current happiness is what really matters at this point, and they are reluctant to impose bad news on her, particularly when there is nothing than can be done about it.

**Therapeutic privilege** is the prerogative sometimes granted physicians to withhold information from patients if they feel that disclosing the information would do more harm than good. For many years doctors withheld information from patients if they thought patients would be unable to understand it or would be distressed by it (Katz, 1984).

Robert Veatch (1991) argues that therapeutic privilege is indefensible because it is counter to the goal of making patients informed partners in their own care. Charles Lund (1995) takes a more moderate view. He asserts that physicians should almost always tell patients the truth, but he warns that blunt honesty is not always the kindest method of disclosure.

In some cultures, people prefer to shield family members from distressing news about their health. In Japan, for example, although people typically want to know the truth about their own health, they often insist that physicians shield family members from distressing diagnoses (Kakai, 2002). Based on cultural ideas about illness and death, they are afraid of destroying their loved one's hope and fearful that talking about adverse outcomes might lead to their occurrence (Kakai).

### What Do You Think?

1. If you were Anna's physician, would you tell her she does not have long to live? Why or why not?
2. If physicians feel certain regimens will help patients but patients are likely to refuse the treatment if they know everything about the diagnosis, are the physicians justified in withholding the information?
3. If physicians withhold information, should they go so far as to lie if patients ask outright about their prognosis?
4. How do you respond to the argument that physicians can never be sure about patients' odds of recovery, so it is sometimes better to withhold information that might diminish patients' hopes?
5. What if you were the physician and a patient told you, "If this condition is terminal, don't tell me"? Would you withhold information even if it meant making treatment decisions on the patient's behalf?
6. What if patients do not say "Don't tell me" outright but their actions seem to suggest that they do not want to know if the news is bad? Would you tell them?
7. Is it ever permissible to give a patient's family information without telling the patient? If so, under what circumstances?
8. If you were the patient, are there any circumstances in which you would wish information to be withheld from you?

short run, it is often counterproductive. Patients who perceive a physician to be domineering talk less than others and are less likely to share information with their doctors (Schmid Mast, Hall, & Roter, 2008). But patients who perceive their physicians to be caring are more at ease than other patients and share their feelings more easily (Schmid Mast et al., 2008). This is an advantage for medical decision making, and it's usually a more rewarding interpersonal dynamic. In a study of physicians, nurses, and genetic counselors, Gail Geller and colleagues (2008) found that practitioners (particularly female caregivers) who felt they were highly engaged with patients considered their work more meaningful and were less likely to experience burnout than other caregivers.

Finally, some people worry that doctors and patients will buy into the dominant–submissive dynamic supported by physician-centered communication. Patients may believe they are helpless and ignorant, and doctors may believe they know what is best, even to the extent of deceiving patients or withholding information (see Box 3.3). And patients who are passive in the doctor's office or hospital may be passive about their health in other ways as well. The reality is that doctors can't do it all. People have the best chance at long, healthy lives if they proactively strive for good health and, when they are ill, work with caregivers to design treatment plans they can and will carry out.

In the face of so much criticism, it may seem that physician-centered communication is a thing of the past. While the tide does seem to be turning, the old model endures in many ways. Morse and coauthors (2008) analyzed doctor visits with people coping with lung cancer. Although they identified 384 opportunities to display empathy with the patients' feelings, physicians actually expressed empathy only about 10% of the time, usually at the conclusion of the interviews. The researchers conclude that physicians' task-orientation can blind them to opportunities for compassionate, biopsychosocial care. By contrast, some health professionals have always been careful to empower and listen to patients, even when physician-centered care was considered

the norm. And many others are beginning to orient themselves toward more collaborative communication, a topic we turn to next.

## COLLABORATIVE COMMUNICATION

**Collaborative communication** establishes patients and caregivers as peers who openly discuss health options and make mutually satisfying decisions (Balint & Shelton, 1996; Laine & Davidoff, 1996). Although collaborative communication is consistent with patient empowerment, it is neither entirely patient-centered nor caregiver-centered. Instead, participants work together as partners. (See Box 3.4 for more about the collaborative interpretation model of health communication.)

This section describes developments in the health industry that make collaborative communication appealing. It also describes communication techniques to encourage patients' active participation in medical dialogues.

### Climate for Change

In an issue of *Health Communication* devoted to "The Patient as a Central Construct," Robert Kaplan (1997, p. 75) forecast a move away from the "find it—fix it" biomedical model to an "outcomes model" that emphasizes long-term quality of life. The goal of the outcomes model is to minimize people's reliance on medicine and to maximize the importance of their everyday health and fulfillment.

Oncologist Jamie Van Roen believes in this. "The first thing I do to try to make the relationship real is teach them [patients] to complain," she says. "I tell them I don't know what it's like to be the patient, to have cancer. It's a matter of control. Patients often feel like they have lost control of everything. I try to give it back" (quoted by Magee & D'Antonio, 2003, p. 202).

Significantly, Kaplan's outcome model (and others similar to it) requires a wide-angle focus, extending far beyond organic indications of illness. Diet, exercise, emotional health, attitude, and similar factors become issues of immediate concern. Caregivers such as nutritionists, exercise physiologists,

## BOX 3.4   THEORETICAL FOUNDATIONS

### Communication as Collaborative Interpretation

*Michelle, a 15-year-old caring for her 5-month-old daughter, seeks emergency care for excessive menstrual bleeding. Although Michelle was hospitalized 2 weeks earlier for asthma and suspects that the asthma and her current problem are the result of stress, she does not mention either the hospitalization or the stress to her doctors.*

This true story, described by Amanda Young and Linda Flower (2002), illustrates what they call a "rhetoric of passivity" supported by participants' assumption that patients should go along with what caregivers say and do. The medical student caring for Michelle asks leading and closed-ended questions that do not encourage her to share her concerns. For her part, Michelle makes only brief replies and is not assertive about sharing her concerns. Consequently, Young and Flower report:

Michelle leaves the hospital with a referral to see a gynecologist with no discussion of what she thinks is causing her problem—a list of stressors that would boggle the mind of a middle-class adult, let alone a 15-year-old single mother in the inner city. (p. 82)

Young and Flower (2002) propose an alternative model of communication based on a "rhetoric of agency" that recognizes patients as coagents in health encounters. Their **model of collaborative interpretation (CI)** proposes that health communication is most effective when patients actualize the roles of decision makers and problem solvers and caregivers function as counselors or friends who work alongside patients to help them achieve shared goals. This rhetorical shift relies on the mutual efforts of everyone involved. It cannot work if patients are unwilling to share their stories and take an active role in health care transactions. Nor will it work if caregivers perpetuate the paternalist notion that they know what is best for patients. With the CI model, patients and caregivers are coagents who establish shared goals and work collaboratively to pursue them.

Importantly, the CI model does not privilege either patients or caregivers. Instead, as Young and Flower (2002) describe it, the goal is "an experience that validates the expertise of both patient and provider and that dignifies the patient's needs" (p. 89). Such a model can be difficult to create, especially since it is a new idea for many people. As a helpful guide, Young and Flower present a list of criteria that define collaborative interpretations. Here are a few criteria on their list.

- Patients and caregivers draw on each other's expertise by asking for details about past experiences with the health concern.
- Discussion includes the patient's views about how the health concern influences his or her lifestyle and physical, mental, and emotional health.
- The patient and caregiver explicitly discuss their interpretations of the health concern and the impact it may have on life, work, and relationships.
- Participants openly share their goals and expectations.
- Patients and caregivers develop a mutual sense of control by identifying strategies that are beneficial, practical, and acceptable.

### Suggested Sources

Emanuel, E. J., & Emanuel, L. L. (1995). Four models of the physician–patient relationship. *Journal of the American Medical Association, 267*, 2221–2226.

Smith, D. H., & Pettegrew, L. S. (1986). Mutual persuasion as a model for doctor–patient communication. *Theoretical Medicine, 7*, 127–146.

Young, A., & Flower, L. (2002). Patients as partners, patients as problem-solvers. *Health Communication, 14*(1), 69–97.

counselors, and others are in a good position to help doctors manage people's overall care.

As caregivers' roles change, so may patients'. Indeed, the very term *patient* becomes problematic when the emphasis shifts to everyday well-being. *Patient* connotes a person in ill health who seeks the services of a care provider. Some theorists suggest that the terms *health citizen* and *health decision maker* are preferable because they acknowledge that people are involved in health care all the time—not just when they seek professional assistance (Rimal, Ratzan, Arnston, & Freimuth, 1997).

As health becomes a way of life, not just an occasional excursion to the doctor's office, many people feel it is insensible to treat patients as passive or incidental components of the process. Patricia Geist and Jennifer Dreyer (1993) apply Eisenberg and Goodall's concept of dialogue to medical encounters. A **dialogue** is a conversation in which both people participate fully and equitably, each influencing the encounter in ways that make it a unique creation. When conversational partners engage in dialogue, they do not simply adopt ready-made roles; they create them to suit their own situations and preferences (for more, see Eisenberg & Goodall, 2004). In the book *On Call: A Doctor's Days and Nights in Residency*, Emily Transue (2004) describes her first conversation with a patient she knew to have terminal cancer. Aware that he had been experiencing depression, Transue asked the man, "How are your spirits?" and he replied, "As good as you could expect them to be, I guess.... Not that I don't have my moments." Rather than brushing his words aside, Transue said, "Tell me about the moments" (p. 13). The patient shared with her that he sometimes considered taking his own life, but he stuck around to have more time with his beloved dog. Transue says such details helped her understand the man better and provide the care he needed. Together, she says, they learned about dying and all the steps along the way.

Researchers suggest that patients and caregivers are typically more satisfied with dialogues than with one-sided conversations, but they may be afraid dialogues will take too long or that others will not wish

**BOX 3.5**

# Can You Guess?

1. Which state ranks highest in terms of health care providers' patient-centeredness?
2. Which ranks lowest?
*Answers appear at the end of the chapter.*

to take part in them (Geist & Dreyer, 1993). Those who take the risk may enjoy profound rewards. For example, even people who are highly frightened about dental care respond well when dentists and dental assistants show a genuine interest in them and work hard to earn their trust (Kulich, Berggren, & Hallberg, 2003).

Likewise, John Suchwalko remembers a doctor's visit that changed his life and that illustrates a patient's perspective on collaborative communication. "My blood pressure was off the charts, but I didn't feel anything," he says (quoted by Magee & D'Antonio, 2003, p. 49). He was also overweight, seldom exercised, was a smoker, and had high cholesterol. It's easy to imagine that a physician might convey disapproval. But Suchwalko's doctor, George Hanna, didn't. As Suchwalko describes it:

> The thing that impressed me about Dr. Hanna was that he didn't come down on me real hard. I didn't feel like I had been sent to the vice principal's office and he was wagging a finger in my face saying, "You better do this" or "You better do that." Instead he came across like he was a very knowledgeable friend.... From then on, I was on a diet, I started walking every day, and I came into his office every two weeks. He would talk to me, encourage me, keep me going. That helped a lot. (p. 49)

Because patient-centered care has been linked to favorable patient outcomes, some funding agencies and health care advocates have begun to measure caregivers' proficiency at it. The Clinical Skills Assessment (CSA) exam, which is required of foreign-educated doctors seeking to practice in the United States, involves interacting with trained (standardized) patients. Physicians earn highest marks if they engage in rapport-building behaviors, are nonverbally attentive, encourage the patients to tell their stories, ask follow-up questions, are tactful and respectful, present information clearly, and show empathy and support (van Zanten, Boulet, & McKinley, 2007). At a more macro level, the Commonwealth Fund ranks each state in the United States on how patient-centered people perceive their health professionals there to be. To establish the rankings, researchers ask Medicare subscribers to indicate the degree to which their health care provider "listens, explains, shows respect, and spends enough time with them" ("State Scorecard," 2007).

Following are several communication techniques useful in initiating and taking part in medical dialogues.

## Motivational Interviewing

We may as well admit it: Most of us *know* about healthy behaviors, but we don't always do them. We know we should work out more, eat less fast food, drink more water, get more sleep, and so forth. But sometimes other options seem more appealing or important. Even when we have the healthiest of intentions, once the day starts, a hamburger is a quick meal on the way to school, it's too hot or too cold to jog, and so on. A whole range of factors seems to keep us from doing what we intended. Theorist Brenda Dervin calls these *gaps*.

Dervin and colleagues propose that life is an enterprise in sense making (Dervin, 1999; Dervin & Frenette, 2001). They use the terms *nouning* and *verbing* to illustrate the point. Nouning implies that things are static and predictable. From this perspective, we decide to drink more water, and we do, as simple as that. But more often, life feels more like verbing, a process in which we are continually making sense of changing circumstances because new information becomes available to us, our perspective changes, circumstances transform, or the like. As this occurs, gaps emerge in what we believe

and in the actions made available to us. To employ a very simple example, perhaps I am determined to drink more water today, but the vending machine is out, a friend surprises me with a latte, or I run out of change. Now there is an unforeseen gap. To visualize what Dervin and colleagues call *gappiness*, imagine walking down a sidewalk, fairly certain about where you are going, and then finding that a significant section of the pavement ahead of you is missing. It may be easy matter to bridge the gap, or it may not. But if you are to keep going in the original direction, you must bridge it in some way. In my example, bridging might mean finding a different vending machine, refusing the latte, or getting change. If I foresaw the gap, perhaps I planned ahead and brought a water bottle with me. Conversely, I might abandon the gappy path for now and resolve to try again tomorrow. This is a simple example. As you might imagine, it's often a lot more complicated. The main point is that life is inherently gappy. We are continually adjusting our goals and behaviors in light of changing circumstances. It's no wonder health professionals want to throw up their hands sometimes! Health (a noun) *is* really important. Yet for a wide range of reasons, our actions (the verbs) don't always support that ideal.

This leads us to another concept that recognizes the verbing side of life—**motivational interviewing (MI)**. Stephen Rollnick and William Miller (1995) conceptualized MI as "a directive, client-centered counseling style for eliciting behavior change by helping clients to explore and resolve ambivalence" (paragraph 3). Let's break that definition down. As the wording suggests, MI was originally designed for use in psychotherapy, but it has since found utility in a variety of settings. It is most frequently applied to health-related behavior choices, but the basic premises of MI work in nearly every setting, including a casual conversation with a friend or an internal dialogue. MI is appealing to many because it is patient-centered and nonconfrontational. The counselor/interviewer does not play a coercive or prescriptive role. That is, he or she doesn't tell the client what to do. In fact, although the

BOX 3.6 **OUCH!**

*Sitting in a quiet reception room you read an article while waiting for your appointment. With little or no warning, a woman walks up to you, extends her hand, and abruptly hits you on the arm. Instantly your blood pressure rises as you become angry and confused....Here's a second scenario. Same setting, but this time, as the woman approaches, she says, "There is a mosquito on your arm, hold still!" Then using the same motion, she gently hits your arm. Is your reaction the same? Most likely not.*

This scenario, presented by Niki Henson (2007, p. 32), reminds dental assistants to tell patients exactly what to expect, even if it will hurt. Her words are right on target. Research is consistent that effective communication can modify people's experience of pain. For one thing, people with realistic expectations about pain are usually better able to cope, and they typically consider the pain less severe than others (N. Adams & Field, 2001).

Another factor is people's reluctance to ask for pain relief. Although 98% of abdominal pain sufferers in an emergency department were in pain, only one-third of them asked for pain medication (Yee, Puntillo, Miaskowski, & Neighbor, 2006). Patients may be afraid of inconveniencing the staff or appearing weak. However, unresolved pain often slows recovery and is stressful for patients, their loved ones, and caregivers. Caregivers can help by educating people about what to expect and encouraging them to ask for relief when they are in pain.

It's hard to imagine a more challenging scenario than managing the pain of people who cannot express themselves clearly. In an attempt to help, nurses who care for people with dementia implemented a pain-assessment checklist to help gauge patients' comfort levels even when the patients could not articulate their feelings. Over 3 months' time the patients showed reduced signs of unresolved pain, and the nurses rated themselves less stressed and less likely to experience burnout than before (Fuchs-Lacelle, Hadjistavropoulos, & Lix, 2008).

interviewer may be knowledgeable about options, he or she doesn't presume to know what is best for the other person. Instead, the interviewer respects that people weigh a variety of factors when making decisions and that consequently they almost always have mixed feelings (ambivalence) about change. The interviewer's job is respectfully and nonjudgmentally to ask questions about (elicit) a person's feelings, to help clarify those feelings, and to assist the person in making choices (resolving the ambivalence).

In one study, nurses used MI to help people experiencing cancer-related pain examine their feelings about various treatment options (Fahey et al. 2008). From a distance it may seem that a person in pain would naturally seek pain relievers, but as you probably know from personal experience (even considering a headache or sore muscle), the decision is

more complicated than that. For one thing, there is no one right way to respond to pain. We might consider it weak to seek relief, or we may be afraid that we will mute our body's natural warning signs. We might fear that we will become addicted to pain killers, believe that they will make us groggy, and so on. (See Box 3.6 for more on the link between communication and pain.) MI practitioners respect this natural ambivalence and try to help people sort through it. MI is a true partnership, say Rollnick and Miller (1995): "The therapist respects the client's autonomy and freedom of choice (and consequences) regarding his or her own behaviour" (paragraph 4).

Following are some common techniques and assumptions of MI, illustrated with questions adapted from Miller & Rollnick (2002), Fahey and colleagues' (2008) work with people experiencing pain, and Gerry Welch and colleagues' (2006) work with diabetes patients.[2]

- *Set a respectful tone.* Explain the basic ideas of MI, and express a sincere commitment to listen to and learn from the other person.
- *Let the decision maker set the agenda.* Ask initial questions to help identify what is important to him or her. "Are you happy with the way things are?" "What's going well?" "Is there anything that could be better?" "Do you have concerns about pain?" "Why do you think you have pain?"
- *Gauge the decision maker's interest.* Keep in mind that change is self-motivated. If the issue isn't important to the decision maker, it's probably not fruitful to focus on it. "On a scale of 1 to 10, how important is it to you to reduce your pain?"
- *Explore ambivalence.* Remember that people almost always have mixed feelings about change, based on values, experiences, confidence level, perceived alternatives, and so on. "It sounds like eating sweets makes you feel unwell, yet you crave them. Is that how it feels?" or "What would change in your life if you had less pain?" or "What factors might prevent you from eating a healthy diet?"
- *Listen.* Let the decision maker do most of the talking.
- *Elicit–provide–elicit.* Ask a question, reflect your understanding of the answer, and ask questions to get a deeper understanding of the issue. "I hear you saying that you would enjoy being around loved ones more if you were in less pain, but you're worried that you might become addicted to the medication. Why does that worry you?"

- *Identify multiple options (including doing nothing) and weigh their merits.* "What options are you aware of?" "What are the advantages of your current diet? What are the disadvantages?" "What are the advantages of changing your diet? What are the disadvantages?"
- *Partner; don't persuade.* If you would like to suggest options or information, make sure they don't sound like prescriptions. "If you'd like, I'll tell you a bit more about…" "Here are a few things that work for some people…"
- *Roll with resistance.* Avoid arguing or convincing. Instead try to understand thoroughly the decision maker's reluctance to change. "It sounds like you are interested in biofeedback, but you're not confident that it will work."
- *Gauge the decision maker's sense of confidence and self-efficacy.* "One a 1-to-10 scale, how confident are you that you can manage the pain by…?"
- *Focus on incremental changes.* "You indicated that your pain level is usually an 8 out of 10. What do you think it would take to get it down to a 6?"
- *Collaborate and empower.* Emphasize that you are partners in the process and that you will work together and adjust the strategy as you go. "I hear you saying that you would like to try sugar-free snacks. Would you like to try that for two weeks, then come back and we'll see how it's going?" "What can I or other people do to help you reach your goal?"

This is but a brief overview of MI. Extensive literature charts its efficacy at helping people quit smoking (Bock et al., 2008), exercise more (A. L. Olson, Gaffney, Lee, & Starr, 2008), seek help when considering suicide (Britton, Williams, & Conner, 2008), and more. See Box 3.7 for more about MI.

### Communication Skill Builders: Cultivating Dialogue

Following are some other techniques for encouraging collaborative communication. Although patients as well as caregivers may use these, the

---

[2] As previously mentioned, our vocabulary is as yet inadequate to describe the partnering roles people play in health scenarios. For clarity's sake, I refer to the people involved as interviewer and decision maker. You could insert a variety of terms in place of decision maker—client, patient, friend, self.

## BOX 3.7 RESOURCES

# More About Motivational Interviewing

Fahey, K. F., Rao, S. M., Douglas, M. K., Thomas, M. L., Elliott, J. E., & Miaskowski, C. (2008). Nurse coaching to explore and modify patient attitudinal barriers. *Oncology Nursing Forum, 35*(2), 234–240.

Miller, W. R., & Rollnick, S. (2002). *Motivational interviewing: Preparing people for change.* New York: Guilford Press.

Rollnick, S., & Miller, W. (1995). What is motivational interviewing? *Behavioural and Cognitive Psychotherapy, 23,* 325–334. Reprinted online. Retrieved October 30, 2008, from http://www.motivational-interview.org/clinical/whatismi.html

Welch, G., Rose, G., & Ernst, D. (2006). Motivational interviewing and diabetes: What is used, and does it work? *Diabetes Spectrum, 19*(1), 5–11.

majority of the literature is addressed to caregivers, recognizing perhaps that patients are traditionally more likely to follow their caregivers' cues than the other way around.

*Nonverbal Encouragement*  Researchers have noted several ways that caregivers can nonverbally encourage patients to take a more active role in medical encounters.

- *Look interested.* Patients respond well when caregivers show interest in what they are saying. For example, the parents of pediatric patients are more satisfied with nurses, doctors, and other health professionals when they show attentive listening behaviors and seem friendly, open, and approachable (Wanzer, Booth-Butterfield, & Gruber, 2004).
- *Touch (cautiously).* People may interpret touch in a number of ways. Subjected to physical contact and proximity usually reserved for intimate relationships, some

patients may feel defensive or violated. Others may regard touch as a sign of comfort or esteem. Nursing home residents perceived nurses who touched a patient's arm to be more affectionate and immediate than other nurses (J. R. Moore & Gilbert, 1995).

- *Allow silence.* Physician Frederic Platt, the author of numerous books and articles on patient–caregiver communication, says that asking the right questions is only half the challenge. The rest is waiting for the answer. "Pausing long enough to allow the patient to find that answer is hard," Platt acknowledges. "Nature and doctors abhor a vacuum; we rush to fill the silences. It works better if we can trust the silence to do its work" (Platt, 1995, p. 13).
- *Pay attention to nonverbal displays.* Partly because patients are so nonassertive verbally, physicians may use nonverbal cues to gauge patients' feelings as well as the severity of their symptoms (Mast, 2007). Patients tend to be more satisfied with physicians who are skillful at understanding body language and are able to display their own emotions nonverbally (Mast).

*Verbal Encouragement*  The challenge has sometimes been to get patients to open up and share concerns. Suchman and colleagues (1997) lament lost opportunities for sharing emotions, asserting that "the feeling of being understood by another person is intrinsically therapeutic" (p. 678). However, many patients feel inhibited, fearing they will seem inappropriate if they share their feelings with a doctor. Some caregivers have overcome patients' inhibitions using open questions, treating people as equals, encouraging self-disclosure, coaching patients, and using humor.

- *Start on a friendly note.* When Gretchen Norling (2005) asked people to describe an experience in which they felt a high degree of rapport with a physician, many said that the first few moments of a medical visit set the tone. They were most likely to feel rapport

## BOX 3.8 RESOURCES

### More on Caregiver Communication Strategies

Branch W. T., Jr., Levinson, W., & Platt, F. W. (1996). Diagnostic interviewing: Make the most of your time. *Patient Care, 30*(12), 68–76.

de Ridder, D. T. D., Theunissen, N. C. M., & van Dulmen, S. M. (2007). Does training general practitioners to elicit patients' illness representations and action plans influence their communication as a whole? *Patient Education and Counseling, 66*(3), 327–336.

Mast, M. S. (2007). On the importance of nonverbal communication in the physician–patient in-teraction. *Patient Education and Counseling, 67*(3), 315–318.

Norling, G. R. (2005). Developing a theoretical model of rapport building: Implications for medical education and the physician-patient relationship. In M. Haider (Ed.), *Global public health communication* (pp. 407–414). Boston: Jones and Bartlett.

Platt, F. W. (1992). *Conversational failure: Case studies in doctor–patient communication.* Tacoma, WA: Essential Science.

Platt, F. W. (1995). *Conversation repair: Case studies in doctor–patient communication.* Boston: Little, Brown.

---

with the doctor if he or she shook hands, smiled, and engaged in a polite greeting and introduction.

- *Use open questions.* Branch and Malik (1993) propose that skillful communicators can address patients' concerns in intense but brief discussions. They observed five physicians who invited patients to expand the scope of medical talk with open questions such as "What else?" By listening attentively, the physicians were able to hear the patients' concerns in 3 to 7 minutes. The patients were satisfied, and the doctors have won accolades as some of Massachusetts' most outstanding general physicians.

- *Don't rush.* Give patients a reasonable amount of time to express their concerns.

- *Avoid abrupt topic shifts.* If you suddenly change the subject, patients may wonder if they have offended you or if you have really been listening. To reduce misunderstandings, strive for smooth transitions, such as: "I appreciate your sharing these things; we're going to have to shift gears now and I'll ask you some different types of questions about your symptoms" (suggested by R. C. Smith & Hoppe, 1991, p. 464).

- *Determine the real issue* before *conducting the exam.* Keep in mind that patients often work up to their main concerns. Do not launch into a physical exam until you are sure of the main point of the visit. ("Is anything else on your mind today?") Ask "What else?" at least three times, or until the patient says that is all.

- *Listen for distress markers.* Remember that patients often stutter and stammer when they are working up to an important disclosure. Do not change the subject before you know what it is. Your reassurance will help them speak openly.

- *Ask for the patient's feedback.* Most patients will not interrupt you to let you know they cannot follow your advice. You must ask, as in "How do you feel about this option?" and "Is there anything that would make this hard for you to do?"

- *Reassure patients.* Keep in mind that patients seek medical attention for many reasons—to be reassured, forgiven, comforted, cured. Words mean a lot ("You needn't feel embarrassed about this." "It's not your fault." "I understand.") Patients typically consider that physicians who are open and reassuring understand them better than doctors who seem controlling (Silvester, Patterson, Koczwara, & Ferguson, 2007). Annette Harres (2008) found that physicians can show empathy and invite response by using friendly tag questions such as "You're in pain, aren't you?" (p. 49).

- *Treat people as equals.* Status differences often inhibit open communication. For example, some physicians earn patients' trust (and gratitude) by disclosing some of their own feelings and reassuring patients who seem nervous or unsure (du Pré, 2002; Smith-du Pré & Beck, 1996).

- *Coach patients:* After researchers trained physicians and the parents of pediatric patients using the PACE model (present information, ask questions, check your understanding, express any concerns), the parents shared more information with the doctor, expressed their concerns more freely, and were more likely than other patients to verify the information the doctor gave them by asking additional questions or restating what they understood (Harrington, Norling, Witte, Taylor, & Andrews, 2007). Physicians trained in the model were more likely than before to encourage parents' questions and to engage them in collaborative decision making. And they accomplished all of this without significantly adding to the length of exams.

- *Consider using humor.* The use of mild, respectful humor seems to be a particularly effective means of minimizing status differences between patients and caregivers (Beck & Ragan, 1992; du Pré, 1998; Ragan, 1990) and helping family caregivers relieve stress (Bethea, Travis, & Pecchioni, 2000). Juliann Scholl (2007) studied communication at MIRTH (Medical Institute for Recovery Through Humor), a skilled nursing unit within a large hospital. Patients in the unit took part in at least two good-humor activities a day, including storytelling, entertainment, cooking, and more. Scholl found that conversational humor helped participants speak candidly without seeming like "bad patients" and created a sense of immediacy and friendliness.

- *Minimize distractions.* James Price Dillard and associates studied medical visits during which parents of newborns who were suspected of having cystic fibrosis found out for sure if their babies were ill (J. P. Dillard, Carson, Bernard, Laxova, & Farrell, 2004; J. P. Dillard, Shen, Laxova, & Farrell, 2008). Even during such important meetings, distractions often made it difficult for the participants to concentrate. The most common distractions were the infants themselves, followed by siblings who were also present. Other distractions included noises from children in nearby rooms, staff and equipment, phone calls, and announcements over the public address system (J. P. Dillard et al., 2008). The researchers suggest meeting in a quiet office, outside of the hospital or clinic if necessary, and providing follow-up information parents can take with them.

For an example of especially pleasing patient–caregiver communication read the mother's story in Box 3.9.

## ENVIRONMENTAL RESTRUCTURING

> *"I wanted to design a building where the healing process begins the moment a patient enters in the front door."*—CÉSAR PELLI

Pelli, a design consultant to the Mayo Clinic, describes the careful attention he and others devote to the clinic's physical environment (Berry & Seltman, 2008, p. 41). Traditionally, medical settings come across as intimidating and sterile. The quarters are usually cramped and the furnishings austere. Some medical centers, such as Mayo, have begun to change the atmosphere, however. The idea is that environments that soothe and uplift can reduce stress (thus reducing pain), keep people's spirits up, and facilitate better communication.

BOX 3.9 **PERSPECTIVES**

# A Mother's Experience at the Dentist

When I first took Kathryn to the dentist, she was very apprehensive. She had never been before due to lack of dental insurance and money, and she only went to the doctor when she was really sick, which was once every 2 years or so. Most illnesses we handled at home, and the idea of preventive care was foreign to her. I knew she needed to go. I knew she wasn't brushing as good as she should, and I also knew that sometimes she lied to me about brushing at all. I couldn't watch her every minute.

When I remarried last year, we were finally fortunate enough to have dental insurance, only we found out there was a 1-year waiting period for anything other than cleanings. So I waited.

Finally, the year was up, and in July I took Kathryn to the dentist for the first time in her life. I tried in advance to make her understand that it was all right to be scared, but that did not mean that it was all right to whine, cry, and generally throw a fit. I told her again and again that I would never take her to anyone I didn't trust or anyone I thought would harm or hurt her unnecessarily.

On a Saturday morning we drove 40 miles to the dental center. Right away, the staff tried to make Kathryn feel at home. The receptionist greeted me and Kathryn by name and asked Kathryn if she was tired from getting up so early on a Saturday. But as I filled out the forms, Kathryn hid behind me, and she spent a lot of time trying to hug me and kiss my cheek. She always does this when she is nervous.

I found I was nervous as well. Not only could I not ease Kathryn's fears, but I found myself feeling like I was a bad parent for not bringing her to the dentist until she was 8. I wasn't sure, as nice as the receptionist was, if she would understand things like no money and no insurance. So we didn't talk about the fact that Kathryn should have been to the dentist years ago; we just talked about easy things, like the nice weather and my wedding pictures.

Soon it was time for Kathryn to go back. After taking x-rays the hygienist led us back to an examination room and found me a small stool to sit on so that I could stay in the same room. She was very friendly and made me feel comfortable. She was also nice to Kathryn and didn't put us down for not coming in sooner.

The cleaning was a little nerve-wracking, since it was a bit uncomfortable, and Kathryn has a wonderful gag reflex. But the hygienist never seemed to get upset, and she even talked to Kathryn as though she understood, asking her questions like "It's a little scary at first, isn't it?" and "Are you okay? We can wait a minute if you want to, but if we go ahead, we'll be done sooner." It was great that she was so understanding.

By this time, Kathryn was less apprehensive about me leaving the room for a few minutes. The dentist and I walked to the other end of the hall, where he explained that Kathryn had a lot of cavities. He recommended a series of four brief appointments to help Kathryn become more at ease as they repaired her teeth. He made me feel at ease, telling me what a pretty girl Kathryn was. Then he got serious and let me know he understood my concerns about not bringing her in sooner, but not to worry. The cavities were not severe, they were all in baby teeth, and although there were several, they would be easy to fix.

I collected Kathryn and stopped by the front desk, where the receptionist pulled out a surprise box and let Kathryn pick out what she wanted. The next visits were not as bad as Kathryn thought they would be. Every time she was a little happier and not so apprehensive about what would happen. Once she had been through the routine, she knew what to expect, and that helped. She said she liked everyone at the dentist's office. Once I brought a newspaper article I had written about Kathryn's school with her picture in it. The staff insisted on reading the whole thing and remarked what a good writer I was and how pretty Kathryn was. They also insisted on seeing my wedding pictures. It wasn't just something to be nice; they really wanted to see them.

I feel good taking Kathryn there because I know, no matter what, we will get the best treatment. Not only that, but we have established friendships with these people that will last. They truly believe they are there to serve, and they show that in everything they do. Just ask Kathryn. She'll tell you.

—Donna

Mayo designers go so far as personally to examine each sheet of marble to be incorporated in floors and staircases to make sure that no unpleasant designs are suggested in the natural color variations. Their goal is to inspire confidence and health from the ground up. The clinic is famous for its art (much of it donated by grateful patients), soaring architecture, large windows, and live music. A grand piano is available in the main lobby of each Mayo campus. James Hodge, who chairs the clinic's art committee, says:

> It is rare that someone is not playing the piano in the Gonda lobby. I've seen patients and visitors join in a sing-along—once patients and visitors were dancing. Another time a diva of opera paused and spontaneously sang. On another occasion, a well-known pop musician sang while a volunteer accompanied him on the piano. (quoted by Berry & Seltman, p. 42)

Even supposed luxuries are considered part of the healing experience. When Serena Fleischaker donated chandeliers for a Mayo grand lobby, she explained that she wanted to provide a beautiful, soothing presence for people coping with hardship. "I want the Chihuly glass chandeliers to pleasantly distract people, to cause them to raise their eyes toward the heavens, to pause in the anxious interludes between appointments, to have a tiny respite from their suffering," she said (quoted by Berry & Seltman, p. 41). The clinic also features large windows, grand staircases, gardens, fountains, and quiet sitting areas.

Research supports that physical environments have a significant influence on health-related communication. Kreps and Thornton (1992) describe the subduing effect of confined spaces (small rooms, low ceilings) versus the stimulation of open spaces and windows. du Pré (1998) observed that communication in a doctor's office tends to be quieter and more private than in the open-air arrangement of most physical therapy units, where conversations are often loud and invite participation from anyone in earshot. With the goal of improving communication and emotional well-being, health practitioners

and researchers are beginning to examine, and in many cases reshape, the environments in which patients and caregivers communicate. In this section we take a closer look at those efforts.

## Soothing Surroundings

One effort to restructure medical environments is led by **Planetree**, a nonprofit organization that helps medical centers establish pleasing and empowering surroundings. Planetree was founded in California in 1978 by Angelica Thieriot, who was dismayed by how "cold, impersonal, and lonely" she found U.S. hospitals compared to those of her native Argentina (Schwade, 1994, paragraph 23). (Planetree is named after the type of tree under which Hippocrates is said to have mentored medical students.)

Hospitals influenced by the Planetree model often offer hotel-style rooms with accommodations for overnight visitors. Patients are encouraged to wear their own clothing, and soothing colors and adjustable lighting help reduce the cold sterility common to clinical settings ("Patient Satisfaction," 2007). Rooms are equipped with thermostats so that patients can control the temperature. Treatment rooms usually allow patients to gaze at colored glass, gardens, or soothing displays as they undergo procedures.

Large windows are a key Planetree feature, allowing access to sunlight and a view of plants, flowers, and fountains. At some hospitals "healing gardens" provide living displays of plants honored through the centuries for their curative properties, complete with labels describing the significance of each.

The Bergan Mercy Medical Center in Omaha, Nebraska, adopted the Planetree model to "humanize and demystify" its emergency services department (Lumsdon, 1996). An administrator remembers that the staff was initially indignant when it was proposed that they institute patient-centered care. They felt they were already patient-centered. But soon, says the administrator, they became excited about ideas they had never considered before. Now the hospital staff keeps clinical equipment in handy closets (not out in the open) whenever possible, plays Disney movies to soothe frightened children, and uses dimmer switches to adjust room lighting. The hospital received only 2 patient complaints the year after changes were implemented, compared to 37 the year before (Lumsdon).

### Easy Communication with Loved Ones

Sometime a healing environment is more virtual than physical. A free online program called Care-Pages provides a way for people coping with health issues to post photos, news, and updates. Loved ones can visit online and post comments of their own. I recently received a CarePage invitation from a former student whose newborn baby was in intensive care. The website allowed the anxious parents to keep loved ones informed without calling everyone individually. They posted pictures of the baby and frequent updates about her condition. When I logged on there were already dozens of messages from loved ones, ranging from "She is beautiful like her mother!" to "We know how worried your are. Our thoughts are with you at this difficult time." CarePages users can also take part in online forums and blogs with people in similar situations. (See Box 3.10 for more about healing environments.)

Sometimes loved ones are close by, but caregivers are not. The following section describes how telemedicine is influencing patient–caregiver communication.

### COMMUNICATION TECHNOLOGY: TELEMEDICINE

From her living room, a physician looks in on patients in the hospital. They are able to see each other and converse through two-way interactive television. A small keyboard allows the doctor to check her e-mail messages, review patient charts, order prescriptions, examine diagnostic information, and read the latest research. This is not science fiction. It's David Bates and Anthony Komaroff's (1996) vision of telemedicine in the not-so-distant future.

The technology is already available to make Bates and Komaroff's vision come true. **Telemedicine** is

**BOX 3.10 RESOURCES**

## More About Healing Environments

Frampton, S., Gilpin, L., & Charmel, P. (Eds.) (2003). *Putting patients first: Designing and practicing patient-centered care.* San Francisco: Jossey-Bass.
Gearon, C. J. (2002). Planetree (25 years older). *Hospitals & Health Networks, 76*(10), 40–43.
Planetree website: www.planetree.org
CarePages website: www.carepages.com/support

the process of communicating across distances for health-related purposes. (*Tele* is Greek for "far.") It may involve the use of telephones, pagers, computers, facsimile (fax) machines, electronic mail, voice mail, Internet links, interactive video, and more. Here are a few examples of how telemedicine can work.

### A Doctor's Visit, Telemedicine Style

A classic example of telemedicine is the program at East Carolina University (ECU) School of Medicine. In the early 1990s, the ECU staff began offering long-distance medical consultations to inmates at Central Prison, 100 miles from campus (Whitten, Sypher, & Patterson, 2000). The patients and caregivers interact via a teleconference link that allows them to see and talk to each other. Medical personnel at the university and prison work together to conduct exams and discuss medical information. Digital cameras and digital stethoscopes transmit detailed information to the off-site physician. Since beginning the program, ECU has expanded it to serve people in rural communities where specialists are not available. The program has been recognized by *Telehealth Magazine* as one of the country's Top 10 Telemedicine Programs.

### Telemedicine in the Future

Glenn Forbes of Mayo Clinic envisions an even more futurist image of telemedicine, in which people have small microchips inserted under their skin or carry digitized medical-information cards that allow medical staffs anywhere in the world to monitor their health. Forbes imagines how the process would work if he were traveling in another country:

> I feel fine, but I check in every once in a while. If I have a chip embedded, I might even be unknowingly "checking in." Every seven days Mayo checks my blood sugar and could send me a message about needing to cut back on the cookies because my sugar level went up from 116 to 124. This information and advice is part of my partnership—part of what I have decided to purchase for my personal benefit. (quoted by Berry & Seltman, 2008, p. 239)

Or, Forbes says, he might have a plastic card he inserts into a "Health Maintenance ATM" anywhere in the world if he has a health concern, such as frequent headaches. The card transmits his health information and location to his home clinic, where the staff might respond, "Your genetics suggest that you are prone to headaches if you've been eating too much pasta" (p. 239). The clinic staff could also recommend a nearby clinic that is part of the network and has access to his online medical records.

Forbes says this futuristic model will not alleviate the need for face-to-face health communication, good listening skills, and sensitivity. Indeed, because patients' information will be so readily available, he says, patients and caregivers might have *more* time to talk about current concerns.

## Telemedicine as Medical Outsourcing

Behind the scenes, telemedicine has made possible a degree of medical outsourcing that might surprise many patients. For example, if you undergo an x-ray, CT scan, MRI, ultrasound, or nuclear medicine scan, there's a good chance a radiologist across the world will evaluate the results—a process called *ghosting*. One of the largest medical outsourcing firms is NightHawk Radiology Service, which provides **teleradiology** (radiology analysis from an off-site location) for more than 1,400 health care organizations in the United States (J. E. Douglas,

2008). More than half of the firm's 100 radiologists live outside the United States. Because health professionals in the United States are licensed by individual states, some NightHawk radiologists have 38 state licenses and privileges to practice at more than 400 hospitals (Singh & Wachter, 2008). The company employees 35 people just to manage licensing and credentialing!

We examine the impacts of medical outsourcing and other forms of telemedicine more in the following section on the pros and cons of technology-based health communication.

## Advantages for Consumers

Many people are optimistic that telemedicine will conserve money and resources. Communication technology offers a number of benefits to patients, especially those who do not live near major medical centers.

First, technology may enable patients and caregivers to communicate more often and more openly, which may improve the quality of care. Patients may also be willing to disclose information via long-distance technology (particularly through e-mail) that they would be uncomfortable sharing face-to-face (Baur, 2000). There is encouraging evidence that e-mail communication between patients and caregivers is as patient-centered, or more, than face-to-face transactions. Debra Roter, Susan Larson, and colleagues (2008) found that—in contrast to in-person visits, during which doctors do most of the talking—patients do most of the "talking" in e-mails, outnumbering physicians' comments 2 to 1. They also report that patients seem to feel more comfortable disclosing emotions and praising and thanking their doctors in e-mails than in person, perhaps because e-mail communication is less intimidating and less constrained by time limits. And physician responses, although briefer than patients', are usually informative, confirming, and reassuring. Doctors displayed empathy and reassurance in 53% of the e-mails Roter and colleagues studied. For example, one doctor told a patient via e-mail: "Please don't ever think of doing so [e-mailing me] as bothering me—I welcome your participation in these decisions!" (Roter et al., p. 83). Overall, coders rated physician e-mails equally as friendly, respectful, and responsive as patients'. Some 60% of U.S. residents surveyed said they would like to have online access to their doctors, their medical records, and their test results ("Online Usage," 2008). And 1 in 4 said they would be willing to pay more for it.

Second, technology may allow people in underserved communities access to the types of doctors and technology usually reserved for big-city dwellers. Doctors, particularly specialists, are disproportionately located in densely populated areas and are relatively scarce in rural ones (Matusitz & Breen, 2007). With telemedicine, a person could conceivably contact a health professional anywhere in the world by phone, e-mail, voice mail, or computer (K. B. Wright, 2008). Participants in the ECU program report that telemedicine has made medical care available to people who would not otherwise have access to it.

Third, better care can mean less expense. Telemedicine reduces the need for each small town to have its own set of medical specialists. Patients in smaller markets can stay close to home rather than transferring to major medical centers. Plus, easier access may mean identifying and treating illnesses before they become severe and more costly to treat (Whitten et al., 2000).

Fourth, patients may become better educated about health matters through long-distance consultations and access to computer databases. The online Medline database, updated daily by the National Library of Medicine, provides online information about more than 750 health topics and includes links to health information presented in more than 45 languages. For many people with health concerns, such information is a way to feel more in control. The majority of participants in Alex Broom's (2008) study of men with prostate cancer say they appreciate the information they found online and feel it helped them manage the uncertainties of treatment decisions. Said one man in the study: "Knowledge is power. I like to be in control of my situation and the way I want to do that is by knowing what is going to happen…I really need that information to feel ok"

---

**BOX 3.11 RESOURCES**

# Journals That Feature Health Communication Research

*Health Communication*
*Journal of Health Communication*
*Communication & Medicine*
*Social Science & Medicine*
*Journal of Qualitative Health Research*
*Journal of the American Medical Association*
*Australian Journal of Communication*
*New England Journal of Health*
*American Journal of Public Health*
*Journal of Health and Social Behavior*
*Communication Monographs*
*Communication Quarterly*
*Communication Research*
*Communication Studies*
*Communication Yearbook*
*Critical Studies in Mass Communication*
*Critical Studies in Media*
*Developmental Psychology*
*Discourse and Society*
*Discourse Analysis*
*Human Communication Research*
*Journal of Applied Communication Research*
*Journal of Communication*
*Journal of Personality and Social Psychology*
*Journal of Sociology*
*Language and Social Interaction*
*Medical Education*
*Medical Economics*
*Patient Education and Counseling*
*Annals of Internal Medicine*
*Annals of Family Medicine*
*Academic Medicine*
*Health Psychology*

---

(p. 98). (See Box 3.11 for a list of journals that feature health communication research.)

Fifth, electronic health records can prevent the hassle of repeating the same information (insurance company, emergency contact, etc.) at every provider's office. Online records can also help doctors share notes and guarantee that a patient's records won't be destroyed in a fire or natural disaster.

Finally, people may enjoy therapeutic support via long-distance communication with others. Computer users can converse electronically with health professionals and laypeople who share their concerns. (We'll talk more about virtual communities in Chapter 7.)

## Advantages for Caregivers

Caregivers may benefit from telemedicine as well. First, being able to communicate with patients and colleagues in remote locations reduces travel time and the demands on office space and staff. There are even benefits closer to home. "E-mail is a timesaver," declares Reese (2008). A physician can e-mail a patient when he or she has time rather than playing phone tag. E-mail also allows doctors to think through patient questions or to research them before replying. One physician Reese interviewed said his staff is able to respond to about 80% of the e-mails he receives. Because e-mails are more detailed than the typical phone message, he can quickly scan the contents to see who should best respond to them. Furthermore, e-mails can reduce the number of unnecessary office visits and after-hours phone calls. Patients who are able to access their physicians via secure e-mail require 7% to 10% fewer office visits and make 14% fewer after-hours calls to their doctors ("The E-Mail," 2007, Reese). E-mails are also time-savers for staff members, who can send out appointment reminders instantly rather than calling patients one by one (Reese).

Second, vital information can be transmitted from one location to another instantly or with only a brief delay, amplifying opportunities for immediate response and medical teamwork. A cardiologist, for example, can monitor a patient's heart activity and direct paramedics' efforts even before the patient arrives at the hospital. At least 64% of the caregivers in the ECU study say they have learned valuable skills and information while participating in exams with other doctors and specialists (Whitten et al.,

2000). Additionally, most doctors now use handheld personal digital assistants (PDAs) to look up prescription drug information and perform other tasks (Terry, 2007).

Third, diagnostic images and patient records can be electronically stored and quickly retrieved, even by people in different locations. Caregivers may be able to access the medical charts of patients they are seeing for the first time. This could save time in emergencies and allow different caregivers to coordinate patient care more effectively. If the systems are well designed, online medical records can also help physicians and researchers collect data on the usefulness of various drugs and therapies (Kush, Helton, Rockhold, & Hardison, 2008).

## Disadvantages

With so many advantages it may seem puzzling that telemedicine is not more prevalent. Although the technology continues to improve, much of it has been available for years.

One reason for the slow beginning is cost. Technology is expensive and quickly outdated. A second concern involves scheduling. Nearly half of the ECU participants studied said it is a hassle to schedule two teams of medical caregivers (one onsite and one remote) to take part in telemedicine consultations (Whitten et al., 2000).

A third reservation concerns privacy. Some people worry about electronic eavesdropping and the possibility that hackers could gain access to confidential patient records. To restrict access, medical networks now rely on encryption (secret coding) and electronic "firewalls" designed to stop unauthorized users from reaching confidential data. Secure e-mail systems endorsed by the AMA and many private insurers are also available (Reese, 2008). By most accounts, these systems are good, although not perfect. But the human component is worrisome as well. Online access means more people would have the chance to view patients' private information than ever before. That worry is compounded in light of international medical outsourcing. Privacy laws apply to people in the United States, but it is less clear if, say, teleradiologists in other countries (some of them with widely different laws and cultural expectations about privacy) can legally be held to those standards.

Fourth, information in patients' electronic health records can be restrictive and hard to use if the formats are not well designed and if physicians are not careful about what they include. One problem is that some online forms require caregivers to fill in lengthy amounts of patient information. For example, a pediatrician may be required to ask every patient a time-consuming list of safety questions (use of bike helmets, seatbelts, etc.). This leaves less time to focus on the patient's immediate concerns (Hartzband & Groopman, 2008). Physicians Pamela Hartzband and Jerome Groopman (2008) describe an additional concern, namely, their frustration with doctors who include inappropriate or too much information in patients' online health records. In some cases doctors plagiarize. "We have seen portions of our own notes inserted verbatim into another doctor's note," say Hartzband and Groopman (p. 1656). In addition to being unethical, this practice results in repetitive, too-long medical records that fail to present each physician's thoughtful analysis of the patient's condition. Another factor that bogs down medical records is a lengthy hodgepodge of test results. If such information is not well organized, more is not better—it's just overwhelming. Write Hartzband and Groopman:

> A colleague at a major cancer center that recently switched to electronic medical records said that chart review during rounds has become nearly worthless. He bemoaned the vain search through meaningless repetition in multiple notes for the single line that represented a new development. "It's like 'Where's Waldo?'" he said bitterly. Ironically, he has started to handwrite a list of new developments on index cards so that he can refer to them at the bedside. (p. 1656)

Fifth, it's still somewhat unclear how caregivers can or should be compensated for services rendered long-distance. Should they charge for phone conversations, e-mail correspondence, and the like? If so, how should those rates compare to the cost of face-to-face visits? Reservations about this issue and the fear of being inundated by patient messages and questions have made some caregivers leery of opening up new lines of communication. The issue is becoming clearer, however, as reimbursement agencies—mindful that a phone call or e-mail can prevent a more expensive outcome—are increasingly willing to reimburse providers for technology-assisted communication. In 2008 a group of health insurance companies launched a pilot project in Pennsylvania in which they pay doctors to keep close tabs on patients using e-mail and websites. Another part of the agreement is that participating physicians will keep a percentage of office hours open so that sick patients can schedule appointments within 48 hours (Goldstein, 2008). The hypothesis is that technology and quick-response protocols will save money in the long run.

Sixth, it's unclear how medical licensing and malpractice laws (both of which are governed by individual states) will apply to medical care that spans state and national boundaries. As mentioned, many teleradiologists are licensed in multiple states. Most physicians are not, so it remains to be determined exactly how state laws will apply to "virtual visits" across state lines. It's also unclear how malpractice laws might apply to medical professionals in other countries who work for U.S. health organizations via electronic means. Furthermore, some physicians worry that they will be sued for malpractice based on information they provide via online forums. Legal experts caution doctors to include disclaimers such as the following if they offer guidance or assistance online, especially if they have not treated the patient personally: "This is not an official medical opinion because I haven't performed an examination. If you need specific medical advice, make an appointment with me or with a physician in the appropriate specialty in your area" (L. J. Johnson, 2007, p. 30).

Seventh, greater use of technology may widen the gap between the well served and the underserved. The cost and complexity of technology suggests that it will proliferate in the households of well-educated and affluent people first, increasing access to those already known to use health resources and systematically excluding underprivileged individuals.

Finally, some worry that telemedicine will become a less effective substitute for face-to-face communication. No one expects (or even wants) telemedicine to replace face-to-face medical visits entirely. Still, the limits of technology may restrict what patients and caregivers are able to convey to each other (Baur, 2000). Some worry that medical decisions will be made on the basis of incomplete or misleading information. Chamberlain (1994) cautions that high-tech methods cannot make up for poor communication: "No amount of technology is going to compensate for an ill-conceived or ill-designed message. The buck stops there...with the communicator" (paragraph 4).

## COMMUNICATION SKILL BUILDERS: TIPS FOR PATIENTS

This chapter looks at health communication from many angles, from the traditional to the futuristic. But the bottom line is that patients and caregivers cannot succeed—in communicating or healing—without mutual effort. Earlier in the chapter, we reviewed ways caregivers can stimulate collaborative communication. Here are a few suggestions for patients.

- *Write it down.* Write down your main concerns and questions as well as any medications you take and any dates that may be important to the diagnosis. Bring two copies so that your doctor can look on and keep a copy for future reference.
- *Rank-order your concerns.* Here's an experience I have had many times. During training sessions with physicians, I tell them that I recommend that patients write down their concerns. Have you ever heard an entire auditorium of doctors groan aloud? They do! But then I add some advice I learned from Branch, Levinson, and Platt (1996). I say: "Before they bring that list to you, I recommend that they rank-order the items from most to least important." Then the doctors cheer. No kidding! The lesson

| BOX 3.12 **RESOURCES** |

# More on Patient Communication Skills

For more on the PACE model, visit: patcom.jcomm. ohio-state.edu/HealthWeb2/w2page1.htm

Cegala, D. J. (2006). Emerging trends and future directions in patient communication skills training. *Health Communication, 20*(2), 123–129.

Cegala, D. J., Post, D. M., & McClure, L. (2001). The effects of patient communication skills training on the discourse of older patients during a primary care interview. *Journal of the American Geriatrics Society, 49*(11), 1505–1511.

for patients is that doctors like a list—*if* it helps them get a succinct overview of all your concerns and *if* the list identifies what you consider most important. (Keep in mind that you may not have time to go through all items on the list in one visit.)

- *Think it through.* Assess your emotions and physical sensations in advance. Rehearse how to state your goals for the interview in a concise and straightforward way (preferably within 1 minute).
- *Prepare for the standard questions.* Be ready with answers to such questions as What does it feel like? When? Where? For how long?
- *State your goals.* Be as clear as possible when making the appointment so that the caregiver knows your concerns and expectations. ("I'm experiencing sharp abdominal pains" and "I'd like an overall physical and a chance to ask some questions.")
- *Talk to the nurse.* Odds are you will speak with a nurse before you speak with the doctor. Let the nurse know your concerns. He or she can help facilitate your visit.
- *Get to the point.* Use the first minute of a medical interview to suggest what you would most like to cover.

## BOX 3.13 CAREER OPPORTUNITIES

# Health Communication Research

Professor
Researcher
Consultant

## Career Resources and Job Listings

Coalition for Health Communication: www.healthcommunication.net

Health Communication Partnership: www.hcpartnership.org

*Chronicle of Higher Education*: chronicle.com

National Communication Association: www.natcom.org

International Communication Association: www.icahdq.org

Graduate programs in health communication: www.gradschools.com/Subject/Health-Communication/74.html

Health Communication Exchange: www.healthcomms.org/comms/index.html

American Academy of Communication in Healthcare: www.aachonline.org

European Association for Communication in Health Care: www.each.nl

Association of American Medical Colleges: www.aamc.org

Society of Teachers of Family Medicine: www.stfm.org/index_ex.html

Society of Behavioral Medicine: www.sbm.org

blog.healthcommunicationresearch.com

U.S. Bureau of Labor Statistics: www.bls.gov

- *Take an active role.* Doctors usually understand patients' goals more clearly and share more information when the patients ask questions and state their concerns, preferences, and opinions (Cegala, Street, & Clinch, 2007).
- *Acknowledge reservations.* If something prevents you from speaking frankly with a caregiver, let that person know ("I'm embarrassed," "I'm afraid," etc.).
- *Be assertive.* If your questions have not been answered or you do not agree with the advice given, state your feelings in a clear and respectful way. Walking away dissatisfied helps no one.
- *Be succinct.* Caregivers have a legitimate need to keep transactions within reasonable timeframes.

## SUMMARY

The traditional power difference between patients and caregivers is manifested in conversations in which patients tend to acquiesce and physicians to dominate. Most studies show that doctors do the majority of the talking and ask most of the questions (questions that stipulate brief responses). Unwittingly or not, patients usually collaborate in the lopsided nature of these medical conversations by speaking hesitantly and abandoning topics when interrupted.

Although it may seem expedient for physicians to keep a tight rein on medical interviews, ineffective patient–caregiver communication is hurtful for everyone involved. Patients who do not have a strong sense of rapport with their physicians are more likely than others to sue for malpractice, to experience heightened pain, to withhold information that may be important to an accurate diagnosis, to switch doctors or avoid medical care altogether, and to distrust medical advice.

Some caregivers, far from being anxious to abuse the power granted them, are frustrated by the barriers it creates. They attempt to empower patients through the use of encouraging words and nonverbal gestures, humor, and more comfortable medical settings. Collaborative communication is neither physician-centered nor patient-centered, but is dedicated to active partnerships. A wide range of verbal and nonverbal strategies is presented for caregivers who wish to build rapport with patients.

Motivational Interviewing is one technique for involving patients as active participants in health-related decisions. The interviewer issues no orders or commands and makes no judgments. Instead, he or she asks questions to help a health decision maker explore the perceived advantages and disadvantages of various options.

Recognizing that the physical environment affects how people feel and how they communicate, some medical centers are restructuring their health care units to include beautiful views, peaceful settings, amenities for family members, soothing music, artwork, and more.

Technology expands the options and the challenges for health communication. Patients and caregivers may have access to more information and more means of message transmission than ever before, but the rules and expectations for telemedicine are still forming. The traditional boundaries of state and nation are blurred as caregiving takes on a virtual dimension. Experts are trying to balance the advantages of cost, convenience, and access with issues of privacy, medical liability, compensation, and information overload.

No matter what the medium or setting, communication between patients and caregivers is most effective when both sides are sensitive to each other's goals. For their part, patients can strive to communicate more clearly and assertively. Caregivers can show that they are sensitive to the challenges patients face in communicating about issues that are personal, fearsome, and uncertain.

## KEY TERMS

transactional communication
physician-centered communication
doorknob disclosures
directives
blocking
patronize
transgressions
therapeutic privilege
collaborative communication
model of collaborative interpretation (CI)
dialogue
motivational interviewing (MI)
Planetree
telemedicine
teleradiology

## DISCUSSION QUESTIONS

1. How could patients and caregivers lessen the likelihood of doorknob disclosures?
2. What factors contribute to the prevalence of physician-centered communication?
3. Traditionally, physicians have had more control over medical conversations than patients have. How do physicians' communication behaviors contribute to this power imbalance? How do patients' behaviors contribute to it?
4. Why might patients and caregivers commit transgressions? What are some methods for handling transgression attempts?
5. What are some reasons for the power difference between patients and caregivers?
6. In your opinion, should doctors and patients work toward greater equity in medical conversations? If so, what could patients do? What could caregivers do?
7. Why is physician-centered communication criticized?
8. What is therapeutic privilege? What guidelines would you suggest for using this privilege?
9. Contrast a "rhetoric of passivity" with a "rhetoric of agency."

10. Based on the model of collaborative interpretation, describe effective patient–caregiver communication. What criteria define collaborative interpretation?

11. Do you feel the term *patient* is accurate when describing well people seeking to maintain their own health? Brainstorm some other terms we might use.

12. Compare the assumptions of physician-centered and collaborative communication. How is the caregiver's role different in each model? How is the patient's role different?

13. What are some common assumptions and techniques of motivational interviewing? Would you enjoy being part of such an interview? Why or why not?

14. In what ways can caregivers use nonverbal communication to encourage patients' communication?

15. How can caregivers use verbal communication to encourage patients' communication?

16. How are some health centers restructuring their environments?

17. In your experience, does the physical environment affect patient–caregiver communication? Why or why not? If so, how?

18. What advantages does telemedicine offer to consumers? To caregivers?

19. What are the potential disadvantages of telemedicine?

20. Would you communicate with professional caregivers via e-mail given the chance? Why or why not?

21. Would you communicate with professional caregivers via two-way interactive television? Why or why not? In what ways might your communication be different than if you were in the same room?

22. What are some tips for better communication on the part of patients?

## ANSWERS TO *CAN YOU GUESS?*

1. Vermont ranks highest, Arizona lowest ("State Scorecard," 2007). To find out how other states stack up, visit www.commonwealthfund.com and search for state scorecard.

# CHAPTER
## 4

# Caregiver Perspective

*I was asked to see Mrs. B, who had just been diagnosed with pancreatic cancer.... Her husband asked numerous questions about the toxicity of the treatment regimen and about difficult quality-of-life issues. I answered his questions, then turned to Mrs. B and asked for her thoughts and feelings. To my surprise, she was engrossed in filing her fingernails and watching television. When she saw me looking at her, she said, "I'm sorry. I wasn't listening to your conversation. What did you say?" (Urba, 1998, paragraph 13)*

After feeling surprised by the woman's conduct, physician Susan Urba (1998) realized what was happening. The patient was overwhelmed by the information, unable to listen anymore. "She was too polite to ask us to leave, so she protected herself the only way she could. With her fingernail file and remote control" (Urba, paragraph 14). In this encounter and others like it, Urba says she has learned a valuable lesson, reflected in the title of the article, "Sometimes the Best Thing I Do Is Listen." She reflects that "the most important healing is done by the patient, and the physician can only have a small role in that process" (last paragraph).

Dr. Urba's experiences bring to mind the privileges and pressures of working every day with human life. This chapter looks at medicine from the caregivers' perspective. Understanding the way caregivers are socialized and the demands and rewards of caregiving provides insight into why caregivers communicate as they do.

The chapter is divided into six sections. The first three describe, respectively, medical socialization, professional influences on caregivers, and psychological influences on caregivers. The fourth section

focuses on stress and burnout among caregivers and reveals the important role communication plays in keeping caregivers healthy. This is followed by a section on communicating about medical mistakes. As we learn more about the way caregivers are trained and the immense pressures they experience, the communication patterns described in Chapter 3 are more understandable. Although caregivers may wish to give more time and attention to each patient, many factors make that hard to accomplish. The last section explores a high-tech process called *knowledge coupling* that may change the way patients and caregivers communicate.

As you read this chapter and the next one, on patients' perspective, remember that, although it is useful to examine one perspective at a time, health communication is ultimately shaped by the way diverse perspectives come together. No one perspective explains the entire process.

## MEDICAL SOCIALIZATION

Becoming a caregiver is not strictly a matter of acquiring technical expertise. It is also a process of **socialization** (learning to behave appropriately within a specific community). By entry into their chosen fields, most health care professionals are expected to be proficient in what Harvard University medical professor Elliot Mishler (1984) calls the **Voice of Medicine**. As the vocabulary of traditional biomedicine, this voice is characterized by carefully controlled compassion and a concern for accuracy and expediency.

The Voice of Medicine does not provide caregivers with much of a vehicle for sharing their emotions or soliciting emotional responses. Instead, it is characterized by medical terminology and attention to physical details. For the most part, patients' individuality is treated as less important than their physical conditions. However impersonal it may sound, the Voice of Medicine answers to the extraordinary demands of time and emotion exacted from caregivers and suits society's image of caregivers (physicians especially) as stoically objective and in control. Let's look at the socializing forces in caregiver education, particularly in medical school.

## Theory of Socialization

A person is said be socialized when he or she can behave with relative ease and appropriateness within a community. But the socialization process is never complete. People and communities change, requiring constant adaptation, and there is no such thing as being perfectly appropriate. (Ironically, it is inappropriate always to be appropriate. People are expected to be unique and break the rules sometimes.)

Communication theorists (e.g., V. Miller & Jablin, 1991) posit that newcomers to a culture attempt to fit in (assimilate) while still maintaining a sense of their own individuality. They learn what is expected of them (including when to misbehave) through official rules and informal conversations. They also witness, and are subject to, rewards and penalties. Rewards may take the form of raises, awards, promotions, friendly behavior, popularity, and so on. However, violators may be regarded as weak, stupid, crazy, or rude and may even be expelled from the community.

As you will see, medical students who do not measure up to expectations may fail or be judged negatively. This may seem a particularly dreadful possibility, considering how much they have invested emotionally and financially. Given these factors, students may go to unusual extremes to meet community standards.

A **speech community** refers to a group whose members share a common set of expectations (Hymes, 1962). Even within one neighborhood, there may be several speech communities with varying degrees of overlap. The distinction between speech communities and geographical communities helps explain why patients and caregivers may seem to have divergent expectations although they transact so frequently. They may live and work in close proximity but be part of different communities by virtue of their expectations. Based on the notion of speech communities, keep a few ideas in mind as you read the following description of medical socialization. First, no two communities are exactly alike; medical schools differ as well. The generalizations given here do not apply equally to all programs. Second, people are active agents in the process. Therefore, even people in the same community may be affected differently. Third, community standards may seem unfair or unreasonable to outsiders, but they usually have a rational basis within the community.

## Selection

An important part of medical socialization is selecting who gets to take part. Those whose abilities and ideals are inconsistent with the caregiver community may be systematically excluded from it, for better or worse.

Entrance requirements may be as simple as a high school diploma for medical aides and nontechnical assistants. Technicians (such as radiology technicians) may be required to have specialized training, serve apprenticeships, and be licensed. Other positions may require a college degree or even postgraduate education.

High rank is usually associated with greater focus on science and technology such that medical school applicants are evaluated in large part based on their aptitude for the sciences. Few people question the value of biology and physiology, but some feel medical schools should be equally concerned about the ethics and social skills of prospective doctors.

Sanford Brown (1995) contends that, far from encouraging social skills, the medical school process actually *inhibits* social development. The pressure to be scientifically competitive discourages premedical students from pursuing broader education in philosophy, art, and history. Individuals who are highly driven to succeed are apt to do well in medical school, but they may be impatient and domineering in dealing with others. Moreover, the rigors of medical school can further inhibit students from developing life experience, social interactions, and personal growth. Brown argues that these are probably as important as science to doctors' personal well-being and success with patients.

## Curriculum

Medicine is both science and art. Creating a curriculum that includes both is a challenging task, however.

*Science* Following the Flexner Report in the early 1900s (see Chapter 2), science became the core of most caregiver education programs. There is still a great deal of science in medical school as well as in nursing school, physical therapy programs, and so on. But many schools are changing the *way* they teach science. Traditionally, medical students have been required to learn massive amounts of scientific material in their first 2 years. In *What Patients Taught Me: A Medical Student's Journey,* Audrey Young (2004) remembers the second year as being "the hardest stretch," with eight classes, her desk stacked 2 feet high with papers, and 35 hours of lecture every week. Regrettably, she says, she "didn't set foot in a real clinic or talk with a practicing doctor for months" during that time (p. 39).

Pressed for time, students may memorize information without understanding it, a process called **rote learning** (Regan-Smith et al., 1994). These students may do well on multiple-choice exams but

be incapable of applying the information to actual situations. Among students in traditional medical curricula, about half (49%) said they did not understand the scientific information they learned for tests (Regan-Smith et al.). One student said that studying science was like memorizing a chant "yet not comprehending a word of it" (paragraph 7).

Another criticism of the traditional medical school curriculum is that clinical experience is limited to the final 2 years. Therefore students have only a delayed opportunity to apply what they are learning. And when they do face actual patients, they may find themselves at a loss to remember everything they crammed to learn. One intern describes what happened when a pulmonologist asked her, "What do you think of when you see a nodulorecticular pattern?"

> *You want an honest answer?* I think to myself. *When I see a nodulorecticular pattern on chest x-ray, I think: nothing.* I know we learned about this in med school, but my mind is drawing a complete blank. Worse, I'm panicking, thinking: *What am I doing here? How am I supposed to succeed as an intern if I can't even remember the differential diagnosis of a nodulorecticular chest x-ray?* (Transue, 2004, p. 16)

Physicians-in-training typically become more comfortable with the knowledge as they use it regularly—and more at ease admitting what they don't know. (See Box 4.1.) This underscores critics' point, that witnessing medicine firsthand is an effective way to learn content and to get a feel for the interpersonal dynamics involved.

Some schools, such as the University of California at San Francisco, are experimenting with integrated medical curricula in which information from various disciplines is woven together along with clinical experiences. This method may help students develop integrated knowledge and apply it immediately in natural contexts. The new method is not without challenges, of course. Faculty who are accustomed to structuring their own classroom experiences are challenged to work, instead, as part of multidisciplinary teams. For their part, students sometimes feel the information is less organized

## BOX 4.1 THEORETICAL FOUNDATIONS

# Talking Like a Doctor

"Being" a doctor is more than using medical jargon and wearing a white lab coat. A large part of professional socialization is learning to talk as doctors talk. Lorelei Lingard and coauthors (2003) studied medical faculty and third-year medical students at a hospital in Canada (Lingard, Garwood, Schryer, & Spafford, 2003). They found that different communication patterns were associated with "thinking as a Student" versus "thinking as a Doctor." These differences were evident in the way students and doctors conducted themselves during **case presentations**, episodes in which health care professionals meet to share information and evaluate the progress of their patients. The communication patterns the researchers observed present theoretical implications about the way doctors are socialized and how communication shapes their identities and attitudes.

## Students Versus Doctors

Although students in clinical practice function much like doctors, that is not their only concern. They must also take care to prove themselves and to fit in. Therefore it is no surprise that they dread seeming incompetent or unprepared. One student in Lingard and colleagues' (2003) study said, "To point out things you don't know is sort of shooting yourself in the back" (paragraph 33).

The students employed a range of face-saving strategies when faced with uncertainty. For example, when a doctor asked them questions they could not answer or challenged decisions they had made, the students typically attempted to (a) emphasize information they *did* know rather than dwell on what they did not know, (b) ask their instructors to provide assistance or suggestions, or (c) deflect criticism by using disclaimers, apologies, and explanations. Lingard et al. (2003) conclude, "For the most part, students in our study approached uncertainty as a condition to be avoided at all costs and, when not avoidable, to be disguised" (paragraph 27).

By contrast, the physicians seemed comfortable acknowledging the uncertainties of medical care. Perhaps because they could admit uncertainty without losing credibility, the doctors spoke openly about the imprecise art of making diagnoses and prognoses. They challenged students to defend their actions and judgments, perhaps to test and develop the students' confidence. However, in larger discussions the same physicians admitted that even experienced professionals often disagree and that scientific evidence is fallible. In short, the physicians communicated in ways that showed them to be both more confident and more tolerant of uncertainty than the students.

Another difference emerged in the students' response to information supplied by patients and their loved ones. The students typically accepted this information as valid and accurate. For example, one student defended a medical judgment by saying, "Well, the mom being, the mom being an MD gave me some terms I took at face value" (Lingard et al., 2003, paragraph 39). In the doctor's eyes, however, even a medical degree did not give the mother unquestionable credibility, as evidenced in his response, "well Mom may not know" (paragraph 39). In other instances as well, the physicians displayed skepticism about what their patients told them.

## Assimilation

Students' communication patterns are understandable, considering the tenuous position in which they find themselves. As Lingard and colleagues (2003) note: "Students are balancing on the threshold of a profession, with one foot inside and one foot outside its activities" (paragraph 23). In that context, owning up to limited knowledge is a risky enterprise. Furthermore, the new students may not be confident (or jaded) enough to question the credibility of physicians or clients.

The students' communication changed, however, as they became more experienced members of the medical community. Their talk began to sound more like doctors', in four ways (Lingard et al., 2003):

- They learned to sound confident even, sometimes, when they did not feel confident.
- They begin qualifying information conveyed by nonmedical sources (e.g., "The parents claim ...").
- They filtered information and presented their interpretations rather than simply relaying what they had seen and heard.
- They began acknowledging greater levels of uncertainty without losing confidence (e.g., saying "I don't know" without a disclaimer).

In short, as students gained experience they began to speak more like doctors. But perhaps more importantly, they began to think and act differently as well. Lingard et al. (2003) reflect that the students had not conquered uncertainty; they had just become more confident in the midst of it. And the students did not just *say* they were more skeptical of patients' accounts. They based their actions on that skepticism. Changes in their communication were matched by changes in their behavior.

As with any form of assimilation, accepting a new identity involves both gains and losses. Explore your reactions to this study by answering the following questions.

## What Do You Think?

1. What are the implications if doctors adopt more confident communication styles? How might this influence their chance of success? How might it influence their interactions with patients? How might their nonphysician colleagues be affected? (Try to think of positive and negative effects within each type of relationship.)
2. In what ways it is advantageous for doctors to be skeptical about what patients tell them? In what ways is it disadvantageous?
3. What are some strategies you might use for managing the immense uncertainties surrounding a person's health status and care?

---

than in the traditional one-subject-per-course curricula, and they are apprehensive about being immersed in complex concepts before they have mastered the fundamentals (Muller, Jain, Loeser, & Irby, 2008). After studying the program, Muller and colleagues suggest that faculty can help by providing an overall "conceptual scaffolding" for students.

Another promising means of reform is the implementation of **problem-based learning (PBL)**. Problem-based learning challenges students to apply information to actual scenarios rather than simply memorizing it. For instance, students may be presented with a case study and asked to analyze the patient's condition and identify factors relevant to the patient's health. PBL is positively correlated with physician competence later in their careers, particularly with physicians' ability to communicate about complex health matters (Koh, Khoo, Wong, & Koh, 2008).

Another useful technique is videotaped role-playing. Students conduct interviews with trained mock patients (sometimes called *standardized patients*), practicing their responses to realistic symptoms and emotional concerns the "patients" present. Usually, students review the videotapes with communication specialists and the mock patients involved.

*Communication Training* The emphasis on science remains. But a new revolution is afoot that expands the traditional model. In a move that Larrie Greenberg (2004) says "could have the greatest impact on medical education as a continuum since the Flexner Report" (p. 1398), the Accreditation Council on Graduate Medical Education (ACGME) announced six new core competencies in 1999. The competencies are medical knowledge, patient care, communication and interpersonal skills, professionalism, PBL and improvement, and systems-based practice.

BOX 4.2

## The Art of Medicine

"The artist knows when the patient needs a warm smile, reassuring words, or a gentle hug. It's the artists who make every patient feel welcome, comfortable, secure, hopeful. The artist sees the anxiety and reassures the new mother that her baby's fever is nothing to worry about....The artist knows when there's nothing more the engineer can do and helps the patient and family cope at the end of life. What the artist does is why I became a physician."

—*Physician Denis Corese*
(quoted by Berry & Seltman, 2008, pp. 1–2)

In this discussion, we'll focus on communication and interpersonal skills—what some might call the art of medicine.

ACGME governs postgraduate education, primarily internships, residencies, and, for some, specialized fellowships. Interns are in their first year of residency (full-time, supervised clinical experience following medical school). Depending on state requirements and medical specialties, residency can last from 2 to 8 years. By the time students become residents they have graduated from medical school, but they are not yet eligible to be licensed practitioners. On the surface, ACGME only controls these experiences, not the medical school curriculum. But the implications of setting new postgraduate standards reverberate throughout the system. This is because, to maintain accreditation, organizations that host medical students, such as hospitals, must screen applicants on the basis of the core competencies and must structure training programs around those learning domains. Therefore students at medical schools who do not also focus on these areas are at risk for hitting a dead end after graduation. And since in 1999 the American Board of Medical Specialties adopted as requirements for physician certification the same six competencies as ACGME, the

list has had a profound impact on medical education at all levels. Greenberg (2004) may be right that nothing has affected the med school curriculum this much since Abraham Flexner filed his report in 1910.

ACGME (2006) proposes that "effective communication skills are at the heart of quality patient care" (p. 20) and that communication is essential to leadership and teamwork (the focus of Chapter 10 in this volume). The council defines competence in interpersonal and communication skills as the ability to:

- create and sustain a therapeutic and ethically sound relationship with patients,
- use effective listening skills and elicit and provide information using effective nonverbal, explanatory, questioning, and writing skills, and
- work effectively with others as a member or leader of a health care team or other professional group. (ACGME, 2006, p. 20)

Research indicates that the most effective communication training programs employ a range of experiential activities (e.g., role-playing, observations, discussion) rather than relying on large, lecture-based formats (Lundine, Buckley, Hutchinson, & Lockyer, 2008). When effective, skills training often improves both patients' and caregivers' involvement in medical encounters. The patients of physicians who take part in communication skills training are more likely than others to feel that they received high-quality care and to recommend their doctors to others (Haskard et al., 2008). Trained physicians typically give more information than other doctors, show more sensitivity, and address a greater variety of patients' lifestyle behaviors (Haskard et al.). Likewise, after communication skills training, nurses are typically more confident about their ability to interact effectively with patients, even in palliative care situations (Wilkinson, Perry, Blanchard, & Linsell, 2008). Many advocates support the creation of more communication courses, including classes on delivering bad news (Zakrzewski, Ho, & Braga-Mele, 2008), working with patients to set medical agendas (Rodriguez et al., 2008), and more.

The emerging emphasis on humanistic aspects of medicine is a welcome change for critics such as Alan Bonsteel (1997), who maintains that "cold, clinical physicians" result from medical education that concentrates on science but neglects interpersonal communication, social issues, and ethics. Traditionally medical students have learned about the human body mostly by using cadavers rather than living individuals. This process is valued as a means of educating students and toughening them up. Cadavers provide valuable opportunities for exploring the human body. But Bonsteel argues that an overreliance on cadavers encourages medical students to regard the body as an inanimate object. There is no need to communicate with a cadaver, treat it gently, or wonder about its feelings. Bonsteel urges medical schools not to portray people as impersonal "biological systems," but as individuals with feelings and emotions.

Medical professor Michael Wilkes reminds medical educators that it isn't enough to design new courses. A great deal of learning occurs via the "hidden curriculum." That is, students are influenced by the attitudes and practices others model. "Think of how young medical students must feel when they witness discriminatory behavior on the part of senior residents and teachers," Wilkes says, adding:

> We can teach extensively about the appropriateness of respecting different cultures, different beliefs and different health practices, but when the student hears a resident dissing a patient's mistaken notions of disease, or hears them making fun of a patient's body, the lesson is clear—to be a part of the "club," this is the expected behavior. (quoted by Lauer, 2008b, p. 50)

Wilkes and others warn that, very often, seeing is doing when it when it comes to shaping new professionals. True change comes through modeling the behaviors we want others to adopt.

## Socialization Process

When students complete their fourth year of medical school, they officially become medical doctors (MDs) or doctors of osteopathy (DOs), but they spend the next years completing residency requirements. Thus, people who enter medical school at age 22 cannot expect to begin licensed practice until they are at least 29. In the intervening years they are surrounded by information and issues foreign to most people. It's said that the average medical student learns 10,000 words that are not in general use outside of medicine. All in all, it's no surprise that most doctors leave medical school with a significantly different perspective—and different vocabulary—than when they began.

Medical school has been called the "longest rite of passage in the Western world" (Bonsteel, 1997, paragraph 3). Few other experiences are so extensive and life-altering. The intensity, uniqueness, and isolation of medical education make it an especially hospitable arena for socialization. In the next section we will examine some of the ways the medical culture is established in medical school.

*Loss of Identity* Medical school has been compared to military boot camp, in that newcomers are apt to feel stripped of their previous identity and doubtful about their self-worth. Like the military, medical school has a strict hierarchy, and those at the lowest levels are reminded in many ways of their lowly status. Interns are referred to as "the dirt on which the ladder stands" (Hirschmann, 2008, p. 59) and as those who get "pimped first, blamed first, and thanked last" (Jauhar, 2008b, p. 201).

The phrase *medical student abuse* appears frequently in published literature. Tales are told of medical students being cursed, slapped, kicked, punished, and worse. Among graduates of 16 medical schools in the United States, 84% said they had been belittled in medical school and 42% said they had been harassed by professors, residents, classmates, or patients (Frank, Carrera, Stratton, Bickel, & Nora, 2006). Only 13% of those surveyed considered the abuse severe, but those who felt abused were more likely than others to regret choosing medicine as a career.

Medical students performing clinical duties are subservient to higher-ranking interns and residents, who are themselves subservient to practicing

## BOX 4.3 CAREER OPPORTUNITIES

# Medicine, Dentistry, and Physician Leadership

Medical doctor
Doctor of osteopathy
Allopathic physician
Medical researcher
Medical school professor
Dentist
Medical director
Physician executive

## Some Medical Specialty Areas

Family and general medicine
Internal medicine
Obstetrics and gynecology
Pathology
Anesthesia
Pediatrics
Psychiatry
Surgery
Cardiology
Oncology
Radiology
Dermatology
Emergency care
Ophthalmology
Cardiovascular care
Neurology
Physiology

## Some Dental Specialties

Oral and maxillofacial surgery
Orthodontics
Prosthodontics

## Career Resources and Job Listings

American Medical Association: www.ama-assn.org
American Board of Medical Specialists: www.abms.org
American Association of Colleges of Osteopathic Medicine: www.aacom.org
American Osteopathic Association: www.osteopathic.org
Association of American Medical Colleges: www.aamc.org/students
American College of Physicians: www.acponline.org
National Institute of Health: www.nih.gov
American Dental Association: www.ada.org
American Dental Education Association: www.adea.org
American College of Surgeons: www.facs.org
American College of Physician Executives: www.acpe.org
U.S. Department of Labor Occupational Outlook: www.bls.gov/oco

physicians. Those of lower rank are reminded of their place with public pop quizzes in which personnel of higher status can publicly challenge them to answer medical questions or make diagnoses. Novices are also called on to do **scut work**, menial chores no one else wants to do. It is commonly accepted that some of these chores are assigned mainly to punish or humiliate the novices, who are referred to in derogatory terms such as "scut monkeys" (Sheehan, Sheehan, White, Leibowitz, & Baldwin, 1990). However, even as they are being cast as peons within

the system, medical school students are induced to see themselves as superior to those *outside* it.

*Privileged Status*   Doctors in the United States are typically granted extraordinary power, prestige, and money. In addition, they witness marvels and horrors unknown to most people.

To be granted access to wonders seldom witnessed can be a heady experience. Perri Klass, whose medical school memoirs were published as the book *A Not Entirely Benign Procedure* (1987), recalls a heady sense of wonder dissecting cadavers, reflecting that she was doing something "normal people never do" (p. 37). Klass compared the sensation to initiation into a priesthood.

Others remember the elation of being addressed as doctor for the first time. This usually occurs during clinicals, when students are less than halfway through medical school. Although they are years away from medical licensing, they are called "doctor" by most patients, who tend to view them as bona fide professionals. In this way, students get an early dose of the prestige, but also the formidable responsibilities, that go with the title.

*Overwhelming Responsibilities* Medical studies are often overwhelming in terms of the amount of work and its critical nature. It's not unusual for students to spend 12 to 18 hours a day in the lab or studying. At least 50% of medical students say they are burnt out, and 10% have thought about suicide (Liselotte et al., 2008). And postgraduate experiences are no easier. Interns frequently report having insomnia, nightmares, and depression. Many are haunted by decisions or oversights that resulted in adverse patient outcomes. Although interns have immense responsibility, they often have less experience than anyone around them. In *Intern: A Doctor's Initiation*, Sandeep Jauhar (2008b) describes the password assigned to him by the hospital staff when he began his internship: "bogus doctor" (p. 45). Transue (2004) describes a similar sense of being out of place. When she found herself lost in the psychiatric ward during her first day as an intern, she says, she was half afraid the staff would think she was not a real doctor, only a delusional patient who had found a lab coat. She soon realized, however, that the staff was accustomed to lost interns, especially in July. She explains in retrospect: "July is when the new interns come, eager and foolish and amusing to everyone else" (p. 6).

On a more somber note, Jauhar (2008b) describes the intense fear and isolation of taking on life-and-death responsibilities for which he felt ill prepared. "It seemed like the only people I wasn't scared of were my patients," he attests. "They were as much at a loss in this place as I was" (p. 113).

The expectation that students will move expeditiously from observers to participants is reflected in the clinical battle cry, "Watch one, do one, teach one" (P. Conrad, 1988, p. 326). Learning on the job can be a frightening experience when human lives (including your own) are at stake. At the same time, there can be an exhilarating sense of being part of the action and learning at a rapid pace. Interns sometimes say that, as much as they long for a day off, when it comes they feel adrift and left out. When things got really tough, Transue (2004) reminded herself: "I will never learn as much in any year of my life as I will in this one. I may never have the same intensity of experience. I intend to make the most of it" (p. 34).

Many physicians-in-training experience a sense of physical and emotional isolation from their loved ones. Transue (2004) recalls the initial shock of clinical work. "I had woken up that morning having never seen a death, and by lunchtime I had been part of one," she says (p. 1). "Nothing in medical school or in life had prepared me for that moment....I felt wrenchingly and terribly alone." As she felt herself being transformed by the experienced, she wondered if people she loved could still relate to her. "Would they understand what I had just seen and done? Would I be inevitably separated from them by this experience and those that would follow it?" (p. 1).

In the past, it was common for residents to work 36-hour shifts and log 90 to 120 work hours per week (Bonsteel, 1997). These rules were begun when most residents lived on-site, however, and had opportunities to grab a nap or some private downtime. They were also established before the age of outpatient care, when at least a portion of hospitals patients were not seriously ill, only recovering from relatively minor surgeries. Sleep deprivation was bad then. It got much worse.

Sleep deprivation typically causes irritability and interferes with people's ability to make decisions, remember details, and solve problems (Lamberg, 1996; L. G. Olson & Ambrogetti, 1998). These deficits can lead to deadly mistakes in medical settings. Residents who are sleep-deprived are more likely than others to experience tension, anxiety, and stress (Rose, Manser, & Ware, 2008). In addition to being impatient and short-tempered, they are prone to accidents and oversights. Compared to residents working 16-hour shifts, those who work 24 hours at a stretch are 300% more likely to make errors that result in a patient's death (Lockley et al., 2007). Sleep-deprived residents performing surgery demonstrate markedly poorer psychomotor skills, memory, and attentiveness than others (Kahol et al., 2008). Sleep-deprived caregivers are also at significantly higher risk for accidentally sticking themselves with soiled needles and other sharps and getting in automobile accidents on the way home (Lockley et al., 2007). And one night's sleep is usually not enough to provide full recovery, so a day off doesn't significantly interrupt the exhaustion cycle (Kahol et al.).

*Withdrawal and Resentment*   Confronted by overwhelming demands, it is not surprising that medical students often begin to regard patients as enemies. Phillip Reilly, author of *To Do No Harm* (1987), remembers the extreme exhaustion during his residency that led him to resent the neediness of a comatose patient: "He was an enemy, part of the plot to deprive me of sleep. If he died, I could sleep for another hour. If he lived, I would be up all night" (p. 226). Another resident recalls hoping that a patient would die so that she wouldn't have to update his chart. She ruefully recounts: "But you know what? I had to write a note anyway, and fill out a death certificate, and deal with the morgue, and call the attending and the family. So it didn't really save me any time at all" (quoted by Jauhar, 2008b, pp. 119–120).

Medical professionals sometimes refer to patients in derogatory terms such as *drain circlers* and *gomers*. The first is a reference to patients who are expected to die (go down the drain) soon. The second, an acronym for "get out of my emergency room," generally refers to elderly patients who have little chance of recovering and are seen as wasting valuable space. Jauhar (2008b), jaded by sleep deprivation and the seemingly endless demands of residency, wrote in his diary:

> Nature did not wire into us the desire to take care of our aged. Maybe that's why the contempt, the frustration, with gomers. They are heavy, dead evolutionary weight. They sap our resources. We don't want to take care of them. Baby shit doesn't smell. But gomer shit smells the worst. (p. 90)

During medical school, students' empathy for patients typically decreases, especially among male students who are not specializing in primary care or psychiatry (Newton, Barber, Clardy, Cleveland, & O'Sullivan, 2008). Empathy typically plummets even more during their internships (Rosen, Gimotty, Shea, & Bellini, 2006). Many graduates report that, by the end of their intern year, they are less overwhelmed than before but also less compassionate and less emotionally available. As an intern, Jauhar (2008b) wrote:

> Do doctors care? I don't know. I don't see a lot of caring. Maybe I myself don't care, or care selectively, which is hypocrisy, which I despise. No, I don't see much attention to the psychosocial aspects of medicine. There is lip service, but by and large, no one seems to pay it much mind. Like this morning. Steve had no interest in holding Camille's mother's hand, in asking her why she was crying.…I myself didn't make an effort, not because I was uncomfortable but because there was so much to do. I thought it best to spend my time doing what needed to be done. (p. 90)

Persuaded by the curriculum (and often by mentors) that disease is best understood in physical terms, it becomes acceptable to depersonalize patients. Who would *not* find it more manageable to think in terms of "the kidney transplant in Room 406" than of the kindly woman whose daughter is weeping at her bedside? Focusing on specific, organic concerns is more familiar and less emotionally exhausting than thinking in terms of unique individuals.

Of course, being emotionally aloof is not trust-inspiring for patients. And caregivers often say they enjoy the job less when they feel cold and removed from their patients.

## Effects of Socialization

It is natural to feel somewhat incensed by the traditionally harsh customs of medical school, particularly from an outside perspective. By the standards of many other speech communities, treatment described as "medical student abuse" would be considered unconscionable. Indeed, efforts are under way at some universities to revamp the way things are done. However, the conditions described here are still common.

Whether justified or not, medical school customs endure partly because they serve several functions. First, the high-pressure environment may prepare students for the actual demands of medical practice. Medicine requires great patience, endurance, and emotional control. Students put to the test early may be better prepared to handle immense pressure later.

Second, a clearly established chain of command may help medical teams make decisions and carry them out. Emergencies are handled most efficiently with decisive leadership, and centralized decision making reduces the likelihood that caregivers' efforts will be disorganized and uncoordinated.

Third, the hardships of medical school may strengthen group membership. Shared activities help shape members' attitudes and unite them in common experience. The result is often an enduring sense of camaraderie.

Fourth, medical school may indeed serve as a long **rite of passage**, a challenge that qualifies one for advancement. Medical students may feel an extraordinary sense of accomplishment as they qualify for higher rank by surviving the harsh years as an initiate (P. Conrad, 1988). They may feel more entitled to the privileges of medical practice than they did on entering medical school.

## Medical School Reform

Reform efforts are under way in some schools to broaden the scope of caregiver education. As mentioned, most medical schools now require some training in psychological and social aspects of illness as well as communication skills training. And many are experimenting with courses in management and business, end-of-life care, and ethics as well.

An innovative program at Harvard Medical School requires students to participate in a 3-year course on doctor–patient relationships (Branch et al., 1991). The program is designed to create "humanistic physicians" who appreciate social and psychological aspects of illness and embody ethics, warmth, and sensitivity. The course makes use of small-group discussions to help students explore their own feelings and philosophies and work together to develop their communication skills.

Pediatric residents at the University of California (UC), Davis, do not just train in hospitals and clinics. They also work as advocates in the community, actively partnering with various groups to improve the overall health of children in the community. "Physicians have a greater responsibility to their patients beyond telling them what will keep them healthy," says Richard Pan, a UC physician who developed the program. "We need to be in our patients' communities and neighborhoods working with families" ("Getting Doctors Out," 2002, paragraph 3). The program has won numerous awards, and research shows that physicians tend to maintain their community focus after they transition into licensed medical practice (Paterniti, Pan, Smith, Horan, & West, 2006).

New rules also limit the work hours of physicians-in-training. In 2003, ACGME decreed that interns and residents must work no more than 30 hours at a stretch, average no more than 80 work hours per week, and have at least 1 in 7 days off. Although organizations that break the rules are in danger of losing their accreditation, many of them continue to exceed the work-hour limits. A study published in the *Journal of the American Medical Association* revealed that 83.6% of interns surveyed had worked hours exceeding ACGME guidelines in the previous year. More specifically, 67.4% had worked longer than 30 consecutive hours, 43% had averaged more than 80 hours a week, and 43.7%

were not given the required days off (Landrigan, Barger, Cade, Ayas, & Czeisler, 2006).

Professionals have mixed reactions to reform efforts. Some physicians feel that working around the clock is important because it allows interns to get to know patients and see how their conditions change. They argue that clocking in and out will give residents naive, snapshot images of illnesses and limit the amount they learn as residents. In a study of Mayo Clinic internal medicine specialists, 87% agreed that the new rules are deleterious. Among them, 75% felt that decreased hours reduce relationship building with patients, and 47% say that their own workloads have become heavier since the clinic has reduced residents' hours ("Residents," 2007). By contrast, some professionals applaud reform efforts and even feel they have not gone far enough. Sleep experts argue that 30-hour shifts are still far too long for safety (Mello, 2007). Others point to improved patient outcomes as evidence that the rules work. Since the new rules took effect, teaching hospitals have experienced a small but statistically significant decrease in medication errors, patient discharges to nursing homes, ICU transfers (Horowitz, Kosiborod, Zhenqui, & Krumholz, 2007), and the number of patient deaths (Kanaka & Bhattacharya, 2007).

## Implications

The intense and isolating nature of medical studies reinforces the realities within the system and largely insulates students from people outside it. Medical students may perceive an important distinction between insiders, who have experienced medical school, and outsiders, who have not. Doctors may come to identify with each other more than they identify with their patients.

Several implications may be derived from the medical school experience. First, it implies that admission to the medical arena is not to be granted lightly. Medical schools pride themselves on admitting an elite portion of applicants and, once admitted, testing their endurance in many ways before authenticating them as doctors. Second, the experience suggests that physicians' authority is

unquestionable and that subordinates should comply with it Third, it implies that doctors should be stoic and self-sacrificing.

These assumptions may profoundly affect doctors' communication with others. For instance, applying the hierarchy of medical school to professional encounters, doctors may regard the people around them as subordinates. Thus, doctors may be especially sensitive to questions and comments that seem to challenge their authority. This assumption sometimes leads patients and coworkers to label doctors as arrogant and bossy. It is more likely, however, that doctors are simply acting according to assumptions instilled in medical school.

Nevertheless, people who expect to be treated as peers may take offense at doctors' attitudes. Others may be intimidated into silence. When people always defer to physicians' judgment, there is room for avoidable errors, and heavy responsibility is placed on doctors' shoulders.

Doctors may also push themselves to extremes that hurt them personally and damage their relationships. Based on the arduous demands of medical school and residency, physicians may feel they should work long hours and stifle personal emotions and discomfort. Anything less may seem weak or inappropriate. However, such a schedule can quickly lead to burnout and loss of family and social interaction. With excessive work and minimal opportunities to relax or vent emotions, physicians may be in worse shape than their patients. When patients' suffering is (or seems to be) less severe than the physicians', doctors may conclude that patients are weak and overly demanding.

Of course schools differ, as do people's reactions. Although it may be inauspicious to begin doctors' careers with experiences that deplete them and cause them to resent patient demands, many doctors bounce back and regain at least a portion of their idealism and compassion. Following the grueling year of internship, it's not uncommon for students to rediscover the reasons they went into medicine. Jauhar (2008b)—who was quite candid about the callousness he and others developed as interns—remembers an awakening experience as a resident when he was cajoled into visiting a patient at home. Jauhar realized, when he arrived at the man's house, that he had forgotten his stethoscope, blood pressure cuff, prescription pad, and all the rest. "Without my tools, I couldn't follow my usual procedures, so I just sat at his bedside, stroking his hand. Afterward, in the kitchen, I sat with his wife and had a cup of tea," he remembers (p. 177). On his way home Jauhar reflected on the sense of peace and satisfaction the encounter had given him. And his kindness was not forgotten. Two years later the patient's wife wrote to thank him again and say she would never forget his thoughtfulness. (Jauhar now directs the Heart Failure Program at Long Island Jewish Medical Center.)

## PROFESSIONAL INFLUENCES ON CAREGIVERS

Once they join the ranks of medical professionals, today's caregivers are influenced by a range of factors, including time constraints, competition, and limits on professional autonomy. Overshadowing it all is managed care, which may either aggravate professional tensions or soothe them.

### Time Constraints

Caregivers are often very busy, and expediency may be the only alternative to turning away patients in need. Time is in short supply. Even adding a few minutes to each patient visit soon adds up. Consider that a doctor who spends 15 minutes with each patient can see 32 patients in an 8-hour day. If the doctor adds just 5 minutes to each visit, however, the number of patients drops to 24 per day. In one month, the doctor will be about 172 patients behind. In one year, 2,064 fewer patients can be seen *by that doctor alone.* Consequently, some doctors feel they must get right to the point with patients if they are to see everyone who needs care. Unfortunately, this game plan often backfires because it results in follow-up visits that might have been avoided, poorly developed relationships, misunderstandings, and other time-intensive outcomes. An ideal strategy is to engage in communication that is open and inclusive but doesn't take longer than the average medical exam. We'll talk about that more later in the chapter.

Caregivers who are employed by hospitals and medical centers face time constraints as well, trying to keep up with a myriad of patient needs and unpredictable caseloads. Short-staffing and emergencies sometimes make it necessary to work long hours under stressful conditions.

Time constraints may affect the amount and type of information patients and caregivers share. Pressed for time, caregivers may seem rushed and impatient. Although it is tempting to blame the caregivers for this less-than-hospitable demeanor, researchers have found that caregivers do not like time constraints any more than patients do. Doctors rate themselves more satisfied when they have adequate time to talk to patients (Probst, Greenhouse, & Selassie, 1997). By contrast, a former Mayo Clinic nurse recalls the luxury of taking time with each patient:

> I called it "Disneyland for Nurses" because finally, after 17 years of nursing, I could be the nurse I always wanted to be. The patient really did come first. . . . I could take an hour to do a dressing change carefully after premedicating the patient for pain and know that I would be able to complete the painful procedure without being interrupted. . . . My coworkers would have time to watch my other patient(s) and would willingly do so because that was our culture. (quoted by Berry & Seltman, 2008, pp. 251–252)

Research indicates that physicians worried about time constraints often limit talk to specific physical indicators. Doctors may reason that people have numerous sources of emotional support—friends, family members, clergy, counselors, and others—but physicians are the only ones qualified to diagnose physical conditions and prescribe treatments. Doctors may devote the brief time available to the physical concerns they are uniquely qualified to assess and treat.

Interestingly, although they may consider the biomedical approach a means of saving time, physicians are typically not satisfied with interviews that focus on strictly biological indicators. Physicians in private practice are most likely to like their jobs if they have good relationships with their patients and feel a sense of professional autonomy (Bell, Bringman, Bush, & Phillips, 2006).

On the bright side, discussing emotional concerns may not be as time-consuming as it seems. A range of studies suggests that patients' emotional concerns can often be addressed in a brief amount of time (Branch & Malik, 1993; du Pré, 2002; R. C. Smith & Hoppe, 1991). An extensive study of medical visits revealed that biomedical visits took about 20.5 minutes each, whereas biopsychosocial visits took about 19.3 minutes (Roter et al., 1997). Jeffrey Rudolph (2008) offers the following tips for bonding with patients when time is limited:

- *Start strong.* Shake hands, look the patient in the eye, inspire trust from the beginning.
- *Don't interrupt, and don't multitask.* Give the patient your full attention.
- *Empower patients.* Provide information, web links, follow-up phone calls and other means of encouraging the patient's active involvement during and after the exam.
- *Don't end the visit before you ask if the patient has other questions or concerns.* You're not actually saving time if the patient leaves without knowing what to do next. And even if you make a note to address some of the concerns on the next visit, it's ultimately more efficient to encourage full disclosure than to remain in the dark about what a patient wants and needs.

Now let's look at another frustration for caregivers.

## Loss of Autonomy

Loss of autonomy is an issue with managed care and fiscal reform. **Professional autonomy** means caregivers work independently, making decisions without much supervision. Traditionally, physicians have had considerable autonomy, and other caregivers, such as nurses, pharmacists, and therapists, have had limited input about treatment decisions. With managed care, even doctors are likely to have supervisors, and their decisions are subject to administrative review and financial oversight. Most physicians' are frustrated with managed care. As you may recall from Chapter 2, only 1 in 10 doctors in the United States feels that managed care is providing good care for patients in financial need (Frank et al., 2008).

Specialists are particularly sensitive to the effects of managed care since they must rely on referrals from primary care physicians, but nearly all doctors are affected. Physician Bhupinder Singh traded private practice for hospital work to get away from the red tape. He recalls:

> I'd write a prescription, and then insurance companies would put restrictions on almost every medication. I'd get a call: "Drug not covered. Write a different prescription or get preauthorization." If I ordered an M.R.I., I'd have to explain to a clerk why I wanted to do the test. I felt handcuffed. It was a big, big headache. (quoted by Jauhar, 2008a, p. 5)

Unfortunately hospital work has not been much better. "Thirty percent of my hospital admissions are being denied. There's a 45-day limit on the appeal. You don't bill in time, you lose everything," Singh says. "You're discussing this with a managed-care rep on the phone and you think: 'You're sitting there, I'm sitting here. How do you know anything about this patient?'" (p. 5). Some physicians who share Singh's frustration have resorted to opening "cash only" practices (see Box 4.4).

Caregivers may also feel constrained by economic pressures and government regulations. They must answer not only to their employers, but also to funding agencies and patients who have strong (but often conflicting) interests in medical decisions. (See Box 4.5 for information about the impact of new privacy regulations.)

## PSYCHOLOGICAL INFLUENCES ON CAREGIVERS

Medicine is an emotional minefield, and research suggests that many caregivers are woefully ill prepared for it. As a result, they may act in ways that puzzle

BOX 4.4

# Cash-Only Medical Practices

Considering the hassles and restrictions of managed care, some doctors (most of them general practitioners) are opting out of the reimbursement game all together and opening **cash-only practices**. As the name implies, patients pay upfront when they visit the doctor. Then, if they are insured (and many cash-only patients are), they file for reimbursement themselves. Physician participation in managed care is down from a high of 90.8% in 2001 to 88.5% in 2006—a small, but statistically significant drop that is expected to increase (O'Malley & Reschovsky, 2006).

Cash-only physicians not only avoid the paperwork hassle, but they and their patients get to decide how things will run. For example, an HMO caregiver might be required to see 20 patients per day. A cash-only doctor might see 10 patients per day but spend more time with each of them.

It's not only a matter of convenience, says one doctor, it's a question of doing what's right for the patient. "Third-party payments are set so low that you're forced to run patients through the office like animals every five to 10 minutes," says physician Robert Berry (quoted by Lowes, 2008c, p. 26). "It's unethical to accept contract terms that aren't good for patients."

And the cost to the patient isn't necessarily any greater. Imagine your cash-only physician charges $80 for an hour-long visit and $20 for a 30-minute visit. If your managed care deductible is $30 per visit, you might appreciate the chance to pay less for a brief concern. And for more serious concerns, you might be willing to pay a little more to guarantee you aren't rushed out after 10 minutes.

One reason cash-only doctors can charge less and see fewer patients is because they need fewer staff members to handle the paperwork and financial side of practice. Vern Cherewatenko, MD, who runs the simplecare.com website and support center for cash-only practitioners, estimates that 25% to 50% of the cost of a managed care visit covers administrative tasks and paperwork required by insurance. Take that away and doctors can provide care for less money, with less stress and rush.

Cash-only isn't for every doctor or every patient. Some conditions, like a major accident or serious health concern, are too expensive for this type of care. But in an arena in which people are increasingly frustrated by the cost and obtrusiveness of managed care organizations, it's something to keep your eye on!

or wound others, even as they are themselves reeling under the pressure. Caregivers' thoughts and feelings, although invisible to most patients, help explain why caregivers communicate and cope as they do. In this section we'll discuss how caregivers are affected by emotional maturity, self-doubt, and satisfaction.

## Maturity

Medical schools have been criticized for allowing students little time to develop and mature as individuals. The intense workload can isolate students from the normal activities and emotional development of young adulthood. As a result, say Wayne

Weston and Mack Lipkin, Jr. (1989), many students progress through medical school "in the throes of delayed adolescent turmoil" (p. 46).

Patients look to caregivers not only for technical advice but also for wisdom and understanding. However, young doctors may have less everyday life experience than the patients who turn to them for guidance. As Weston and Lipkin (1989) put it, a physician "may know precise drug treatment but stand empty-handed and mute before the patient who desperately needs counsel and support" (p. 45).

Doctors may avoid emotional matters or offer stiff platitudes (such as "I'm sure it will all be fine").

**BOX 4.5 ETHICAL CONSIDERATIONS**

# Privacy Regulations Incite Controversy

In recent years some people have been outraged to learn that health care providers have sold or carelessly leaked their "confidential" medical information to others. For example, a Florida state worker was able to download the names of people diagnosed with AIDS (Barnard, 2003). Companies, including Eli Lilly pharmaceuticals and CVS Pharmacy, have been charged with selling the names of patients on Prozac and other drugs (D. Ho, 2002; "Medical Records," 2001). The problem has grown since the advent of computer databases that make it easy to transmit medical data that was once stored only in doctors' filing cabinets (Conan, 2002).

New federal regulations went into effect in 2003 to prevent these types of privacy violations. The Health Insurance Portability and Accountability Act, better known as HIPAA, provides patients increased access to their own medical records and regulates who else may see them. The new regulations—which present a number of implications for health communication—have provoked a good deal of controversy.

One area of controversy involves the mandate to inform patients of privacy regulations. HIPAA requires health care providers to give every client a written copy of the organization's privacy policies. As a consumer, you have probably encountered this in the form of *HIPAA Alert* or *Patient Privacy* statements that doctors, pharmacists, health plans, dentists, and others ask you to sign. On the surface, this seems like a positive measure. Patients are informed upfront about the measures being taken to protect their privacy and their right to file a grievance if the rules are not upheld. However, the process is less than perfect.

For one thing, the forms can be lengthy and difficult to understand, especially for people with limited reading skills. Compounding this is the implied or explicit demand that patients sign the forms whether they understand them or not. According to the U.S. Department of Health and Human Services, it is not necessary

for patients to sign this form to receive care or services (Health Privacy Project, 2003). However, based on confusion about HIPAA standards (the act is about 400 pages long) and fear of incurring costly fines for noncompliance, a number of health care providers have refused to treat patients who do not sign the privacy notices.

The most serious complaint about the privacy notices is that they do not give patients a choice about how their medical information will be used. Early on, legislators envisioned the forms as consent letters. Patients could say yes or no to receiving information about the latest drugs or treatment options associated with their medical needs. For example, if you are on a drug commonly used to treat AIDS, you might appreciate receiving updates and promotional information about related drugs. However, you might feel that putting such information in the mail is a violation of your privacy. Says one physician, "When my postman knows what diseases my wife has, that's not appropriate" (Barnard, 2003, paragraph 19). Others worry that if these mailing lists are in circulation, the information will be used to discriminate unfairly against them. One man, who mistakenly receives information meant for people with hepatitis C, wonders:

> What happens now with—my wife and I are going to be refinancing our house, and what if somehow the erroneous information that I have hepatitis C finds its way from an insurance company or a pharmacy, a manufacturer, something like that, into someone's financial database and they say, "Well, jeez, we don't want to lend money to someone who has hepatitis C"? (Conan, 2002, transcript p. 7)

Under HIPAA regulations, health care providers cannot sell their mailing lists to others. However, they can accept money to send information to patients themselves as long as the information is health related. Either way, the information is in the mail. Janlori Goldman, director of the Health Privacy Project, says: "They don't have to tell the customer they're doing it, and they don't have to give the customer the chance to opt out" (quoted by Conan, 2002, transcript p. 6).

Despite HIPAA's shortcomings, it does emphasize providers' legal responsibility to maintain privacy. In 2008, Lawanda Jackson, an administrative specialist who had previously worked for the UCLA Medical Center, was indicted for selling celebrities' medical information to the media. If convicted, Jackson faces a maximum 10-year jail sentence and $250,000 fine ("Former UCLA," 2008). Less obvious breaches of confidentiality are harder to identify and eliminate. Perhaps the most common breaches involve overheard conversations about patient care and leaving patient paperwork (such as registration forms) where others can see it (Brann, 2007). In one study, 81% of patients interviewed expressed concern that their medical information would be inappropriately shared with people in the organization not responsible for their care (Brann & Mattson, 2004).

There isn't room enough to outline all the provisions of HIPAA or to describe the pros and cons of each, but here a few of the mandates.

- Health care clients must be assured of confidential environments.
- Health care clients around the country have the right to see their medical records and suggest changes.
- People who feel their medical privacy has been violated can register a complaint with the U.S. Department of Health and Human Services. Some people feel this regulation should have included the provision for patients to sue for breaches of confidentiality. That right is not guaranteed under HIPAA.
- HIPAA requires that health care providers adopt a standardized set of codes, train staff about privacy

regulations, and appoint a staff member to oversee implementation of HIPAA. The benefits are that medical information will be easier to share and compare and privacy will be a top agenda item. The drawback is that the transition is costly and time intensive. Some medical professionals say the regulations allow even less time for patient care in already short-staffed medical units.

## What Do You Think?

1. Have you been asked to sign HIPAA Alerts? Did you understand the information provided? Did you feel you had to sign?
2. Under what circumstances, if any, would you like to receive health-related information through the mail? Do you feel it is important that people have an opportunity to opt out of such mailing lists?
3. Have you ever felt that you had to discuss confidential medical information within earshot of others (e.g., at a pharmacy counter or during a medical visit)? Do you feel this is a serious problem? If so, what would you do to fix it?
4. Some people feel the private environment regulations are too strict. For example, an orthodontist who previously encouraged patients and families to move throughout the clinic and get to know staff members issued an HIPAA Alert saying, "We must now regretfully restrict all patients and friends to the reception seating areas only." What is your opinion of this?
5. How far do you think the federal government should go to enforce privacy regulations? Do you agree with adding staff members, more paperwork, and oversight committees? Would you suggest other or additional measures?

---

Patients are likely to sense doctors' insincerity and feel their concerns have been brushed aside as unimportant. Seldom do patients realize that doctors may not *know* how to respond, having never experienced or been prepared for the situation at hand.

Caregivers may have emotional hot buttons. When one of these sore spots is touched, the emotional response can surprise the doctor and the patient, although neither may understand it (Novack et al., 1997). For example, a physician may feel resentment, disgust, or sexual attraction for a patient, become overly protective, or wish to have nothing to do with a patient. Novack and coauthors point out that personal biases are unavoidable, but caregivers will have a hard time putting their feelings in perspective if they do not take time to acknowledge and understand them.

On the positive side, a sense of being "in this together" often fosters important friendships in medical school and beyond. During observations and interviews with 14 male first-year medical students, Theodore Zorn and Kimberly Weller Gregory (2005) found that the men did not consider themselves especially close to their medical school friends, but they relied on them for assistance, companionship during long hours of studying and lab work, and diversion from the stress of their studies.

### Self-Doubt

Caregivers sometimes feel like frauds. They may doubt their capacity to cure and understand the people they treat, and they may wonder what gives them the right to make decisions and know others' most intimate secrets. Their confidence may also be shaken by mistakes, a topic we'll cover later in the chapter.

Socialized to be confident and in control, physicians may hide their self-doubt behind a protective gruffness or arrogance (Bonsteel, 1997). The message is "Don't get too close," not because the doctors dislike people but because they are intimidated by their appraisals. Patients are likely to misinterpret the physicians' behavior as cold and distant.

Caregivers' self-doubt may become more of an issue as patients become more knowledgeable and assertive. While it was once assumed that patients could not understand the details of their conditions, today patients may know more than their doctors about particular experimental procedures and the latest research. Primary care providers, particularly, cannot be expected to know offhand the latest details of every medical condition they encounter. Still, they may feel defensive or inadequate when they do not. Later in the chapter we'll learn how knowledge coupling provides physicians

---

### BOX 4.6

## Can You Guess?

1. What is the average salary of a general surgeon in the United States with at least one year of experience?
2. Is the job outlook for physicians expected to improve or decline?
3. In which medical specialties are shortages expected to occur?

*Answers appear at the end of the chapter.*

---

and patients immediate access to up-to-date medical information, which may ease the expectation that physicians know everything.

Physicians may restrict patients' communication because it's difficult to refuse their requests even when the doctor does not agree with them. Tanya Stivers (2002) studied what happened when parents of pediatric patients suggested "candidate diagnoses" rather than asking the doctors' opinions. In most cases (82%), the parents suggested conditions that could be treated with antibiotics, apparently eager to secure prescriptions for them. It often worked. Even when the physicians disagreed with the diagnoses and believed the children's conditions would not be improved with antibiotics, they prescribed antibiotics 62% of the time. Stivers concludes that doctors, like other people, are not immune to interpersonal pressure.

### Satisfaction

Research to date has largely considered caregivers' satisfaction as secondary to patients'. Most people seem to take it for granted that caregivers' satisfaction is either guaranteed or irrelevant. However, unsatisfying communication is linked to stress and burnout and to high employee turnover rates. Physicians who are dissatisfied are two to three times more likely than others to leave the profession (Landon, Reschovsky, Pham, & Blumenthal, 2006). For this reason and others, scholars such as Ashley Duggan (2006) urge researchers to give more attention to caregivers' emotional well-being and its link to communication skills and health outcomes.

Evidence suggests that doctors are usually quite satisfied with medical visits, sometimes more than their patients. Although patient needs are often demanding, patients who are friendly and upfront about their needs can help physicians avoid burnout (Halbesleben, 2006). This may be because 88% to 94% of medical students say they want to be doctors so they can "make a difference" ("Minorities," 2005). Even when patient care is highly challenging, the sense that they are helping others is energizing and rewarding.

Dealing with the nonmedical aspects of medicine is another story, however. Of 2,400 physicians surveyed, only 3% said that they are *not* frustrated by the "business" aspects of being doctors ("Physicians Report," 2008). Their frustrations involve hassles over reimbursement, medial liability issues, being overworked, and feeling overwhelmed by regulations and policies.

Grace Terrell (2007) proposes that physicians may be especially disappointed when things do not go well because they have invested so much in becoming doctors. She writes:

> Doctors have sacrificed. They have suffered. They really have. For a profession built upon delayed gratification it is not fair that, at the end of all the hard work and sacrifice and all that training and achievement, we go up against managed care, Medicare, six-figure student loans and malpractice. (p. 14)

Terrell argues that, since doctors are motivated primarily by the desire to help others, they go to extreme lengths to accomplish that. But, like anyone else, they have an interest in being appreciated and rewarded, and they can become depleted by excessive demands and threats. In the current health care climate, she says, it's no wonder if physicians feel that managed care and malpractice have tipped the balance—reducing the rewarding aspects of the job (helping people) while increasing the negative aspects (oversight, hassle, threats, limitations, and so on).

It's a testament to caregivers' commitment that most stay in the profession even with the intense pressures levied on them. Although they are almost universally frustrated by the hassles, 72% of physicians surveyed said they would choose medicine all over again, knowing what they know now ("Physicians Report," 2008). Pamela McKemie, who supervised the study, said that most doctors surveyed stay in the profession because of "the satisfaction of doing something that matters, the intellectual stimulation of solving clinical challenges, or the thrill of actually implementing medical procedures" ("Physicians Report," last paragraph).

Like patients, caregivers are discouraged by the loss of long-term patient–caregiver relationships. Doctors often feel betrayed or cheated when patients switch doctors. (Ironically, at the same time patients cry that doctors should not make decisions based strictly on costs, patients themselves are now likely to switch doctors based on that very consideration.) Physicians interviewed by Geist and Dreyer (1993) said they were gratified by patients who remained with them even when less expensive medical plans were available.

Nurses are most satisfied when they have a reasonable workload and feel a sense of personal satisfaction. Nurses are also sensitive to issues of autonomy and respect. Nurses are most likely to stay in the profession if they feel that people recognize and honor their efforts and involve them in decision making. Many report feeling dissatisfied because doctors or supervisors do not give their opinions much credence (Tourangeau & Cranley, 2005).

## STRESS AND BURNOUT

Health care is emotionally demanding, as evidenced by high substance abuse and suicide rates among professional caregivers. Stress and burnout threaten to deplete caregivers' energy and reduce their capacity for compassion. In the United States, 300 to 400 physicians a year commit suicide, which is two or three times the average number of students in a medical graduating class (American Foundation for Suicide Prevention [AFSA], 2008; "Struggling in Silence," nd). (See Box 4.7 for related resources.) Suicide and substance abuse are more prevalent among health care professionals than in any other profession, mostly because of the intense emotions, stress, and a high incidence of depression ("Exposure to Stress," 2008). When medical professionals abuse drugs, it may be difficult for coworkers to know what to do. (See Box 4.8 for a true story about one staff member's response to a physician's substance abuse.) Nurses are also prime candidates for burnout, as you will see in this section, which focuses on stress and burnout among health professionals.

**Stress** refers to physical and psychological responses to overwhelming stimuli. Stress is considered a major cause of burnout among caregivers, but other factors (like boredom and feeling unappreciated) also contribute.

**Burnout** is actually a combination of factors. In her 1982 book *Burnout: The Cost of Caring*, Christina Maslach describes burnout as emotional exhaustion, depersonalization, and a reduced sense of personal accomplishment. In Maslach's words, **emotional exhaustion** is the feeling of being "drained and used up" (p. 3). People experiencing emotional exhaustion feel they can no longer summon motivation or compassion. **Depersonalization** is the tendency to treat people in an unfeeling, impersonal way. From this perspective, people may seem contemptible and weak, and the individual experiencing burnout may resent their requests. A **reduced sense of personal accomplishment** involves feeling like a failure. People who feel this way may become depressed, experience low self-esteem, and leave their jobs or avoid certain tasks.

### Causes

There are several common causes of stress among health care employees. Stress is a major cause of burnout, but it is not the only cause.

*Conflict* Stress can result from many factors, including competing and ambiguous demands. Nurses report feeling stressed when they have more tasks than they can complete, when they must work holidays or weekends, when their efforts are frequently interrupted by phone calls and conflicting demands (Gelsema et al., 2006), when physicians behave inappropriately and disruptively (Rosenstein & O'Daniel, 2008), and when they perceive that the organization does not reward and support them (McGowan, 2001). Nurses also report a high degree of stress when they are required to carry out treatment decisions they believe to be inappropriate or harmful to patients (Catlin et al., 2008). These situations place them in a **double bind**, meaning there are negative consequences no matter which option they choose. Employees who must choose between family time and work are in a double bind. Likewise, nurses who believe their actions are hurting patients' health are likely to feel bad, but they may be reprimanded or lose their jobs if they do not carry out orders. (This topic is covered more fully in Chapter 9's discussion of organizational conflict.) By contrast, nurses report less stress when they perceive that coworkers and supervisors are supportive and when they feel that they have some control over their work environments and procedures (Gelsema et al., 2006).

Robert J. Wicks (2008) proposes that our energy and compassion aren't knocked out of us with one

## Blowing the Whistle on an Impaired Physician

As manager of a small community clinic, having to identify an impaired physician was not on my agenda. Clinic operations were going smoothly and patients seemed to like the clinic and the physician, Dr. Havard (not his real name). I knew things about Dr. Havard, such as his turbulent relationship with his ex-wife and his constant financial difficulties. However, he seemed to be a caring and sensitive doctor. Several months into his employment at the clinic, I started noticing strange behavioral changes in Dr. Havard, such as being chronically late for work and his inability to account for missing narcotic samples.

I thought Dr. Havard's actions were suspicious, but did not know they were signs of an impending problem until I received a phone call from a representative of an Internet pharmaceutical company. The woman on the other end of the phone explained to me that large quantities of a prescription narcotic had been ordered for the clinic. I explained to her that the physician does not dispense narcotics on the premises because of the potential of robbery. After several similar phone calls from various companies, I approached Dr. Havard with the information. He said, "It's all a mistake. I'll take care of it."

I knew that he was not going to resolve the situation, and the phone calls became more frequent, demanding payment in excess of $20,000. I notified the clinic administrator, whose office is in a neighboring city. When I originally reported the problem, the administrator told me to "watch and listen." A week later, while working in my office, I received a phone call from a local pharmacist, who explained to me that a clinic patient presented a prescription for the same narcotic with authorization for three

refills from Dr. Havard. She called because she knew it was rare for Dr. Havard to write prescriptions for such a large quantity of narcotics. When I asked for a description of the patient, she described Dr. Havard to a "T." After my initial shock, I called the administrator back and explained the situation. The next day, the administrator confronted Dr. Havard and asked if he had written the prescription. He denied it and said he didn't know who the patient was. I was given the "go-ahead" to treat the prescription as stolen and contact the Sheriff's Department.

Soon after the incident, Dr. Havard was drug tested and suspended from employment because he tested positive for narcotics and could not produce a legitimate prescription. When sheriff's deputies caught up with him, he confessed to writing the prescription for a "relative." He was offered assistance through the state's impaired-practitioners program. The program offers confidential counseling and assistance and the chance to resume practice.

I felt that I was ruining Dr. Havard's career by turning him in. However, I had an ethical and moral obligation to report him to his superiors to protect his patients.

—Denise

### What Do You Think?

1. If you discovered your doctor was abusing narcotics, would it change your opinion of him or her?
2. Do you believe patients should be informed if their doctor is found to have a drug addiction, or should this information be kept confidential? Why?
3. Would you want the doctor to undergo counseling and have a second chance to practice medicine? Why or why not?

---

punch. More likely, they drain slowly, almost unnoticeably. "The causes of burnout are often so quiet and insidious that we fail to notice them until they have caused a great deal of harm," Wicks says (p. 18). He quotes psychiatrist James Gill, who observes

that, "helping people can be extremely hazardous to your physical and mental health" (p. 21).

*Emotions* Intense emotions can cause stress and lead to emotional exhaustion. Although caregivers

**BOX 4.9 COMMUNICATION SKILL BUILDERS**

# Dealing with Difficult Patients

Some patients bring out the best in their caregivers. Others—a small percentage but powerful nonetheless—evoke defensiveness and anger. Transue (2004) recalls the brother of a dying patient in the hospital who brushed her off as "only an intern" and demanded to speak to a "senior doctor" instead. Although Transue remained polite and cool on the outside, her inner sense of defensiveness, compounded by exhaustion and frustration, was exacerbated by the man's contemptuous tone and his demand that she call the doctor on his behalf. He belligerently taunted her: "Are you willing to do it, or aren't you?" And when Transue agreed to call and asked the man for contact information so that the doctor could easily reach him, he exploded with: "Why don't you pay some attention to what's easier for *me* for once?" (pp. 54–55). There's no doubt about it. Some patients, and some families, are difficult.

Experts offer the following tips for communicating effectively with patients who are stressed, tired, and worried, without becoming too frustrated yourself.

- *Treat complaints as opportunities.* Frustrated patients and family members may want or need something they are afraid to ask for outright. Their emotion can be a signpost calling your attention to it. Physician Calvin Martin recalls an aggressive patient who threw things at the staff and yelled at everyone around him. "He knew he was dying, but everyone else was denying it," he says. Once the doctor learned the problem and was honest with the patient, his entire demeanor changed. "He was wonderful after that," Martin recalls (quoted by Magee & D'Antonio, 2003, p. 163). He says, "In medical school they tell you that 75% of the people you are going to see have nothing really wrong with them. That's not true. I think they all have something real, but we are just not finding it" (p. 164).

- *Empower your staff to handle problems before they grow.* Most nonclinical problems start as minor annoyances—a phone call not returned, an appointment mix-up. A quick and thoughtful response (even if the patient doesn't complain out loud) can usually save a great deal of time and stress down the line.

- *Invest in patient relationships.* In *The Field Guide to the Difficult Patient Interview,* Platt and Gordon (2004) propose that "engaging our patients in a partnership with us" and "enlisting them in following our recommendations" are the hallmarks of effective caregiver communication (p. 3). They encourage caregivers to take the time to know patients and establish mutual trust and rapport. "Spending more time early in our patient encounters saves time in the long run," they maintain (p. 3).

- *Show empathy.* Demonstrate through words and nonverbals that you understand what the patient is experiencing. Platt and Gordon (2004) recommend listening attentively, paraphrasing to check your understanding, and asking for clarification until the patient confirms that you understand what he or she is trying to express.

- *Display curiosity.* If a patient hints at a grievance or a concern that he or she is reluctant to share, show a gentle and encouraging interest in hearing more. Platt and Gordon (2004) use the example of a patient who refuses to say how much she smokes. They propose a few responses: "OK, that's fine. But can you tell me why you don't want to tell how much you smoke? That interests me," or "That is really interesting! Of course you don't have to tell me. But I an enormously curious to understand why you don't want to tell me. Can you help me understand that?" (p. 118).

- *Try a little humor.* If the patient shows an inclination toward it, you can sometimes use gentle humor to clear the air. Transue (2004) recalls a hospital patient who did nothing but complain about the food, the service, and the interruptions. She recalls thinking to herself: "I'm pretty sure there's humor under his crabbiness, but I can never quite pin it down" (p. 100). One day the man declared that he wouldn't leave the hospital until the food there improved. Several days later, after checking his lab results and vital signs, Transue was prepared to discharge him, but she asked first, "Has the food gotten any better?" She recalls:

He stares at me for a long moment. Finally he bursts out laughing. "How do you think I'll answer that…Has the food gotten any better. You get out of here—"…I wave and walk away, listening to him laugh" (p. 101)

---

work in an emotionally charged atmosphere, they are expected to remain calm most of the time (Pincus, 1995). It can be difficult to be caring and compassionate yet keep personal emotions in check. (See Box 4.9 for tips on dealing with difficult patients.) Caregivers often develop what Harold Lief and Renée Fox (1963) call **detached concern**, a sense of caring about other people without becoming emotionally involved in the process. Some degree of detachment is useful to keep from feeling overwhelmed. However, the expectation that health professionals will squelch or avoid their own emotions may lead them to become apathetic, cynical, and confused (Novack et al., 1997).

In "Blood, Vomit, and Communication" Krista Hirschmann (2008) describes what she learned following medical interns through several 24-hour hospital shifts. At one point she asked the interns how long it took to become cynical. "A week," said one. "About a day," said another (p. 64). It may sound like an exaggeration, but Hirschmann had much the same experience herself.

Hirschmann (2008) was emotionally affected by the first death she witnessed, that of a 76-year-old man named Sumner. As staff members rushed into the man's room, Hirschmann looked at Sumner stretched out on the bed, "completely naked, except for his black nylon socks," restrained hand and foot as the room became a "jungle of IVs and wires" (p. 67). Watching the drama, she created an imaginary life story for him:

Sumner has a wife, whom he sent daily love letters while they were separated by war; he has three children for whom he played Santa every year until they had children of their own; five grandchildren who now are in college but still receive cards from him containing crisp 20s. (p. 67)

When the medical team was unable to save Sumner and he was pronounced dead, Hirschmann tried to remember his last words but was dismayed to realize they were lost in the confusion.

By contrast, during her second observation, a month later, Hirschmann (2008) was exposed to a patient she dubbed Turkey Woman. The woman was rushed into the ER, near death. Although she had requested DNR (do not resuscitate) status the previous day it was not yet in her paperwork, and the medical team was obligated to try to keep her alive. As Hirschmann watched, the team quickly stripped the woman of clothing so that they could more easily insert needles and catheter, but thick roles of body fat inhibited their efforts. Then the unconscious woman began to vomit up the Thanksgiving dinner she had eaten earlier, filling the air with a thick, unpleasant order, and making it difficult to insert tubes down her throat. Hirschmann, who was weary of dealing all day with nameless "unconscious bodies" and was too tired to imagine their lives outside the hospital, found herself thinking: *"Come on lady, just get it over with, and die"* (p. 69). Later she reflected on her "2-day transformation" from an idealist to a detached observer and her very different emotional response to the two patients.

Hirschmann's honest account forces us all to consider how we would think and behave in similar circumstances. It is tempting to imagine that we would remain as compassionate on day 2 (and year 2 and decade 2) as we were on day 1. But none of us are entirely immune to emotional hot buttons and fatigue.

Ironically, the very qualities that draw people to careers in health care make them especially prone to burnout. The **empathic communication model of burnout** proposed by Katherine Miller and associates suggests that health care is appealing to people who are concerned about others and are able to imagine others' joy and pain (K. I. Miller, Birkholt, Scott, & Stage, 1995; K. I. Miller, Stiff, & Ellis, 1988). These people are typically responsive communicators (able to communicate well with people in distress), but they may easily feel overwhelmed by constant exposure to emotional situations. Regrettably, caregivers typically receive little instruction on how to care for themselves or manage their own stress and burnout.

*Communication Deficits*  Communication plays a significant role in stress and burnout. Caregivers are affected by the amount of information they receive, their confidence as communicators, and how involved they are in decision making. Too much information can make people feel overwhelmed. Too little information can make them worried and uncertain (Maslach, 1982).

Other evidence suggests that people are more susceptible to burnout if they do not feel they are skillful communicators. A good deal of research (e.g., Ramirez et al., 1996) suggests that physicians who feel their communication skills are below par are more likely than others to treat people in impersonal ways and to perceive a low sense of personal accomplishment. But other data paints a more complex picture of the issue. When Ratanawongsa and colleagues (2008) studied actual patient–caregiver interactions, they found that physician communication practices were not correlated with the doctors'

self-reported burnout levels. The difference may be one of confidence and perception. That is, physicians who *perceive* themselves to have communication deficits are more likely to burn out than others, even if their actual communication behaviors look the same to observers.

*Workload*  An excessive workload or a highly monotonous one can cause stress. Because overnight hospital stays are now limited to people who are very sick or badly hurt, nurses and residents may be continually involved in difficult, intense situations. On the other end of the spectrum, some caregivers must cope with monotonous, repetitive tasks. Laura Ellingson (2007) studied staff members at a dialysis care center, where they are required to perform the same unpleasant routines over and over. Many of the caregivers said they break the monotony by focusing on the unique qualities of each patient. As one put it: "Our job is repetitious, but the patients are not. Yeah, they all have the same illness, they have kidney failure, but each person is different, so that's what makes it different every day" (p. 109).

The sense of being constantly responsible for people's lives can be emotionally draining in itself. Perri Klass (the same Klass whose 1987 memoirs of medical school are cited earlier in this chapter) continues to use her remarkable writing talent to describe the dilemmas she faces as a physician today. In a 2008 article called "The Moral of the Story," Klass describes a fairly routine ER visit by a mother with a 20-month-old who was feverish, vomiting, cranky, and lethargic. Klass and her colleagues diagnosed an ear infection and were ready to send the child home when the worried mother worked her way up to an anxious disclosure. She said the child had fallen down some stairs the night before. "So we had a problem," Klass says (p. 2313). Some of the symptoms attributed to the ear infection (vomiting, lethargy) could be from head trauma. But the child showed no bumps or bruises, and the symptoms of head trauma do not usually wait 24 hours to present. Eventually Klass sent the mother home with instructions to watch for other signs of head injury and call immediately if they surfaced. Klass wrote the mother's phone number on a scrap of paper towel and took it home with her and then called later in the evening to check on the boy. The child was fine. It was a rather routine and benign condition after all. But Klass kept returning to the incident in her mind:

> Why did this boy get me so worried? Maybe precisely because the head trauma wasn't the reason for the visit.... I hadn't asked the right question, I had been pursuing the wrong story. I had almost missed this history altogether—didn't that make it more likely that I'd missed something serious? Wouldn't that turn out to be the "teaching point" if you were telling this story to medical students? Listen properly, and don't overtake the patient's narrative with your own, or you'll miss the most important information. (p. 2313)

Klass mentally reviewed other cases she had heard of in which people experienced a bump on the head, seemed fine, and then collapsed and died from undetected internal bleeding. Klass even looked up a preceptor who had told her such a story 20 years earlier, and they shared a still-profound sense of grief over a 10-year-old patient the preceptor lost decades ago. "You can't let all the what-ifs terrorize you," Klass concluded. Yet she also vowed to continue honoring the haunting stories that "tug on her sleeve" in unexpected moments and remind her "to watch out, to think again, or at least to scribble a cell-phone number on a piece of paper towel and call later just to be sure that everything's truly okay" (p. 2313).

Klass's story is a powerful reminder of the immense, nearly crushing responsibility that health care professionals bear on a regular basis. In the clamor for doctors and others to be more patient-centered, it's worth pausing to spare some compassion for the professionals themselves.

**Other Factors** Stress does not affect everyone in the same way, nor does it always lead to burnout. People are able to tolerate different levels of stress before they experience burnout (Fagin et al., 1996; Ray, 1983). Studies show that stress is more bearable if people feel they are appreciated and are performing important services. A British study (Ramirez et al., 1996) found that surgeons had higher stress levels than most doctors. But because surgeons were highly satisfied and publicly respected, they were less likely to experience burnout than other professionals, such as radiologists. Radiologists were the least stressed but also the least satisfied of those surveyed. They experienced the highest burnout rate, apparently because they felt isolated and unappreciated.

### Effects

Stress and burnout affect people physically and emotionally, causing sleeplessness, fatigue, weight changes, digestive disorders, headaches, and more (Hanlon, 1996). People experiencing burnout are also are at elevated risk for heart disease and other stress-related conditions (Ornish et al., 1998). Psychological symptoms include reduced self-esteem, depression, defensiveness, irritability, and a tendency toward accidents, anger, and emotional outbursts (Hanlon, 1996). Burnout also makes it more likely that employees will be apathetic, miss work, and quit their jobs (Ellis & Miller, 1993; K. I. Miller, Stiff, & Ellis, 1988). What's more, there is exploratory evidence linking physician burnout with patient outcomes. In one study, patients of high-burnout physicians were less satisfied than other patients. They tended to recover more slowly and to leave the hospital later than patients of physicians who were not burnt out (Halbesleben & Rathert, 2008), perhaps because the emotionally exhausted physicians were less attentive to details and because their relationships with patients were not as open and trusting as they could have been.

**Healthy Strategies** Caring for patients all day can be draining. But patients and friends can offer remarkable insights about life and happiness as well. Many analysts suggest that gratifying patient–caregiver relationships are the best antidote for burnout. "Being a doctor is stressful," attests George Hanna. "It can be exhausting. But don't let anyone tell you it's not rewarding....It's worth it to put in the time and to let yourself care. It's better for the patients, but in the end, it's a lot better for you, too" (quoted by Magee & D'Antonio, 2003, pp. 53–54).

With a similar conviction, Wicks (2008) remembers visiting a dying friend in the hospital who asked him about the "good things" he had been doing.

> As I started to launch into an obsessive (naturally well-organized) list of my recent academic and professional accomplishments, he interrupted me by saying, "No, not that stuff. I mean what really good things have you done? When have you gone fishing last? What museums have you visited lately? What good movies have you seen in the past month?" (Wicks, p. 45)

Wicks reflects that, in dying, his friend understood life better than he—in the "arrogance of good health"—did. Here are a few of Wicks' suggestions for avoiding burnout, from his book *The Resilient Clinician.*

- *Hold daily debriefings with yourself.* Honestly assess your own emotions and hot buttons. Reflect on such questions as: "What made me sad? Overwhelmed me? Sexually aroused me? Made me extremely happy or even confused me?" (p. 31).
- *Resist the urge to put off the "good stuff."* Wicks recommends making time for quiet walks, meditation, laughter, listening to enjoyable music, having friends over for dinner, daydreaming, being in nature, making love, and journaling.
- *Be mindful about what makes you happy.* Frequently consider your answers to the following questions: What is my heart's desire? What is truly important to me? How do I most want to live?
- *Design your own time pie.* Too often, our time is gobbled up by outside demands so that nothing seems left. Wicks borrows the notion of a time pie from Alice Domar and Henry Dreher's (2000) book *Self-Nurture.* He challenges us to visualize and actualize our ideal time pie. What size slice would you give to serving others, learning new things,

spending time alone, being creative, relaxing with family, and so on?

- *Seek the company of people whose presence replenishes you.* A good friend who listens without judgment or helps you find the humor in a tense situation can ward off burnout. Transue (2004) remembers a playful conversation with a fellow intern who asked her, "Do you really want to be a doctor for the rest of your life?" Laughing, Transue responded, "I don't even want to be a doctor for the rest of the week, especially" (p. 75).

## MEDICAL MISTAKES

### "Doctor Amputates Wrong Leg"

The headlines foretold a shocking story. A Tampa surgeon, Rolando Sanchez, had mistakenly removed Willie King's left leg rather than his right one. It's easy to imagine the anguish of a patient with one good leg and one bad leg, awakening to realize the good leg is gone. "Now he'll be without any legs at all," mourned the patient's brother ("Florida Hospital," 1995, paragraph 4).

### Why Mistakes Happen

The Willie King case is horrifying. But the public didn't hear the whole story. In his book *Medical Errors and Medical Narcissism,* clinical ethicist John Banja (2005) relates the behind-the-scenes facts of the case. First, King did not have one good leg and one bad leg. He suffered from diabetes and related vascular diseases to such an extent that open sores on both legs had developed gangrene, his skin was cold to the touch, and it was nearly impossible to detect a pulse in either leg. The left leg (which was mistakenly amputated) was actually worse than the right, and King was aware that he would lose both legs before long. He chose to have the right leg amputated first because it was the more painful of the two. So it wasn't an easy choice between good leg and bad leg. But a cascade of communication errors contributed to the mistake as well.

Someone dropped the ball. Who? There's no easy answer, says Banja (2005). The public might imagine a distracted, careless, or bumbling surgeon. However, Dr. Sanchez was anything but. He was "at the height of a sterling medical career" (Banja, p. 9), having served as chief resident among his colleagues at New York University School of Medicine and professor at Albert Einstein College of Medicine before returning to practice in his native Tampa. The mistake ended with him, but it began much earlier.

Because of a miscommunication between Dr. Sanchez's office staff and the surgery department at the hospital, the surgical staff incorrectly listed the procedure as a left-leg amputation. A hospital nurse detected the error and told another nurse about it. That nurse put a surgery-schedule correction notice on a clipboard, which she gave to another nurse. Each nurse began a sequence of remedial events. But the sequence was somehow interrupted. The correction never made it to the official surgical log or to the blackboard in the surgery unit. The next day, a surgical technician consulted the blackboard, saw "left leg amputation," and prepped King's left leg.

Yet another correction opportunity arose just prior to surgery, when King told a nurse that his right leg was to be amputated. She noted this on his record but his left leg remained prepped. When the surgeon entered the room, King's body was draped, except for the left leg, which was braced and ready for the operation. Sanchez confirmed, by looking at the blackboard, that this was the intended leg, and he was nearly done with the surgery before the medical team realized the error.

It is easy to see, in retrospect, that the mistake might not have happened if people had communicated more clearly with each other or if the surgical team had consulted King's consent form (which correctly indicated his right leg) rather than relying on the blackboard or surgery schedule. But at the time, people were following standard procedure, and the error occurred because of system and communication breakdowns that were beyond any one person's control (Banja, 2005).

Banja (2005) points out the systemic nature of this mistake and others like it. "Well-trained, well-motivated people make errors all the time" he says (p. 11). Medical mistakes are often the result of ineffective communication—sloppy handwriting, forgotten or delayed instructions, busy shift changes in which there is not time to talk about everything in a patient's chart, and so on. Small omissions and misunderstandings can quickly lead to critical breakdowns.

In 2007, another high-profile case hit the news when three newborns at Cedars Sinai Medical Center in Los Angeles (two of them twins born to movie star Dennis Quaid and his wife, Kimberly) were mistakenly given 10,000 units of the blood thinner Heparin rather than the 10 units they were supposed to have. The error occurred because a technician mistakenly put prepackaged vials containing adult dosages in the infant nursery cabinet. Because the packaging was similar to that of infant dosages, a nurse administering the drug to newborns didn't notice the discrepancy. The California Department of Health fined the hospital $25,000 for the mistake, and the Quaids sued the drug manufacturer for negligence in packaging. (Fortunately, the babies recovered.)

## What Happens After a Mistake?

People who are hurt by medical mistakes often say they just want an apology, to feel that they are getting the full story, and reassurance that the organization is taking steps to avoid similar errors in the future. It can be agonizing not to know exactly what caused a loved one's death or suffering. Dale Ann Micalizzi (2008) recalls her own bewildered grief when her 11-year-old son died following a relatively minor surgery to treat an infected cut on his ankle. Micalizzi says the family didn't want to sue. She works for an HMO herself and understands the intricacies of medical settings. But otherwise, no one would tell them what happened. "We were owed the truth," she says. "Money wasn't an issue for us" (paragraph 12). Micalizzi describes sitting in a courtroom 3 years later, seeing the defense team consult a 6-inch-thick binder containing her son's medical records and reports from the hospital investigation. "This was information that I had begged to see for such a long time and have still never seen," she says. "In the intervening time I had searched for the truth, only to hit my head against walls of silence" (paragraph 8).

Errors can happen in any organization, in or out of health care. But medical mistakes are particularly hard to handle because the stakes are so high and because caregivers are not expected to commit errors. When doctors' mistakes are brought to light, they may suffer more than most professionals with feelings of guilt and inadequacy, recriminations from others, and legal action. Even if others are involved in medical mistakes, it is typically physicians who are sued. And they may feel personally responsible, even when events were out of their control.

On the one hand, it is hard for doctors to deal with guilt and self-blame in isolation. Ethical guidelines and a sense of fair play encourage them to make full disclosure to patients and their loved ones, apologize, and take corrective action. Likewise, hospitals' contracts with insurers typically stipulate that the hospital will promptly report medical errors when they occur. However, professionals may be discouraged from admitting mistakes by their own sense of distress, by fears about their reputation, by ego needs that make them loathe to admit fallibility, and by reluctance either to blame others or to accept blame for what is often a systemic chain of events involving numerous people (Banja, 2005).

Of 39 physicians who described medical mistakes in Joyce Allman's (1998) study, the doctors' most common emotional reactions were remorse and anger. Several said they considered giving up medicine in the wake of a mistake. Most of the doctors had disclosed the mistake to another physicians, but two had told no one at all, afraid their peers would think less of them and/or they would be sued.

Mistakes do happen. In a survey of 53 family physicians, the doctors recalled an average of 10.7 significant mistakes each, and the average number of deaths from their mistakes was 1.2 per physician (Ely et al., 1995). Several doctors experienced grief over their mistakes, even when the results were not serious. One remembered making a serious mistake because he was ashamed to ask for help: "I think in medical school and often through your training programs is the time when you're most made to feel that asking and calling on people for help is an error" (Ely et al., paragraph 42).

Banja (2005) proposes that physicians may rationalize not saying anything because they believe no permanent harm was done, the error probably didn't change the outcome (e.g., "The patient would have died anyway"), knowing about the mistake would only make the family feel worse, or the mistake wasn't anyone's fault, just something that happened.

Added to people's natural reluctance to admit mistakes are more tangible considerations, such as "Who will be held responsible?" and "Who will pay?" Malpractice insurance policies often include a clause that revokes coverage if the physician admits culpability (Banja, 2005, p. 22). Thus, although patients yearn for an apology and explanation and physicians may desire to give them, physicians may realize that if they own up to mistakes, they are on their own if lawsuits ensue.

The issue is not only who will pay for a malpractice judgment. It's also who will pay for remedial care. For example, if a hospital stay is extended or a patient is transferred to an intensive care unit because of a medical error, who pays for the extra care? In recent years, many insurance companies have declared they will not pay costs associated with what they call *never events*. **Never events** are loosely defined as clear, preventable errors with serious consequences. "Think wrong-side surgery," says Dennis Murray (2007, p. 18). The idea is that hospitals with a strong financial incentive to avoid never events will be even more diligent about preventing them, identifying their root causes if they do occur, and avoiding future tragedies.

But the issue isn't black and white. A gray zone surrounds less obvious avoidable outcomes such as infections. If a patient contracts an infection in the hospital, was the staff negligent? In many cases, it's hard to say what constitutes negligence versus a reasonable (but imperfect) standard of care. David Burda (2008) worries that insurers will become so stringent that medical professionals will live in fear of trying new procedures. Even if the standard options are not working, professionals may feel they cannot step out of bounds, for fear of being either sued or refused payment. And Burda warns that caregivers terrified of making mistakes won't learn very much, and they will probably order so many precautionary tests that precious medical resources will be squandered. (Already doctors are caught between the competing agendas of saving money and covering their bases.)

Medical mistakes (and perceived mistakes) aren't only expensive. They can be demoralizing and humiliating. Although many new residents consider that doctors are likely to be sued at least once (Noland & Walter, 2006), it can be devastating when it happens. Family physician Steven Erickson (2008) remembers being sued over a difficult birth that resulted in the baby's having brain damage. In the courtroom, he weathered aggressive questioning by the plaintiff's attorney, all the while worrying that his colleagues, family, and friends would think less of him and doubt his judgment. Erickson won the case, but embarrassment and fear of future lawsuits shadowed him for a year, until he met a new patient, Roger. Roger had just moved to town and he and his wife had chosen Erickson to be their doctor based on their son's recommendation. A year earlier, their son was on the jury that heard the malpractice case against Erickson. Roger said that, as a farmer, his son had explained to fellow jurors that births do not always go perfectly even when the doctor is honest, competent, and doing his or her best. Writes Erickson:

> I thanked him for his candor and finished up the visit, all the while fighting to maintain my composure. But as I walked back to my office, my eyes welled up and I was crying. After all the embarrassment and self-doubt my malpractice case had engendered in me, there was a juror who not only believed my defense, but trusted me enough to refer his elderly father and mother to me. (p. 33).

Erickson's words remind us that—while we should guard citizens' right to reasonable legal recourse if they have been badly treated—lawsuits have many costs, emotional and financial. Very often, patients wish to avoid lawsuits just as much as doctors do, but a variety of human and systemic restraints may stand between them. When it comes down to it, the factors that lead to mistakes—and the factors that determine what will happen afterward if mistakes are made—involve mostly one thing: communication. If by communicating more effectively we can save lives and prevent some of the anguish that bereaved families and guilt-ridden professionals feel, surely it is worth the effort.

## Communication Skill Builders: Managing Medical Mistakes

Following are some tips from the experts on how to avoid misunderstandings, disappointments, and lawsuits.

### From the Beginning

- *Establish trust.* Invest in open and trusting relationships with patients from the very beginning. Be sincere, polite, friendly, and engaging. Patients are less likely to sue doctors they like and trust (Boodman, 1997), and it is easier to share decisions and to admit mistakes with people one knows and trusts.
- *Invite feedback.* Patients who play an active role in deciding on treatment options are more likely to consider them worthwhile, even if things don't work out perfectly.
- *Respond to complaints and requests as quickly as possible.* Patients who perceive that you don't care or aren't paying attention are likely to assume you have neglected other aspects of their care. When you are unavoidably delayed, apologize, explain why, and express your sincere concern.
- *Show that you care.* Don't assume that patients know this. Be explicit, as in "It

sounds to me like your number one goal is to be you pain free. I don't know if we can eliminate 100% of your pain. But I think, if we work together, we can do a lot. It would make me happy to see you smiling and walking again."

- *Create realistic expectations.* Brushing aside patients' concerns, as in saying "There's nothing to worry about," may set them up to be disappointed and even to file lawsuits, down the line. Says attorney S. Allan Adelman (2008): "You can't always prevent undesirable outcomes, but you can help create realistic expectations" (p. 14). He recommends taking the time to build relationships and openly discuss what outcomes—good and bad—might result from treatment options.

- *Put it in writing.* "Document, ad nauseam," recommends Ralph Caldroney (2008), a family physician who has never been sued in 30 years of practice. He reminds doctors that judges and juries consider that "if it isn't written down, it wasn't done" (paragraph 5). And a quick note such as "chest pain; plain stress test ASAP" won't suffice, Caldroney says. A better, more specific alternative is: "I doubt it's ischemic, but in light of the multiple cardiac risk factors, we'll proceed with a stress test ASAP; in the interim, if the patient's symptoms intensify and/or he develops symptoms at rest, we're to be notified immediately" (paragraph 5).

- *Don't be shy about giving referrals.* If another doctor can help or the patient wants a second opinion, be supportive. Don't cast yourself as the roadblock that kept the patient from exploring all avenues (Caldroney, 2008).

- *Don't forget the family.* Keep in mind that family members often have opinions and fears of their own. Invite their input, and nurture those relationships as much as possible.

- *Own up to small mistakes.* Showing that you have nothing to hide can engender trust.

When my father was in the hospital following a stroke, we arrived one day to find bruises on his arms. We didn't suspect it was anything serious until the nurses reacted evasively when we asked them about it. I still think it was probably a small matter, and a brief explanation would have put it to rest. Dad was unsteady. Probably, he nearly fell over, and they caught him. But by not admitting that, the staff put many family members on edge. They became hypervigilant, almost expecting something worse to happen. They have never returned to that hospital.

*If An Error Does Occur* Banja and Geri Amori (2005, p. 178) recommend the following five-step guide to telling a patient or his or her loved ones about a medical mistake:

1. Rehearse how you will disclose the information.
2. Deliver it as simply, truthfully, and economically as possible.
3. Stop talking.
4. Assess how the news is being received.
5. Respond empathically.

Banja and Amori recommend using the word *error* or *mistake* rather than blurring the issue with a term such as *unintended outcome* or *unexpected occurrence*. They also coach health professionals to tell the people affected: (1) when and where the error occurred, (2) what harm resulted, (3) what actions have been taken to offset the harm, (4) actions being taken to prevent future errors, (5) who will be caring for the patient and how, (6) a description of systemic factors that contributed to the error, (7) the costs of responding to the error and how they will be handled, and (8) information about counseling and support resources. They also recommend that the speaker "apologize profusely" and mean it (p. 185).

Finally, don't let doubt and remorse cripple your confidence. It is easy to obsess about what might have happened—if only you had stopped by one more time, ordered one more test, put a request in writing rather than called it in, and so on. These are not necessarily errors, just limitations in the amount a person can do.

Now we switch to a subject with the potential for easing some of the pressure on health care professionals.

## COMMUNICATION TECHNOLOGY: KNOWLEDGE COUPLING

By now, many people are getting used to an additional presence in the patient–caregiver relationship—a computer. **Knowledge coupling** is a form of medical informatics in which patient information is entered into a computerized data bank, where it is matched (coupled) with extensive information about diagnoses, treatment options, the latest research, and more (Weaver, 2003).

Here is how knowledge coupling works. When someone makes a doctor's appointment, the computer generates an extensive list of questions relevant to the patient's health concerns. The lengthier questionnaires include hundreds of items covering much more information than a patient could convey during a regular medical visit (Weaver, 2003). The patient fills out the questionnaire and submits it prior to the medical visit. The medical staff enters the information into the computer database and reviews the result—a descriptive report that suggests what additional questions to ask, what physical factors to investigate, what risk factors, disease, or illnesses seem to be indicated, and possible therapies to help the patient.

The process will not make doctors or medical visits obsolete. With knowledge coupling—instead of spending a majority of the medical visit collecting health information—patients and caregivers can use their time together to "interpret, discuss, and evaluate" the results suggested by the computer (Weaver, 2003, p. 63). In other words, the computer finds and presents relevant information, but the decisions are still left up to the people involved. Their job is to "weigh the pros and cons associated with various options; and to agree to a plan to address the problem" (Weaver, p. 63). Information and decisions from the medical exam are entered

into the computer, and patients leave with a printout of "office notes" describing the information and decisions reached.

Although some people are put off by the use of computers in patient care, a good deal of evidence suggests that the majority of patients respond favorably. They like the thoroughness of the questionnaires, which often ask for information they might not have supplied during a doctor's visit. "They help me think that things aren't being missed," reported one respondent (Weaver, 2003, p. 66). Patients also report greater confidence with diagnoses and treatment recommendations, and they appreciate leaving medical exams with a written record they can study and share with others.

Some patients feel it is distracting if the computer is actually in the examination room. They prefer that the doctor not type during the medical visit. But most patients feel that the computer, by doing its job, frees them up to spend more time being "heard and understood" by their doctors (Weaver, 2003, p. 74).

## SUMMARY

People dissatisfied with health communication may assume that caregivers do not know how or do not care to communicate well. However, it is probably much closer to the mark to say that caregivers are sometimes overwhelmed, unsure, exhausted, or oriented to different goals than their patients.

Medical school serves as a powerful socializing agent, preparing students to accept the immense privileges and responsibilities of medical practice. As students become professionals, they typically adopt the communication styles, logic, and attitudes of their mentors. In many ways they begin to think and talk like the professionals they model. This can have positive and negative consequences for communication. Guidelines established in 1999 that include communication as one of six core competencies in medicine are changing the way that medical schools operate.

Medical school often deprives students of family, personal, and social time. Shielded from life experience of this sort, physicians may have a difficult time understanding their patients or reacting to them with patience and wisdom. The extraordinary demands placed on medical students and residents encourage them to see patients as weak and contemptible. Overall, caregiver-education programs are considered more successful at instilling technical competence than at preparing caregivers to deal with the diverse emotions and personalities they will encounter. The academic emphasis on physical matters, for instance, often persuades students to think of patients as mere bodies to be fixed. This may reduce the emotional burden on caregivers, but it may be very unsatisfying for patients and caregivers. Medical school reform efforts that focus on integrated knowledge, communication skills training, and clinical experience in addition to science may help change that.

The way caregivers communicate is, in part, a reflection of professional pressures. Patients may be quick to assume that caregivers do not want to spend time with them, when caregivers may have little say in the matter themselves. Indeed, time constraints seem to bother doctors as well as patients. A loss of professional autonomy is another factor. Doctors accustomed to making their own decisions may be required to follow new guidelines, cut spending, and justify their actions. The added scrutiny may add to job stress. Sometimes a gruff demeanor hides a caregiver's feelings of burnout, uncertainty, and self-doubt.

In short, caregivers find themselves managing a host of demands that are often at odds with each other. They are expected to be quick but thorough, strong but emotionally accessible, always available but never tired, and honest but infallible. Understanding these conflicting demands may help people understand why caregivers communicate as they do. Considering the pressures they face, it is no wonder caregivers experience higher-than-average rates of suicide and substance abuse. It is vital that we identify healthy solutions.

To some degree, medical mistakes are inevitable. But effective communication can help minimize their occurrence. A great deal of evidence suggests that doctors are least likely to be sued if they build strong and trusting relationships with patients, take time to discuss treatment options and consequences carefully, and thoroughly describe their decision processes in writing. When mistakes do occur, disclosing them compassionately and fully can actually prevent lawsuits, provide comfort to those affected, and relieve some of the guilt that caregivers feel.

Knowledge coupling makes it possible to collect extensive information about a patient and couple it with the latest medical data. This may relieve caregivers of the pressure to know everything there is to know about medicine. It remains to be seen how widespread knowledge coupling will become and whether this will free patients and caregivers to engage in better-informed partnership behaviors.

As stressful as it is, medicine can also be richly rewarding, and most caregivers consider it immensely gratifying to help patients. Doctors' satisfaction hinges largely on the amount of time they have, patients' input, and a sense of accomplishment. Nurses' satisfaction is linked with rewarding patient contact and the sense that their ideas are valued by others.

In the next chapter, we'll look at health communication through the eyes of patients. As you explore health care from another perspective, remember what you know about caregivers. The richest insights come from understanding several angles at once.

## KEY TERMS

socialization
Voice of Medicine
speech community
rote learning
case presentations
problem-based learning (PBL)
scut work
rite of passage
cash-only practices
professional autonomy

stress
burnout
emotional exhaustion
depersonalization
reduced sense of personal accomplishment
double bind
detached concern
empathic communication model of burnout
never events
knowledge coupling

## DISCUSSION QUESTIONS

1. How is a speech community different than a geographical community?
2. Compare the communication patterns of students and physicians in Lingard et al's (2003) study. In what ways did the students become socialized to think and communicate as doctors? In your opinion, in what ways are these changes positive? In what ways are they negative?
3. How is science taught in traditional medical school curricula? How does rote learning differ from problem-based learning? Would you rather have a doctor who learned via rote or PBL?
4. In what ways is medical practice a science? An art?
5. What are the implications of ACGME's six competencies for postgraduate medical education? Do you feel the six competencies adequately summarize what makes a good doctor? Why or why not?
6. How does sleep deprivation typically affect people? On the whole, do you think it is a good idea or a bad one to limit the work hours of medical residents? Why?
7. What are four main effects of medical school socialization?
8. How are some medical schools reforming their curricula?
9. What are some implications of the way physicians are socialized? Do you see evidence of these in the doctors you know?
10. How might time constraints affect patient–caregiver communication? How do you respond to some physicians' argument that they must limit patient's input so they can keep exams within a particular time limit? How can patients help with this?
11. What are some tips for bonding with patients when time is limited? Which of these do you consider most important? Why?
12. Would consider seeing a primary care doctor in a cash-only practice? Why or why not?
13. What are some of the "business" aspects of medicine that frustrate doctors and contribute to burnout?
14. Describe the provisions of the Health Insurance Portability and Accountability Act (HIPAA). What are the implications for health communication?
15. What are emotional hot buttons, and how might they influence patient–caregiver communication?
16. What factors are linked to caregiver satisfaction?
17. What factors contribute to stress and burnout among caregivers?
18. Does high stress always lead to burnout? Why or why not?
19. What are the effects of stress and burnout among caregivers?
20. What are some communication techniques for dealing with difficult patients?
21. What is your reaction to residents' admission that they sometimes yearn for a dying patient to go ahead and die so that they can finally get some rest? Can you imagine feeling a similar way under the same sorts of pressures?
22. In the case of Willie King, who do you believe should be held responsible for amputating the wrong leg? Why? Who, if anyone, should be sued? Who should pay the extra medical bills?
23. Who do you think should be held responsible in the Cedars Sinai case? Why?
24. Many people hurt by medical errors say they just want an apology, the full story, and assurance that future errors will be prevented. If a family

member of yours nearly died from a medical error, do you think these factors would influence your desire to sue for malpractice? Why or why not? What other factors might influence how you felt?

25. What do you say to doctors who are devastated by a mistake and want to apologize yet are afraid that doing so will invalidate their malpractice coverage and possibly destroy their careers?

26. How does knowledge coupling work? In what ways is knowledge coupling appealing to you? In what ways is it unappealing? What are the implications for health communication?

## ANSWERS TO *CAN YOU GUESS?*

1. General surgeons typically earn about $282,500 a year in the United States ("Physicians and Surgeons," 2008). On average, medicine is the highest-paying occupation in the country.

2. Careers in medicine and surgery are expected to grow faster than the national average, at a growth rate of about 14% ("Physicians and Surgeons," 2008).

3. Shortages are expected in general and family practice, internal medicine, and obstetrics/gynecology, particularly in rural areas of the country ("Physicians and Surgeons," 2008).

# CHAPTER
# 5

# Patient Perspective

*I remember, as a child, the distinct smell of the doctor's office. It is different than any other odor, and it leaves a lasting impression. The smell of rubbing alcohol, the smell of medicines, and the smell of antibacterial soap on the doctor's hands. As a child, you don't know what to make of it.*

These musings by a college student evoke vivid images of patienthood. Whatever else people may remember of childhood, most will never forget the sensory alert of waiting anxiously to be seen by a doctor.

Being a patient can be a frightening experience, even as an adult. Uncertainty is guaranteed, and pain is a strong possibility. At the same time, though, there is the promise of relief, a cure, or a reassuring health assessment. (See Box 5.1 for a true story about one patient's experience managing uncertainty.)

In this chapter we look at health care situations through patients' eyes. We'll investigate the socialization process that helps patients learn how to behave appropriately, what patients like and dislike about caregivers, and what motivates people to follow (and, just as often, to ignore) medical advice. The chapter concludes with a discussion of narratives, illness, and personal identity.

## PATIENT SOCIALIZATION

Being a patient often means suspending the rules of everyday interaction. In medicine, the touch and physical exposure usually reserved for intimate relationships occurs under bright lights in the company of strangers. The contrast can be challenging for both patients and caregivers. Recalling her early experiences as a doctor, Transue (2004) remembers a moment when it dawned on her that touching a patient had become something very different than it used to be. As she administered CPR compressions to a hospital patient in distress, she struggled to compare it to other forms of touch:

> I think, irrationally, of lovers whose skin I have delighted in, clasped beneath my fingers, massaged, caressed. What framework can I find to encompass both these concepts, the thrilling touch of beloved flesh, and this strange doughy substance beneath my hands? What is skin, what are bodies?—these fragile, mortal shells that house us, all so much the same. (p. 45)

In one sense, it may be comforting for patients to realize that most caregivers learn early on to separate intimate and professional touch. But patients are unlikely to find the distinction easy to make, particularly since it is their bodies that are being viewed and touched.

## BOX 5.1 PERSPECTIVES

# The Agony of Uncertainty

It all began one day when I was in eighth-grade physical education class. As the class began to warm up and stretch, I noticed a knot on my knee. A month passed and the knot did not go away. In fact it grew from the size of a pencil eraser to the size of a quarter. My mother made an appointment with our family doctor, and I began to panic. I personally gave myself one year to live.

During my appointment the doctor asked questions like "Have you fallen down recently?" I was so distraught I felt like screaming "I did not come in here for a bump and scrape!" But I just said no.

After ordering x-rays, the doctor said he could not tell if the knot was a cyst or a tumor and referred us to a bone and joint specialist. I was beyond scared. I was only 13 and had never had anything worse than the flu. I had so many questions, but there wasn't much chance to ask them. Every question I asked got a brief response, when what I really wanted was a full explanation and, above all, reassurance. The conversation went something like this.

> DOCTOR: It looks like you have a cyst or a tumor. I'm going to refer you to a specialist.
> ME: What does that mean?
> DOCTOR: It means he will look at your knee and figure out what is going on.
> ME: Is it serious?
> DOCTOR: That's what he'll be able to determine.
> ME: Well, OK.

I wasn't sure about the difference between a cyst and a tumor, and both sounded horrible. I was afraid the doctor would laugh if I said I was afraid of having cancer. Or had he just told me I *did* have cancer? I left not knowing, and I had to wait a month to see the specialist.

On the day of the appointment with the specialist, Dr. Benze, we waited 2½ hours to see him. However, his personality and gentle manner made up for the wait. Dr. Benze compassionately and carefully told me the lump (now the size of a small orange) was a tumor. When I began to cry, he explained that not all tumors are cancerous. He arranged to surgically remove the tumor in two days, and he promised to tell me everything about the surgery in advance and to share the lab results with me as soon as he received them.

On the day before surgery my mother and I visited the hospital to make arrangements. The admitting attendant was detached and unfriendly, but the nurses and doctors were wonderful. They tried to make me feel comfortable and relaxed. An outpatient nurse sat down with us and described in detail what would happen before, during, and after the surgery. I felt comfortable asking every question I did not feel safe asking the first doctor.

Suffice it to say that the surgery went well. The tumor was not cancerous, and I have had no more tumors. Overall, the experience was a positive one. The worst part was leaving the first doctor's office with so many fears and questions I never got to voice. Although the surgery was frightening, I felt better once people started telling me what was going on.

—*Sarah*

## What Do You Think?

1. Do you think the first doctor could have communicated more effectively with Sarah? If so, how?
2. Do you think Sarah could have communicated more effectively? If so, how?
3. Sometimes doctors feel they will alarm or confuse patients (especially young patients) by giving them medical details. Do you agree?
4. How can patients help ensure that they get the information they want?

In emergencies or especially intense circumstances such as childbirth, modesty may not be on anyone's mind. But during routine exams, there is a fine line to walk, and evidence suggests that patients and caregivers walk it together, demonstrating in subtle ways that the body-as-examined is more an object than an intimate landscape. In a microanalysis of exam-room behaviors, Christian Heath (2006) described the process with which patients present themselves as clinical objects during potentially embarrassing or painful examinations. They typically lower their eyelids, turn their heads aside, and gaze into the middle distance—behaviors quite distinct from those we would expect in a personal, intimate encounter. At the same time, health professionals typically avoid direct eye contact during sensitive exams, focusing instead on particular parts of the patient's body. This "body work," as Heath calls it, is a sophisticated, collaborative performance in which participants display that what might otherwise seem to be an intimate or callous infringement is—by mutual consensus—an acceptable, clinically approved interaction with its own rules of appropriateness.

As patients we are invested in avoiding embarrassment and pain as much as possible. We are also involved in securing the good opinions of our caregivers. With our very well-being hanging in the balance, we are loath for caregivers to view us as whiny, crazy, annoying, stupid, or so on.

How is it, then, that people come to understand what behaviors will distinguish them as "good" patients? Unlike caregivers, patients are usually in medical situations only briefly and occasionally. Moreover, whereas caregivers are allowed, even required, to watch other caregivers, patients seldom get to observe other patients, and few training programs are available to patients about communicating in medical settings (Cegala & Broz, 2003). Thus, socialization into patienthood is an imprecise process. Patients may feel they have been thrust center stage but do not know the script.

People apply their everyday knowledge to the patient role and generally display all the hesitancy you might expect. This section describes the Voice of Lifeworld, the typical power difference between patients and caregivers, and the dilemma patients face when they disagree with caregivers.

## Voice of Lifeworld

Quite naturally, patients interpret their health within the arena most familiar to them—everyday life. In contrast to the scientific Voice of Medicine that physicians use, patients speak what Mishler (1984) calls the Voice of Lifeworld. The **Voice of Lifeworld** is concerned with health and illness as they relate to everyday experiences. For example, a physician may understand back pain in terms of specific discs and muscles, but from a lifeworld perspective, the main issue is that the pain interferes with a person's ability to pick up a child or perform tasks at work. Patients are usually most concerned with how they feel and how their health affects their regular activities. When asked by a doctor what is wrong with them, patients typically describe sensations and events, as in "I get a horrible pain behind my eyes when I try to read the newspaper. It really scares me."

As the following analysis shows, the Voice of Lifeworld and the Voice of Medicine differ in two main ways: One is primarily oriented to feelings and the other to evidence, and one is precise and the other specific.

*Feelings Versus Evidence* Doctors and patients tend to have different philosophies about health. That is, they make sense of it in different ways. Patients "know" they are sick (or healthy) based on how they feel. Through experience, comparisons with others, and gut instinct, they distinguish between feeling well and feeling ill (Mishler, 1981, 1984).

Physicians, however, are taught to be empirical. Science holds that feelings can be distorted and unreliable. Doctors "know" someone is sick based on observation and tests. You may recall from Chapter 2 that this emphasis on physical indicators has roots in the Renaissance principle of verification, the nineteenth century discovery of germs, and scientific means of detecting illness using microscopes and other technology.

As a general principle, patients trust feelings, but physicians trust evidence. Depending on which perspective the participants take, health care encounters may sound very different. Predictably, lifeworld talk is more emotional, social, and contextual, while medical talk is more technical.

Howard Waitzkin (1991) proposes that lifeworld concerns can be problematic from a medical perspective. Lifeworld troubles may seem irrelevant to the medical condition, they may be relevant but outside the physician's power to control, or they may be uncomfortable to discuss. "Under these circumstances doctors typically interject questions, interrupt, or otherwise change the topic, to return to the voice of medicine," Waitzkin says (p. 25).

*Specific Versus Diffuse* One result of their disparate philosophies is that doctors are often precise while patients are diffuse. To illustrate, a doctor hears "pain behind the eyes" and wants to know exactly where, how strong, how long. Patients, however, may be concerned with surrounding issues, such as the scariness of the pain (Will I die? Can I still be a good parent? Am I going blind? Do I have a tumor? What have I done to deserve this?). Although both mean well, doctors may be frustrated when patients "go on and on," and patients may feel rebuffed when doctors seem uninterested in their feelings.

Patients are also more diffuse in their perception of what causes illness. Unlike doctors, who typically strive to find the cause of an illness, patients often perceive that it has multiple causes, common among them stress and relationship issues (Helman, 1985). Consequently, physicians' scientific specificity may seem sorely deficient in explaining illnesses as patients perceive them. People may leave exams wondering if their doctors really understood their problems at all.

Patients may also have numerous goals that take precedence over purely physical healing. They may wish to vent emotions, confess, or be reassured, forgiven, or comforted during a medical visit. These goals may be in direct opposition to doctors' efforts to eliminate situational factors and to focus on measurable ones.

All in all, patients tend to interpret illnesses in the broad context of everyday life, whereas physicians are usually taught to reduce diseases to their simplest, most measurable parts. Of course, the differences described do not hold true for all patients or all medical professionals. Some caregivers are very sensitive to their patients' emotions and life experiences, and some patients are precise and oriented to biomedical concerns. Even so, understanding that patients and caregivers have traditionally been socialized to regard illness differently may help both sides understand each other better.

The Voice of Medicine and the Voice of Lifeworld overlap to a large extent when the goal is *preventing* disease and injury rather than just *treating* them. Prevention is, by nature, a diffuse topic involving an array of risk factors and lifestyle decisions. Furthermore, talking about prevention is usually not as emotionally intense as talking about existing illness. Some speculate that a third voice will emerge that is both diffuse and informative. For example, in the book *YOU: The Smart Patient,* Michael Roizen and Mehmet Oz (2006) coach patients to focus on the overlap between what we might call medical and lifeworld voices. Following are some of their suggestions.

- *Create a one-page health history*. In an easy-to-read format, present information about your health (medications, illnesses, hospitalizations, allergies, surgeries) and any diseases diagnosed in your immediate family. Bring a copy to all doctor's visits and hospital stays.
- *Bring your medications*. Also bring a bag (preferably a clear plastic bag) filled with all the medications you take—both prescribed and over-the-counter—in their original bottles.
- *Choose your doctors carefully*. Find a doctor who is well respected by his or her peers and who listens well and makes you feel comfortable. Patients' thoughts and feelings are as legitimate as their medications and health histories. Find a doctor who pays attention to both.

- *Know what treatment you're supposed to get, and make sure your caregivers know it too.* As we saw in Chapter 4, medical mistakes do happen. Tell caregivers why you are there (e.g., for an appendectomy), and make sure everyone agrees. This might prevent a wrong-side surgery or medication error.
- *Make a phriend.* Get to know a local pharmacist and ask his or her advice. Pharmacists are among the most knowledgeable but underutilized health experts.
- *Wash away germs.* Wash your hands well and often. This applies to daily life and is doubly important in medical environments. When in the hospital, bring hand sanitizer and clean everything (the TV remote control, the phone, and so on.) Ask your guests to sanitize their hands when they enter the room and when they leave.

Next we turn to some factors that define particular patient experiences, including the nature of the health concern, the personalities involved, and participants' communication skills.

## PATIENT CHARACTERISTICS

Although patients would like to maintain their caregivers' positive regard, they may have goals that are at odds with their caregivers' preferences. For instance, a patient may doubt the validity of a diagnosis or wish to reiterate information the caregiver has dismissed as unimportant. Other patients may not be well educated, assertive, or skillful enough to participate as they would like to in health care transactions.

### Nature of the Illness

A patient whose condition is chronic or hard to define may feel like a nuisance to the doctor. Situations such as this present a dilemma. The patient must either risk the caregiver's disapproval or leave feeling that nothing much was accomplished. Either choice has negative consequences.

What do most patients do? Evidence suggests they usually abandon or delay pursuit of their own goals rather than challenge their caregivers (Dyche & Swiderski, 2005). This may be because a damaged identity is hard to mend, but specific goals can usually be pursued at a later date. Whatever their rationale, patients may hint at their feelings, but seldom do they assert them. Instead, dissatisfied patients are known to switch doctors or to come back again and again, perhaps hoping for the right conditions in which to accomplish their goals. All the while, physicians may be unaware of the patients' dissatisfaction.

The problem is especially difficult for people with multiple concerns. For example, a patient with depression may feel that other concerns are brushed aside as psychosomatic even when they are legitimate. Gillespie (2001) describes the frustration of low-income patients experiencing depression and chronic health problems:

> They resented feeling as though they had to prove or stress how sick they "really" were, especially since they felt this account might also label them as neurotic. They had to hide their upset because showing it only leant further evidence to potential neuroses. (p. 109)

### Patient Disposition

Patients' backgrounds and personalities also influence how they communicate in medical settings. After reviewing patient–caregiver literature, Jeffery Robinson (2003) concluded that a number of factors persuade patients to temper their participation in medical dialogues:

- Patients may think it is appropriate to be passive.
- They may be too fearful or anxious to be assertive.
- They may not know or understand enough to participate in medical discussions.
- They may be discouraged by caregivers' communication styles.
- Socioeconomic factors such as education level may influence how actively patients participate.

## BOX 5.2 RESOURCES

## Patient Self-Advocacy and Willingness to Communicate

Brashers, D. E., Haas, S. M., & Neidig, J. L. (1999). The patient self-advocacy scale: Measuring patient involvement in health care decision-making interactions. *Health Communication, 11*(2), 97–121.

Hermansen-Kobulnicky, C. J. (2008). Measurement of self-advocacy in cancer patient and survivors. *Support Care Center, 16*, 613–618.

Walsh-Burke, K., & Marcusen, C. (1999). Self-advocacy training for cancer survivors. The Cancer Survival Toolbox. *Cancer Practice, 7*(6), 297–301.

Wright, K. B., Frey, L., & Sopory, P. (2007, March). Willing to communicate about health as an underlying trait of patient self-advocacy: The development of the Willingness to Communicate about Health (WTCH) measure. *Communication Studies, 58*(1), 35–49.

- The nature of the medical visit (routine or symptom-specific) may influence their behavior.
- The length of the visit and the people present may influence patients' involvement.

A number of studies support these ideas. Patients are more likely to be **self-advocates**—actively seeking health information, comfortable talking about health concerns, and assertive about seeking care—if they are well educated (Street, Gordon, Ward, Krupat, & Kravitz, 2005) and/or they are confident they can make a difference in their own health (Curtin et al., 2008). Cultural factors play a role as well. African American patients are typically less likely than European Americans to self-advocate about health concerns (Street et al., 2005; Wiltshire, Cronin, Sarto, & Brown, 2006). (See Box 5.2 for related resources.)

### Communication Skills

Patients may benefit from skills training programs that prepare them to communicate effectively with medical providers. Although the results are mixed and patient education programs are scarce, there has been modest success in this area. During training sessions, patients are usually instructed and encouraged to ask questions, provide information, and verify their understanding of information (Cegala & Broz, 2003). One reason skills training has not been more effective is that, even if patients are trained *how* to pose questions, they may not know *what* to ask. Donald Cegala and Stefne Broz (2003) reflect:

> Most patients do not formulate questions until they have had time to process what the physician has said or do not realize their lack of understanding until they try to follow the recommended treatment or explain their illness to someone. (p. 10)

Even well-educated patients with good communication skills may find themselves out of their depth conversing about medical topics on the spot. Nevertheless, Cegala and Broz (2003) conclude that even modest improvements can enhance medical care and reduce the length of medical visits.

In his book *How Doctors Think*, Jerome Groopman (2007) offers behind-the-scenes insights for patients so that they can more actively assist their doctors. A physician himself, Groopman attests: "Doctors desperately need patients and their families and friends to help them think. Without their help, physicians are denied key clues to what is really wrong" (pp. 7–8). Following are some of his suggestions.

- *Keep in mind that doctors' emotions may sometimes influence their judgment.* As Groopman (2007) puts its, "Patients and their loved ones swim together with physicians in a sea of feelings" (p. 58). Sometimes, he says, patients can help doctors put things in perspective. He cites an example during which a patient told his doctor, "Don't save me from an unpleasant [medical] test just because we're friends" (p. 58). His gentle remark helped the doctor realize that she had been tempted to do just that. In another

---

BOX 5.3 **CAREER OPPORTUNITIES**

## Patient Advocacy

Patient advocate
Patient navigator
Social worker
Case manager
Patient care coordinator or consultant

## Career Resources and Job Listings

Patient Advocate Foundation: www.
   patientadvocate.org
National Patient Advocate Foundation:
   www.npaf.org

Patient Navigator Outreach and Chronic Disease
   Prevention Demonstration Program: bhpr.hrsa.
   gov/patientnavigator/default.htm
National Association of Social Workers:
   www.socialworkers.org
Council on Social Work Education:
   www.cswe.org
Case Management Society of America: www.cmsa.
   org
National Organization for Human Services: www.
   nationalhumanservices.org
U.S. Bureau of Labor Statistics Occupational
   Outlook Handbook: www.bls.gov/OCO

---

case a middle-aged woman whose previous doctors had written off her symptoms to menopause helped her new doctor see beyond that stereotype by saying:

I know I'm in menopause, and all five doctors have told me that's the cause of my problems. And two told me that I'm crazy. And, frankly, I *am* a little crazy.... But I think this is something else, that what I'm feeling is more than just menopause. (Groopman, p. 56)

Her doctor listened, and the patient was right. She had a rare tumor that, if left untreated, might have threatened her life. Groopman concludes that patients can help doctors by acknowledging emotions out loud rather than leaving them unspoken.

- *Recognize the limits of emergency medicine.* An assessment in the ER is typically only a snapshot attempt to find a major problem. ER doctors do not usually have the benefit of long-standing relationships with patients or full access to their medical records. Thus, their evaluation is incomplete at best. Groopman declares, "The last thing I want is a patient to leave the ER and say, 'The doctor

said there is nothing wrong with me'" (p. 74). If the concern is serious, follow-up care and further assessment are essential.

- *Beware of your own stereotypes.* Physicians are sensitive to discrimination, just as patients are. Groopman tells of doctors whose patients take one look at them and, based solely on the doctor's skin color, demand a different doctor. JudyAnn Bigby, an African American physician who oversees residents, recommends that residents who are female or from minority cultures always wear their lab coats and name badges and keep their stethoscopes visible. Even so, she says, "they will sometimes be asked if they have come to take the meal tray" (p. 96). Patients are responsible for showing their doctors the same respect they would wish to be shown themselves.

- *Be patient with medical uncertainty.* Patients often find comfort in believing their doctors know exactly what is wrong with them, but that isn't always the case. Sometimes the underlying causes of an illness are revealed only gradually with patient investigation over time. A false sense of certainty can blind

## BOX 5.4

# Can You Guess?

The U.S. health care system ranks last in many areas, compared to Germany, New Zealand, Australia, Canada, and United Kingdom. But it excels at one thing in particular. What do you think that is?

*The answer appears at the end of the chapter.*

both physicians and patients to the real or multiple causes of an illness. Groopman encourages patients not to criticize doctors for uncertainty or pressure them into acting more certain than they feel.

- *Ask questions.* Physicians, like all of us, are subject to cognitive errors and limitations. Groopman admits, "Sometimes I come to the end of my thinking and am not sure what to do next" (p. 264). He encourages patients to stimulate physicians' thinking and communication by asking such questions as: What else could this be? What's the worst-case scenario? What should I expect next? Is it possible I have more than one problem? and Is there any evidence that doesn't fit?

In the next two sections we look at factors that contribute to patient satisfaction and patient–caregiver cooperation.

## SATISFACTION

Patients seem to have many grievances about medical care, but they are moderately satisfied overall. A study by the physician-rating program DrScore.com found that Americans give their doctors an average overall score of 7.4 out of 10 and their physicians' office staffs a 7.5 out of 10 (Feldman, 2008). Yet the same patients have a number of serious complaints. Slightly more than half of them said they are unhappy with the doctor's level of caring,

rude staff members, and cumbersome check-in and checkout procedures. Their greatest complaints concern time:

81%—I wait too long in the doctor's lobby.
50%—I wait too long in the exam room.
58%—My doctor doesn't spend enough time with me.
62%—My doctor doesn't answer all my questions and seems rushed.

Some countries do better. In a survey of patients in Germany, New Zealand, Australia, Canada, the United Kingdom, and the United States, the United States ranked last in terms of perceived quality of physician communication, patient engagement, and responsiveness to patient preferences and last in terms of overall efficiency and equitable access to health care (K. Davis et al., 2006). (We'll talk more about these issues later in the book.)

Satisfaction with nursing home and hospital care in the United States is marginal. Among U.S. residents who received nursing home care or witnessed a loved one in a nursing home, between 16% and 41% felt the staffing, environment, or quality of care were substandard ("Patient and Family," 2006). About 28% were very satisfied, and 32% were somewhat satisfied. The numbers are better in U.S. hospitals, but there is plenty room for improvement. Some 63% of U.S. hospital patients rate their care 9 or 10 on a 10-point scale (Jha, Orav, Zheng, & Epstein, 2008). Only about 67.4% say they would recommend the hospital to a friend (Jha et al.). The most frequent complaints are ineffective pain management and unclear communication at discharge. On the other hand, satisfaction is positively associated with low nurse–patient ratios and positive health outcomes. Overall satisfaction is significantly higher at not-for-profit hospitals than at their commercial counterparts.

Researcher Ashish Jha encourages hospital staff to do better. But he also encourages patients to be more assertive about asking questions and voicing their discontent. "The more engaged patients are, the better the care they will receive and the better the care all of us will receive, because they will drive the change for better systems of health care" (Jha quoted by Reinberg, 2008, paragraph 6).

Patients have strong opinions about doctors and nurses. They know what they like—attentiveness, lots of information, and no hassles. They want to know they can speak freely, and they want to feel confident their doctors will not turn against them if they seek second opinions (Jadad & Rizo, 2003). In operational terms, they like health professionals who listen, ask questions, keep them well informed, and encourage them (Jadad & Rizo). In the next section we take a closer look at what patients like and dislike about health care experiences.

## Attentiveness and Respect

Patient satisfaction is more closely linked to caregivers' communication than to their technical skills (Tarrant, Windridge, Boulton, Baker, & Freeman, 2003). This may be because it is hard to judge technical skills and because patients automatically assume caregivers are technically competent. It may also reflect how important communication skills are to diagnosis and treatment. In their article "I Am a Good Patient Believe it or Not," Alejandro Jadad and Carlos Rizo (2003) describe a series of interviews with patients. They conclude: "In most cases it would not take fancy technology, extra time, or increased costs to satisfy what patients 'want.' It would take only an assertive patient and a confident healthcare provider who is willing to listen" (paragraph 6).

There is some evidence that pediatricians lead the pack in terms of patient/parent satisfaction. When researchers ("Patient Perceptions," 2006) asked people if their doctors (or their children's doctors) "listened carefully, explained things clearly, showed respect, and spent enough time" with them, about 73% of patients' parents said yes, compared to young adults (51%), middle-aged adults (56%), and people 65 and older (61%).

People of all ages like doctors who seem to take them seriously and like them back (Grant, Cissna, & Rosenfeld, 2000). This impression is enhanced when doctors are courteous and nonverbally expressive, maintain eye contact, ask about patients' coping strategies, and encourage patients and their families to participate in medical decision making (C. N. Hart, Kelleher, Drotar, & Scholle, 2007; Koermer & Kilbane, 2008).

Physicians also get high marks for listening attentively and acknowledging patients' emotions without trying to control them (Grant et al., 2000). Conversely, patients are displeased when they feel their dignity has been compromised (Milika & Trorey, 2008). Some of the most commonly perceived threats to dignity include the following (from Milika & Trorey):

- *Invasions of privacy.* Patients feel dishonored when staff members allow them to be physically exposed to others or carelessly allow others to read or overhear their confidential information.
- *Curt, discourteous, or disrespectful communication.* Patients resent it when caregivers neglect to introduce themselves or when they ignore them, don't listen attentively, or talk down to them. Some patients also prefer not to be addressed by first name. Before he retired, physician John Egerton (2007) had a rule for his front-office staff: "Avoid mentioning the patient's name and diagnosis in the same sentence" (Milika & Trorey, paragraph 6.) For instance, never say, "John Smith has prostatitis again" or "Helen Will has head lice" (paragraph 6). Naturally, caregivers will need to discuss patients and their conditions in private. But making such statements where others might overhear them threatens patients' privacy and reduces them to symptoms rather than treating them as complete persons.
- *Compromised appearance.* Patients typically report feeling most dignified when they are allowed to wear their own clothing and jewelry.

Satisfaction may vary by health concern. Overall, the least satisfied patients are those with chronic, hard-to-cure conditions, such as headaches and back pain (Tan, Jensen, Thornby, & Anderson, 2006). By contrast, obstetric, cancer, and heart patients are more satisfied than average, perhaps because these conditions are treated by doctors as more serious and legitimate.

## Convenience

Patients also like it when things run smoothly. Satisfaction is enhanced when there is good news about their health, when the wait is not long, and when their health plan is covering the costs (Probst, Greenhouse, & Selassie, 1997). Hospitals in recent years have begun efforts to streamline paperwork and admitting procedures, realizing that patient satisfaction relies on more than skillfully performed medical procedures. Some hospitals are experimenting with check-in centers at which patients arriving for surgery or emergency care can key in their information (health history, payment information, health concern) at one of several private computer kiosks rather than waiting for staff members to interview them (Huvane, 2008). In many cases this has reduced overall wait times. (Patients who prefer can still register with a staff member.)

Convenience is also a factor in the creation of retail clinics in drugstores and department stores across the country (see Chapter 9), as well as extended-hour clinics, and open-access clinics available to people who haven't made appointments in advance (Lowes, 2008b).

## A Sense of Control

Patients appreciate being well informed and actively involved in their care. Although patients appreciate doctors' advice, only about 20% want their caregivers to make decisions without them ("Reality Check," 2008). This applies to everyday decisions as well as major treatment options. One hospital patient interviewed said he appreciates it when nurses who bathe him wash body parts he can't reach and then ask, "Would you like to do the rest for yourself?" (quoted by Milika & Trorey, 2008, p. 2713). He says he feels respected when he is given choices, and this one allows him to maintain dignity and take care of private needs himself.

Other patients echo the same sentiment. A man with diabetes in Ciechanowski and Katon's (2006) study describes his favorite doctor this way:

He doesn't just come in, do your treatment and leave. He kind of talks, you know, "How are things going? Tell me about yourself," and he has a fabulous memory. He remembers about those things that you tell him.... I don't know if it's just a really good memory, or he puts notes in the chart, or whatever, but it's just...he makes you feel comfortable coming in...I feel like I can be my weird, twisted self and my doctor understands that. (p. 3074)

This leads us to the next discussion of how patients define interpersonal warmth.

## Genuine Warmth and Honesty

When Susan Harris and Edith Templeton (2001) conducted focus groups involving women with breast cancer, they asked participants to rank-order the most positive elements of communication with their doctors. Beginning with the most important quality, the women listed: (1) physicians' active listening, (2) physician awareness about the depth of the patient's knowledge, (3) honesty, (4) partnership, (5) interest in the patient as a person, and (6) touch. Focus group participants said they appreciate it when doctors encourage them to audiotape medical sessions and when they offer them photocopies of lab results. Said one woman in the study: "It was helpful for me to get the information, important to have the hard copy in my hand. It gave me a sense of 'power.' I could question and read it through" (p. 446). Many women said they appreciate it when their doctors don't "mince words" but instead are honest and upfront about their conditions. They say they are deeply grateful when doctors don't seem rushed and when they extend human kindness and encouragement. Said one woman: "I'm very grateful my GP didn't feel he had to maintain some kind of professional distance. I was freaking out. I needed a hug" (p. 446).

## COOPERATION AND CONSENT

Let's go back to a summer day in 2008 when Tiger Woods limped up the sloping hill of Torrey Pines golf course to where his ball lay on the green. He made the final shot to finish one stroke ahead of his nearest competitor after a grueling playoff in a golf tournament that included 91 holes. Woods won the 2008 U.S. Open, thrilling fans but confounding his doctors, who had urged him not to play because of a knee injury.

In this respect Woods isn't so different from the majority of people. Although patients are unlikely to challenge their doctors' advice in person, only 50% to 60% of patients follow medical advice completely or most of the time (Martin, Williams, Haskard, & Dimatteo, 2005). This includes patients' decisions to engage in dangerous and unhealthy behaviors, not to undergo recommended health screenings or see recommended specialists, not to make regular doctors' appointments, not to take prescribed drugs, not to exercise or eat as recommended, and so on.

As Michael Burgoon and Judee Burgoon (1990) observe, it is curious that patients do not follow medical advice more closely, considering that patients pay for the advice, presumably stand to benefit from it, and typically revere the expertise of medical professionals. In the next section we explore some of the reasons patients may not follow through. Then we'll examine caregivers' stake in getting patients to perform medical regimens and look at policies concerning informed consent for medical treatment.

## Reasons for Nonadherence

People who do not follow medical advice are not necessarily lazy or indifferent about their health. A number of more legitimate concerns may affect their decisions.

For one, medical recommendations may be impossible or impractical to carry out, considering patients' circumstances. They may be unable to afford prescribed medications or be physically incapable of performing suggested routines (Frankel & Beckman, 1989). For example, patients who miss dialysis treatments often report that no one is available to drive them to and from appointments (E. J. Gordon, Leon, & Sehgal, 2003). Likewise, low-income patients may have little choice concerning

their exposure to "avoidable" health threats. As Gillespie (2001) describes it:

> Low-income families live in older homes filled with lifetimes of dust and molding timber. They breathe the air polluted by factories that never cease production and by the cars of daily downtown professionals who sleep in clean, suburban air each night. Often depressed, they are more likely to smoke and less likely to eat well. Many sleep on the floor, knowing that the asthma this triggers could kill them, but afraid that a stray bullet shot through the window will do so sooner. (p. 114)

In other situations, recommended regimens may be so foreign to patients that they cannot integrate them into their lifestyles. For instance, some people consider it inconceivable to remove red meat completely from their diet. Or, like Tiger Woods, they may feel that some goals and obligations are too important to miss, even if it means risking a personal illness or injury.

Second, patients may not agree with the doctor's assessment or treatment recommendations. Research suggests patients are apt to distrust diagnoses and thus to ignore medical advice if they are unable to describe their concerns during the medical visit (Frankel & Beckman, 1989). People may also deny diagnoses that threaten their self-image. It may be difficult to admit obesity, hearing loss, depression, sexually transmitted diseases, and the like.

Third, patients may stop medical routines prematurely if they perceive no effect or if their symptoms cease (Forrest, Shadmi, Nutting, & Starfield, 2007). For example, it is difficult to get people to remain on treatment for conditions such as high blood pressure because they cannot directly perceive that the medicine has a positive effect.

Finally, patients may stop taking medication if they experience unpleasant side effects (Löffler, Kilian, Toumi, & Angermeyer, 2003). Rather than contact the physician for alternate instructions, they may try other methods or conclude that the cure is worse than the disease.

These factors are exacerbated when physicians do not encourage patients to express their concerns

BOX 5.5

## Cash for Cooperation?

Communication is important, but can it stack up to cold, hard cash? Maybe not. Some medical centers are having success with innovative cash-for-compliance programs that reward patients for healthy behavior. An overview of 11 programs suggests prizes and coupons may work well and actually save health agencies money (Giuffrida & Torgerson, 1997).

Incentives include cash or cash coupons (usually $4 or $5 or a chance to win from $25 to $100) for keeping appointments, maintaining healthy blood pressure (for hypertensive patients), reaching weight-loss goals, immunizing children, or abstaining from drug abuse. In all but one program, cash incentives were more successful than reminder phone calls and warnings. Incentive programs were even more successful than a program to offer more convenient appointment times.

Program sponsors say it is less expensive to offer cash prizes than to pay staff to work overtime or call patients, and everyone stands to gain if incentives reduce unnecessary care and keep serious health concerns from escalating. It is not clear, however, if patients will develop motivation to continue the behaviors without the rewards.

and reservations at the time they give medical advice. Evidence suggests many people leave their doctors' offices knowing they cannot or will not follow through with advice given, but they do not feel free to say so. Doctors who assume that patients should follow orders regardless of their circumstances may be discouraged when treatment outcomes are less than optimal. What's more, patients who do not feel comfortable talking with the doctor in person may be reluctant to be honest about treatment failures later on.

### Caregivers' Investment

It may be tempting to assume that, if patients do not follow medical advice, they have only themselves to blame. But caregivers may (justly or unjustly) be blamed as well. Lack of patient–caregiver cooperation often results in harmful health outcomes. Nonadherence is linked to diabetes treatment failures (Joy, 2008), increased hospitalization for heart failure (Fonarow et al., 2008), and asthma-related complications and deaths (Gillisen, 2007), to name just a few. These are not just patients' problems.

Caregivers' careers may be damaged by excessive treatment failures. With capitation and restricted reimbursements, health care organizations lose money on patients who do not improve as expected.

Consequently, hospitals may refuse to grant doctors privileges if their treatment outcomes are below par, and medical groups may deny them employment for the same reason. Doctors' reputation among patients may suffer as well. Physician Wesley Sugai of Kailua-Kona, Hawaii, says he doesn't treat patients who chronically ignore medical advice without explanation.

> As a rural solo pediatrician, I have neither the time nor the desire to try to convince parents about the importance of childhood immunizations, follow-up with specialists, or medications. . . . I tell parents that I have to be able to trust them to carry out the treatment plan, just as they must trust me to prescribe the proper therapy. If neither of us trusts the other, then the patient–doctor relationship is nonexistent and we must go our separate ways. (Sugai, 2008, p. 14)

Sugai says that he does work with patients who are upfront about reservations or limitations that affect their health behaviors. All in all, it is important for patients who cannot follow treatment advice or who don't agree with it to be upfront in negotiating more suitable options with their doctors.

Public health is at stake as well. Good communication and healthy behaviors can avert pandemics and reduce spending on preventable illnesses and

## BOX 5.6 ETHICAL CONSIDERATIONS

# Patients' Right to Informed Consent

During the infamous Tuskegee Syphilis Study, which began in 1932, some 600 African American men were enrolled without their knowledge in a medical experiment. They were patients of the Public Health Service in Macon County, Alabama, and the experiment was conducted by the U.S. government through the Tuskegee Institute in Alabama.

Although medical researchers knew that 399 of the men had syphilis, the men were not told. Doctors simply told all the men they had "bad blood" and provided them with medicine, meals, and burial expenses. However, the medicine was not really medicine at all. It was a harmless but ineffectual placebo.

The study was designed to help medical researchers learn more about the effects of syphilis among African Americans. Syphilis is a sexually transmitted disease that affects the bones, liver, heart, and central nervous system. In advanced stages, it can cause open sores, heart damage, tumors, blindness, insanity, and death. When the study was begun, there was no effective treatment for syphilis. However, by 1940 penicillin was known to be very effective at treating and even curing it.

The syphilis patients in the Tuskegee experiment were not given penicillin. Instead, researchers continued to watch the disease progress until the experiment was called off in 1972, some 40 years after it began.

When details of the Tuskegee study were made public, there was an angry outcry. Some likened it to the Nazis' medical experiments on Jewish prisoners during World War II. The courts eventually ordered the federal government to pay the men and their families a total of $10 million for the injury and indignity they had suffered. Twenty-five years after the experiment (in May 1997) President Bill Clinton publicly apologized for the government's behavior.

Now, before patients are given medical treatment (experimental or otherwise), they must be fully informed, give consent, and be aware that they can

cease treatment at any time. It is hoped that informed consent will prevent atrocities such as the Tuskegee Syphilis Study. But informed consent is sometimes hard to apply. Jauhar (2008) describes the ethical challenges of informed consent in some instances:

> [An] issue I continue to struggle with today is how to balance patient autonomy with the physician's obligation to do the best for his patient. As a doctor, when do you let your patient make a bad decision: When, if ever, do you draw the line? What if a decision could cost your patient's life? How hard do you push him to change his mind? At the same time, it's his life. Who are you to tell him how to live? (p. 233)

Jauhar (2008) describes a particularly difficult case when a hospital patient, Mr. Smith, began to cough up blood and have trouble breathing. His condition quickly deteriorated, and doctors knew they would have to act quickly to save his life. Their only hope was to insert a temporary breathing tube. But the patient adamantly refused. In his mind, being intubated seemed a worse fate than death. Mr. Smith's fear seemed irrational, yet he was coherent and capable of communicating, thus he was capable of giving (or refusing) informed consent. As the doctor responsible for Mr. Smith's care, Jauhar faced a dilemma. He could honor the patient's wishes and allow him to die, or he could overrule the patient and insert the breathing tube by force. What would you have done?

Jauhar chose to insert the breathing tube, although the staff had to restrain Mr. Smith physically to do it. During the procedure Jauhar worried that the patient would be hate him for disobeying his wishes. "'If you live through this,' I whispered to Mr. Smith, 'I hope you can forgive me'," he remembers saying (Jauhar, 2008, pp. 236–237). Two weeks later, as Mr. Smith neared recovery, Jauhar stopped by his room and told the patient he was responsible for the decision. The patient considered his response for a moment. "I've been

*(continued)*

**BOX 5.6** *(continued)*

through a lot," he finally said, his voice still hoarse from two weeks of intubation....But thank you" (p. 237). This is an extreme case, but it illustrates some of the ethical dilemmas involved in informed consent.

## What Do You Think?

1. Do you agree with Jauhar's decision? Why or why not? What would you have done in his shoes?
2. Sometimes medical information is difficult to understand fully. How do you establish if the consenting person is informed enough to give consent?
3. Some people, such as those with terminal illnesses, are willing (even anxious) to try untested therapies. Researchers may not know what results to expect, and they may even anticipate negative outcomes. Who should decide whether

the patient undergoes untested therapies? Should public money be used in these cases?
4. In medical research, is it ever justified to deceive people (as in giving placebos) to make sure they are not just responding to the power of suggestion? If so, under what conditions?
5. Sometimes it is in the best interest of society or health care workers to know if a person has a contagious disease (such as AIDS). If the person does not consent to a test for that disease, do you think it should be permissible to perform the test without the person's knowledge? (A vial of blood may be used for a variety of tests without the patient's knowledge.)
6. On what grounds, if any, should health professionals judge whether a patient is emotionally capable of making a life-or-death judgment about emergency treatment?

---

injuries. In the United States, the cost of preventable hospitalizations is about $29 billion per year, equal to about 10% of total health costs (Russo, Jiang, & Barrett, 2007). Analyst Bill Clements (1996) advises: "Make no mistake about it: Bad communication costs you money" (paragraph 3).

Considering these factors, how far should caregivers go to gain patients' cooperation? Some doctors are trying cash rewards (see Box 5.5). Others are trying to involve patients more in medical decision making. As the next section illustrates, over time, public policy has changed concerning patients' role in medical decisions.

### Informed Consent

For centuries physicians considered it wise to tell patients only as much as they could understand (in the doctors' opinion) and nothing that might dissuade them from following medical advice. For example, if a doctor judged that the potential advantages of a drug outweighed its possible side

effects, the doctor might not tell the patient about side effects, for fear the patient would not take the drug (Katz, 1995). Likewise, although doctors have always been required to get patients' permission before they operated on them, they have not been required to tell patients about the risks involved.

In most cases physicians were presumably following their best judgment. In some cases, however, patients were subjected to risks, even to deadly medical experiments, without their knowledge. One example is the **Tuskegee Syphilis Study** conducted in Alabama (Box 5.6).

Public outrage over the Tuskegee Syphilis Study and others like it led the U.S. government to pass informed-consent laws. **Informed consent** means patients must (a) be made fully aware of known treatment risks, benefits, and options; (b) be deemed capable of understanding such information and making a responsible judgment; and (c) be aware that they may refuse to participate or cease treatment at any time (Ashley & O'Rourke, 1997).

When patients are children or are otherwise unable to make decisions, close family members may be allowed to consent on their behalf.

Informed-consent requirements are designed to allow patients enough information so that they can make knowledgeable judgments about their own care. Some theorists believe health care should go even further toward including patients in treatment decisions. As early as 1973, medical analyst Harold Walker predicted that doctors would become less authoritarian and more persuasive. The difference is subtle but important. From an authoritarian perspective, patients are expected to *comply* with doctors' orders. From a persuasive perspective, however, patients take an active role in decision making. They *cooperate* in the process as informed and influential participants.

If patients are included in decision making, it may be possible to overcome or accommodate many of the factors that now keep them from following medical advice. The caregiver aware of a patient's financial and physical limitations, cultural reservations, denial, or discouragement is better able to negotiate more acceptable options with the patient or provide information that may assuage the patient's reservations. At the very least, patients and caregivers can establish outright what each is willing to do. This may ultimately be less frustrating than allowing their differences to go unspoken.

Informed consent is a victory for patient empowerment. However, the terms are sometimes hard to apply, even when people try hard to do so. For example, a long list of complications (many of them extremely unlikely) might result from a simple procedure. It may be impractical or impossible to list every possible outcome. However, physicians may be accused of negligence if an unlikely outcome results and the patient was not warned about it in advance. Partly because complete disclosure is so difficult to define, the courts have been somewhat reluctant to hold physicians responsible for informed-consent violations except in clear-cut cases. See Box 5.6 for ethical implications concerning informed consent.

Acknowledging that patients make decisions based on a number of factors outside formal medical settings, in the next section we examine how illnesses can affect people's sense of identity.

## ILLNESS AND PERSONAL IDENTITY

To understand the effects of illness on personal identity, consider for a moment who you are. A few words might come to mind: student, son, daughter, parent, athlete, kind, smart, energetic, and the like. To the extent that you and the people around you agree on these roles and descriptions, the roles and descriptions make up your identity. They define who you are, and you are not likely to change in unforeseen, significant ways. **Personal identity** is a relatively enduring set of characteristics that define a person.

At first consideration, having an identity may seem easy. You simply are who you are. However, the deeper reality is that you work hard to "be" who you are. People generally want to be viewed favorably and to feel good about themselves. Therefore, they act in ways that are consistent with the positive image they wish to portray (Goffman, 1967). Like other people, you are probably invested in maintaining the qualities and talents that make you unique. Very often, this requires a great deal of work (studying, listening, practicing, rehearsing, exercising, etc.). These behaviors are not "you," but they do support the identity that helps you and others understand you.

What if you were suddenly unable to maintain the behaviors that seem to make you who you are? What if you lost your memory and could no longer pass a test? What if your looks or your ability to talk or walk changed substantially? These are extreme examples, but even minor illnesses and injuries can interfere with people's ability to "be" who they are. If the effects are short-lived, people probably do not experience a serious crisis of identity. However, long-term effects can change how people see themselves and how others treat them (Vanderford, Jenks, & Sharf, 1997).

Michael Arrington (2003) interviewed men with prostate cancer, the treatment of which may render men impotent and incontinent. One man in the study, Walsh, describes his struggle to reconcile his sense of self and manhood with his inability to have an erection:

> And the final thing was to know myself. Do I know what's happening to me? Do I understand, in my own anxieties, how important, as I look back on it, the whole sexual experience of my own sexuality has been to me? Have I overloaded myself with that or not? Have I given it too much value in life? Are there things in life that are maybe more important to me personally than that? I think that evaluation and that process is one that I have given a lot of time and attention to, being the kind of a person I am. (p. 35)

Some men in the study chose various methods (pumps, injections, pills) for simulating erections, but others felt that such solutions were phony and inauthentic. Said one man:

> Come on. That's not sex. That's, forget that stuff; that's not gonna cut it with me. I'm just done with it, that's all....It's not a natural thing when you do that. I just don't, uh, want to be an artificial man. (p. 38)

Thus, the men either found new ways to achieve or define sexual performance or they redefined its importance in their lives (Arrington). For example, one participant in the study said that men who cannot find other ways to please their partners sexually are "piss-poor lovers" anyway (p. 39).

In addition to personal identities, we have **social identities,** characterized by perceived membership in societal groups such as "teenagers," "Hispanic Americans," and "retired persons" (Harwood & Sparks, 2003). Based on the groups with which we identify, we may expect ourselves (and others like us) to think and behave in particular ways. For example, we may be surprised when a youthful friend reveals she has a serious heart condition and we may thereafter view her as "older" than her peers (Kundrat & Nussbaum, 2003).

When we are diagnosed with an identity-threatening illness, it may become part of our identity as well. Jake Harwood and Lisa Sparks (2003) call this a **tertiary identity**—a label that defines simultaneously the illness and one's alignment toward it. For

example, during a leadership retreat, a colleague of mine introduced herself to the group as, among other things, a "breast cancer survivor." The group responded with applause and hugs. Surviving cancer was treated as courageous and admirable, and I believe group members felt a sense of intimacy that she had shared this news with them. Harwood and Sparks propose that a number of tertiary identities are available to people with the same health conditions. For example, my colleague might have said, "I'm a cancer victim" rather than a "survivor." I believe the crowd would have been sympathetic, but their reaction (and their image of her) would have been somewhat different. Perhaps even more important, different wording would reflect something important about the way she viewed her *own* circumstances.

This section examines how people manage their identities in the life-altering circumstances of ill health. It reviews common responses to illness and describes the role of patient narratives.

### Reactions to Illness

Patients' reactions to illness may be surprising and unexpected, even to the patients themselves. Kathy Charmaz has studied the way people with long-term illnesses seek to reconcile their previous identities with the changed circumstances in which they find themselves. In a 1987 report, she identified four stages common to the process. First, people typically take on a **supernormal identity**, determined not to let the illness stop them from being better than ever. This stage is usually followed by a sense of **restored self**, when people are not quite as optimistic but typically deny that the illness has changed them. The third stage is **contingent personal identity**, when people admit that they may not be able to do everything they could previously do and begin to confront the consequences of a changed identity. The final stage, **salvaged self**, represents the development of a transformed identity that integrates former aspects of self with current limitations. Of course, not everyone goes through every stage or spends the same amount of time in each stage. However, Charmaz's model illustrates that illness and identity are sometimes intertwined and that people actively try to manage their identity when illness threatens their ability to behave as they normally would.

In the case study "I Want You to Put Me in the Grave with All My Limbs" (Sharf, Haidet, & Kroll, 2005), a woman with a family history of diabetes says she would rather die at age 60 than experience amputation. Many of us shudder at such a choice, but for her the devastation of losing a limb is familiar and distinctly identity-threatening. She explains:

> My grandfather had no legs; my dad has no legs, and part of his chest is missing, and part of one hand is missing, and he can only see out of one eye, but not very good. Also, my dad's brother has one hand missing, and one leg missing and so forth. And so it goes in the family. (Sharf et al., p. 43)

Sometimes people's abilities are not substantially altered by their health conditions, but they may be surprised or dismayed to have a condition that seems to clash with their established beliefs. For instance, an unmarried high school teacher may be horrified to learn she is pregnant and may wonder if her pregnancy will affect students' image of her or cost her job.

It can be useful to ascertain whether people consider their health conditions to be identity-threatening and how they react to that possibility. Patients may feel determined, ashamed, victimized, or even relieved by diagnoses. Some respond to illness with a zealous determination to "beat" it, as if it were an enemy. Others interpret illness as punishment. For others, it is comforting to have a name for the illness and perhaps a plan for dealing with it.

Leigh Ford and Brigitte Christmon (2005) illustrate this diversity well with narratives from women who have had breast cancer or feared that they might. One woman, Helen, described the nausea and fatigue of undergoing chemotherapy while doing her best as a wife and mother. She says, "It was a terrible time for us, but when I look back at it now, I feel nothing but pride in our resilience as a family and in the love that allowed us to make this work"

(p. 160). Another woman said she put her faith in God when she didn't know what lay ahead. A third challenged the "corporatization of breast cancer," saying:

> Breast cancer is now part of the market economy. We have pink ribbons and scarves and bears and T-shirts and coffee mugs and wind chimes and breast cancer candles and tchotchkes galore. There is something offensive about this. Most of these items advertise that "part of the proceeds go to breast cancer research." I wonder how much—and to what end? I prefer a straight business transaction—at least the motives and agenda are clear. (p. 165)

She also questions the pink-ribbon movement's emphasis on feminine beauty, optimism, and survival—to the extreme of ignoring the deadly and devastating aspects of breast cancer. "If you refuse to enact the role of the noble survivor," she says, "you are invisible and marginalized, not just by mainstream society but also by most other women who have experienced this disease" (p. 163).

These diverse reactions can be informative. People may assume that people who are upbeat are "taking it well" or are "strong." But in some instances they are hiding deeper feelings or harboring unrealistic expectations. Others may feel their illness is degrading or is unfair. Patients who seem relieved may have expected something worse (it might be helpful to know what), or they may simply be glad to escape part of the dread and uncertainty of not knowing. In the case of extended illnesses, reactions are likely to vary considerably even within one person.

## Narratives

Anne had seen a lot of doctors over the years, but Dr. Falchuk was different. She could barely believe her ears as he sat before her:

> Falchuk offered a gentle smile. "I want to hear your story in your own words." Anne glanced at the clock on the wall, the steady sweep of the second hand ticking off precious time. Her internist had told her that Dr. Falchuk was a prominent specialist, that

there was a long line waiting to see him. Her problem was hardly urgent, and she got an appointment in less than two months only because of a cancellation in his Christmas-week schedule. But she detected no hint of rush or impatience in the doctor. His calm made it seem as if he had all the time in the world. (Groopman, 2007, p. 12)

Actually, Anne's condition *was* urgent. As Groopman relates her story, although she was eating 3,000 calories a day, she was unable to keep food down and she had become critically underweight. They problem had persisted for 15 years, and although Anne was only in her 30s, her body's systems were crashing. Of the 30 or so doctors she had consulted before Dr. Falchuk, none had asked to hear her whole story the way he did. Instead, most doctors had asked only brief, closed-ended questions. Their subsequent diagnoses ranged from depression, to bulimia, to irritable bowel syndrome, and more. Some felt the illness was all in her head. Most urged her to eat a high-carbohydrate diet of cereals and breads to gain weight. But her health kept deteriorating.

After listening carefully to Anne's story from beginning to end, Falchuk was the first to identify her disease correctly. He suspected, and confirmed, that she had celiac disease, a severe allergy to the gluten found in many grain products (notably the same products other doctors were urging Anne to eat). Falchuk's diagnosis and her subsequent diet change saved Anne's life. When Groopman (2007) interviewed Falchuk about the episode, he denied doing anything extraordinary. Listening to patients' stories *should* be a doctor's first priority, Falchuk said, avowing that "once you remove yourself from the patient's story, you are no longer truly a doctor" (quoted by Groopman, p. 2007).

People are natural storytellers. One person tells another what it was like to undergo surgery, have a baby, go on a blind date, or so on. Nearly any time people gather, even for a few moments, they tell stories of this sort. According to narrative theorists (e.g., Beach & Japp, 1983; S. Fisher, 1984), people tell stories for some very compelling reasons. (A **narrative** is a story.) At a surface level, narratives are informative. They tell people of specific goings-on and perhaps prepare them to take part in similar circumstances. But at an even deeper level, narratives shape interpretations and viewpoints—some would say they shape reality.

The essence of narrative theory is that people use storytelling to help establish common values and interpretations. An example may help to clarify this idea. A 58-year-old cardiac patient told his doctor:

It's been tough. I've gone from being a man who is really healthy and has no problems to having a bad heart attack and a big operation and being a real weight watcher. It has been a big change, and it has had its tough moments, but I'm alive and I guess that is what matters. (quoted by J. B. Brown, Weston, & Stewart, 1995, p. 39)

In this simple account, the man suggests an identity for himself. Despite the unusual occurrence of his ill health, his words imply that he is by nature a strong man, physically and emotionally. This characterization sums up a series of events and may shield him from being typified as self-pitying or sickly.

People may not be fully aware of what their narratives imply. The cardiac patient might say he was just telling his story as he saw it, with no particular intention of creating an image for himself. Nevertheless, stories tend to leak cues about people's viewpoints, and they are often persuasive in suggesting certain interpretations. Especially when different narratives reinforce the same themes and morals, they help solidify expectations about the world and shape people's identities.

Narratives are important to health communication, for two main reasons. First, patients naturally speak in narrative form (Eggly, 2002). Patients typically describe their health concerns within a sequence of events they consider relevant. Although these narratives may seem simple or irrelevant on the surface, they can address a sophisticated number of goals simultaneously. In the telling of a story, a speaker might disclose concerns he or she wouldn't otherwise blurt out. For example, Timothy Halkowski (2006) observed that patients sometimes present a "sequence of noticings" rather than coming straight to the point about a health concern.

The "noticings" typically involve emerging indications of a potential health problem and what the patient did about them at each step, leading up to the current visit. These narrative details may seem superfluous to a physician, who may wonder, as one doctor I know puts it, why patients don't just come to the point and "bottom-line it." But for a patient, Halkowski says, they are a means of managing the dilemma of simultaneously impressing the doctor that one's concerns are legitimate while avoiding being typed as melodramatic or overly self-concerned. The patient is able to present a number of indicators that are demonstrated as being relevant to the current concern, underscoring its status as real rather than imagined. Patients can also display that they were not actively looking for things to go medically wrong and can share useful information about what has or has not worked so far. This sequential narrative, Halkowski says, gives patients a mechanism for presenting their concerns in an informative and identity-supporting way.

This leads to the second reason narratives are important: They are loaded with information. A sensitive listener can detect cues to a person's hopes, fears, doubts, future intentions, and more. Particularly since patients are often nonassertive about expressing these feelings, caregivers may find that narratives offer valuable insights. Subtle cues may be the only indications that a patient is dissatisfied, in despair, reluctant to cooperate, overly anxious to please, or so on. All of these factors can be directly relevant to the success of medical care.

Janice Brown and Julia Addington-Hall (2007) identified four types of narratives in the stories told by people with motor neurone disease (MND), a neurological disorder that gradually diminishes people's ability to move and speak. Most people with MND die in 3 to 5 years. Some of the people Brown and Addington-Hall studied used **sustaining narratives**, that is, storylines that emphasize hope and positive thinking. For example, one mother of two young children said she was grateful for what she could still do, even though her ability to walk and talk were ebbing. "I mean, I still feel I could be a lot worse off. I mean I know everything's hard work, but there's no pain it" (p. 204). The researchers also

identified **enduring narratives**, which describe a process of stoically living through one's suffering, ambivalent about whether it would be better to live or to die. One man in the study, who could no longer move his hands or arms, said, "They say there's not much they can do about it, you have just got to take it" (p. 205). He said he had instructed caregivers not to resuscitate him if he had a heart attack because dying would be better than "sitting here like this" (p. 205). In **preserving narratives,** people describe illness as something to be conquered, with varying levels of confidence in their ability to do so. One participant in the study had turned to holistic therapies in addition to pharmaceutical prescriptions, changed his diet, and eliminated chemicals from his home. "I am just willing to try anything," he said (p. 205). Finally, **fracturing narratives** describe fear, loss, denial, and threats to self-concept. Said one woman with MND: "I try and remain optimistic and fear that if the day comes when I have to fully embrace this illness, possibly because of increasing symptoms, then I will totally fall apart. I am trying to postpone that moment" (p. 206). The researchers reflect that caregivers can better understand people by listening to their narratives and appreciating that the narratives are likely to evolve over time.

If the move toward patient empowerment continues, narratives are likely to become more influential components of patient–caregiver communication. Geist and Gates (1996) describe it as "movement from biology to biography" (p. 221). When caregivers listen and ask open-ended questions, they can learn a great deal, not only about patients' physical conditions, but also about their expectations and values (Eggly, 2002). How relevant are such factors to personal health? Very relevant, according to the integrative health theory (Box 5.7), which proposes that health is not an isolated condition, but alignment between multiple factors.

## SUMMARY

In contrast to the well-established ways caregivers are socialized, people learn how to be patients mostly through life experience and watching others (including their caregivers). Patients often communicate in

## BOX 5.7 THEORETICAL FOUNDATIONS

# Integrative Health Model

Health cannot accurately be reduced to a failure of body, identity, or behavior, say the creators of integrative health theory (Lambert, Street, Cegala, Smith, Kurtz, & Schofield, 1997). Instead, **integrative health theory** proposes that health is alignment between interpretive accounts (assumptions and explanations), performance (activities and behaviors), and self-image (understanding of one's own identity).

Ideally, alignment is stable and enduring (the person is healthy), but a change in any one force can upset the alignment. Lambert and colleagues (1997) present the example of a man who feels healthy despite undiagnosed high blood pressure. However, once his condition is diagnosed and he begins taking medication for it, the man experiences a side effect (impotence). His interpretive account—that as a healthy male and husband (his self-image) he should have a sexual relationship with his wife—is threatened by his inability to engage in intercourse (performance). In short, "the impotence is a resistance that destabilizes his healthy alignment," write Lambert and associates. "When he realizes he is impotent, he no longer feels healthy" (p. 34).

Lambert and colleagues (1997) use the term **resistance** to describe factors that threaten alignment. The effects of resistance are not predictable or universal. The man in the previous example might respond by altering his self-image, redefining his ideas about being a good husband, or resuming sexual activity by ceasing the medication (Lambert et al.).

People may have a difficult time adjusting to resistance factors that seem small to others. By the same token, over time, people sometimes achieve alignment others would not think possible. Marianne Brady and David Cella (1995) described the resiliency with which some cancer patients ultimately adapt to their illness: "Many even say they are strengthened by the experience and note an improved outlook on life, enhanced interpersonal relationships and a deepened sense of personal strength" (paragraph 13). Although their physical abilities may be compromised by the disease, these people apparently adjust other factors to achieve a new (even an improved) sense of alignment.

The integrative health model presents several implications for health communication. For one, it sets aside the centuries-old question of whether health is fundamentally a matter of mind or body. By rejecting reductionistic notions, it provides an inclusive definition of health that relies more on alignment between factors than isolation of any one element. From this perspective, a health examination would not be focused on identifying the "cause" of a health concern but in considering how it is situated within broader contexts.

Another implication is that restoring alignment may be simple or complex. Sometimes there is primarily one form of resistance. Lambert and coauthors (1997) give the example of an appendectomy that restores a young woman to full health. In her case, alignment is disrupted but quickly restored. In other situations, however, focusing on one resistance point may not help (or may even worsen) overall alignment. For example, amputating a limb may remove physical danger but plunge the patient into personal crisis. Considering this, the biomedical model may be appropriate for some medical encounters but woefully insufficient for others.

A third implication is that outcomes are neither static nor definitive. Lambert and colleagues (1997) write: "It is never known in advance which accommodations will be successful, nor is it known whether accommodations will themselves lead to the emergence of new resistances" (p. 35). Even when alignment is present, there is no guarantee it will stay that way. In fact, it almost certainly will be challenged. Because of this, health is viewed more productively as a process, as a temporal emergence, than as an outcome.

Finally, in the midst of this complexity, Lambert and colleagues (1997) argue that there is one constant: The patient is always central in the process. As an individual involved in the ongoing work of balancing identity and performance, a "patient is at the center of the aligned elements" and is "also the one doing the work of interactive stabilization" (p. 31).

## What Do You Think?

1. In what ways do your daily activities support your self-image? How would you feel if you lost the ability to perform these activities?
2. Think of the last time you felt unhealthy. What resistance factors were involved? Was alignment restored? If so, how?

## Suggested Sources

Integrative health is based on the collective ideas of a number of theorists. For the rich background behind this theory, see the following.

Charmaz, K. (1987). Struggling for a self: Identity levels of the chronically ill. In J. Roth & P. Conrad (Eds.), *Research in the sociology of health care* (pp. 283–321). Greenwich, CT: JAI Press.

Corbin, J., & Strauss, A. L. (1988). Experiencing body failure and a disrupted self image. In J. Corbin & A. L. Strauss (Eds.), *Unending work and care: Managing chronic illness at home* (pp. 49–67). San Francisco: Jossey-Bass.

Goffman, E. (1974). *Frame analysis: An essay on the organization of experience.* New York: Harper Colophon.

Pickering, A. (1995). *The mangle of practice: Time, agency, and science.* Chicago: University of Chicago Press.

hesitant and nonassertive ways, probably because they are uncertain what is expected of them and are afraid to seem rude or ignorant.

Although a caregiver may conceive of health as a biological phenomenon to be identified by its physical manifestations, patients usually interpret illnesses in light of their effects on everyday activities. The Voice of Lifeworld is concerned with feelings and events. Patients' communication and their willingness to self-advocate are influenced by a variety of factors, including the nature of their illness, their personality, and their communication skills. Throughout the chapter, experts offer suggestions for patients on how to be more active participants in medical encounters.

Patient satisfaction is often based more on how caregivers listen and empathize than on perceived technical competency. Doctors who seem interested, genuinely caring, and sympathetic rate highest in patients' assessments. Patients also appreciate having a sense of control and being treated with dignity. Interestingly, patients tend to have serious complaints but still consider themselves as satisfied overall with their doctors' care. Nursing homes and hospitals usually get lower satisfaction scores than doctors, mostly because patients perceive that their pain is not adequately managed and that they are not kept well informed.

Patients' adherence to medical advice is notoriously low for a range of reasons, including limited money and resources, mistrust of the diagnosis or treatment plan, a sense that the illness is cured, and a perception that the treatment (including drug side effects) is worse than the disease. Although patients may have good reasons for not following medical advice, the results can be disastrous for patients, doctors, and the public. Many health advocates urge patients and caregivers to be more explicit about negotiating treatment options that are practical and acceptable.

Ethical principles and U.S. laws stipulate that patients be well informed about health choices and allowed to decide for themselves what care they will and will not receive. Informed-consent laws protect people from atrocities such as the Tuskegee Syphilis Study, but some cases fall within a gray zone in which it is difficult to determine when patients are too distraught or fearful to make informed choices.

Illness can affect people's very identity. Evidence suggests that people work to maintain their identities, even when illness changes their patterns of behavior. Narratives are a key component of patient talk and may reveal much more than factual details. Storytellings usually reflect how people view the world, how they see themselves in relation to others, and what events are most significant to them. Information of this sort can give caregivers valuable insight.

Patients may respond to illness in many ways—from relief to terror—and may experience changes in their personal identity as a result of illness. The integrated health theory describes the importance of alignment and resistance in maintaining good health.

Now that you have an overview of patient issues, read Chapter 6, in which you will learn how health and health communication are influenced by diversity in age, race, income, ability, language, sexual orientation, and more.

## KEY TERMS

Voice of Lifeworld
self-advocates
Tuskegee Syphilis Study
informed consent
personal identity
social identities
tertiary identity
supernormal identity
restored self
contingent personal identity
salvaged self
narrative
sustaining narratives
enduring narratives
preserving narratives
fracturing narratives
integrative health theory
resistance

## DISCUSSION QUESTIONS

1.  What is the Voice of Lifeworld?
2.  How is a patient's philosophy of health and illness traditionally different from a doctor's?
3.  What suggestions do Roizen and Oz (2006) present for being a smart patient?
4.  Have you ever found yourself unable to tell a doctor what you wanted to say? If so, what held you back? What factors would make it easier for you to communicate openly?
5.  How do patients typically behave when their goals are different than their doctors'?
6.  What advice does Groopman (2007) offer to patients for helping their doctors?
7.  What are some career opportunities in patient advocacy?
8.  What factors are linked with patient satisfaction? What communication behaviors are associated with these factors?
9.  What are some factors that patients tend to associate with a loss of dignity?
10. What reasons might patients have for not following medical advice?
11. Have you ever not followed medical advice? Why or why not?
12. Would you be more likely to follow medical advice if you were to get a cash prize for doing so? Why or why not?
13. How does patient–caregiver cooperation affect patients and caregivers?
14. What are the stipulations of informed consent? What are some ethical considerations associated with informed consent?
15. What are the four stages in Charmaz's (1987) model of identity management during chronic illness?
16. What do you think of Dr. Falchuk's approach? Why do you think more doctors do not take this approach?
17. What is the significance of what Halkowski (2006) calls a "sequence of noticings"?
18. Why are narratives important to health communication?
19. Describe the four types of narratives identified by J. Brown and Addington-Hall (2007).
20. Describe integrative health theory. What is meant by *alignment*? By *resistance*?

## ANSWER TO *CAN YOU GUESS?*

The United States excels in terms of how quickly sick patients with insurance are able to see their doctors (K. Davis et al., 2006).

# CHAPTER
# 6

# Diversity Among Patients

*She was in a motorized wheelchair that she controlled with her only usable finger. I could not understand her guttural speech or her facial contortions. She could not consistently hold her head up or control her drooling. After a few desperate moments, I asked her if she knew how to use a typewriter. She managed to make me understand a "yes" answer, and I ran out of the room to locate a typewriter on a movable stand. Pleased with my ingenuity, I stood next to her expecting some limited request. My smugness gave way to sheer awe as she painstakingly, letter by letter, tapped out with her left fourth finger the question: "What are the risks for me taking the birth control pill?" (Candib, 1994, p. 139)*

In this account, Lucy Candib (1994) recalls a young woman who taught her to respect each patient as an individual. In the scope of health care, it is easy to group patients within impersonal categories. However, there is extraordinary diversity among the people who seek care. This chapter explores patient diversity in terms of status, gender, sexual orientation, race and ethnicity, language, disabilities, and age. As you will see, each has an impact on health communication. *Skill Builder* sections provide tips on overcoming status barriers, interacting with people who have disabilities, talking to children about illness, and reaching members of marginalized populations.

## STATUS DIFFERENCES

A basic law of communication is that people who are similar are likely to understand each other better. In a study of pediatrician and parents (T. N. Brown, Ueno, Smith, Austin, & Bickman, 2007), when parents and doctors were of the same race, they shared

more laughter during the exam. When they were of the same gender, the parents asked more biomedical questions than other patients. And when doctors and parents were both highly educated, they shared more laughter, more expressions of concern, more self-disclosure, and more biomedical information. The authors speculate that similarities increased the participants' sense of comfort and affinity.

Conversely, when high-status caregivers communicate with poor and illiterate patients their life experiences are likely to be so different that they have a hard time understanding and warming up to each other. Patients of low **socioeconomic status** (SES is a combined measure of such factors as income, education, and employment level) are consistently less satisfied with medical care than other patients (Becker & Newsom, 2003).

### Misunderstandings
Research supports that misunderstandings occur for several reasons when caregivers interact with low-SES patients. First, low-SES patients typically

131

ask fewer questions than others and reveal less about their health concerns (B. A. Fowler, 2006). This occurs despite evidence that they are typically more fearful about their health than most people and less able to judge the severity of their illnesses themselves (James et al., 2008).

Second, although low-SES patients are more likely than others to follow doctors' advice, they may not be receiving as much information or guidance. In Bao, Fox, and Escarce's (2007) study of 5,978 patient interactions, physicians were more likely to discuss cancer screening with patients of high, rather than low, SES, particularly if the high-SES patients were well educated. For all tests except mammograms, doctors were twice as likely to discuss cancer screening with patients who were college graduates than with patients who had not finished high school. Race and ethnicity also played a factor. White and black patients were significantly more likely than Hispanic or Asian patients to take part in detailed discussions with their doctors. Bao and colleagues speculate that the difference lies partly with patients and partly with doctors. Low-SES patients may initiate fewer discussions because they are not knowledgeable about the issues, they are intimidated by doctors, and/or cultural mores dissuade them from questioning their doctors. For their part, doctors may perceive (rightly or wrongly) that low-SES patients will not be interested in—or capable of understanding—many details about their health.

Third, low-SES patients are less likely than others to benefit from written materials. About one in two adults in the United States is unable to read above an 8th-grade level (National Commission on Adult Literacy, 2008), and some adults who can read are not proficient in English. Some U.S. hospitals report a 300% increase in the number of Spanish-speaking patients since 1998 (Brice, Travers, Cowden, Young, Sanhueza, & Dunston, 2008). Worldwide, about 774 million adults (two-thirds of them women) cannot read (UNESCO, 2008). In the United States, literacy is a special challenge for non-English-speaking patients, many of whom cannot read medical consent forms or instructions on a medicine bottle.

Unlike other patients—who may be exposed to health information via pamphlets, cable television, newspapers, computers, and other means—low-income and literacy-challenged patients are likely to rely strictly on their doctors and advice from people they know. (We'll talk more about language and health literacy later in the chapter.)

Fourth, it may be especially tricky to negotiate treatment decisions when patients have limited means. Physicians surveyed by Susannah Bernheim and associates (2008) said that, ideally, SES should not be a factor when making treatment decisions, but practically speaking it often *is*, because the patient's work schedule limits what he or she can do (e.g., get physical therapy three times a week), because some medications are too expensive for low-income patients to afford, and because it is difficult to find specialists or therapists who will care for patients of limited financial means. Said one doctor in the study:

> He [a patient] was a trucker…we really had to tailor the medication. He did not have any proper time to eat, and you know, he did not have time to come to his appointments. We have to tailor his appointments according to his travel schedule. It is not optimal, but we do the best we can. (p. 56)

In this and other ways, physicians surveyed say they try to do their best, but they are often constrained by factors outside their control (Bernheim, Ross, Krumholz, & Bradley, 2008).

Finally, preconceived notions can be a stumbling block to communication between caregivers and low-SES patients. Many of the general practitioners Sara Willems and colleagues (2005) interviewed consider that people are impoverished mostly because they don't try hard enough to overcome their circumstances. Said one doctor: "They don't want to change their situation,…they are used to it. They no longer have the courage to change it" (p. 179). Physicians interviewed also tend to view low-SES patients as indifferent about staying healthy. As one doctor put it, "They are not interested in their health. They don't see the advantage of, for example, healthy food" (p. 180). Although these were common viewpoints, some doctors in the study *were* vigorous advocates of seeking care for impoverished patients and actively trying to help them improve their neighborhoods and living conditions.

## Health Literacy

About 90 million people in the United States suffer from health literacy challenges and the consequent health risks ("Health Literacy," 2003). Health literacy involves reading and understanding health information, but it's more than that. As defined by WHO, **health literacy** "represents the cognitive and social skills which determine the motivation and ability of individuals to gain access to, understand and use information in ways which promote and maintain good health" ("Health Promotion Glossary," 1998, p. 10). This definition emphasizes that it is not enough to read and write. To be literate about health, people must also:

- Understand the language in which information is conveyed (be it English, Spanish, statistical jargon, legal talk, or some other language variant),
- Have access to reliable and relevant information,
- Be interested in health-related information,
- Have the social skills to discuss health matters with others,
- Have adequate hearing and/or vision to get the information,
- Understand how to apply the information, and
- Be willing and able to put health information to effective use.

Regarded this way, it is clear that none of us is entirely health literate. Medical information is often baffling, even to well-educated individuals. A study by J. D. Power and Associates (2008) revealed that less than half (45%) of people across the United States fully understand their health plans. About one in five Americans is unable to read a prescription bottle, one in two cannot understand a medical brochure, and three in five cannot understand a

consent form (AMA, 2003). For some people, reading is a challenge, but other factors include math skills, the ability to see and hear well, and English proficiency. Emotions also play a role. Otherwise highly literate people may feel so overwhelmed by what they are hearing that they cannot pay attention to medical information. And sometimes information is so complex that people cannot be expected to understand it. When we consider that 8 in 10 people cannot understand a Medicaid application (AMA, 2003), it seems that the real problem is the form rather than the readers.

Low literacy is masked by embarrassment. People are often too ashamed to admit they are unable to read or understand medical information (Bernhardt & Cameron, 2003). Even friends and family members may not realize it. At a briefing to launch the AMA's new health literacy initiative, physician David W. Baker said:

> We find that a lot of people have gone through their lives and listen to the radio, watch television and don't read their newspapers too often but can get by pretty well with minimal reading skills.... They come into the health care setting and they are all of a sudden faced with medications and instructions and all of this information written at too high a level for easy comprehension. (AMA, 2003, paragraph 7)

Embarrassment and frustration may discourage people with literacy challenges from pursuing medical care and may lead them to take medicine incorrectly, overlook health risk factors, and miss out on important information.

These factors contribute to worsening health and higher expenses. In the United States, costs incurred because of health literacy challenges are estimated at $106 billion to $238 billion a year (Vernon, Trujillo, Rosenbaum, & DeBuono, 2007). That's enough money to insure all 47 million uninsured residents of the country!

About 90% of patients with literacy challenges say it would be helpful if their doctors understood their limitations (Wolf et al., 2007). Clearly, compassionate communication is required to help people

BOX 6.1  **RESOURCES**

## More About the Health Literacy Initiative

AMA's *Ask Me 3* health literacy materials and
video: www.npsf.org/askme3

Health Literacy: A Prescription to End Confusion:
http://www.iom.edu/?id=19723&redirect=0

Low Health Literacy: Implications for National
Health Policy: http://www.gwumc.edu/sphhs/
departments/healthpolicy/chsrp/downloads/
LowHealthLiteracyReport10_4_07.pdf

with literacy challenges feel comfortable asking for help.

The AMA and cosponsors have launched *Ask Me 3*, an effort to minimize the literacy gap. *Ask Me 3* is a simple program that encourages patients to ask questions and seek clarification when they talk with medical professionals. Patients are encouraged to ask their doctors, nurses, and pharmacists these three questions:

- What is my main problem?
- What do I need to do?
- Why is it important for me to do this?

Simple and attractive *Ask Me 3* materials reassure people that "Everyone wants help with health information. You are not alone if you find things confusing at times." Handouts suggest options for patients who feel confused. For example, if they do not understand answers to the suggested questions, patients are encouraged to say, "This is new to me. Will you please explain that to me one more time." (For more about the Health Literacy Initiative, see Box 6.1.)

Other promising avenues include using interactive computer modules (some of them multilingual) to teach patients about antibiotic use (Leeman-Castillo et al., 2007) and medical decision making (Jibaja-Weiss & Volk, 2007) and videos about treatment options so that people with literacy challenges can better understand the risks and benefits before they consent. Because these formats present information both visually and verbally, they help overcome many communication barriers, particularly when designers take into account that some users will have limited reading and computer skills.

### Communication Skill Builders: Surmounting Status Barriers

The unfortunate result of status-related communication barriers is that the neediest people receive the least amount of information and attention. Experts offer the following ideas for improving communication between caregivers and patients with low health literacy.

- *Caregivers: Be attentive and respectful.* Try to identify patients' needs and respect their contributions. Double-check patients' understanding of verbal information, listen attentively, and do not be put off by colloquialisms. In an article titled "All I Really Need to Know About Medicine I Learned from My Patients," physician Dwalia South (1997) says most patients do not have large medical vocabularies. They describe unfamiliar lumps and bumps as "hickeys" and "doodads." Nonetheless, people know a lot about their own bodies, and smart caregivers take patients' knowledge seriously.

- *Caregivers: Let patients know what is expected.* Bochner (1983) suggests that low-SES patients may be tongue-tied by intimidation or may simply be unaware of what is expected of them. He encourages doctors to socialize patients into the medical context by explaining routines and encouraging them to participate in discussions.

- *Patients: Be explicit about feelings and questions.* Do not assume caregivers understand your concerns. Instead, make an extra effort to express your feelings and questions. You can improve communication by overcoming your reluctance to speak up.

## GENDER DIFFERENCES

It is naive to assume that all women or all men communicate in the same way. Neither are males and females always different in how they communicate. Whether male, female, young, or old, patients tend to want the same things, namely, caring and respect. Studies do indicate some general differences and similarities, however.

Research has typically indicated no significant difference in emotional intelligence between male and female medical students (Stratton, Saunders, & Elam, 2008). But men and women typically display different affective styles. Compared to men, female patients and caregivers tend to be more nonverbally expressive in health care situations, engage in more partnership-building behaviors, and reveal more personal information about themselves (Gabbard-Alley, 1995, 2000). Females in the United States are also more knowledgeable than males about health issues. This may be because women are most often targeted as consumers, they utilize medical services more than men, and they typically feel more responsible for the health of family members ("Women Most Active," 2003).

A New Zealand study presents evidence that rapport with female patients is typically greater if the doctor is a woman rather than a man (Gross et al., 2008). The researchers found that male doctors were more likely than female doctors to assume that female patients had a hidden agenda and were exaggerating their symptoms. For their part, female patients were more timid when interacting with male doctors than with female ones. Again, familiarity seems to foster trust and openness.

Research in the United States indicates only slight differences between the preferences of male and female patients. Men typically have no strong preference concerning the sex of their doctors, whereas women indicate a slight preference for female caregivers and women's clinics as compared to traditional clinics (Bean-Mayberry et al., 2003; Piper, Shvarts, & Lurie, 2008).

In the next section we discuss **heterosexism**, the assumption that people's romantic relationships involve members of the opposite sex.

## SEXUAL ORIENTATION

In the article "Do Ask, Do Tell," physician Jennifer E. Potter (2002) asserts that gay and lesbian individuals often receive substandard care because doctors are not aware of or misunderstand their sexual orientation and behaviors. Potter recalls her own experience as a teenager, when, after telling her family physician she was attracted to girls, he laughed it off as a "phase a lot of girls go through" (p. 341). Later, a psychiatrist tried to "cure" her of homosexual tendencies, and doctors urged her to use birth control, never considering that she might be sexually active with women rather than men. Although Potter regarded the prescription for the pill "absurd," previous experience told her to keep the truth to herself. Even as a student at Harvard Medical School, Potter was encouraged to keep her lesbianism secret.

Fear of social rejection can rob homosexual individuals of comfort and acceptance. Potter (2002) describes the temptation to "pass" as heterosexual: "On the face of it, maintaining silence makes almost everyone happy" (p. 342). But pretending to be heterosexual felt like lying by omission. She says that pretending to be something she wasn't eroded her self-respect, unwittingly put her in cahoots with people who wished to ignore and invalidate homosexuality, and made her feel isolated. She could not introduce her long-term partner to friends or invite her to professional and social gatherings. Now, although Potter is open with her close friends and associates, other people still make erroneous assumptions about her lifestyle. Although it may seem inappropriate or awkward to reveal her sexual orientation to new acquaintances, misunderstandings can make people feel embarrassed or deceived. Potter reflects: "Coming out is a process that never ends. Every time I meet someone new I must decide if, how, and when I will reveal my sexual orientation" (p. 342).

Discrimination is a particularly threatening possibility when one's health is at risk. For example, some homosexual women with cancer say they fear they will receive substandard care if they reveal their sexual orientation to their doctors (Matthews,

1998). However, keeping quiet about homosexuality presents risks as well. Although a vaccination against hepatitis A is recommended for men who have sex with men, a study in Birmingham, Alabama, revealed that only 34% of gay African American men there had been vaccinated (Rhodes, Yee, & Hergenrather, 2003). The researchers found that men who had open communication with their caregivers were more likely than others to be aware of the hepatitis risk and to seek the vaccination.

The tell-or-not dilemma may be especially difficult for older adults. A Canadian study reveals that homosexuality among older adults is largely ignored by society and by health care providers (Brotman, Ryan, & Cormier, 2003). Moreover, older adults who are homosexual may be especially sensitive to societal stereotypes and lack of acceptance, although they may be in long-term relationships that are important to their happiness.

In the United States (although not in other countries), a disproportionate number of HIV/AIDS cases have occurred among homosexual males, adding to the stigma and stress they may already feel. In a study of homosexual couples in which one or both partners has HIV/AIDS, Haas (2002) found that primary relational partners provided the majority of support during the illness, followed by friends and family members. Ignoring or minimizing the importance of these relationships can have serious consequences for people's coping abilities.

Caregivers who avoid talking about sexuality are not necessarily prejudiced against it. They may be embarrassed or uncomfortable with the subject or feel that it lies outside their expertise. Richard Gamlin (1999) proposes that nurses should strive to become more comfortable with their own sexuality and should use role-playing to gain experience talking about sexuality with patients. Caregivers who are comfortable discussing sexuality are more likely to help patients feel comfortable. In one study, adolescents said they think it is important for their caregivers to know their sexual history, and they are most comfortable revealing this information when the caregivers asks about sexual issues directly (Rosenthal et al., 1999).

---

**BOX 6.2**

## Can You Guess?

1. Which country has the longest average life expectancy?
2. Which country has the shortest average life expectancy?
3. How does the average life span for men and women in the United States compare?

*Answers appear at the end of the chapter.*

---

In summary, like everyone else, homosexual individuals are adversely affected when they feel they cannot be open with their caregivers. As you will see in the next sections, a similar fear of discrimination influences people of different races.

## RACE

Racism can make you sick. That is the conclusion of studies linking race to everyday well-being, medical care, and life expectancy. As this section shows, people of nondominant races and ethnicities are at a disadvantage where health and longevity are concerned.

**Racism** is discrimination based on a person's race. People belong to a certain race if they share a hereditary background or common descent, such as European or African (Merriam-Webster, 1999). Practically speaking, people often judge race by visible characteristics such as skin color. Because the black/white distinction is so visible, it is the basis for a great deal of racism, with direct and indirect effects on health.

In the United States, race is associated with life expectancy. The average life span of an African American male is 69.5 years, which is 6.3 years shorter than the average white male (National Center for Health Statistics, 2007a). Likewise, African American women live an average of 76.5 years—4.31 years shorter than most white women.

Research shows that the link between health and race is social rather than biological. In other words, people of minority status do not suffer ill health because of the genes they are born with but because of what occurs during their lifetimes (Bhopal, 1998).

## Different Care and Outcomes

Some researchers suggest that people of color receive different medical care than others. In its 2003 report "Unequal Treatment: Confronting Racial and Ethnic Disparities in Health Care," the Institute of Medicine summarized research about health disparities (Smedley, Stith, & Nelson, 2003). Among the findings: Hispanic Americans are twice as likely as others to die from diabetes and African Americans are significantly more likely than others to die from cancer, heart disease, and AIDS. Part of the reason is that they receive different care. For example, African Americans are less likely than European Americans to receive advanced cardiac therapy while they recover from a heart attack (Peterson et al., 2008). Similarly, in an extensive study of 20,915 people with cancer in the head or neck, Molina and colleagues (2008) found that white patients lived an average of 40 months, compared to 21 months for African Americans. The difference was significant even when researchers controlled for age, income, and other health concerns.

Only slightly more promising is evidence that black patients live about as long as white patients (about 6 years) following their first hospitalization for heart failure (Croft et al., 1999). However, black patients are typically younger than white patients, so, although their response to initial treatment is roughly the same, they experience ill health sooner in their lives and often die at a younger age.

## Explanations

There are several explanations why people of different races seem to receive different medical care and may respond differently to it. Overall, differences seem rooted in distrust, high risk, lack of knowledge, limited access, and ineffective patient–caregiver communication.

*Distrust* One explanation for the link between race and health is that people of color are less likely to pursue medical attention, because they distrust the medical establishment. Based on historic patterns of discrimination (like the Tuskegee Syphilis Study described in Chapter 5), members of minority races may distrust medical personnel (Meredith, Eisenman, Rhodes, Ryan, & Long, 2007).

In the United States, members of racial and ethnic minorities are more likely than European Americans to feel that their doctors fail to listen, show respect, and explain things clearly ("Doctor–Patient Communication by Race/Ethnicity," 2008). About 14% of Asian Americans feel this way, 12% of Hispanic Americans, and 11% of African Americans—compared to 9% of white Americans.

Distrust may cause people to underutilize health services and to doubt the validity of medical advice (Armstrong et al., 2008). This could contribute to the comparatively low number of medical interventions among African Americans and Hispanics. They may be approved for prescriptions they never fill or may decline to undergo medical procedures if they distrust their doctors' judgment. Or they may never see a doctor at all.

*High Risk, Low Knowledge* A second explanation is that members of minority races are not well informed about health issues, despite the fact that they are often at high risk for disease. African American men are significantly less knowledgeable about prostate cancer warning signs than white men, although African American men are twice as likely to die of prostate cancer (Weinrich et al., 2007). Members of minority races may also be at high risk for disease because a disproportionate number of them are of low socioeconomic status. With limited resources, they may suffer from poor living conditions, unhealthy diets, and insufficient access to health information and health services (Baldwin, 2003). For example, people with limited resources are often forced to live in violent and polluted neighborhoods (Ahmed, Mohammed, & Williams, 2007).

There is also evidence that everyday discrimination threatens people's health. A survey of black, white, Hispanic, and Asian individuals shows that ill health is higher among people who are subjected to everyday discrimination, such as poor service, insults, and being treated as inferior or stupid (Gallo, Smith, & Cox, 2006). The researchers conclude that the stress of dealing with negative social feedback takes a significant toll on people's health.

Despite their high-risk status, members of minority races may be relatively unaware of health issues because they do not use or trust mainstream media as much as white audiences and because many health messages are not designed to appeal to minority audiences. Individuals who are not well informed about health services and disease warning signs are more likely than others to become seriously ill before they seek medical attention (J. A. Ferguson et al., 1998). If African Americans are sicker than others when they seek medical care, that might explain (in part) why they do not respond to treatment as well and why they do not undergo the same procedures as other patients.

*Access*  A third explanation is that members of minority groups have comparatively low access to advanced medical facilities. In the United States, more than three out of four (78%) uninsured residents do not undergo recommended health screenings (Cantor, Schoen, Belloff, How, & McCarthy, 2007). Table 6.1 shows health statistics related to gender and ethnicity. As you can see, infant mortality rates are dramatically higher among African Americans than among other groups, and Hispanic Americans are more than twice as likely as white Americans to be uninsured and to lack a regular source of medical care (Cantor et al.).

Low-income individuals may not qualify for care in high-tech medical centers, and such centers are not likely to be located within low-income, minority neighborhoods. Consequently, they are less likely than other patients to end up in hospitals that offer advanced-care treatments such bypass surgery and chemotherapy. Even emergency response time may differ by social class. Canadian researchers report that residents of affluent neighborhoods usually get quicker ambulance service than people in poor neighborhoods and that the best paramedic crews are dispatched to rich neighborhoods (Govindarajan & Schull, 2003).

Moreover, patients who cannot pay their initial medical bills may be discouraged from returning. Sora Chung (2008) says she has seen patients who felt they couldn't return to see their doctors because they still owed $25 on their bill. And the access gap grows. Between 500 and 1,000 physicians in the United States have converted to **concierge medical practices**, which offer better-than-average patient–staff ratios and longer exam times, but only to patients who can afford to pay more than their insurance will cover. Concierge practices are one way around the frustrating limitations and reimbursement tables of managed care. The special attention is nice for patients who can afford it, but many worry that concierge practices will widen the gap between the health rich and the health poor (Lowes, 2008a). In short, low-income individuals may receive care that is less advanced and less personalized because the medical facilities available to them do not offer it.

*Patient–Caregiver Communication*  Finally, medical care may differ because of poor communication across racial and ethnic lines. Patients and caregivers may be uncomfortable with people of other races, may misinterpret communication cues, or may allow stereotypes to interfere with their judgment. Members of racial and ethnic minorities often feel that medical personnel are reluctant to implement costly procedures they might use to treat other patients. An African American participant in Meredith Grady and Tim Edgar's (2003) study remembers being diagnosed with diabetes and the diagnosing physician's reaction:

> He said, "I need to write this prescription for these pills, but you'll never take them and you'll come back and tell me you're still eating pig's feet and everything.... Then why do I still need to write this prescription?" And I'm like, "I don't eat pig's feet." (p. 393)

**Table 6.1  U.S. Statistics Relevant to Health Care, Race, and Ethnicity**

| | Percentage of Members in Each Category Who Fit the Description at Left | | |
|---|---|---|---|
| | **White Americans** | **Black Americans** | **Hispanic Americans** |
| Uninsured | 13.2% | 19.3% | 34% |
| Have not visited a doctor in 2 years | 17% | 9.4% | 18.7% |
| Needed to see a doctor in last year but were unable to afford it | 11% | 18.9% | 17.9% |
| Over age 50 who did not undergo recommended health screening | 58.1% | 63.8% | 64.3% |
| Without a usual source of medical care | 17.2% | 22.5% | 35% |
| Infant mortality per 1,000 live births | 5.9 | 13.7 | 6.3 |

Source: The Commonwealth Fund Commission on a High Performance Health System (Cantor, Schoen, Belloff, How, & McCarthy, 2007).

The patient was left to wonder how the doctor's prejudicial assumptions affected other decisions as well.

The idea that stereotypes affect physicians' judgment is supported by research. Some 55% of doctors surveyed say they believe white patients receive better care than minority patients, and nearly two out of three have personally witnessed such episodes ("Physicians Are Becoming," 2005). To put this idea to the test, Schulman and colleagues (1999) videotaped actor/patients describing chest pains using the same words and gestures, wearing identical clothing (hospital gowns), in the same setting. The patients differed only in terms of age, sex, and race. Doctors who viewed the patients' videotaped presentations of symptoms were significantly more likely to recommend heart catheterization for male and white patients than for female or black patients. This suggests that—all other things being equal—racial and sexist stereotypes do influence physicians' judgments. These stereotypes are likely to affect how doctors perceive patients' conditions and the treatment they recommend. (See Box 6.3 for a discussion of ethical principles when allocating health resources.)

In summary, research shows that racism affects health and health care in varying degrees depending on the level of patients' trust, their knowledge and health risk, access to medical information and services, and stereotypes affecting patient–caregiver communication. Many of these issues can be addressed with more effective communication. Verbal and nonverbal signs of acceptance are appreciated. In one study, African American and Latino-American patients said they felt more comfortable with caregivers who had culturally sensitive artwork, reading material, and music in their offices (Tucker et al., 2003).

What's more, a new type of discrimination—based on health conditions that haven't even surfaced yet—may loom ahead. See Box 6.4 for information about the pros and cons of genetic testing results.

## LANGUAGE DIFFERENCES

"Every day, I jotted [Spanish] vocabulary words on index cards and studied them before each shift," says physician Harold Jenkins (2008, p. 42). "Commuting to work, I recited road signs and license plate numbers in Spanish. I even rolled my Rs." Spanish-speaking nurses have encouraged Jenkins. They are not put off that he can only speak in present tense and that his pronunciation is sometimes a bit off. (One nurse was amused when Jenkins asked a patient to "vacuum deeply" instead of inhaling.) They give him a thumbs-up for trying. His patients appreciate the effort as well. Jenkins says he feels like a better doctor when he can understand and speak at least a bit of the patients' language.

## BOX 6.3 ETHICAL CONSIDERATIONS

# Who Gets What Care?

"Doctor, do everything you can!"

Is it ever justified for a doctor to do less than everything possible? Conventional American wisdom says no. Americans have come to expect that physicians will provide the best possible care, cost notwithstanding. However, it has become too expensive to do everything possible for every person.

For example, after Oregon officials decided to remove organ transplants from the list of procedures covered by Medicaid, media stories abounded about people who were being allowed to die. One of the highest-profile cases was 7-year-old Colby Howard, whose life depended on a $100,000 bone marrow transplant. His family went public asking for donations, and they raised $700,000, but Colby died before they could raise enough. Floyd McCay, a spokesperson for the Oregon governor's office at the time, said:

> We are rationing health care on the basis of price. The state shouldn't have to pay for these things to begin with. But as long as they are forced to make decisions, you will have children with names and faces that will die or have severe difficulties. (quoted by Egan, 1988, paragraph 10)

An Oregon physician explained that, for the price of one organ transplant, the state could fund prenatal care for about 25 pregnant women, an investment with broader implications and the potential to avoid expensive care for premature and unhealthy newborns.

Many people feel that if the U.S. health system is to survive, it is necessary to make judgments about who gets what care. Health care is being called on to eliminate excessive and unnecessary procedures. The question is: Where is the line between necessary and unnecessary?

One option is to provide care to those people who can afford it. This option places underprivileged persons at a disadvantage and may create a deeper schism between people of high and low socioeconomic status. All in all, few people are willing to allow low-income citizens to suffer in ill health.

Another option is to give priority to procedures that are known to have high success rates. For instance, a procedure that gives patients a 30% chance of survival may be granted priority over one with a 20% survival rate. This seems logical, but it is difficult to allow patients to go untreated when there is even a 1 in 5 chance of saving their lives. As Norman Levinsky (1995) points out, statistics are merely generalizations, and every patient is unique. There is no guarantee that a risky procedure will fail or that a tried-and-true one will succeed. Moreover, statistics vary, and sticking with well-established procedures diminishes the chances of developing new, better treatments.

Still another option is to provide care for people who are likely to enjoy the highest quality of life as a result. From that perspective, it might be more important to fund expensive treatment to help a young child walk than to help an 85-year-old use his legs again following a stroke. Levinsky (1995) warns that such judgment calls are likely to lead to unfair discrimination. He wonders how it is possible to judge people's quality of life, and warns that such judgments are likely to be biased against people who hold values different from the medical decision maker's.

As you can see, deciding how health resources will be allocated is no simple matter. To get an idea of how difficult it is, try answering the following questions.

## What Do You Think?

1. If one person can afford expensive treatment but another cannot, is it OK to refuse care to the less affluent person?
2. If there is a slight chance that an expensive experimental drug will prolong a dying person's life, should the insurance company or health organization pay for use of the drug?
3. If two patients suffer from the same condition, should they be treated differently? What if one is a child and one is very old? What if one is famous and the other is unknown? What if

one is homeless and the other is a community leader?
4. If you could fund only two of the following procedures, which would you choose? On what criteria would you base your choices?
   a. Surgery to help an infertile couple conceive a child
   b. Plastic surgery to improve the appearance of a person born with a facial deformity
   c. Chemotherapy for a very sick person
   d. Drug therapy that might prevent a person from getting AIDS
5. Who should decide which care will be funded? Doctors? Funding agencies? Community members? Patients? Legislators?
6. If research is able to develop improved treatment options but the cost of the research significantly raises health care costs, should the system continue to fund research? What if higher costs mean some people will lose their insurance?
7. Doctors say one reason they overtreat patients is because they may be sued for malpractice if they do not do everything possible. How would you resolve this dilemma?

---

He's right. It's hard to offer quality care across a language gap. A physician at Maimonides Medical Center in New York asserts:

> It is great training for your young residents to understand that when you walk up to a person from another country who speaks another language, that is a risk—period. It's as much of a risk factor as diabetes or anything else…if you had an internal point system to admit the patient, you should add 25% of risk. (quoted by Salamon, 2008, paragraph 5)

Cognizant of the risk, Maimonides employs more than 30 patient representatives who help families and interpret when needed. And medical center President and CEO Pamela Brier has implemented a "Code of Mutual Respect," complete with staff training sessions on communication and diversity appreciation. The extra effort is worth it, says Brier:

> Communication problems are what cause mishaps that can harm patients. I mean communications between doctor and nurse, nurse and clerk, housekeeper to nurse or doctor, everybody. The idea of the "Code of Mutual Respect" for me was to make the place safer and medical care better. (quoted by Salamon, paragraph 9)

It's her conviction that good communication is good medicine and good business.

Nearly 21 million people in the United States do not speak or understand English proficiently (Gany & Ngo-Metzger, 2008). Non-English speakers are predictably less satisfied than others with medical care (Weech-Maldonado et al., 2003), and parents of Spanish-speaking children are more likely than other parents to fear that their children will be misdiagnosed or given the wrong medicine (Flores, Abreu, Olivar, & Kastner, 1998). (Box 6.5 describes the experiences of a Spanish-speaking woman in a U.S. hospital.)

Language barriers can be frustrating for patients and caregivers. It's difficult to make an accurate diagnosis if the caregiver can't fully understand what the patient is experiencing. And even if the diagnosis is correct, it's hard to ensure that patients are fully informed concerning their medical options.

For the most part, the U.S. health system hasn't kept pace with the rising number of Spanish-speaking residents. At one urban children's hospital, 68% of residents speak little or no Spanish, yet most say they care for patients with limited English proficiency "often" or "every day" (O'Leary, Federico, & Hampers, 2003). Most of the residents feel that Spanish-speaking families understand the diagnosis only "sometimes" or "never," and 80% of the residents say they avoid caring for these patients whenever possible.

BOX 6.4

# Genetic Profiling: A View into Your Health Future

*"The crystal ball says you will live a long and healthy life."*

It's hard to put much stock in such a prediction. But scientists have come up with something better. They did it by unlocking the codes that make up our genetic blueprints. To understand how, let's review some basic biology.

The cells in our bodies are home to DNA (deoxyribonucleic acid) molecules. Sequences of DNA, called *genes*, serve as a living instruction book for cellular activity. Genes determine our eye color and other physical features we inherit from our parents, how our bodies react to the environment, how we metabolize food, what diseases we are likely to get during our lifetime, and more. There are 20,000 to 25,000 genes in the human body.

In 2003, scientists around the world completed the Human Genome Project, a 13-year odyssey during which they catalogued nearly all of the genes and chemical base pairs (about 3 billion of them) in the human body ("Human Genome," 2008). For example, the gene Zbtb7 (rather cleverly code named Pokémon) enables other cells to become cancerous, but when inactive, it seems to inhibit cancer (Maeda et al., 2005). Scientists are still investigating what makes genes such as this seem to turn on and off.

Sophisticated knowledge of genetics better enables medical scientists to look into our future— or at least the future to which we are genetically predisposed. For example, you might have genetic testing done early in life to find out if you are predisposed to various forms of cancer, liver disease, Alzheimer's disease, or other conditions known to have a genetic link. Being predisposed to these diseases doesn't mean you will necessarily get them. In fact, that's the main promise of genetic testing. You might find out in time to lower your odds. For example, you might engage in more preventive behaviors if you know

you are at high risk. Your doctor might start screening you for the identified conditions earlier than usual and, in some cases, begin preventive therapies. Focusing on genes might also help medical scientists design new ways of treating and preventing diseases. So far, the cost of a complete DNA workup is costly (at least $100,000), but scientists hope to reduce the cost to $1,000 a person by 2014 (Hall, 2006).

## Religious Perspective

But there are potential downsides. For one, some people see genetic testing as overstepping the boundaries between science and religious faith. In a series of focus groups, participants expressed a great deal of ambivalence about the issue. Some participants who believe in God said they feel that God's role ends at creating the genes that make a person unique, therefore genetic testing is not contradictory to their values. But some focus group members were openly apprehensive that, in deciphering the genetic code, scientists are "trying to do God's work" or "making changes to something that you are not supposed to be bothering" (Harris, Parrott, & Dorgan, 2004, p. 112). Participants were especially inclined to feel this way if they believe that God plays a role in illness and healing to the extent of changing a person's genetic structure after birth and/or if they feared that genetic profiling would be used to identify some people as worthier or superior to others (Harris et al.).

Another conflict between genetics and some people's religious faith lies in scientists' efforts to chart human history through genetic markers. In a *National Geographic* article titled "The Ultimate Family Tree" (2005), scientists with the Genographic Project describe genetic evidence that they believe links people around the world to African ancestors 60,000 years ago. Some people consider this evolutionary prospective contradictory to their religious beliefs.

For the most part, however, people seem not to consider genetic profiling to be a direct challenge to religion. After a survey of 858 people, a research team led by Roxanne Parrott (2004) concluded that respondents' religious faith did not predict most people's attitudes about genetic testing. Media exposure was a more powerful antecedent. Religious faith was not wholly irrelevant, however, because intrinsic religiosity (the degree to which an individual bases his or her worldview on religious beliefs) is often related to the type of media that person uses and trusts. The researchers suggest continued investigation to better understand the overlap between religion and health (Parrott, Silk, Krieger, Harris, & Condit, 2004).

## Fears of Discrimination

Another reservation concerning genetic testing is people's fear that the results will be used against them or their family members. So great is this fear that scientists sometimes have a hard time finding participants for research projects on the subject (Hudson, Holohan, & Collins, 2008). The issue is likely to become even more prominent when genetic testing is made available to the public.

To help ease those fears, U.S. lawmakers approved the Genetic Information Nondiscrimination Act of 2008 (better known as GINA). GINA stipulates that health insurance companies cannot refuse health coverage on the basis of genetic test results, nor can they require people to undergo genetic testing. By extension, GINA rules out informal genetic profiling, such as basing a person's insurance rates on a family history of heart disease. In the past, health insurance companies could figure family history into the price of your coverage. GINA now forbids that practice, although it does allow consideration of a person's current health status.

GINA also stipulates that employers cannot judge job applicants or current employees on the basis of genetic profiles. That is, they cannot hire, fire, promote, or refuse to promote anyone because of genetic propensities. Nor can employers require, request, or purchase genetic test results on any employee. (This does not apply to tests designed to monitor the effects of workplace exposure to dangerous materials. Those are still allowed.)

"GINA is the first major new civil rights bill of the new century," said Senator Edward Kennedy, a cosponsor of the bill, along with Olympia Snow (quoted by Hudson, Holohan, & Collins, 2008, paragraph 6). Many applaud the forward-thinking nature of the legislation, which was passed before the issue became a widespread concern.

It is important to note what GINA does not cover, however. The stipulations do not apply to life insurance, long-term care insurance, or disability insurance. And GINA does not apply to the U.S. military, the Veterans Administration, or Indian Health Services, because they are governed by a different set of laws.

## What Do You Think?

1. If it were affordable, would you undergo genetic testing? Why or why not?
2. Are you worried that genetic test results may be used to discriminate unfairly against individuals or groups of people? Why or why not?
3. Suppose your test results show a genetic propensity for a disease that, so far, we do not know how to prevent. Would you want to know? Why or why not?
4. Do you think genetic test results would strengthen your resolve to engage in healthy behaviors?

## Suggested Resources

To view an interview with Francis Collins, director of the National Human Genome Research Institute of the National Institutes of Health, visit: http://content. nejm.org.ezproxy.lib.uwf.edu/cgi/content/ full/358/25/2661/DC1

Humane Genome Project information: http:// www.ornl.gov/sci/techresources/Human_ Genome/faq/faqs1.shtml

## BOX 6.5 PERSPECTIVES

# Language Barriers in a Health Care Emergency

Picture yourself in Mexico at a hospital trying to get someone, anyone, to help make a terrible pain in your stomach go away. You hear: "Tu no hablas Español, y nadien te puede entender." In other words, "You don't speak Spanish, and no one can understand you." Finally, you find a first-year English student, a schoolboy, who attempts to translate. Next, you find yourself in a room, half-clothed, wearing a hospital robe, wondering: Did the boy understand me? Did the doctors understand him? What is wrong with me? What is happening?

Perhaps this will give you some idea what is like for Spanish speakers in the United States health care system. This is a true story about my mother, Maria, and her mother, Consuelo, Cuban Americans trying to deal with the frustrations, anxieties, and fears of communicating with medical professionals who speak a different language.

## The Story

Consuelo had been showing symptoms for some time before finally agreeing to see a doctor. Now that she had moved to a new city with little to no Hispanic culture, she wondered fearfully if she would be able to communicate with doctors. But this time the pain was intense, and at least she had her daughter, Maria, to help her communicate. Consuelo wanted very much to be understood, and maybe this time she would be. That thought finally gave her the courage to see a doctor.

At the doctor's office Consuelo could tell something was wrong. She was now in her early 60s and knew her diabetes was not getting any better. She understood enough of the conversations between the doctors and her daughter to gather that she needed a heart catheterization. Maria was not giving her all the details, but Consuelo could sense from her body language that the procedure was serious. She was right. A few moments later she found herself being wheeled

off to the operating room for an emergency catheterization—without Maria. Now she felt more scared and afraid, knowing she had no means of communicating with the people around her and unsure what they were doing or why.

Before the procedure the surgeon needed Consuelo to understand the process and answer some questions. This was no easy task. Once again, as Consuelo had feared, she was unable to communicate. By this time, she began feeling extremely anxious and frustrated that neither the surgeon nor any of his assistants could understand what she was saying. Finally, after what seemed decades, the surgeon summoned Maria to the operating room after finding no one else who could translate.

For Maria, the experience involved mixed emotions. She had accompanied her mother many times before to the hospital but had never been allowed inside the operating room. Now that she was there, she felt more anxious than ever. First, she wanted to do a good job because she felt her mother's life depended on it. Second, she felt uneasy being in the room because she was unfamiliar with the environment. Consequently, Maria did not know how she should act, what she should say, or what was expected of her. She also had to fight her emotional reactions at seeing her mother on the operating table. However, Maria was relieved to be able to be with her mother and decided to concentrate on positive feelings to get them both through the experience.

When Consuelo was back in a hospital room after the procedure, the doctor broke the news that Consuelo needed open-heart surgery and would soon be transferred to a larger hospital. Once again, Consuelo could tell something negative was being conveyed, but knew she would have to wait until the conversation was over to get the full story from Maria. Waiting only added to her anxiety. A few times, Consuelo tried to interrupt, but was only chastised by Maria for interfering with her efforts to understand the implications of what the doctor was trying to tell her.

Unfortunately, although the larger hospital was located within a predominantly Hispanic community, few doctors and nurses there could speak Spanish. That meant that Maria and her husband, Jesus, would have to take turns staying at the hospital to translate for Consuelo. But the difference in Consuelo's outlook was remarkable. After only a few hours in the new hospital, she started to feel better about herself and less depressed. This was because the new physicians, regardless of whether they spoke Spanish or not, attempted to speak to her in Spanish and to understand what she was saying. Consuelo recalled one young physician who would walk into her room saying, "Buenos dias," bringing a smile to her face, and then leave saying, "Buenas noches," despite the time of day, making her laugh. These small gestures made all the difference to Consuelo.

Maria noticed that her mother began to light up whenever a doctor entered the room. She also noted that the doctors were no longer looking at her but talking directly to her mother instead. Maria was still translating, but she was no longer the focus of their conversation. In return, she noticed that her mother seemed more attentive and willing to follow the doctors' advice. A few times, Consuelo even answered the physicians in English with responses such as "Yes" when she understood what they were saying. This in turn would make them laugh and rub her hand as a sign of acceptance and reward. And if this were not enough, Consuelo was introduced to a Spanish-speaking nurse at the hospital who would occasionally visit, making her feel even more at home.

The surgery went well, but following it, Consuelo was paired with a therapist who could not speak Spanish and made no effort to communicate with her. She began to feel depressed and frustrated again. But she learned to get over this new obstacle quickly after talking about her feelings with her family. They found a way to make her realize that her good experiences at the new hospital far outweighed the bad ones, and soon Consuelo was able to ignore the therapist's behavior and move on with her treatment.

Consuelo was in the hospital for about a month. In that time she learned a lot about what she liked and did not like. As a result, she asked Maria to help her look for doctors who would be as attentive with her as the hospital doctors had been. Now Consuelo has at least one doctor she likes very much who speaks Spanish.

—*Marie*

## What Do You Think?

1. How might you have acted if you were Consuelo? If you were Maria?
2. Do you think hospitals should do more to accommodate non-English speakers? Why or why not?
3. How could Consuelo have eliminated some of her anxiety?
4. What could the first surgeon have done to help both Maria and Consuelo feel more at ease?
5. Researchers have found that people are more fearful about medical visits if they feel socially alienated and disconnected from their environments. What might we do to ease these feelings?
6. Have you ever been in a situation in which you have had to communicate with someone who did not speak the same language as you? How did you handle the situation?

In many medical settings, family members and bilingual employees fill in as untrained interpreters. It's not uncommon for members of the housekeeping staff to do most of the interpreting, although they may speak English poorly themselves and have little knowledge of medical terminology. Medical centers may be hesitant to incur the expense of professional interpreters because guidelines for reimbursement are

## BOX 6.6 CAREER OPPORTUNITIES

### Diversity Awareness

Diversity officer
Health care interpreter
Equal Employment Opportunity (EEO) officer

### Career Resources and Job Listings

American Hospital Association's Institute for
Diversity in Health Management: www.
diversityconnection.org
"What is a Chief Diversity Officer?": www.
insidehighered.com/workplace/2006/04/18/williams

"Wanted: Bilingual Healthcare Workers":
http://career-advice.monster.com/business-
communication/healthcare/nursing/diversity-
inclusion/multicultural-workers/Wanted-
Bilingual-Healthcare-Workers/home.aspx
National Council on Interpreting in Health Care:
www.ncihc.org
Registry of Interpreters for the Deaf: www.rid.org
U.S. Equal Employment Opportunity Commission:
www.eeoc.gov
U.S. Bureau of Labor Statistics Occupational
Outlook Handbook: www.bls.gov/oco

---

unclear in many states. California has led the nation in this regard. Based on a new state law, health insurers there are now responsible for making sure patients have adequate language assistance (Vesely, 2008). Interpreter services in California say they expect hundreds of new requests every month (Vesely).

Other efforts are under way as well. Wake Forest University School of Medicine has piloted a training program to help physician assistants work effectively with interpreters and Spanish-speaking patients. After a four-hour training session, 94% to 97% of students were able to demonstrate proficiency in role-play scenarios that involved interpreters and non-English-speaking patients (Marion, Hildebrandt, Davis, Marin, & Crandall, 2008). Other organizations report success using trained interpreters who are either present in the exam room or linked via telephone or videoconference technology (D. Jones, Gill, Harrison, Meakin, & Wallace, 2003). There is even promising use of remote simultaneous interpreting similar to that used at the United Nations, which is particularly quick and accurate (Gany, Kapelusznik, et al., 2007).

For useful resources on becoming a diversity officer or medical interpreter, see Box 6.6 and read Elaine Hsieh's (2006) excellent article "Understanding Medical Interpreters."

## DISABILITIES

Joanne had time for a cup of coffee and a chance to read the newspaper. Friday was the day that the personal ads ran in the paper. Joanna reads these ads without fail, trying to picture what kind of man would write advertisements to find dates. Although she sometimes thought about answering one of these ads, she never did. What would she say? "Woman, 28 years old, math whiz, attractive, red hair, green eyes, like movies, jazz, loves to cook, uses a wheelchair to get around." No, she just couldn't picture it. (Braithwaite & Japp, 2005, p. 175)

Individuals with disabilities are often confronted with frustrating dichotomies. For one, people tend either to treat their disabilities as the most important thing about them or self-consciously to avoid the issue entirely. Health professionals have typically not received much training on how to communicate with people who have disabilities. Consequently, when treating these individuals, physicians often focus on the disability and ignore medical concerns that are not directly related to it (Braithwaite & Thompson, 2000). On the other hand, well-meaning acquaintances may consider it taboo to talk about the disability. A woman described by Dawn Braithwaite and Lynn Harter (2000) said she initially appreciated it when her future husband did not make a big deal about her disability when they met. But after several months getting to know each other, she was exasperated that he never even mentioned the subject. Eventually she brought it up, to end the awkward silence.

Another dichotomy concerns the way persons with disabilities are regarded by society. Sally Nemeth, a health communication scholar who is blind, reflects that people with disabilities are often cast "either as heroic super crips or as tragic, usually embittered and angry, unfortunates worthy only of pity and charity" (Nemeth, 2000, p. 40). The reality is that people with disabilities are much like anyone else.

It is frustrating to be treated as helpless or unsophisticated. Health professionals (and others) tend to treat individuals with disabilities as if they are childlike—speaking slowly and loudly to them even when that is not necessary and giving instructions rather than asking for their opinions. People may avoid talking to children with disabilities about sensitive subjects such as sex. I remember attending the wedding of a friend, Melissa, who had been deaf since age 6. Although Melissa was well into her 20s when she married, her family realized on the eve of her wedding that she knew nothing about birth control. The school Melissa attended did not provide sex education to students with disabilities, and her parents had always considered her too sheltered to need such information.

People whose disabilities are invisible to others may encounter unique difficulties. They face the dilemma of either keeping their illnesses a secret or revealing them to others and risking a changed social identity. Some individuals, particularly men, may be loath to admit disabilities they think will make them seem dependent or pitiful (L. W. Moore & Miller, 2003). A study of people with heart disease revealed that they consider themselves older than their same-age peers, largely because of physical limitations and attention to end-of-life issues typically associated with older people (Kundrat & Nussbaum, 2003). (For more about the frustration of invisible disabilities, see Box 6.7.)

These challenges have an effect on health communication. Individuals with disabilities are typically less satisfied with managed care providers than with doctors they choose themselves, mostly because doctors on a provider list may not be knowledgeable about or comfortable dealing with disabilities (Kroll, Beatty, & Bingham, 2003). And because of the need for trust and familiarity, it may be particularly stressful for persons with disabilities to change doctors (O'Connell, Bailey, & Pearce, 2003). Physicians admit that they *do* often feel uncomfortable caring for people with disabilities, particularly if they involve mental impairments (Aulagnier et al., 2005). On the bright side, even brief training sessions tend to help caregivers interact more confidently and sensitively (Tuffrey-Wijne, Hollins, & Curfs, 2005).

### Communication Skill Builders: Interacting with Persons Who Have Disabilities

- Talk to people with disabilities directly, not to their interpreters or companions.
- Remember to identify yourself to sight-impaired persons.
- Treat adults with disabilities as adults.
- When a person with a disability is difficult to understand, listen attentively, and then paraphrase to make sure you heard correctly.
- Whenever possible, sit down when speaking to people in wheelchairs so that you can communicate at eye level.
- Relax! For example, do not become embarrassed if you accidentally say to a blind person, "See you later."
- Do not insist on helping people with disabilities. If they do not ask for help or if they decline your offer of assistance, respect their wishes (Soule & Roloff, 2000). Keep in mind that it is discouraging regularly to "owe" people gratitude for their assistance, especially when the assistance is unnecessary. (It is okay to extend the same common

## "My Disability Doesn't Show"

Dear Editor,

Since receiving my handicapped hangtag two years ago, I have been rudely approached by so many people that I've lost count.

I am a 44-year-old female, tall, thin, and do not walk with a cane, nor am I in need of a wheelchair. My handicap is internal, from two major back surgeries, and although I do have pain while walking, I walk with confidence. By simply looking at me, one would not know that I have a handicap.

Since using my handicapped hangtag, I have been rudely approached by, not only people off campus, but from just as many students on campus. I have heard it all, from "You sure look handicapped" or "You must really be handicapped from driving a car like that (a 1992 Firebird)," to "How can I get one of those (a handicapped hangtag)?" These comments not only hurt my feelings but are truly insulting, especially since I received my back injuries from serving my country while in the military, and the scar on my back extends from my neck to my buttocks.

I would like to educate everyone on campus, as well as people off campus, that not all handicaps are visible. Not everyone with a handicap is over 60, nor do they have to walk with a cane, nor do they have to be in a wheelchair.

In order to receive a handicapped hangtag, the Department of Motor Vehicles requires that one must have limitations of walking because of arthritic, neurological or orthopedic (which I have) conditions, and one must have a disability rating of 50% or greater. My disability rating is 80% and is permanent.

The last comment came January 28th by a student getting into his blue truck, which was parked next to me in front of the campus police station. The young man made the normal comment that I did not look handicapped. Normally I usually just tell people if they have a problem with me to take my license plate number and report me, but this time, I lost it and told this guy to mind his own business, and added a few explicit words to boot.

I would like to see people stop stereotyping others based on their looks and think before they inadvertently insult someone, because it really does make me feel bad, and I have every right to use my handicapped tag.

—*Beverly Davis*

*Source:* Copyright © 2003 by *The Voyager*, the student newspaper at the University of West Florida. Reprinted by permission from *The Voyager* and Ms. Davis.

---

courtesies you would offer an able-bodied friend, such as holding a door open.)

- Heed the wisdom of Thuy-Phuong Do and Patricia Geist (2000), who remind us: "Everyone is othered to some extent; we all possess disabilities, whether visible or invisible" (p. 60).

As you are probably gathering by now, the concept of being "othered," treated as if you do not belong, is demoralizing in everyday life and particularly in medical transactions. As the following section shows, age can be a source of "othering" as well.

## AGE

*"Aging alone is rarely viewed in a positive light and thus has led many to depict aging as a time of great loss and decline."*

—NUSSBAUM (2007, P. 1)

In his presidential address to members of the International Communication Association, Jon Nussbaum (2007) challenged scholars to reconsider social assumptions about aging. "Aging alone has also been a favorite of the great poets, playwrights, and novelists, who love to make us feel the 'horribleness' of our lonely human existence," he said (p. 1). But that idea, he argued, is more cultural myth than objective reality: "My mission is to spread the news that we are not purely or even remotely organisms that exist only within our own skins" (p. 1). Nussbaum proposed that it is possible to age successfully and happily and that the nexus of sustained quality of life is effective communication, as evidenced by people's ability to manage interpersonal conflict, develop relationships, manage uncertainty, share thoughts and ideas, and more.

Researcher Douglas Friedrich, author of *Successful Aging,* agrees. "Successful aging is within the grasp of most of us, especially if we develop coping or preventive strategies early in the life span and maintain them" (Friedrich, 2001, p. 157). Based on his own research and an extensive review of the literature, Friedrich concludes that lifestyle choices with the greatest influence on aging involve diet, exercise, safety precautions, healthy relationships, and a positive attitude. Many or all of these rely on communication—being well informed and interpersonally skillful.

In this section we examine the communication practices that affect people throughout their lives. We focus first on children and then more extensively on older adults. As you will see, both groups use health care services a great deal, and their communication is profoundly affected by the assumptions of people around them.

## Children

*"She gots bad monsters inside her tummy that try to eat her up."*
—FOUR-YEAR-OLD SOPHIA EXPLAINING HER MOTHER'S BREAST CANCER

This quote, from Jenifer Kopfman and Eileen Berlin Ray's (2005) case study "Talking to Children About Illness" (p. 113), helps illustrate the way children make sense of illness. Although their conceptualizations may seem naive, children are often remarkably attuned to the ramifications of illness experiences. When Sophia's young friend Ethan asks her what color the monsters are, she says, "I think they're orange 'cause orange's a gross color"

(p. 113). She goes onto to explain what happens when her mother receives chemotherapy:

> She always gives me lots of hugs and kisses before she gets her medicine from the doctor 'cause she says it makes her throw up and be tired after she takes it, and I hafta be quiet and let her sleep and not ask for too many hugs and kisses until she feels better again. (p. 113)

After that, Ethan shows Sophia his "scary monster face" and they dash off to play.

Communicating with children can be challenging because their perceptions are often different from adults'. For example, children may perceive that painful medical treatments are a means of punishment (Hart & Chesson, 1998). Moreover, children may be unsure of how to express their feelings or be afraid to speak freely in front of people they do not know.

Bryan Whaley and Tim Edgar (2008) outline the phases of development in which children conceptualize illness with increasing degrees of sophistication. In the **prelogical conceptualization** phase (roughly ages 2 to 6), children define illness as something caused by a tangible, external agent, such as a monster or the sun. In the **concrete-logical conceptualization** phase (ages 7 to 10), children begin to differentiate between external causes, such as wind and cold, and internal manifestations, such as sneezing and talking funny. In the **formal-logical conceptualization** phase (ages 11 and older), children are remarkably adept at envisioning the complex influence of agents they cannot readily see. Whaley and Edgar share the following example of formal-logical conceptualizing from Bibace and Walsh's (1981) study, in which they asked children to explain various illnesses:

> Have you ever been sick? "Yes." What was wrong? "My platelet count was down." What's that? "In the bloodstream they are like white blood cells. They help kill germs." Why did you get sick? "There were more germs that platelets. They killed the platelets off." (Bibace & Walsh, p. 37)

This is clearly a far more sophisticated explanation than Sophia's concept of orange monsters, which is a good reminder that children's ideas typically evolve over time.

Parents can be both a help and a hindrance in caring for young patients. Many times, parents have valuable information about their children's conditions and are able to comfort them as no one else could. Parents may become especially frustrated if their concerns are not taken seriously or if they do not feel well informed about their children's health needs (Kai, 1996). And rightly so. Parents are the children's principle caregivers, and their responsibility does not end at the doctor's office or hospital. However, it can be difficult for caregivers to attend to young children *and* manage the complex emotions of their parents. Parents tend to be especially anxious, guilty, and uncertain where their children's health is concerned.

When children are hospitalized, parents and professional caregivers may have conflicting ideas about what care each of them should provide. It may be unclear who is to feed the child, change bandages, and perform other tasks. With nurses' input, R. J. Adams and Parrott (1994) drafted a list of tasks parents should perform for their hospitalized children. By sharing the list with parents (orally and in writing), the nurses were able to reduce parents' uncertainty and their own. As a result, the nurses were more satisfied with their jobs, and the parents were more confident in the care their children received.

### Communication Skill Builders: Talking with Children About Illness

*Communication Skill Builders: Talking with Children About Illness* Bryan Whaley, who has conducted extensive research about children in health situations, and his colleagues offer this advice for explaining illnesses to children:

- *Let children set the tone.* Determine what the child wants and needs to know before launching into explanations the child may find incomprehensible, distressing, or simply irrelevant to his or her concerns (Nussbaum, Ragan, & Whaley, 2003; Whaley, 1999; Whaley & Edgar, 2008).

- *Pay attention.* Notice how the child conceives of illness and medical care. Ask questions and invite children to describe (and perhaps draw) their images of medical care and illness (Whaley, 2000).
- *Go easy on medical terminology.* Usually, children are more interested in how an illness will influence their lives and activities than the precise germs, tests, and scientific names involved. As Whaley (1999) puts it, "Disease and etiology appear inconsequential or of negligible concern to children" (p. 190).
- *Talk about illness as something normal.* Children are typically reassured to know their illnesses are normal and manageable. Speaking of an illness as a crisis or mystery may interfere with the child's coping ability (Whaley, 1999).

Buchholz (1992) adds that children benefit from honesty. Like adults, children usually cope better if they have a realistic idea of what to expect from health care experiences. Adults should also keep in mind that prior experience with medical procedures may not diminish children's fear and anxiety (Buchholz). Experienced youngsters may be all too aware of how frightening and painful procedures can be.

### Older Adults

Experts predict that the number of U.S. residents over age 85 will triple between 2008 and 2050. By 2030, one in five people in the United States will be over age 65 (U.S. Census Bureau, 2007). Population shifts will likely change health care needs and transform our understanding of the aging process. The outdated notion that "growing old cannot possibly be a positive experience and surely will be a time of great sadness, depression, and failing physical capacities" is likely to be revealed as more stereotype than reality (Nussbaum, Ragan, & Whaley, 2003, pp. 187–188). As with all stereotypes, the belief that all members of a group are alike in some way (e.g., sad, fun, weak, jovial) rarely holds water. **Ageism** is discrimination based on a person's age. It occurs when people judge others by preconceived notions about their age group, as when managers refuse to hire employees over age 65 because they believe people of that age are not productive.

Ageism results largely from negative stereotypes of older adults, which are common among U.S. residents of all ages. Physicians sometimes reinforce these stereotypes by referring to older patients in such derogatory terms as "coffin dodgers" and "digging for worms" (C. Fowler & Nussbaum, 2008). Ageism is also reinforced by media portrayals of older adults as unhealthy, lonely, unhappy, and irritable (T. Robinson, Callister, Magoffin, & Moore, 2006).

People with ageist beliefs are unlikely to regard elders as unique individuals who can change, learn, react, and grow physically stronger. Instead, they tend to patronize the elderly by speaking very slowly to them, using baby talk, and restricting conversations to happy subjects (Hummert & Shaner, 1994). They may even avoid communicating with older adults (H. Giles, Ballard, & McCann, 2002). Young people in Japan, the Philippines, and the United States tend to feel that older adults are less accommodating than their peers and that communication with older adults is based on obligatory signs of respect (Ota, Giles, & Somera, 2007). Youth in all three countries said they are likely to avoid communicating with older adults who are not part of their families. American youth rated their obligation to show elders respect the lowest, but they were more willing than youth in the other countries to talk with older adults.

Social beliefs about growing older often have profound implications for one's identity. When Laura Hurd Clarke and Meredith Griffin (2008) interviewed women ages 50 to 70, many of the women said they actively engage in beauty work to maintain a youthful appearance because they believe that, if they don't, they will become "invisible" in society's eyes. As one woman in the study put it: "Be young or you're not counted" (p. 660). Another expounded:

We won't love women if they're not lovely. Our society says that from the beginning. And for women who are older, we're invisible anyway. If you're considered ugly and old, ageism is awful and it's so prevalent. As a woman, we always look to someone else to see if we're okay. And as you get older, you get less and less okay, and people look at you less and less.... It gets down to "Well, you're old. You can't look good anyway." So, I think it's about trying to look young, youthful, perky, and put on this "See I'm lovely, you can love me" kind of thing. (pp. 660–661)

Women in the study said they feel immense pressure, both from the idea that women's worth is inherent in their appearance and the notion that feminine beauty is inherently youthful.

Based on the idea that getting older is a process of decline, people often assume that natural signs of aging (hearing loss, vocal changes) indicate cognitive decline. Young adults tend to underestimate the cognitive abilities of older adults with known hearing loss, although they do score them highly on wisdom and visual memory (Ryan, Anas, & Vuckovich, 2007).

But despite Western society's cynical views about aging, many older adults enjoy good health, rewarding relationships, and a positive outlook on life (Nussbaum, Ragan, & Whaley, 2003). And life's milestones are not what they used to be. Physicians report that baby boomers have different health needs than their parents at the same age. For instance, because they are more athletic, middle-aged people today have more sports injuries than prior generations ("Getting Old," 2003).

Not all older adults accept ageist beliefs about their health. My grandmother, for one, once stomped angrily from a doctor's office after being told she "was just getting old." As she left, she declared, "I don't owe you a cent. I knew how old I was when I came in here." James McCague, a columnist for *Medical Economics,* uses his 85-year-old aunt as an example of changing attitudes among older adults. When his aunt insisted on having bypass surgery despite her age, her doctor told her she was "quite functional" for an 85-year-old and was not a candidate for the surgery. To this she retorted, "I am the sole caretaker of my 90-year-old sister. I can't be just 'functional.' I want to be as healthy as I can be"

(McCague, 2001, p. 104). The physician finally performed the procedure, and McCague reports that last time he checked, his aunt was out applying for a passport! A physician himself, McCague reflects on changes among elderly patients:

> The elderly patient does not report symptoms with resignation; the questions ask for a solution. The elderly patient does not want his [or her] questions taken within the context of his age and, more important, is angry when the physician does so. Elderly patients today see medicine like everyone else—as a commodity to which they have the right to equal access.... That hope, that wonderful "great expectation" of the human species, is the crux of the demand of the elderly and, while we physicians need to moderate or shape it, we must never ignore or ridicule it. (p. 104)

*Effects of Ageism*  Despite changing trends, reconciling Western society's negative view of aging with new ideas about getting older is still a challenging enterprise with numerous implications for health communication. (See Box 6.8 for more on communication accommodation and overaccommodation.)

For one, older adults are usually treated by caregivers who are significantly younger than they are. Relatively unfamiliar with the diversity in the older generation, young people are likely to rely on stereotypes. They may lump elders into simplistic categories, such as frail, mild-mannered grandparents, and, worse, cantankerous grumps.

Second, people may not try very hard to maintain or restore older people's health. Research indicates that people expect older adults to be ill and confused. This expectation is common even among doctors and among adults themselves (Nussbaum, Thompson, & Robinson, 1989). As a result, people tend to shrug off elders' illnesses and emotional distress as unavoidable and untreatable. In short, because they do not believe older people can change, many people do not try to help them.

Third, studies support that treating people as if they are helpless encourages them to believe it. Margaret Baltes and Hans-Werner Wahl (1996) found that, at home and in nursing homes, caregivers encouraged elders to be dependent by being attentive and supportive when the elders needed help, but caregivers discouraged or ignored them when they seemed independent. The authors conclude that caregivers are sometimes overresponsive in ways that encourage learned helplessness among older adults.

Fourth, caregivers tend to underestimate older patients' desire for information. Caregivers may assume older patients are not interested in medical details, are incapable of understanding them, or will be unduly frightened by risk factors. However, research suggests most older adults are interested and are capable of understanding and assessing risks. In fact, because of long-standing experience, older adults often have more extensive medical vocabularies than younger laypersons. Reflecting this, seniors' satisfaction with medical care is most closely linked to how well caregivers listen, how concerned and attentive caregivers are, and how actively they, as patients, are included in decision making about their own care (Atherly, Kane, & Smith, 2004).

*Communication Patterns*  Although older and younger adults are not as different as caregivers (and others) may imagine, it is worth noting several communication patterns that distinguish older adults' behavior in medical contexts.

One is many older adults' reluctance to ask questions and assert themselves with doctors, despite their desire to participate and be well informed (Nussbaum, Ragan, & Whaley, 2003). Older adults' silence may mask their desire for complete information.

Conversely, some older adults become what C. Fowler and Nussbaum (2008) call *extreme talkers*, chatting incessantly about topics that may seem irrelevant to their health concerns. Given time constraints in medical organizations, "it is quite easy to imagine communication with patients who have a tendency to stray from the matter at hand being quite frustrating" to doctors and others, say Fowler and Nussbaum (p. 165).

**BOX 6.8 THEORETICAL FOUNDATIONS**

# Communication Accommodation

When people believe (rightly or wrongly) that older adults have diminished capacities, they tend to change their behavior toward them. For instance, people may speak more loudly to accommodate a hearing loss or move closer to accommodate an elder's shortsightedness. To **accommodate** is to adapt to another person's style or needs.

In some cases, accommodation is useful and appreciated. According to **communication accommodation theory**, people tend to mirror each other's communication styles to display liking and respect (Coupland, Coupland, & Giles, 1991). It is called **convergence** when partners use similar gestures, tone of voice, vocabulary, and so on. On the other hand, **divergence** is acting differently than the other person, as in whispering when the other shouts. Divergence implies that the partners are socially distant. They may be asserting uniqueness, pursuing different goals, or displaying that they do not understand or do not like each other.

To illustrate, patients who are baffled by their doctors' rapid explanations may converge by speaking rapidly themselves or by being silent to accommodate the physicians' speech. However, patients may diverge by paraphrasing the explanations more slowly to make sure they understand them. Socially speaking, divergence is risky, in that it shows the participants to be somewhat out of sync. Extreme divergence may seem disrespectful or rude.

People often mirror the behaviors of their conversational partners without really thinking about it, especially if they like each other. Accommodation can spiral, however, so that feedback encourages people to escalate their behaviors toward each other. For instance, when a dear friend speaks loudly and slowly to an elderly person, the elder may respond in a similar way, which may reify the friend's belief that the elder is a bit slow and hard of hearing. In turn, the friend may accommodate even more, and so on. Thus, what was

intended to be accommodation has become **overaccommodation**, an exaggerated response to a perceived need.

Especially if the overaccommodation is pervasive (everybody seems to do it), elderly individuals may begin to believe they are indeed of diminished capacity, and they may behave in line with that expectation (Ryan & Butler, 1996). In short, they start to "do" being old, as society has defined it.

Elderly individuals usually have no control over the cues that suggest to others that they are aging. Indeed, they may have a hard time dealing with these cues themselves, although the cues may not be signs of significantly reduced ability at all (Nussbaum, Pecchioni, Grant, & Folwell, 2000; Ryan & Butler, 1996).

An older-sounding voice is one example. In one study, people whose voices sounded old were perceived by others to be older than their contemporaries and even perceived *themselves* to be older (Mulac & Giles, 1996). An "old" voice is quivery and breathy, with prolonged vowel sounds and extended pauses between words. These characteristics are certainly not signs that the speaker is less intelligent or is physically impaired in any significant way, but they may be enough to spur accommodation and overaccommodation.

Ironically, a great number of accommodating behaviors are unnecessary. Contrary to the assumption that older people are worse communicators than others, they are sometimes better. Mark Bergstrom and Jon Nussbaum (1996) found that respondents over age 50 handled conflict more cooperatively and productively than young adults, who were apt to be confrontational and judgmental. There is also evidence that older adults compensate for deficiencies in some areas by becoming stronger in others. For example, many become especially good at reading nonverbal cues if their hearing diminishes (Fowler & Nussbaum, 2008).

Older adults' physical abilities are not as compromised as people suspect, either. Significant hearing loss only occurs in about one-third of people ages

(continued)

**BOX 6.8** (*continued*)

65 to 74 and in about one-half of people over age 85 ("Hearing and Older," 1998). Likewise, only one in four people experiences significant vision loss by age 75 (Desloge, 1997). These conditions are worth note, and they are more prevalent among older persons than others, but they by no means apply to *all* older adults. In fact, 62% of people over age 65 who live at home have no limitations that prevent them from living ordinary lives (Joyce, 1994). This means that accommodating behaviors are largely unnecessary.

### What Do You Think?

1. To test the effects of communication accommodation, try altering your speech and observing how your conversational partners react. Do they converge (e.g., whisper if you whisper) or diverge?
2. How would you react if everyone started speaking unusually slowly or loudly to you?
3. Do you tend to change your communication patterns around older adults?

---

Third, caregivers may be put off by the presence of loved ones who often accompany older adults to medical visits. According to Nussbaum, Ragan, & Whaley (2003), "The companion will ask more questions, will cause the medical encounter to last significantly longer, and will expect more information regarding the health of the older patient than the older patient normally seeks" (p. 192).

Finally, the fast pace of medical contexts may be incompatible with older adults' health needs, which (although they are not necessarily debilitating) are likely to be more numerous and chronic than younger patients', making it infeasible to cover them during a quick visit (Nussbaum, Pecchioni, Grant, & Folwell, 2000).

**Promising Options**  Even brief training sessions have been effective in dispelling ageist assumptions among medical students and health professionals (Christmas, Park, Schmaltz, Gozu, & Durso, 2008). Although not yet widespread, such educational programs may help change the way elders are treated in medical situations.

Technology provides another resource. The next section discusses communication technology as it affects older adults. And the chapter concludes with communication skill builders for reaching marginalized populations.

*Communication Technology and Older Adults*
Advanced technology can be a benefit or a liability for older adults. From one perspective, access to online health information and interaction expands opportunities for adults with limited mobility. On the other hand, older adults who do not keep up with technology may have difficulty finding and keeping jobs and staying in the mainstream of a technology-savvy society (McConatha, 2002). There is some evidence that older adults are rising to the challenge. "It's clear that older adults, like their younger counterparts, don't want to be left behind on the information highway," writes Donald Lindberg (2002, p. 13). Around the world, individuals over age 55 make up the fastest-growing segment of Internet users (Hopkins, 2007).

Older adults who are proficient at using online resources may benefit from a greater sense of control over their environment and personal fate. They may also feel less isolated and more informed about choices and options. Based on these ideals, Douglas McConatha (2002) proposed what he called the **e-quality theory of aging**, which posits that older adults benefit as both teachers and learners when they "use, contribute to, influence, and express themselves" in electronic environments (p. 38).

Based on experience working with older adults in an assisted living facility, David Lansdale (2002) says residents experienced a new sense of freedom when they learned to use an online computer made available to them. Lansdale applies the metaphors of "driving" and "going back to school." He writes:

> *Driving* is the antidote to helplessness. One of the most exciting events in adolescence comes with access to the keys to the car, and the freedom it promises. At the other end of life's continuum, an elder is often forced to relinquish the keys, often one of the more trying transitions of a lifetime. (p. 135)

Lansdale says older adults who begin using the computer are free again to "go" where they please and choose their own paths and experiences. At the same time, they can relieve boredom and feel that they are participating in life beyond the facility's borders. Similarly, by "going back to school" via the Internet, many older adults find pleasure in expanding their knowledge and skills. This provides a striking contrast to the view of aging as a steady decline in intellect and abilities. (For more resources about health communication and older adults, see Box 6.9.)

The Internet may even serve as a modern equivalent to a house call. In their study of Internet use among people ages 63 to 83, Wendy Macias and Sally McMillan (2008) report that many seniors are "bringing the physician and health information into their homes through the Internet" (p. 38). The Web allows them to take their time, learning as much or as little as they like about a health concern without being constrained by someone else's timetable. One woman in the study said:

> When my husband had his shoulder replacement, he could not get in to therapy right away, and that's when I went in to the websites and was able to print actual diagrams and information about what...for him to do, so then when we finally got in to the therapy and back to the doctor, he said this was very good. (p. 38)

Although participants in the study sometimes felt overwhelmed by the volume of online information and unsure what information to trust, they generally appreciated the opportunity to research their own concerns and issues affecting their friends and family members.

---

**BOX 6.9  RESOURCES**

# More on Health Communication and Older Adults

Coupland, N., Coupland, J., Giles, H., & Coupland, D. (2003, March). *Language, society, and the elderly: Discourse, identity, and aging* (Language in Society, No. 18). Malden, MA: Blackwell.

Hummert, M. L., & Nussbaum, J. F. (Eds.), (2001). *Aging, communication, and health*. Mahwah, NJ: Lawrence Erlbaum.

Morrell, R. W. (Ed.). (2002). *Older adults, health information, and the World Wide Web*. Mahwah, NJ: Lawrence Erlbaum.

Nussbaum, J. F., & Coupland, J. (Eds.). (2004). *Handbook of communication and aging research* (2nd ed.). Mahwah, NJ: Erlbaum.

Nussbaum, J. F., Pecchioni, L. L., Robinson, J. D., & Thompson, T. L. (2000). *Communication and aging* (2nd ed.). Mahwah, NJ: Lawrence Erlbaum.

Sparks, L., O'Hair, H. D., & Kreps, G. L. (Eds.) (2008). *Cancer communication and aging*. Cresskill, NJ: Hampton Press.

AgePages sponsored by the National Institutes on Aging and the National Library of Medicine: www.healthandage.net/html/min/nih/entrance.htm

WHO Active Ageing: A Policy Framework 2002: www.who.int/hpr/ageing/Active Ageing PolicyFrame.pdf

Williams, A., & Nussbaum, J. F. (2001). *Intergenerational communication across the life span*. Mahwah, NJ: Lawrence Erlbaum.

---

## COMMUNICATION SKILL BUILDERS: REACHING MARGINALIZED POPULATIONS

As this chapter has shown, people may be marginalized on the basis of many factors, including status, gender, race, sexual orientation, language, disability, and age. All have implications for health and health communication. Leigh Arden Ford and Gust A. Yep

(2003) offer the following suggestions for understanding and improving health-related communication with members of marginalized populations.

- *Do not impose your worldview.* Instead, seek to understand and work within the worldview of the people involved. Allow for multiple meanings.
- *Establish open dialogues in which people can communicate openly and honestly.* Strive for understanding. Allow meanings to emerge.
- *Strive to communicate in culturally acceptable ways.* Develop new skills and awareness.
- *Listen to people rather than telling them what do or think or how to act.* Seek opportunities for open-ended interviews, focus groups, and casual interactions.
- *Empower people to use their own skills and resources.*
- *Allow members of the population to emerge as leaders of the health effort.*
- *Help to unite community groups into broader-based coalitions.*

## SUMMARY

Patients are quite diverse. It is tempting to stereotype what is unfamiliar, but categorizations are often barriers to communication. Status differences can intimidate people into silence, outmoded ideas about old age can typecast the elderly as grumpy and sick, and language differences can create frustration and misunderstandings. In other ways as well, stereotypes contribute to inequitable patterns in which people may be undervalued and misunderstood.

Patients of low socioeconomic status are typically more fearful and less informed than others, but they talk less during medical exams and are likely to be treated within a strictly biomedical model. In addition to the communication challenges, practical considerations such as financial constraints, inflexible working schedules, and lack of transportation may limit the care they are able to receive.

Unfair discrimination is especially worrisome in the current climate, in which medical services are being rationed to save money. Decision makers are cautioned not to make assumptions based on social prejudices.

Low health literacy is an invisible epidemic affecting one in two American adults in the United States and 774 million people worldwide. The consequences of health literacy challenges include hundreds of billions of dollars of avoidable expenses, unnecessary suffering, frequent misunderstandings, reduced productivity, shame, and premature death. Better communication is the answer. Patients and caregivers can most effectively bridge literacy gaps if they develop trust, acknowledge and reconsider stereotypes, make the most of face-to-face communication, and encourage questions and open dialogue.

Female patients and caregivers in the United States are typically more expressive and self-disclosive than their male counterparts. There is some evidence that female patients and female physicians are especially trusting and comfortable together. But although women indicate a slight preference for female physicians, both men and women typically say that a doctor's qualifications are more important than his or her sex.

Sexual orientation can be a difficult subject for both patients and caregivers. Caregivers may feel out of their depth discussing sexual issues, although ignoring them may compromise medical care because some health risks are related to sex and because close relationships are crucial to coping. Patients may be reluctant to bring up the issue for fear of being negatively judged.

Although members of racial minorities are often at high risk for disease, their health may suffer because they do not trust doctors and because they have limited access to medical facilities and health information. Some evidence suggests that doctors treat African Americans and Hispanics differently than white patients.

A new source of health information (and potential discrimination) looms ahead in the form of genetic profiling. Emerging knowledge about human genes is expected to foster breakthroughs in medical science. Already, people who understand their genetic predisposition for various diseases may be able to offset their risks and take part in early screening procedures. The Genetic Information Nondiscrimination Act of 2008 is designed to minimize the risk that genetic risk factors will be used to penalize people in terms of employment and health insurance.

Some risk factors are not genetic, but social and linguistic. People in the United States who do not speak English well are at a disadvantage as patients. One physician estimates that their risk level is elevated 25%. Patients baffled by language differences may agree to procedures they do not understand or be so frustrated they do not return for further care. Caregivers can be frustrated also and may be held liable if adverse outcomes result. The good news is that community interpreters and long-distance interpretation services have mostly pleasing results if they are used. Still, people who are not proficient in English may wish to bring a friend or relative along, since interpreters are sometimes not available.

Many people treat individuals with disabilities as if they are childlike or incapable of contributing to conversations and decisions. These assumptions may seriously limit communication between individuals with disabilities and their caregivers. Moreover, the same attitudes can make it difficult to cope on a daily basis. Although people mean well, their actions may stigmatize and isolate individuals with disabilities. Suggestions are presented to make communication more equitable and respectful.

Children frequently undergo routine exams and emergency care, but they may have a difficult time dealing with the foreign atmosphere, strangers, and threat of pain that medical care poses. Parents can help, but their role is somewhat ambiguous. Caregivers may feel that parents are either too demanding or not helpful enough.

Finally, older adults may be typecast in ways that affect their personal identities and the health care they receive. Ageist assumptions that older people are less healthy and less intelligent than others may cause people to write off legitimate health concerns as unavoidable signs of old age. Communication accommodation behaviors are often unnecessary and can be stigmatizing, especially if carried to extremes.

## KEY TERMS

socioeconomic status (SES)
health literacy
heterosexism
racism
concierge medical practices
prelogical conceptualization
concrete-logical conceptualization
formal-logical conceptualization
ageism
accommodate
communication accommodation theory
convergence
divergence
overaccommodation
e-quality theory of aging

## DISCUSSION QUESTIONS

1. Why might misunderstandings occur between patients and caregivers of different socioeconomic status?
2. Have you ever felt that you were regarded as having lower social status than a physician who was treating you? If so, what cues gave you this impression? What was the result? What would have improved the situation?
3. What abilities are included in health literacy?
4. Experts point out that we all have literacy challenges to some extent. What factors might affect your ability to understand complex medical information?
5. How prevalent is low health literacy in the United States? What are the consequences?
6. Describe the AMA's *Ask Me 3* program.
7. What are some tips for improving communication between patients and caregivers of different socioeconomic status?
8. Describe typical style differences between the way men and women communicate in health care settings.

9. Do you prefer that your caregivers be either male or female? If so, why?

10. Why is discussion of sexual orientation important yet challenging in medical transactions?

11. What are some explanations of why people of different races seem to achieve different health outcomes?

12. Have you ever felt unfairly discriminated against because of your sex, sexual orientation, appearance, race, gender, ability, or ethnicity? If so, how?

13. What guidelines do you suggest when deciding who gets medical care (see Box 6.3)?

14. Are you concerned that your genetic profile might be used against you? Why or why not? Are you interested in knowing your genetic profile? Why or why not?

15. What are some promising options for bridging the language gap?

16. What did you learn from the case study "Language Barriers in a Health Care Emergency" (Box 6.5)?

17. What are two frustrating dichotomies people with disabilities often face?

18. What are some tips for communicating effectively with people who have disabilities?

19. Describe the three phases of conceptualization that children experience as they mature.

20. What are some tips for communicating with patients who are children?

21. What preconceived notions do you have about growing older? Are you as willing to talk to older adults as to people your own age? Why or why not?

22. Do you think people typically become less attractive as they age? Why or why not? What are the implications for older adults' social status and their appeal as relationship partners and community members?

23. How do ageist assumptions affect health communication?

24. Describe communication accommodation theory.

25. What are some tips for communicating with members of marginalized populations?

## ANSWERS TO *CAN YOU GUESS?*

1. The longest-living people in the world are women in Japan, who live an average of 86 years.

2. The shortest average life span occurs among men in Sierra Leone and women in Swaziland, both of whom live an average of 37 years.

3. In the United States, men live an average of 75 years and women 80 years. *Source: Health Status: Mortality, 2007.*

# PART III

# SOCIAL AND CULTURAL ISSUES

# CHAPTER
# 7

# Social Support

---

*Struggling to be strong after the death of his young daughter, Alonzo is hurt and mystified when friends' first question is "How is your wife?"*

*Margie misses the normal times, when people talked to her about the weather, boys, and school. Now they just hold doors for her and try not to stare at her wheelchair.*

*Everyone knows Drew's illness is very serious, but no one speaks of it to him. Drew wonders how he is supposed to cope with such an emotional topic in silence.*

*Lucy spends two hours each morning and three hours each evening caring for her three children and her elderly mother. In between, Lucy maintains a full-time job outside the home. She is glad she can help, but she wonders how many years it will be before she can take a vacation or spend a quiet day alone. Such thoughts make her feel sad and guilty.*

*Mario is pleased with life and himself. Things have not been easy, but he appreciates the pleasures of life like never before. Friends and loved ones are closer and he is at peace with himself. He marvels that dying has brought about some of the best days of his life.*

As these scenarios suggest, the majority of communication about health does not occur in a doctor's office or hospital. It occurs at home, at the grocery store, on the telephone, and in other settings of everyday life. Spouses, children, friends, and coworkers often have as much influence as doctors and nurses.

Social support includes a broad range of activities, from comforting a friend after a romantic disappointment, to listening while a grieving father tells and retells his story, to performing an Internet data search, to acknowledging that a handicapped individual is a normal person.

Most people perform more supportive behaviors than they realize and, as a consequence, have positive effects on people's health and moods. Research shows that supportive communication can help speed healing, reduce symptoms and stress, lessen pain, and build self-esteem (see, e.g., S. Cohen & Wills, 1985; Metts & Manns, 1996). And the benefits go both ways. People who provide social support often feel an increased sense of worth and personal strength themselves.

This chapter is divided into five sections. We'll begin with a conceptual overview of coping and social support and then explore the idea of health crises as transformative experiences before examining social support in two contexts—lay caregiving and end-of-life experiences. The final section cautions that, although social support is invaluable, inappropriate or excessive amounts of it can be counterproductive.

## CONCEPTUAL OVERVIEW

In the simplest sense, **social support** is people helping people. Melanie Barnes and Steve Duck (1994) define social support as "behaviors that, whether directly or indirectly, communicate to an individual that she or he is valued and cared for by others" (p. 176). Some theorists (e.g., Albrecht & Adelman, 1987) consider that the central function of social support is increasing a person's sense of control. Their viewpoint is substantiated by research (covered in this chapter) that people cope best when they feel well informed and actively involved. This section describes different coping mechanisms and the role social support plays in helping people through crisis situations.

### Coping

To understand social support, it is useful to begin with the phenomenon of **coping**. As Sandra Metts and Heather Manns (1996) define it, coping is "the process of managing stressful situations" (p. 356). Everyone is affected by stressful situations, which range from everyday hassles to life-threatening occurrences.

Coping usually involves two efforts: changing what can be changed (**problem solving**) and adapting to what cannot be changed (**emotional adjustment**) (Tardy, 1994). Of course, it is not always easy to know when to solve a problem and when to adjust. The options vary according to the people and the circumstances involved. Often, coping strategies depend on how much control people believe they have over their situation.

Sometimes attaining a sense of control requires reevaluating ideas about one's body. Canadian researchers Jennifer English and colleagues (2008) interviewed women about the strategies they used to heal emotionally and physically from the effects of breast cancer. From the respondents' stories, the researchers conceptualized the body as a

"therapeutic landscape." Often, they say, that term is used to describe places and physical environments, such as spas, gardens, and nature, that foster a sense of peace and well-being. In this case, English and colleagues applied the same idea to the body, regarding it as a place of illness but also of healing and recovery. Breast cancer is particularly relevant to the landscape image, of course, because mastectomies represent a physical redefinition of the body-physical. Although the women interviewed were unaware of the landscape concept, their stories naturally illustrate the concept. For example, one woman described her body as a damaged object:

> It was feeling like I had been broken....My body was cut up and I took all these chemical drugs and I was radiated, and you know what I mean. I just sort of in my mind felt like I was coming from a not very good physical place. (p. 71)

Another described the realization that radiation was permeating the very cells of her body. She felt the experience was simultaneously taking her into the depths of her unconscious. The women also spoke of the physical changes in their bodies—hair loss, weight gain, and new awareness of the food, air, and other elements that were affecting their bodies. In a therapeutic sense, they spoke about the healing properties of time spent with friends, exercising, and enjoying nature. Many said such pleasures are more intense because life has lost some of the taken-for-granted quality it used to have. The authors conclude:

> The body, being the smallest and most personal landscape, represents the embodiment of illness for women living with breast cancer. In other words, the body is both an everyday sight of illness but also an everyday landscape of healing. (English, Wilson, & Keller-Olaman, 2008, p. 76)

In this way and many others, illness, coping, and healing occupy the same spaces in human experience.

When people believe they can manage their health successfully, they are said to have **health self-efficacy** (Bandura, 1986). Efficacy is derived from the Latin term for "change-producing." People with high self-efficacy are more likely than others to maintain healthy lifestyles. A sense of self-efficacy may be fostered by positive experiences in the past, encouragement from others, and an **internal locus of control**, the belief that people control their own destinies. Locus of control is more general than health self-efficacy, although the two are often related. Many North Americans have an internal locus of control. As a result, they are change-oriented and hard working, but they may be frustrated by failure and may feel baffled and betrayed when things do not work out as they had planned (Marks, 1998). People who believe they control their own fate may be reluctant to ask for help and may believe they are responsible for what happens—both good and bad. Faced with ill health, they might ask, "What did I do to cause this?" Even assured that no one is to blame, these people may feel guilty and ineffectual.

Sometimes making sense of a health event involves comparing it to something familiar. In a study of American and Puerto Rican male veterans recovering from stroke, many of the men compared having a stroke to experiencing a crash or a natural disaster such as a hurricane (Boylstein, Rittman, & Hinojosa, 2007). This is a fitting metaphor, they said, because both strokes and disasters are unexpected and destructive. But the men typically chose a different metaphor—war—to describe their recovery. Like war, they said, recovery requires immense courage, determination, and active engagement. "I've always been a fighter," said one man (p. 284). Another said, "You quit, they're gonna win. Now where's the fight in you?" (p. 284). The researchers note that, in the men's stories, the "enemy" is typically a body part (an arm, a leg, or a hand) that does not work like it used to and that requires diligent therapy and exercise. The men's explanations reveal that, although their strokes seem to have come from out of the blue, they consider themselves active agents in getting well again.

By contrast, people who do not believe they can change their health for the better have low health self-efficacy. This is common in cultures in which people have an **external locus of control**, that is, the belief that events are controlled mostly by outside forces. Because of their belief in fate, these people are sometimes characterized as fatalistic.

They are likely to regard events as God's will or the natural order of things.

People with low health self-efficacy may not be motivated to take personal action regarding health matters. For example, even if they are aware of healthy dietary recommendations, they may not change their diet because they do not feel they have control over their health (Rimal, 2000). In fatalistic cultures people may reason: "It makes no sense to change my lifestyle. I will die when it's my time, no sooner or later," or "I'm sick because God willed it. Therefore, it is not right to seek a medical cure."

People with a fatalistic worldview are significantly more likely than others to feel that cancer is unpreventable and to avoid seeking information about the subject (Ramanadhan & Viswanath, 2006). And, as you might expect, adolescents with an external locus of control are more apt to "follow the crowd" and smoke if their friends do (Booth-Butterfield, Anderson, & Booth-Butterfield, 2000).

Our locus of control may also influence how we interpret other people's actions and health. For example, do people become overweight because of behavioral choices or because of factors beyond their control? As information surfaces about a genetic tendency toward obesity in some people, the public is likely to feel more sympathetic toward overweight people (Jeong, 2007). But at the same time, people may become more lax about health behaviors, concluding that obesity either is or isn't their genetic destiny and that there's not much they can do about it (Jeong).

As with most things, the extremes are typically dysfunctional. People at either extreme of the internal/external locus-of-control scale are likely to have trouble coping. One moderating effect, at least for the fatalists, is a healthy dose of confidence. Some researchers have found that people are less likely to avoid threatening health messages if they are well informed and confident about prevention methods (Fry & Prentice-Dunn, 2005).

Coping strategies may be affected by cultural beliefs and perceptions of self-efficacy. People with high self-efficacy are typically problem solvers, highly motivated to protect their own health.

However, they may be at a loss when illness reduces their sense of control. In some situations people are powerless to change their health status or to repay their caregivers' kindness (Metts & Manns, 1996). One man adapting to physical limitations after a stroke described his frustration this way: "It's hard to depend on other people to take you places. Because, you know, they have things they have to do, and they need to get done, and you don't want to interfere with their schedule" (Egbert, Koch, Coeling, & Ayers, 2006, p. 49). Forced dependence may be especially demoralizing for people who have always believed they can control their health. In these situations, a belief in fate may help people accept what they cannot change. All in all, effective coping seems to combine elements of both problem solving and acceptance.

## Crisis

A **crisis** is an occurrence that exceeds a person's normal coping ability. The first sign of crisis is usually a sense that events are out of control. This may give rise to panic or denial. For example, the parent of a seriously ill child remembers: "I didn't want to talk about it because it was something I wanted to shut in the back of my mind and have go away" (Chesler & Barbarin, 1984, p. 123).

People in crisis are also likely to feel that things have changed, perhaps forever. During difficult times, people often yearn for the simple routines that characterized everyday life (Wartik, 1996). It may seem that life will never be that way again. Following a death, for example, grieving loved ones may wonder how they will ever resume daily activities when they feel so sad and disconnected to the things that used to seem normal. It is common for people in intense grief to forget momentarily how to perform simple routines such as using an ATM and driving from one place to another (Wartik).

A major crisis may serve as a turning point or dividing line. People affected by serious illnesses often feel their life has two parts, before the diagnosis and after it (Buckman, Lipkin, Sourkes, Toole, & Talarico, 1997). Circumstances are so radically altered that nothing seems the same. The change is

not always negative. People who learn to cope with terminal illnesses or near-death experiences sometimes say they are happier than before, appreciating pleasures they used to disregard (McCormick & Conley, 1995). A cancer survivor interviewed by Anderson and Geist Martin (2003) reflects on the strength and courage she has discovered while undergoing surgery and radiation treatments:

> I wear my scar as a badge of courage but I've never thought of myself as a courageous person. But I am, I am a courageous person. People notice the scar. But you know, I don't mind the scar. Years ago, I decided that I wanted to change my name, to pick out who I wanted to be. Ivy came to mind because I liked the plant. It's a vine, it is strong, you can cut it down and it comes back. There's a lot of strength in Ivy. (p. 138)

We'll talk more about transformative health experiences later in the chapter.

## Normalcy

A sense of crisis doesn't usually abate until it seems that life is normal again. **Normalcy** is essentially the sense that things are comfortable, predictable, and familiar. Being normal is not always as easy as it sounds. It requires the cooperation of other people, even strangers (Barnes & Duck, 1994). Consider the dilemma of individuals with physical disabilities. Often, their toughest challenge is not learning to use wheelchairs or other appliances. Their toughest challenge is resuming a sense of life as usual. Without this, they are trapped in a crisis-like state, excluded from the comfortable give and take of everyday transactions with people (Braithwaite, 1996). Persons with disabilities may be inundated with people willing to help them but with very few who engage them in casual conversation or friendly debates over politics or sports. When people behave as if individuals with disabilities are unlike other people (even by being unusually kind or helpful toward them), they perpetuate a sense of crisis and alienation (Braithwaite).

While doing research about support groups, I once heard a young woman who had recently become blind say she longed to do favors for friends again. As she put it: "You appreciate people's help, but it's not the way life really is. You want to help back and no one lets you do that." In short, it is hard to lead a normal life when everyone treats you as if you are abnormal.

## COPING STRATEGIES AND SOCIAL SUPPORT

Coping strategies and social support often look very much alike. For instance, people may cope with stress by taking steps to improve their situation, learn more about it, seek the company of loved ones, have a good cry, or talk it out. These activities fall into two main categories, which also characterize the two main types of social support. As Carolyn Cutrona and Julie Suhr (1994) describe it, social support may be categorized as **action-facilitating support** (performing tasks and collecting information) or **nurturing support** (building self-esteem, acknowledging and expressing emotions, and providing companionship). Here is a description of social support based on Cutrona and Suhr's categories.

### Action-Facilitating Support

Two types of action-facilitating support are performing tasks and favors and providing information. For instance, people might support someone trying to lose weight by sharing fitness information, buying healthy foods, and serving as exercise companions.

Tasks and favors are called **instrumental support** (Cutrona & Suhr, 1994). Research shows that instrumental support is most appreciated when care receivers feel they are active participants and are involved in decision making (Bottorf, Gogag, & Engelberg-Lotzkar, 1995). **Informational support** might involve performing an Internet data search, sharing personal experiences, passing along news clips, and so on. Information can help people increase their understanding and make wise decisions. As Kreps (2003) points out, "Information is the primary process for promoting cancer prevention" (p. 164), and it is an important part of coping

effectively with cancer as well. In a book about her experience as a breast cancer survivor, Susan Ryan Jordan (2001) described her quest for information and the ways that knowledge made the disease seem less fearful, reflecting that "fear is worse than death."

Even when people cannot change their circumstances, those who are knowledgeable about what is happening usually feel more in control, experience less pain, and recover more quickly than others (Roter & Hall, 1992). Margo Charchuk describes the sense of hopelessness and impotence she felt as the mother of a seriously ill child (Connor) in a neonatal intensive care unit (NICU). "I felt that I was an outsider looking in with no voice in the care of my child," she writes (Charchuk & Simpson, 2005, p. 198). Her sense of being uninformed was associated with a loss of hope. Charchuk urges health providers to foster hope, even when the outcome is uncertain:

> In my experience, health care providers can help
> parents to enjoy their child and find hope in
> the moment even if the child will not ultimately
> survive....I hoped that he would live, but I also had
> hope that I was being a good mother and that I was
> doing all that I could to ensure his health and safety.
> When I was involved in his care, my hopes increased,
> as this enabled me to feel I was being a good parent.
> I did not lose hope when the information was bad;
> I only lost hope when I was given no information at
> all. (pp. 194–195)

Charchuk describes a dilemma that many people feel in health situations. She sensed that, if she showed emotion, Connor's caregivers would consider that she was incapable of hearing the hard truths and making important decisions, but if she didn't show emotion, they might overlook her fervent concern and desire to know more. One of the most hope-enhancing events of Charchuk's account occurs when a NICU nurse invites her to rub the baby's back to soothe him. "The importance of this small amount of control that I was able to take helped restore my hope," she remembers (p. 199).

Although most people, like Charchuk, say it feels better to be well informed, sometimes too much information can feel overwhelming and compromise our coping ability. The theory of problematic integration (Box 7.1) describes how and why we manage ambiguous, contradictory, and complex information.

Partly as a result of problematic integration and partly because of other factors, people differ in terms of the type and amount of information they seek and the information to which they are incidentally exposed. Jeff Niederdeppe, Hornick, and colleagues (2007) differentiate between **health information seeking,** which involves an active search for information, and **health information scanning**, which includes information that comes up in conversation or in the media and sticks in the memory. They have found that information gained while health *seeking* is usually of greater depth and of more direct assistance in making medical decisions. However, people are exposed to far more information incidentally than purposefully, making health *scanning* very important as well.

Information exposure isn't enough. Experts point out that another crucial element in becoming well informed is **health information efficacy**, in other words, confidence in our ability to get and understand health information. Health information efficacy is highest among people who are well educated, those who are active in their communities, and people who keep up with health stories in the news (Basu & Dutta, 2008). Women are typically more likely than men—and older adults more likely than younger ones—to have high health information efficacy and to be actively oriented to seeking health and prevention information (Basu & Dutta). Confidence and health information seeking can be a bonus both in coping and in making health-related decisions.

## Nurturing Support

Nurturing typically involves three types of support: esteem support, emotional support, and social network support. These are not directly oriented to task goals but, rather, to helping people feel better about themselves and their situations.

*Esteem Support* **Esteem support** involves efforts to make another person feel valued and competent. Here's a beautiful example from Maria Carpiac-Claver and Lené Levy-Storms' (2007) study of a long-term care facility:

> A nurse aide stands next to the resident after delivering her tray of food and says in a soft and moderately pitched voice, *Hi [resident's name]. Okay. Want a spoon?* The resident, with laughter in her voice, says, *Thank you* and smiles broadly at the nurse aide. The nurse aide gives the resident a spoon and says, *Here you go.* The resident thanks the nurse aide while shaking her head and pulling the nurse aide down to give her a kiss on the cheek. (p. 61)

The researchers observed other nurse aides laughing and singing with residents and helping those with cognitive impairments keep their memories active. In one episode a smiling aide said to a resident, "Remember your daughter? You remember you're a grandma? She's coming to visit you, you know. And she's bringing a little boy" (p. 62). Another aide sat close to a resident, touched her arm, and looked into her eyes while asking: "Tell me. What's your name?" The nurse aide responded warmly when the patient was able to tell her. Carpiac-Claver and Levy-Storms identified four themes of the nurse aides' affective communication: *personal conversation*—pleasantries and talk not directed to any particular task, *addressing the resident*—using the person's name or a term of endearment, *checking in*—asking and looking to see if the resident is feeling okay or needs anything, and *emotional support/ praise*—as in saying "You look beautiful today!" or "Congratulations!"

Encouraging words may ease feelings of helplessness and despair (Wills, 1985). People often report that unconditional approval is the most helpful form of support. Statements such as "We're behind you no matter what you decide" are comforting reminders that loved ones will not leave just because the situation is difficult to handle. Listening is also important. Studies show that most distressed individuals are not looking for advice; they just want to talk and be heard (Lehman, Ellard, &

## BOX 7.1 THEORETICAL FOUNDATIONS

# Theory of Problematic Integration

Imagine that you will go through life knowing with relative certainty what to expect and how to feel. Perhaps you will graduate, establish a rewarding career, stay healthy and fit until retirement, and enjoy your later years with the money you have wisely saved along the way. At least this is what you expect and what you hope for.

The theory of problematic integration is based on the idea that we orient to life in terms of *expectations* (what we think will probably happen) and *evaluations* (whether occurrences are good or bad) (Babrow, 2001). However, our expectations and values are challenged almost constantly in large and small ways. (Although this sounds regrettable, the challenges are actually opportunities for greater development, a point to be discussed presently.)

As defined by Austin Babrow and colleagues, the **theory of problematic integration** describes a process in which communication serves to establish a relatively stable orientation to the world but also to challenge and transform that orientation (Babrow, 1992; Brashers & Babrow, 1996; Ford, Babrow, & Stohl, 1996). *Problematic integration* (PI) occurs when expectations and evaluations are at odds, uncertain, changing, or impossible to fulfill. The disruption may be relatively minor (perhaps a setback that delays graduation) or major (someone close to you is diagnosed with a life-changing illness). Whatever the case, communication will play a pivotal role at every stage of your experience. As Babrow (2001) puts it:

> Communication shapes conceptions of our world—both its composition and meaning, particularly its values. [Problematic integration theory] also suggests that communication shapes and reflects problematic formulations of these conceptions and orientations to experience. (p. 556)

In recognizing that communication helps to define, challenge, and transform our experiences, Babrow (2001) makes the point that uncertainty is not inherently bad or good, and we are not always able to extinguish uncertainty by dousing it with information. Sometimes uncertainty exists because we have too little or too much information or because we are not sure what to make of the information presented us. Uncertainty and ambivalence may also be inherent in the information we receive about health conditions. Scientific findings change, and every promise of relief is accompanied by some degree of risk and side affects (Gill & Babrow, 2007). Furthermore, resolving one uncertainty may produce others. Babrow writes that "PI permeates human experience" (p. 564), although it is difficult to predict when and how uncertainties will arise. Going back to Babrow's first point, the notion of uncertainty is not necessarily undesirable. Indeed, he suggests that uncertainty presents an "opportunity for self-exploration" (p. 563). (For exploration of a similar idea, see the Box 8.4, on health as expanded consciousness.)

Consider the example of advance-care planning provided by Stephen Hines (2001). Medical professionals have typically been disappointed by patients' disinclination to specify what care they wish to have (or forgo) should they become too ill to express their wishes. Hines suggests that people shy away from the issue because health care professionals, in their desire to reduce their own uncertainty in end-of-life situations, have not been very sensitive to the uncertainties experienced by prospective patients and their loved ones. In short, people may neglect to file advance-care directives, not because they are indifferent or stubborn, but because the uncertainty they present feels unmanageable.

This brief review does not encompass all the facets of problematic integration theory, but hopefully it does illustrate something about the way people constitute, challenge, and transform their understandings, particularly in health-related crises.

*(continued)*

**BOX 7.1** *(continued)*

## Suggested Sources

Babrow, A. (2001). Uncertainty, value, communication, and problematic integration. *Journal of Communication, 51*(3), 553–573.

Babrow, A. S. (1992). Communication and problematic integration: Understanding diverging probability and value, ambiguity, ambivalence, and impossibility. *Communication Theory, 2,* 95–130.

Bradac, J. J. (2001). Theory comparison, uncertainty reduction, problematic integration, uncertainty man-

agement, and other curious constructs. *Journal of Communication, 51*(3), 456–476.

Ford, L. A., Babrow, A. S., & Stohl, C. (1996). Social support messages and the management of uncertainty in the experience of breast cancer: An application of problematic integration theory. *Communication Monographs, 63,* 189–208.

Hines, S. C. (2001). Coping with uncertainties in advance care planning. *Journal of Communication, 51*(3), 498–513.

---

Wortman, 1986). Following are some tips from the experts on listening well.

*Communication Skill Builders: Supportive Listening* Brant Burleson, a leading authority on social support, offers the following tips for being a supportive listener (based on Burleson, 1990, 1994).

- *Focus on the other person.* Give the person a chance to talk freely. Focus on what he or she is saying rather than on your own feelings and experiences.
- *Remain neutral.* Resist the urge to label people and experiences as good or bad. Likewise, encourage the speaker to describe experiences rather than label them.
- *Concentrate on feelings.* Focus on feelings rather than events. It is usually more supportive to explore why someone feels a certain way than to focus on events themselves.
- *Legitimize the other person's emotions.* Statements such as "I understand how you might feel that way" are typically more helpful than telling the other person how to feel (or how not to feel). A friend of mine who suffered the death of two family members within a few months said the

most comforting thing anyone told her was, "I know there's nothing I can say that will make this any better for you. But I'm here." That statement, she said, let her know she wasn't alone, and, unlike many, it gave her permission to grieve.

- *Summarize what you hear.* Calmly summarizing the speaker's statements can help clarify the situation and help the distressed individual understand what he or she is feeling. As Burleson (1994) explains: "Due to the intensity and immediacy of their feelings, distressed persons may lack understanding of these feelings" (p. 13).

*Emotional Support* **Emotional support** includes efforts to acknowledge and understand what another person is feeling. This support is particularly valuable when people must adapt to what they cannot change (Albrecht & Adelman, 1987). In a health crisis it is common to feel angry, baffled, afraid, depressed, or even unexpectedly relieved or giddy.

Emotions are a natural part of coping with health crises, yet many people are not comfortable with emotional displays (theirs or others people's). They may be afraid to appear weak or be reluctant to upset others (Zimmermann & Applegate, 1994). The result is that people tend to present the appearance that things are going well, even when they are not.

No one can deny the power of positive thinking. But problems may arise when people find themselves feigning a cheerfulness they do not feel or avoiding subjects they actually wish to discuss. Suppressing emotions commonly leads to depression and moodiness (Metts & Manns, 1996). When asked, people (patients, caregivers, and others) often say they avoid sensitive topics because they do not wish to distress the people around them (Gotcher, 1995). However, when interviewed individually, the same people usually express the private wish that those topics be brought into the open. In the long run it is usually easier to cope when emotions can be expressed and discussed without trepidation. Following are some tips for accomplishing this.

### Communication Skill Builders: Allowing Emotional Expression

- *Look for "affective moments."* Frederic Platt (1995) encourages caregivers to stay tuned for signs of strong feelings such as anger, sadness, fear, and helplessness. These are opportunities to understand something important about the other person and his or her coping status, he says.
- *Do not assume people are okay because they do not seem emotional.* Quiet people are at greatest danger for being ignored and misunderstood. When people are quiet or apprehensive about communicating, people around them are less likely to share concerns with them and less likely to understand their feelings (Ayres & Hopf, 1995). In interviews, fathers of children with cancer said they were reluctant to discuss their feelings because they might be overcome by emotion (Chesler & Barbarin, 1984). These fathers received less emotional support than the mothers did and were often expected to act "strong" when others were emotional.
- *When necessary, give yourself a moment.* Emotions often flood out other thoughts,

making it difficult to respond effectively. A helpful strategy is to say, "Let me stop and think about what you've been telling me for a moment" (Platt, 1995, p. 25).

- *Keep in mind that people usually benefit from opportunities to talk openly and honestly.* Cancer patients who feel they can talk about subjects like death and pain with their loved ones typically cope better than people who consider those topics taboo (Gotcher, 1995).
- *People in grief often find it insensitive and unhelpful when others try to minimize their losses or get them to cheer up* (Lehman, Ellard, & Wortman, 1986). Ivy, the cancer survivor interviewed by Anderson and Geist Martin (2003), put it this way: "The emotions went up and down, up and down. I talked to Jack and he listened. There was a point where Jack's optimism got to me. It was like stop, you're not listening to me. I could die, stop" (p. 137).
- *Acknowledge and respect emotions.* Branch, Levinson, and Platt (1996, paragraph 15) suggest the following communication tools for responding to emotions: (1) Acknowledge the emotion: "I can understand how upsetting it must be"; (2) show respect: "You've been doing your best to cope"; (3) reflect: "It sounds as though you are really feeling overwhelmed"; and (4) support and partner: "Maybe we can work together on these things."

All in all, it's important to remember that emotions are a natural part of the coping process and that the person who displays strong and even conflicting emotions may be coping more effectively than the one who keeps a stiff upper lip.

**Social Network Support**  Social network support involves ongoing relationships maintained even when no crisis exists. Companionship of this sort helps people feel valued and is a reassuring reminder that friends' support is always available (Barnes & Duck, 1994).

Friendships are important at every stage of life, but the nature of friendship tends to change as we mature. Whereas our social networks tend to be extensive in our younger years and involve many casual acquaintances, after age 70 or so we are likely to put more stock in a small number of very close friends and family members (Nussbaum, Baringer, Fisher, & Kundrat, 2008). According to Nussbaum and colleagues (2008), these smaller, more intimate networks are well suited to later life, when we may have limited mobility and when changes in hearing and vision may impact our communication abilities. These networks are also a valuable source of day-to-day support. It's common for loved ones to help older adults with complex health issues that might overwhelm any one person. For many reasons, in ways that change throughout our lives, having strong social ties is good for our health.

Unfortunately, health concerns can interfere with social interaction and friendships, particularly when an individual's ability to communicate is affected. When researchers led by Jennifer Bute (2007) interviewed friends and loved ones of people with compromised communication abilities, they found that some of them continued to feel an easy and even improved camaraderie despite communication limits. But many experienced it as a profound loss, particularly if dementia was involved (Bute, Donovan-Kicken, & Martins, 2007). Said one woman in the study: "It is a different relationship....I have lost the friend I used to have before" (p. 239).

In a sense, social support is like money in the bank. It's nice to know it's there, even if we don't spend it. When Joann Reinhardt and colleagues (2006) interviewed adults age 65 and older experiencing vision loss, they found that participants were least likely to be depressed and most likely to adapt well to lifestyle changes if they perceived that they had strong affective support. For them, actually receiving support was less important than knowing it was there if they needed it (Reinhardt, Boerner, & Horowitz, 2006).

Strong networks can enhance our confidence and coping abilities. For example, teens are most likely to negotiate safer-sex options with their partners if they come from families that display a problem-solving orientation. However, teens accustomed to conflict avoidance are more reluctant to bring up sexual protection, and they subsequently put themselves (and their partners) at elevated risk (Troth & Peterson, 2000). Likewise, eating disorders are more prevalent among people whose fathers are oriented to conformity and whose parents have expected personal perfection and conveyed that expectation to their children (Miller-Day & Marks, 2006). Conversely, teenage girls who regularly engage in mutually satisfying conflict resolution with their fathers are less likely than other girls to develop eating disorders (Botta & Dumlao, 2002).

A good deal of evidence links strong social networks with a long and healthy life. Lonely individuals are more likely than others to have high blood pressure (Hawkley, Masi, Berry, & Cacioppo, 2006). Conversely, resting blood pressure and blood glucose levels are lower (healthier) among people who express a great deal affection as compared to those who don't (Floyd, Hesse, & Haynes, 2007). Health benefits are also associated with humor use (Alston, 2007) and an overall sense of strong social support (Gallagher et al., 2008). Social support is even associated with longevity. In an Australian study of people ages 70 and older, those with the most active social networks (in the top third as compared to their peers) were 22% more likely to live another 10 years than those with the least active networks (the bottom third as compared to their peers) (Giles, Glonek, Luszcz, & Andrews, 2005). This is no surprise to older adults who have experienced the death of a spouse. They typically say the best coping strategy is to keep busy and interact with others, and the worst coping strategy is to isolate oneself at home (Bergstrom & Holmes, 2000).

Friends and romantic partners may even be able to talk us out of unhealthy behaviors when we won't listen to anyone else. Rachel Malis and Michael Roloff (2007) found that teenagers are most likely to be effective when confronting their peers about alcohol abuse if both parties perceive that they are good friends and that the concern is legitimate. Likewise, romantic partners with whom we share a

## BOX 7.2

## Can You Guess?

1. Of every 10 people who provide care for their frail parents, how many are sons and how many are daughters?
2. What is the most needed organ, based on the number of U.S. residents on transplant waiting lists?

*Answers appear at the end of the chapter.*

high sense of intimacy are more likely than others to convince us to improve our diets and engage in other healthy behaviors (M. R. Dennis, 2006). All in all, we usually benefit most from having a number of friends and family members who stay in close contact, display liking and respect, and seem genuinely interested in our well-being. Following are some reasons and strategies for nurturing social-network involvement, whether we are a loved one or a health professional.

*Communication Skill Builders: Keeping Social Networks Healthy* Common sources of social support include family members, friends, professionals, support groups, virtual communities, and self-help literature. Each source is likely to provide a somewhat different form of assistance. Here are some suggestions for facilitating social support in a variety of contexts.

- *People need social support even when they seem okay.* Although women give and receive more social support than men, men may need it just as much. Likewise, people with limited education usually receive more support than highly educated individuals, probably because people assume highly educated people are self-sufficient (Choi, 1996).
- *Friends are important.* Friends' attention is flattering because it is so freely given (family members are more obliged). Friendship

also offers a pleasing sense of continuity, entertainment, and a gentle reminder that other people have joys and concerns too (Rook, 1995). In some instances, friends are even more helpful than family members. When individuals studied by Metts and Mann (1996) told loved ones they had HIV or AIDS, friends were typically more supportive than family, perhaps because the family members were more overwhelmed by their own emotions.

- *Emotional support can be as important as doing favors or running errands.* A study of people with chronic fatigue syndrome (CFS) revealed that emotional support was more helpful than favors and tangible assistance, even though people with CFS are often too weary to do much on their own (K. S. Kelly, Soderlund, Albert, & McGarrahan, 1999).
- *Even simple gestures mean a lot.* Experts suggest that friends drop by for brief visits and make their willingness to help known. When uncertain what to do, they can provide services like mowing the lawn and leaving a casserole without fear of being in the way.
- *Keep family members well informed.* When a loved one is in the hospital, family members may be especially anxious if they do not feel well informed. This is hard on the families, and it may compromise their ability to cope and provide support (Cross et al., 1996). Health professionals are encouraged to share information often and freely. It's good medicine.
- *Make family members and loved ones feel welcome.* Presbyterian Hospital Matthews in Matthews, North Carolina, has expanded its critical care unit so that a family room adjoins each patient room (Daniels, 1996). Every family room is equipped with soothing artwork, a sofa bed, a recliner, a telephone, and a window to provide a view of nature and allow in sunlight. A kitchen and showers are also available to guests. Nurses report that patients are less agitated and experience

fewer symptoms of stress and anxiety when loved ones are near. The arrangement also gives nurses a chance to educate patients' families and answer their questions. (The hospital requests that each family choose a spokesperson so that nurses are not flooded with the same questions from different people.)

- *Health professionals can assist with communication strategies as well as treatment regimens.* Because of their regular experience with health dilemmas, health professionals may be able to suggest strategies people would not think of on their own. Consider the dilemma of people who have had unprotected sex while cheating on their romantic partners. Health counselors in Marifran Mattson and Felicia Roberts' (2001) study helped people find acceptable ways to insist on condom use while they awaited the results of HIV tests. The counselors first encouraged clients to be honest with their partners, but if it became clear that clients would rather expose their unsuspecting partners to a health risk than admit their infidelity, the counselors helped people devise stories to tell instead. In one instance, a counselor suggested a man could tell his girlfriend he had urethritis ("kind of like a male yeast infection") and must use a condom for several months (at which point results of the HIV test would be available). Such deceptions may seem questionable, but the alternative (risky sex) may be worse.

## Support Groups

**Support groups** are made up of people with similar concerns who meet regularly to discuss their feelings and experiences. As defined by Schopler and Galinsky (1993), support groups may utilize a range of formats, from informal self-help groups (with an emphasis on shared concerns and minimal intervention by the facilitator) to treatment groups (providing a form of psychological therapy with active guidance by a trained professional). In recent years, online support groups and virtual communities have joined the list.

In their various forms, support groups are popular around the world. More than 24,000 Al-Anon/Alateen group meetings are conducted in 30 languages in 115 countries (Al-Anon.Org). There are also support groups for people dealing with grief, codependence, an enormous variety of illnesses and addictions, and other concerns.

The effort may be justified. Support group members tend to experience fewer symptoms and less stress, and they may even live longer than similar people who are not members ("Living With Cancer," 1997; K. Wright, 2002). Similarly, involvement in support groups has been shown to reduce depression and anxiety among cancer patients (Evans & Connis, 1995).

Support groups have several advantages. Being around similar others may make people feel that they are not alone or abnormal. Similar others can also give firsthand information on what to expect and how to behave. At the same time, support group members may feel better about themselves because they are able to help others (S. E. Taylor, Falke, Mazel, & Hilsberg, 1988). Another advantage is the convenience and low cost of support groups. Because they are made up mostly of laypersons, there are few or no fees and (for the most part) members can schedule meetings where and when they wish.

The greatest dangers are that support groups will become counterproductive gripe sessions or that members will develop an us-versus-them viewpoint (J. D. Fisher, Goff, Nadler, & Chinsky, 1988). They may begin to feel that no one outside the group understands them as well as they understand each other (a form of oversupport described later in the chapter).

## Communication Technology: Virtual Communities

Communication technology has expanded the options for supportive relationships. Telephones and computers have given rise to **virtual communities**, groups of people with similar concerns who communicate via information technology.

Online support groups allow people to communicate about key issues, sometimes with the guidance of professional facilitators. Consequently, expertise in communication technology is becoming a useful skill for health professionals.

Research shows that people are most likely to participate in online health support groups if they are intrinsically interested in health issues or if extrinsic factors (e.g., a diagnosis or a perceived health risk) motivate them to learn more (Dutta & Feng, 2007) and if the postings are easy to read and relevant to their daily concerns (Donelle & Hoffman-Goetz, 2008). Tamar Ginosssar's (2008) analysis of more than 1,400 e-mails between members in one online cancer community revealed that women posted about 75% of the messages and that most messages were oriented primarily to information exchange and only secondarily to emotional support. Family members were less active in the online community than patients themselves, who typically sent more e-mails and engaged in more interactive discussions than their families did.

T. Ferguson (1997) surveyed therapists to gauge the quality of advice typically offered on computer bulletin boards. In one instance a grieving man who shared his story online received dozens of immediate replies. People said they understood how he was feeling and advised him to continue therapy, find solace in his religious faith, be kind to his wife, accept others' help, and resist any temptation to abuse drugs. The therapists Ferguson surveyed applauded the people's kind efforts, and most said they would not have been able to help the man in such an "immediate, compassionate, and practical way" themselves (paragraph 8).

Although there are many benefits to online community membership, there are also potential drawbacks. On the good side, online interaction is helpful for people who are short on time or transportation, have disabilities or responsibilities that prevent them from leaving home, or find comfort in the relative anonymity of technology-mediated conversations (Braithwaite, Waldron, & Finn, 1999; Galinsky,

---

## BOX 7.3 **RESOURCES**

# More About Coping and Social Support

Here are some additional sources of information about supportive communication.

Green, J. O., & Burleson, B. R. (Eds.) (2003). *Handbook of communication and social interaction skills*. Mahwah, NJ: Lawrence Erlbaum.

Lewis, M., & Haviland-Jones, J. M. (Eds.) (2000). *Handbook of emotions*. New York: Guilford Press.

Miller, J. F. (2000). *Coping with chronic illness: Overcoming powerlessness*. Philadelphia: F. A. Davis.

Reinhardt, J. P. (Ed.) (2001). *Negative and positive support*. Mahwah, NJ: Lawrence Erlbaum.

Ryff, C. D., & Singer, B. H. (Eds.) (2001). *Emotion, social relationships, and health*. New York: Oxford University Press.

Stroebe, M. S. (Ed.) (2001). *Handbook of bereavement research: Consequences, coping, and care*. Washington, DC: American Psychological Association.

---

Schopler, & Abell, 1997). For example, people with HIV/AIDS who make use of Internet information are found to have greater knowledge of the condition, more success coping, and larger support networks than similar people who do not go online (Kalichman et al., 2003). And women in an online breast cancer support group who engaged in insightful disclosures (using words such as *understand*, *realize*, *feel*, and *think*) reported better moods and greater emotional well-being than others. However, overreliance on technology-mediated communication may prevent people from developing relationships in their own communities, ultimately robbing them of the types of social support that cannot be transmitted via fiber optics. Other disadvantages include difficulty using and obtaining technology, potential threats to privacy, lost nonverbal cues, and hurtful remarks people might *not* make were they face-to-face (Galinsky, Schopler, & Abell, 1997).

All in all, coping and social support go hand in hand. Social support is essentially a concerted effort to help people cope with difficult circumstances. Even a relatively minor health event can constitute a crisis if the people involved do not have adequate skills or resources to cope with it. (For more about coping and social support, see Box 7.3.)

## TRANSFORMATIVE EXPERIENCES

Carol Bishop Mills remembers the day her daughter Maren was born:

> Dr. Jacobs, the NICU doctor, approached my bed about 15 minutes later and handed me a gorgeous baby girl. He was very pleasant and smiled when he told us all about her. "Mr. and Mrs. Mills, your daughter is quite healthy. She seems to have a strong heart, and her kidneys will be fine. There was some fluid pooled, but it will eliminate itself naturally. Her APGAR scores [used to measure a newborn's health] were 8 and 9 [out of a possible 10]. She's a beautiful little girl. There are some preliminary indicators in her features that she might have trisomy 21, Down syndrome, but we need to run some blood work to confirm that." (Mills, 2005, p. 198)

The Mills were not surprised; they suspected their baby might have special needs. But they *were* deeply grateful—grateful that the doctor had not said "I'm sorry" or labeled their daughter "abnormal." Instead he saw, as they did, a unique, perfect little girl in radiant good health with a condition not all children have.

Good health is often defined in terms of what is "normal" or "expected." A deviation from that can feel like a tragedy—meaningless and unfair. In reality, however, what looks on the surface like a "bad outcome" can turn out to be one of life's most valuable and important gifts. Mills (2005) attests that, although no one hopes to have a child with Down syndrome, "it is simply a gift we were given that we would have never known to ask for and probably would never have understood before our Little Miss Magic captivated our hearts" (p. 196).

In this section we explore instances in which, in the midst of what might seem to be great hardship,

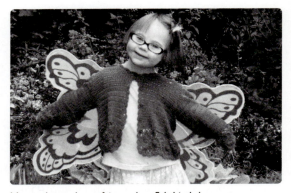

Maren dressed as a fairy at her 5th birthday party.

people discover unexpected rewards. I adopt the perspective of social constructivists (e.g., Berger & Luckmann, 1966) as well as other philosophers and theorists who put forward that life is defined largely by a quest for meaning, a quest that is shaped both by our own experiences and by our interactions with others. To illustrate the powerful effect of social interaction, let's return to Mills' (2005) case study but this time, look through the eyes of Kate, another mother, who has just given birth to Joshua:

> We heard a cry, we saw our boy, and then heard the following from Dr. Lee, "I am so sorry to tell you this. This baby looks like a Down's. I'm so sorry....In 20 years, I've never delivered a Down's. Didn't you have tests? ...I'm sure it's a Down's. I am so, so sorry." (quoted by Mills, p. 199)

As you might imagine, Kate's experience was much different than the Mills'. "In my heart, I knew the Down syndrome was my fault, and it was clear the doctor was angry," Kate remembers thinking. "I didn't have a boy, in my mind, I had an 'it,' a Down's, one of those short, funny, retarded kids that work at grocery stores. My mind flooded with thoughts of drooling, retardation, the little yellow buses, the teasing, and the problems" (quoted by Mills, p. 199).

Mills (2005) reports that Kate and her husband, Chris, have come to realize that Down syndrome is only one feature—a relatively insignificant one—in the myriad of qualities that make their son Joshua

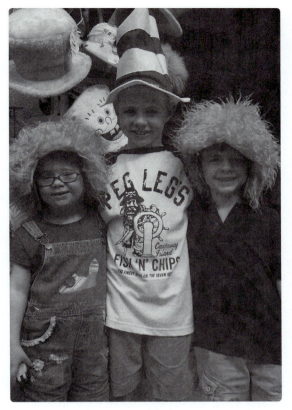

Maren with brothers Jonah and Archie on a recent vacation.

wonderful. But they have often had to overcome health professionals' hurtful comments in the process. Considering what people may learn from her experiences, Mills says, "I really hope that students realize that, often, it is not the diagnosis that is so scary, but the language we use to talk about it that is so embedded in cultural disdain that taints our view about it."

We may all sometimes fall into the hurtful trap of believing, as Kate and Chris's doctor did, that there is a norm—a normal way to look, a normal life span, a normal reaction, and so on—and that what is "normal" is the "good" or "right" way to be. Most people who experience a crisis initially feel the same way, wondering: *Is this my fault? What did I do to deserve this? Why did this happen? Can I make it okay again?* In short, if the norm is right, a deviation

means something has gone dreadfully wrong. This is a common assumption because the unknown is often frightening and because, as humans, we are continually involved in sense-making and an unexpected occurrence can rob of us our sense of safety and meaning. For this reason, I believe it's especially important to learn more about diverse ways of being (in other words, shrink our distrust of the unknown) and to remind ourselves continually that, although it takes courage to embrace them, some of life's most enriching gifts lie beyond the status quo.

You might be surprised how frequently people who have been part of health crises (even to the extent of learning that they do not have long to live) ultimately consider themselves grateful for the experience. du Pré and Eileen Berlin Ray (2008) examined such episodes in a study of **transcendent experiences**, which they define as episodes in which people come to perceive an overarching meaning, or supra-meaning, within experiences that might otherwise seem senseless or unthinkable (p. 103). The term *supra-meaning* comes from psychologist Victor Frankl's (1959) reflections about life in a Nazi concentration camp during World War II. In the midst of suffering more horrific than most of us can imagine, Frankl observed that some of his fellow prisoners still found a reason to value life and be optimistic about the future, largely because they perceived a meaning in life that was not bounded by the chain-link fences that kept them physically captive. Frankl came to believe that a quest for meaning is the primary motivation of human nature. From his perspective, write du Pré and Ray, "transcendence is not denial of one's circumstances, but an awareness that those circumstances exist within the framework of something more meaningful than one might previously have imagined" (p. 103). In a similar way, people who don't have long to live sometimes say life takes on a new, larger meaning that makes everyday concerns seem trivial. As one cancer survivor put it:

> I am no longer concerned that someone might see me in the same outfit and I no longer have to have the same sweater in every color. I can now not finish

a book if I don't like it. Every day is a guessing game. But that's okay. I'm still here to talk about it. (Brett, 2003, p. B1).

Others say they have been able to lay old grievances to rest and have developed a heightened appreciation for nature and loved ones. Many people facing life-altering circumstances say they have found larger meaning in a spiritual quest that involves helping others, dedicating themselves to a cause larger than themselves, allowing themselves to be creative and have fun, and seeking to live up to their full awareness and potential (Egbert, Sparks, Kreps, & du Pré, 2008). Some people say the loss of a loved one was relieved in part by the knowledge that his or her organs helped save lives. (See Box 7.4 for more on this topic.)

This is not an easy or guaranteed process. Transcendence often happens when we least expect it. But being aware that what appears tragic on the surface may eventually yield something beautiful is a good start toward coping when things seem their darkest.

## LAY CAREGIVING

It is important to remember that patients are not the only ones in need of social support. Loved ones and caregivers experience grief, uncertainty, and exhaustion as well, and their needs are frequently overlooked in concern over the ill individual. This section focuses on **lay caregivers**, nonprofessionals who provide care for others. Lay caregivers are an important source of social support, but they also need support themselves.

### Lay Caregivers' New Role

The number of lay caregivers has risen in recent years, mostly because the older-adult population is growing and because hospital stays are shorter than they used to be. Many surgeries are now conducted on an outpatient basis. Patients recuperate at home rather than in the hospital. As Donna Laframboise (1998) puts it: "Good news! You can go home from the hospital tomorrow. Bad news! You'll have to do everything yourself, even though you're still on crutches or full of stitches" (p. 26).

Someone must help ill or hurt individuals while they are at home. Home health professionals provide a portion of this care, but researchers estimate that unpaid caregivers provide at-home care for three out of four older adults with severe disabilities (R. W. Johnson & Wiener, 2006).

### Profile of the Lay Caregiver

Most lay caregivers in the United States are women, and most care receivers are older-adult relatives. As you can see in Table 7.1, the vast majority of unpaid at-home caregivers in the United States are wives and daughters. Most work about 201 hours per month as caregivers, which exceeds a 40-hour workweek by 29 hours (Johnson & Wiener, 2006). However, frail older adults who are female receive about 63 hours less monthly care than men in the same boat (Johnson & Wiener).

Lay caregivers are in demand like never before. The average cost of a private room in a nursing home is $77,745 a year, and the average monthly cost of an assisted living apartment is $2,969—with an additional $1,110 per month if dementia-related care is required ("The MetLife Market Survey," 2007). Medicaid may cover some of the costs, but only if the nursing home resident is out of money. Most states require that people be down to their last $2,000 to qualify (R. W. Johnson, 2008). The percentage of the U.S. population who lives in nursing homes is down from 10.2% in 1999 to 7.4% in 2006, partly because of the rising expense and partly because today's older adults are healthier than their parents were (El Nasser, 2007; U.S. Census Bureau, 2004).

### Stress and Burnout

Caregiving is no simple task. By some estimates, young adults today will spend more time caring for their parents than they will raising their own children. In addition to providing medical care and assistance, lay caregivers are frequently responsible for maintaining the household and budget, working

BOX 7.4

# Organ Donations: The Nicholas Effect

*"Recently I strolled through a park in Rome with Andrea Mongiardo, a 23-year-old Italian whose heart once belonged to my own son."*

With this comment, Reg Green (2003) introduces the Nicholas Green Foundation website, named in honor of 7-year-old Nicholas, who was killed near Naples by robbers who mistook the Green's car for their own and fired into the vehicle. Even in their shock and grief over the sudden attack, Reg Green recalls, he and his wife agreed that Nicholas' organs should be donated to others. The family has since befriended the seven people whose lives were changed as a result. Reg Green remembers when he and his wife met these organ recipients for the first time:

> Our grief was still agonizingly raw. But that meeting, which both us had to steel ourselves to attend, was explosive. A door opened and in came this mass of humanity, some smiling, some tearful, some ebullient, some bashful, a stunning demonstration of the momentous consequences every donation can have. We now think of them as an extended family. We've watched the children grow and leave school and get their driver's licenses and the adults go back to work. One of them, 19 year-old Maria Pia Pedala, in a coma with liver failure on the day Nicholas died, bounced back to good health, married and has since had a baby boy. And, yes, they have called him Nicholas. (paragraph 11)

Reg Green's (1999) book *The Nicholas Effect: A Boy's Gift to the World* and a video of the same title tell the family's story.

Another advocate for organ donation is Lisa Slinsky, whose 42-year-old husband Bill died of a brain aneurysm in 2002. She says she had no particular opinion about organ donation at the time, but she knew he was a registered donor, so she complied with his wishes. His organs were transplanted into 27 people (Somma, 2008).

In the United States, an average of 19 people a day die waiting for an organ transplant (Organ-Donor.Gov, 2008). The waiting list is more than 100,000 people long, and the greatest need is for kidneys (accounting for 76% of all transplants).

The issue of organ donation is an emotional one, and not everyone agrees with the Greens and Lisa Slinsky. Following are some common attitudes and misperceptions about organ donation.

- *Mistrust of medical establishment.* Some people fear medical professionals will be less vigilant about keeping them alive if they are eager to harvest their organs (Frates, Bohrer, & Thomas, 2006; Morgan, Harrison, Afifi, Long, & Stephenson, 2008).
- *Suspicion of underground market.* Some people, influenced by horror movies and fictional TV dramas, fear their organs will be sold for a profit (Morgan et al., 2008).
- *Concerns about recipients' worthiness.* For some people, the possibility of a "bad person" receiving one's vital organs is off-putting. Several participants in Morgan and colleagues' (2008) study said they wished they could specify who would receive their organs. As one person put it: "Ideally, I'd like to be able to be like, 'I'd like a 12-year-old to have my heart....I don't want some old man who needs everything in his body to have everything out of mine" (p. 29).
- *Religious/spiritual considerations.* There is mixed evidence about the influence of religious convictions. For the most part, it seems that altruism (which is sometimes linked to religious beliefs) is a factor. "Why [should] two people have to die if you can help one live?" asked a participant in Morgan and colleagues' (2008) study. On the other hand,

*(continued)*

BOX 7.4 (continued)

the strongest deterrent to organ donation is the belief that one's body should be kept "complete" after death (Stephenson, Morgan, Roberts-Perez, Harrison, Afifi, & Long, 2008).

Many misconceptions surround the issue of organ donation, partly because of sensationalized accounts on TV and in the movies (Morgan, Harrison, Chewning, Davis, & DiCorcia, 2007). In reality, physicians who care for a patient are not involved in decisions about his or her organ donation. That is handled by an entirely different staff and medical team. Concerns about conflict of interest are unfounded. Moreover, although there is often a great deal of publicity when rich and famous people receive donated organs, they actually do not receive preferential treatment, and strict U.S. laws prohibit the sale or purchase of organs as well as bribery for desired organs ("Organ Donation," 2008, paragraph 3). Another common myth is that organ donation will mar a deceased person's appearance such that the family cannot have an open casket at the funeral. This is not true. Physicians are able to maintain the person's appearance so that people cannot tell the difference ("Organ Donation").

A variety of other concerns also affect people's decision to donate their organs or not. Studies show that people typically resist registering as organ donors if they feel others are pressuring them into it (Bresnahan et al., 2007a). They also resist if they feel that a donation will interfere with their death or afterlife (Bresnahan et al., 2007b). On the other hand, people are inclined to register if they feel that people they like and admire support the decision, if they perceive that there is a serious need for organs, and if they feel comfortable talking about the decision with their families (Bresnahan et al., 2007a; S.W. Smith, Kopfman, Lindsey, Yoo, & Morrison, 2004). People are also inclined to donate their organs if they feel that doing so signals a spiritual connection in which one is able to "live on" in some fashion or to have a spiritual link with the organ recipient (Bresnahan et al., 2007b). The issue may be weighted by cultural values, as well. For example, Koreans, although they may express favorable inclinations to register as donors,

are far less likely than Japanese and American citizens actually to register, probably because of cultural reservations (Bresnahan et al., 2007a).

## What Do You Think?

1. What factors make you more (and less) inclined to register as an organ donor?
2. What is most fearful about the prospect? What is most appealing?
3. Would you have made the same decision if you were Nicholas Green's parents? Why or why not?
4. If you knew that, like Bill Slinsky, your organs could improve the odds for 27 people, would that affect your decision about whether to register as a donor?
5. Unlike the Greens, who live in Italy, people in the United States are not usually given the opportunity to meet the people who receive a loved one's organs. Would you want to meet them? Why or why not?
6. Have you seen TV programs or movies in which people's organs are misused? Were the depictions realistic, in your opinion? Do you think such depictions affect people's attitudes about organ donation?

## Suggested Resources

*Journal of the American Medical Association* on Organ Donation: http://jama.ama-assn.org/cgi/reprint/299/2/244.pdf

U.S. Department of Health and Human Services: OrganDonor.gov

National Kidney Foundation Facts About Organ Donation and Transplant: www.kidney.org/news/newsroom/fs_new/25factsorgdon&trans.cfm

Mayo Clinic: "Organ Donation: Don't Let These 10 Myths Confuse You": www.mayoclinic.com/health/organ-donation/FL00077

The Nicholas Green Foundation: www.nicholasgreen.org

YouTube video The Nicholas Effect: see http://www.youtube.com/watch?v=SHBV-TcF1iI

### Table 7.1 Portrait of Lay Caregivers in the United States

| | |
|---|---|
| Of people who rely on unpaid caregivers at home... | 2/3 rely only *one* caregiver |
| Of adult children who provide care for frail parents... | 7/10 are *daughters* |
| Of unpaid caregivers in the United States... | 2/3 are *female* |
| Among frail older adults who are married... | 9/10 caregivers are *spouses* |
| Among spouses who care for frail partners... | 1/3 are in poor health *themselves* |

*Source:* R. W. Johnson & Wiener (2006)

at a career outside the home, and providing information and support to others.

Legislation was passed in the 1990s to help career people provide care for needy family members. The **Family and Medical Leave Act of 1993** guarantees that people can take up to 12 weeks off work to care for ailing family members, seek medical care themselves, or bring new children into their families (through birth, adoption, or foster parenting). However, the act does not require that employers *pay* workers while they are on leave, and it does not apply to all companies or all employees. To be eligible, employees must have worked at the company at least 1 year for an average of 25 hours or more per week. Only companies with at least 50 employees are obligated to provide medical and family leave.

Although most people juggling careers and caregiving say they feel good about what they do overall, it's easy to feel stressed, exhausted, and resentful at times. Said a 31-year-old caring for her ill mother: "Your parents have given you so much that the last thing you're ever going to do is not help them out. But at the same time, it's so hard. I get resentful sometimes" (quoted by Laframboise, 1998, p. 26).

Part of the strain is emotional. Caregivers may grieve over future plans that no longer seem possible. A 76-year-old woman caring for her ailing husband lamented: "This isn't how we planned to spend our retirement years....Why did this happen to us?" (quoted by Ruppert, 1996, p. 40).

It's also painful to see a loved one suffer or change. The progression of Alzheimer's disease is particularly heart-wrenching to witness. Caregivers may watch sadly as the individual's personality and awareness gradually change. Sometimes

Alzheimer's patients become belligerent or unable to recognize the people around them (see Box 7.5). To make matters worse, caregivers may feel guilty about their own frustration and resentment. It may seem wrong to be angry with a person who is ill and needy.

Lay caregivers may also feel unprepared to perform the tasks delegated to them. Although they now perform many services once carried out by health professionals, lay caregivers often receive only minimal instruction on what to do and what to expect. As a result, they may feel overwhelmed and may worry that they will do something wrong or miss important warning signs. When a loved one's life is at stake, the pressure can be as exhausting as the physical demands of caregiving.

Caregivers may jeopardize their own health if they overextend themselves. People are like elastic, says Geila Bar-David of the Caregiver Support Project in Toronto (Laframboise, 1998). If they are stretched too thin for too long, they will lose strength and may even snap. Caregivers who are reluctant to leave their posts may need reminding that they will be of no use unless they remain healthy (emotionally and physically) themselves.

### Caring for Caregivers

Community resources are expanding somewhat to serve the needs of people who care for loved ones at home. Many medical centers now sponsor lay caregiver support groups and skills-training programs. A program at Salem Hospital in Salem, Oregon, helps lay caregivers establish diet and exercise regimens and teaches them skills such as how to move patients without hurting themselves (Ruppert,

BOX 7.5 **PERSPECTIVES**

# A Long Goodbye to Grandmother

A few years ago, I lost my grandmother to Alzheimer's disease. Until she died, I saw my grandmother every week of my life. We had a very close relationship.

Alzheimer's is not a disease that just appears one day and kills you. It causes gradual deterioration of a person's memory and sense of being. Minutes and days and years all seem the same or don't exist at all. My grandmother's condition started about 1 year before her death.

Before Grandma got Alzheimer's, our extended family was fairly close. No one wanted to put Grandma in a nursing home, but caring for her was not going to be easy. Her three daughters (including my mother) decided Grandma would stay with each of them for one week at a time.

Grandma and I had always enjoyed playing Scrabble and working crossword puzzles together. She always tried to get me to use my thinking skills. My favorite times were when she would tell me stories about when she was a young girl or a teenager. She was a very flirty girl, although she had a prissy attitude as an elderly person.

As Grandma's forgetfulness worsened, she often forgot what year it was. She would also forget to eat. Soon she could no longer remember conversations we had had. I could answer a question and 5 minutes later, she'd ask it again. I would tell her every week why and where I was going to school. We would talk about the world now compared to the world in her day. Sometimes she would talk out loud to her parents, who had been dead 50 or 60 years.

Her worst times were at night. She stayed up most of the night talking to people she thought were there. As much as I loved Grandma, I would get aggravated with her during those nights of constant talking. Several times a night, we'd go into her room to comfort her. She'd whine and cry like a child. It was difficult for me to deal with this. I started distancing myself from her during the day because she made me angry with the things she did at night. Even though I knew she had no idea what she was doing, it still aggravated me.

The stress started wearing on other family relationships as well. The daughters started finding fault with each other. No one said anything out loud, but the frustration was there under the surface. I was sad to see relationships start to disintegrate. I asked my grandmother to forgive me even if she didn't quite understand why.

Over the months, Grandma's condition deteriorated. She lost touch with reality and she lost trust in her family. One day she and I were home by ourselves and I got her a glass of water. When I gave it to her, she smelled it. Then she looked at me and said, "I never thought you would do this." I asked what she meant, and she said, "Of all people, I didn't think you would poison me. I expected the others, but not you." This hurt me very much. I took the glass of water and poured it down the sink and let her watch me pour a new glass. But she continued to believe I was trying to kill her.

By the time she died, Grandma weighed less than 95 pounds. The times that I could talk with her were over. She stayed with us for the last month of her life. She was in such bad condition we didn't want to move her. The night of her death my mom and dad left for church and I stayed behind. I read her the Bible and sang her some songs while I played my guitar. As I did this she began to cry a little. I didn't expect her to respond, but that was a special moment. About 5 hours later, she died in her bed, with her family in the room with her.

—*Nicholas*

1996). Members also learn about caregiver stress and emotions and have a chance to express their feelings. Good communication skills can help. In a study of 76 older adults and lay caregivers, Jim Query Jr. and Kevin Wright (2003) found that participants with high communication competence were less stressed and more satisfied with the social support they received than others.

Friends and families remain the most promising source of support for lay caregivers. In a meta-analysis of 50 studies about lay caregiving, a prominent theme was that caregivers missed opportunities to socialize with others (Al-Janabi, Coast, & Flynn, 2008). Whenever possible, caregivers say they also value expressions of love and appreciation from the person they are caring for. Said one man who cares for his wife at home:

> Sometimes she'll look up to me and give me such a priceless lovely smile, which says it all and then the other morning she laid down for a bit and looked up to me and said, "You're lovely. I love you." It came out clear as a bell. Well, you can't put a price on that, can you? (Al-Janabi et al., pp. 116–117)

In one social support effort, 40 people in Fairfax, Virginia, organized themselves to help a dying friend and her family ("What Her Friends Did," 1997). Lynn Mazur was inspired by the book *Share the Care* (Capossela, Warnock, & Miller, 1995). She organized a group effort to help her friend, Karen Hills, who was dying of cancer at age 34. Mazur called everyone in the Hills' family address book and found 40 people anxious to help out. They met at the Hills' home and filled out questionnaires suggesting what they could each contribute to the effort. They chose team captains, and soon volunteers were in place to drive Karen's young daughter to school, clean house, prepare meals, read to Karen, help with her physical therapy, and so on. The assistance allowed Karen and her husband and child to spend more relaxing time together. The tasks were simple and quick enough that burnout was not a problem. In fact, Mazur says, people were relieved to know they could help, and caregivers turned to each other for support when they were tired or sad.

All in all, it is important to remember that caregivers need care too. Assistance can sweeten the rewards of caregiving and lessen the demands.

## END-OF-LIFE COMMUNICATION

Death is an unpleasant topic to people in many Western cultures. "Death is un-American. It doesn't square with our philosophy of optimism, of progress," wrote Herbert Kramer, a terminally ill cancer patient (Kramer & Kramer, 1993, paragraph 21). Nevertheless, dying is inevitable, and it marks a stage of life during which social support is crucial. What's more, end-of-life experiences can be more meaningful and beautiful than many people realize.

To some people, the phrase "a good death" seems like an oxymoron. They do not believe there is such thing. However, many people argue that dying can be a special (albeit emotional) experience with many positive aspects. This section analyzes these two perspectives, which are characterized as "life at all costs" and "death with dignity." It also explains advance-care directives and offers experts' advice for dealing with death.

### Life at All Costs

Have you ever walked past a hospital morgue? Probably not. Most hospitals locate the morgue in an out-of-the-way area where people will not chance upon it. What's more, the morgue staff may be regarded as somewhat weird and eccentric based on their choice of occupation. This may seem perfectly understandable if you grew up in a society in which death was regarded as something gross and ghoulish.

Today's Grim Reaper is a modern-day version of Thanatos, the merciless and malicious Greek god born of "darkness" and "sleep." In Greek mythology, Thanatos is often depicted as a rival of Bios (Greek for "life"). The lessons of such tales are easy to divine: Death is the enemy of life. Life is victory, death a merciless and permanent defeat. In modern terms, medicine is associated with Bios. Health professionals are considered, quite literally, to be in *mortal* combat with the enemy, death. Hence we entertain such notions as "battling cancer" and "fighting for one's life." These conceptualizations thrive in an atmosphere in which death is considered taboo and unknown and medicine the ultimate savior.

If you are a caregiver pledged to maintain life, death may be more than creepy; it may represent failure (Hyde, 1993). Caregivers have several incentives to keep patients from dying. For one, they are typically trained to preserve life, not allow it to end. Most physicians approach medicine as detectives and problem solvers—endeavors that are successful only if they solve the mystery and fix the problem (Ragan & Goldsmith, 2008). Moreover, death is frightening, even to professionals who have encountered it before (Hegedus, Zana, & Szabó, 2008). Saving a life is usually a rewarding experience, whereas a patient's death may bring feelings of guilt and grief. Finally, caregivers (doctors especially) may be harshly criticized or sued if a patient dies. Physicians' decisions are often intensely scrutinized by family members, lawyers, insurance companies, quality assurance and risk management personnel, administrators, and others (McCue, 1995). Jack McCue attests: "It is little wonder that physicians engage in inappropriately heroic battles against dying and death, even when it may be apparent to physician, patient, and family that a rapid, good death is the best outcome" (paragraph 2).

Medicine's dedication to preserving life has many benefits. Caregivers' devotion and talent, along with their access to medical technology, has helped to increase the average American's life expectancy from 47.3 to 77.8 years since 1900 (National Center for Health Statistics, 2007a). But a "life at all costs" approach can rob people of the opportunity for a good death. Susan Block (2001) calls a good death "The Art of the Possible." The means of realizing this possibility, she says, lie in making people physically comfortable and helping them nurture caring relationships, maintain a sense of self, find meaning, feel a sense of control, and prepare for death. One man at the end of his life attested: "What this last year has provided me with is the occasion to be deliberately open to receiving other people's love

and care…and I'm delighted when it happens" (quoted by Block, p. 2902).

Many caregivers who become comfortable with death say it's a privilege to be with people at the end of their lives. A physician Block (2001) interviewed said of one dying patient:

> I really like seeing him because no matter how distraught I am about that particular day or feeling overwhelmed…I feel so much better after each visit with him. It's almost like he's a doctor to me. (p. 2903)

Loved ones often feel the same way, that they have learned something precious by being present at the end of a cherished individual's life.

Conventional wisdom says we are likely to lose faith or be angry at God when someone close to us dies. But this occurs mostly when death is sudden or when people have not accepted its inevitability. Participants in Maureen Keeley's (2004) study of "final conversations" say their loss was tempered by a renewed sense of comfort, meaning, and spirituality. Said one, "You can't go through this…witnessing death, without that awe of what life is. Where it comes from and where it goes" (quoted by Keeley, p. 95). In another episode, a survivor remembers asking a loved one, "When you get to heaven, you know, keep an eye out for my girls," and her reply, "I will, you know. I'll be their guardian angel" (p. 97). In these episodes, the dying individual was able to help others find peace and comfort.

Proponents of a good death remind us that that might *not* involve preserving life as long as possible. As McCue (1995) proposes, "a rapid, good death" is sometimes preferable to a prolonged, painful end. Prolonging life sometimes means prolonging death. And caregivers and others who perceive death to be a frightening enemy are not equipped to help with end-of-life care. Dying individuals sometimes feel forgotten and ignored because their caregivers are uncomfortable with death, reluctant to become emotionally involved, and uncertain how to act around dying people (Hyde, 1993).

Unfortunately, the opportunity to die peacefully among loved ones is sometimes lost in a confusion of tubes, wires, monitors, and hospital restrictions (Cohn, Harrold, & Lynn, 1997). Most people (68.9%) receive hospital care in the last 48 hours of their life and 92.1% of those individuals die in the hospital (Teno et al., 2004). It may be comforting to have professionals on hand, but it is hard for loved ones to be present and difficult to maintain a sense of intimacy and individuality in an institutional setting such as a hospital. Communication scholar Sandra Ragan reflects on the difference between her father's death and her sister's:

> Dad's death was a conflicted one: He died in a hospital, connected to various machines, and in constant fear, until his last 48 hours, when he entered a morphine-induced semiconsciousness, that his doctors would not give him adequate medication. (Ragan, Wittenberg, & Hall, 2003, p. 219)

In contrast, her sister died at home under hospice care:

> Sherry died peacefully in her own home with no medical intervention other than oxygen, a catheter, and the blessing of morphine and ativan. Her family and loved ones surrounded her, and throughout her last night, she was cradled by her daughter and her beloved cocker spaniel. (Ragan et al., pp. 219–220)

## Death with Dignity

In Japan, a metaphor for the ideal death is *pokkuri shinu*, which translates roughly into "popping like a bubble." People in many cultures share the same wish, of living fully and then dying without languishing slowly away. In the United States, a good death is often described as one in which people maintain dignity and die surrounded by loved ones and familiar, comforting surroundings.

The motto of death with dignity is attributable mostly to **hospice**, an organization that provides support and care for dying individuals and their families. Hospice provides **palliative care**, that is, care designed to keep a person as comfortable and fulfilled as possible at the end of life but not designed to cure the main illness once it has been determined that medical care will not improve it.

About half of all dying patients in the United States now receive hospice care at home. Of those, nearly 71% consider their care to be "excellent," a figure that is 20% higher than people who die in hospitals and nursing homes (Teno et al., 2004). The bad news is that about 36% of people who die at home receive no hospice or other nursing care (Teno et al.). Consequently, they and their families are more likely to feel alienated and to feel that their pain was not managed effectively (Teno et al.)

Central to hospice's philosophy is the belief that death is a natural part of life, thus personal and unique (McCormick & Conley, 1995). People are encouraged to die as they have lived, surrounded by the people and things they love most. Hospice volunteers and professional caregivers visit with terminally ill individuals and their loved ones to talk with them about death (if they wish), make sure the dying person is not in pain, encourage spiritual exploration, and provide many forms of assistance. In this effort, hospice is more oriented than conventional Western medicine to personal expression, emotions, spirituality, and social concerns. Loved ones are considered important participants in the dying process.

Beth Perry, a hospice nurse, recalls an especially rewarding experience helping a dying patient. "Roman, a handsome man in his mid-50s, seemed too well to be a patient on a palliative care unit," she remembers (Perry, 2002, paragraph 5). But Roman *was* dying, and he was bored and tired of the process—ready for the tedium to end. Although Roman's caregivers knew his death was near, they sought a way to rekindle his sense of purpose. Someone remembered that he and his wife had bought a new home just before he became ill, and the grounds were not yet landscaped. They suggested that the couple plan the garden and grounds together. "The result was amazing," writes Perry:

> The next time we visited the pair, gone was the stony silence, the painful watching of time tick by. Instead, we found the two of them with their noses in the same magazine, eagerly debating annuals versus perennials, tulips versus delphiniums. (paragraph 7)

Although Roman did not live to plant the garden, his last days were filled with enthusiasm rather than boredom. Julie, another nurse caring for Roman, says, "People can take almost anything, but they can't take being forgotten. They want to know that something they have done will live on after they die, and sometimes it is part of my role to help them" (quoted by Perry, 2002, paragraph 8).

Hospice volunteers play a vital role in the organization. A beautiful account of this is available in Elissa Foster's (2007) book *Communicating at the End of Life: Finding Magic in the Mundane*. In the book, Foster chronicles her year as a hospice volunteer and shares the stories of other volunteers and the patients she meets along the way. Threaded throughout the narrative is Foster's relationship with Dorothy, a petite, energetic woman with "lively blue-green" eyes and white, close-cropped hair. Dorothy is under hospice care because doctors recognize that she is in the final stages of chronic obstructive pulmonary disease (COPD). Foster describes her initial sense of uncertainty and nervousness meeting Dorothy and her family, as well as the warmth and camaraderie that develop between them during weekly visits and outings. Foster captures the confusion and concern she feels as Dorothy's condition seems alternately to deteriorate and improve over time. She also reveals the mutuality of their relationship. Dorothy is not simply the recipient of Foster's care; the caring goes both ways. In a particularly poignant passage, Foster values Dorothy's level-headedness during the September 11, 2001, terrorist attacks. For Dorothy—who has lived through world war and lost a son to Vietnam—the violence is less shocking, less surreal, than it is to many. On a day when the world seemed to turn upside down, Foster remembers thinking: "I can hardly wait to arrive at Dorothy's apartment, to cocoon myself in her world, if only for a couple of hours. I will feel safe" (p. 140). Foster also describes her own sense of loss when Dorothy dies. She visits Dorothy's family in the hours after her death, shares hugs and tears with them, and thanks them for "sharing" their mother with her. She later reflects: "My relationship with Dorothy taught me that I could connect with someone whom I hardly

know, simply by being there and being willing to let it happen" (p. 210).

We turn next to the concept of slow medicine. Slow medicine does not necessarily involve palliative care, but the two have something in common—a commitment to taking our time and developing caring relationships.

### Slow Medicine

As physician Dennis McCullough (2008) explains in *My Mother, Your Mother*, the "slow medicine" concept draws inspiration from Italy, where some communities have decided to resist the urge to eat, drive, talk, and live quickly. In some slow cities, cars are no longer allowed downtown. This permits people to walk more safely and leisurely and visit with neighbors along the way. McCullough, a geriatrician, has adapted a similar philosophy of care that emphasizes deep, rich understanding, wisdom, patience, and flexibility. The central tenets of slow medicine include: (1) taking time to understand older adults as individuals with rich histories, wisdom, and challenges, (2) working to develop a healthy, trusting balance between independence and assistance, (3) communicating with warmth, caring, and patience, (4) steadfast advocacy for people who are in need, and (5), as McCullough puts it, "kindness, no matter what" (p. 12).

The idea behind slow medicine is not to compromise the quality of medical care, but to imbue it with warmth, patience, and gentleness. McCullough (2008) compares a slow medicine annual review to the traditional medical workup:

> Unlike the battery of lab tests and screenings a doctor might order for you at middle age, in late life it is rather an exercise in attentive listening. Most questions focus on medical problems certainly, but also include asking how an elderly man, say, spends his time, searching for clues about his emotional state, observing how his mind works, and inviting him to share his own insights about these important aspects of successful aging. (p. 23)

He encourages the families of older adults to adopt the same slow style. "Over the course of three full days, just go and be with your parent without escaping into your own preferred activities," McCullough encourages (p. 27). Observe their routines and rituals. This intimate time is likely to be more enjoyable and more intimate than a jam-packed itinerary. It also better equips you to notice "slow slips" in health that might be reversed with early care and to differentiate between the preferences of youth and the pleasures of later life.

The experience of slow medicine also enables us to learn from the people in our lives whose experiences far exceed our own. They have a lot to teach us about life and death, McCullough (2008) says:

> An elder, ending life with both identity and dignity intact, is at the center of everyone's attention—forgiven for what he or she did wrong or was unable to do, celebrated for a known public or lesser-known private life, and cherished in the memory of those who knew the breadth and depth of his or her being....An elder's well-supported death invites a celebration of his or her living. (p. 202)

## Advance-Care Directives

**Advance-care directives** describe in advance the medical care a person wishes to receive (or not receive) if he or she becomes too ill to communicate. These directives take some of the pressure off caregivers and loved ones, who might otherwise be forced to make those decisions on their own.

Despite the advantages, the majority of U.S. residents have not written advance-care directives or even conveyed their wishes about end-of-life care to their physicians. By most estimates, fewer than 26% of U.S. residents have filed advance-care directives with their doctors. The percentage may be as high as 70% among the nation's nursing home residents, but they constitute less than 10% of the population. That leaves an overwhelming number of people without written instructions about their end-of-life care, even though communicating one's preferences for end-of-life care is central to the idea of a good death (Borreani et al., 2008).

Advance-care directives have become more specific through the years. When they were first

conceptualized as "living wills" in the 1960s, they typically referred in vague terms to "heroic" life-saving measures (Emanuel & Emanuel, 1998). This presented obvious difficulties in interpretation (e.g.: Is a feeding tube heroic? Is intravenous therapy heroic?). It is now common for advance-care directives to include a person's preferences regarding specific procedures and circumstances, to endow someone with decision-making authority, and to describe the person's philosophy of life and death to help guide decisions during unanticipated circumstances. (See Box 7.6 for a discussion of the right-to-die issue.)

Some of the ambivalence about advanced-care directives stems from terminology and some from the factors people weigh when considering the value of life. Amanda Young and Keri Rodriguez (2006) asked veterans about their interpretation of terms such as *life-sustaining treatment* and *state of permanent unconsciousness*. They identified the following main themes in the veterans' responses.

- *Life should be judged by quality rather than quantity*. Most respondents said they would not be in favor of prolonging life if the individual had no chance of regaining consciousness. In those cases, they said, life support was more a comfort to the living than a kindness to the patient. Said one participant in the study: "I don't think anyone who cares for you would want you to just exist. If you're just existing, you're just existing for someone else's benefit in most cases because you certainly don't have any chance at a life" (p. 55).
- *People should weigh costs and benefits*. Most people interviewed felt that suffering is worthwhile if the person is still able to enjoy life or make a contribution to others, as in undergoing experimental treatments to help with medical research. But they felt that it was wasteful to spend money and other resources on life support that would not restore a person's quality of life.
- *It's a matter of control*. People's attitude about life-sustaining measures often hinged

## BOX 7.6 ETHICAL CONSIDERATIONS

# Do People Have a Right to Die?

In 1997, Oregon made history by legalizing physician-assisted suicide for terminally ill patients. Under the law, a doctor may help a person commit suicide if at least two physicians verify that the person has less than 6 months to live and the patient requests help with suicide at least once in writing and twice verbally, with at least 15 days between requests ("Oregon Begins," 1998).

**Physician-assisted suicide** refers to instances in which, at the request of a terminally ill person, a doctor provides the means for that person to end his or her own life (Krug, 1998). The doctor does not actually kill the patient. This is different from **euthanasia** (also called *mercy killing*), in which a physician or family member intentionally kills the patient to end his or her suffering. The distinction lies in who does the killing—the patient or another person.

The person most commonly associated with physician-assisted suicide is Jack Kevorkian, a physician who, by his own estimate, has assisted in the suicides of 130 people since 1990 (Robertson, 1999). Kevorkian was tried for murder five times, but he was not convicted until the fifth trial, which concluded in April 1999. Kevorkian was declared guilty of second-degree murder by a Michigan jury and sentenced to 10 to 25 years in prison. The conviction was based on an assisted suicide that Kevorkian videotaped and allowed to be broadcast on *60 Minutes* (Willing, 1999). Kevorkian, who was released on parole in 2007, argues that he is motivated by compassion for people dying slow, painful deaths. His opponents charge that he is a medical "hitman" operating outside the law (Robertson).

Controversy over physician-assisted suicide is likely to continue for quite some time, with people vigorously arguing both sides of the issue. Proponents of physician-assisted suicide include Dax Cowart, who was badly burned in an explosion in 1973 (Cowart & Burt, 1998). Two-thirds of Cowart's body was burned in the accident, and he lost his eyesight and his fingers.

For more than a year Cowart begged doctors to let him die. Despite his pleas, medical teams continued to treat his burns. The treatment kept Cowart alive and eventually helped him regain the ability to walk. But for more than a year he was in nearly unbearable agony. He recalls: "The pain was excruciating, it was so far beyond any pain that I ever knew was possible, that I simply could not endure it" (paragraph 21). Cowart supports physician-assisted suicide. However, even if a law such as Oregon's had been in place when his accident occurred, he would not have qualified for lawful physician-assisted suicide because he was not dying.

Cowart is now an attorney in Corpus Christi, Texas, and describes himself as "happier than most people." But he maintains his conviction that people should not be forced to undergo treatment they do not wish, even if that treatment is needed to keep them alive (Cowart & Burt, 1998). Faced with the same ordeal again, he feels he would wish to die and should be allowed to do so. Cowart's views are captured in his videos *Please Let Me Die* and *Dax's Case*.

On the other side of the issue, some argue that people in intense pain and grief may not see things clearly enough to make life-ending decisions. They point out that Cowart has changed his mind about living with his disabilities. Although he initially felt life would be empty, he now is happy and successful (Cowart & Burt, 1998). Other critics say ill (even terminally ill) patients may request death for the wrong reasons. They may be afraid about the future, feel out of control and scared, or believe they are a burden to loved ones (Muskin, 1998). For these reasons, they feel it is wrong to help someone commit suicide, even if the person requests it.

## What Do You Think?

1. Under what circumstances, if any, do you feel patients should be assisted in killing themselves?
2. Should it make a difference whether a patient is terminally ill or not?

3. If you were in Dax Cowart's place, do you feel you would want to die? What would you have done if you were Cowart's caregivers and loved ones?
4. What do you think of the argument that people who are scared and in pain may be not thinking clearly enough to make life-or-death decisions?
5. What do you think of the counterargument—that people should not second-guess the patient's wishes because they cannot fully understand the extent of his or her personal suffering?

## Suggested Sources

Cowart, D., & Burt, R. (1998). Confronting death: Who chooses, who controls? *The Hastings Center Report, 28,* 14–24.

Kenny, R. W. (2001). Toward a better death: Applying Burkean principles of symbolic action to interpret family adaptation to Karen Ann Quinlan's coma. *Health Communication, 13*(4), 363–385.

Kenny, R. W. (2002). The death of loving: Maternal identity as moral constraint in a narrative testimonial advocating physician assisted suicide. *Health Communication, 14*(2), 243–270.

Krug, P. (1998). Where does physician-assisted suicide stand today? *Association of Operating Room Nurses Journal, 68,* 869.

Muskin, P. R. (1998). The request to die: Role for a psychodynamic perspective on physician assisted suicide. *Journal of the American Medical Association, 279,* 323–328.

on issues of control, whether that control was perceived to lie with God, the medical establishment, the patient, or loved ones. One man described how his mother asserted control by refusing to eat after she lost her will to live. "She wanted to go, she just wanted to die. She did" (p. 57). Others considered that the decision rightfully rests with God or fate. As one man put it: "I don't think I should take that kind of thing into my own hands. That's another human being. That's not my kind of decision. It's God's decision" (p. 57).

## Communication Skill Builders:
### Delivering Bad News

One of the most difficult communication challenges anyone faces is sharing devastating news with another. The consequences are profound for the news recipient as well. Karen Belk, who has diabetes and a number of other health concerns, remembers one of the most difficult moments of her life. "When the doctor said, 'I don't think I'll be able to save your left eye. I'll try to save your right eye,' those were the worst words I had ever heard," she says. Her fears were heightened because she didn't know what to expect and didn't know if her lack of insurance would dissuade doctors from doing everything they could to save her sight. "I didn't know how long I was going to keep my sight," she recalls. "It was always in the back of my mind: I'm going to be blind. There's so much I want to do before that happens."

Bad news is never easy to give or to receive. But there are a number of communication strategies that help optimize people's coping ability. Here are some suggestions from the experts on how to share bad news compassionately.

- *Build caring relationships from the beginning.* In a study of recently diagnosed cancer patients, Pär Salander (2002) found that patients did not describe one distinct event during which they learned their diagnosis. They considered that it occurred within the context of ongoing relationships with the medical staff. Said one woman: "The kindness, the support, and the help I received from the entire staff when treatment started is what I appreciate the most" (p. 724).

- *Foreshadow the disclosure.* A simple statement such as "The news isn't as good as we hoped" may help prepare people for what's to come.
- *Invite the recipient to bring along supportive others.*
- *Talk in a quiet, private place.* Resist the temptation to deliver bad news in a hallway or semiprivate space. Likewise, avoid delivering bad news over the phone whenever possible (Sparks, Villagran, Parker-Raley, & Cunningham, 2007).
- *Tell the truth.* People typically cope better when they know what is happening and what to expect. This is true even when death is to be expected. A participant in Thomas McCormick and Becky Conley's (1995) study said, "That's one of the things that I like my doctor for, because he was plain with me that I was incurable" (paragraph 38). She explained that people who do not know they are dying cannot prepare for it emotionally or practically. They lose the chance to settle financial affairs, communicate with loved ones, set new priorities for their limited time, and adjust emotionally to what is occurring.
- *Avoid medical jargon.*
- *Acknowledge and legitimize emotions.* Emotions are a natural part of the coping process. Ignoring them may make the news recipient feel foolish or inappropriate. Instead, acknowledge emotions with statements such as "I know this is very hard to hear," "I understand this can feel overwhelming," and "It's natural to feel a range of emotions when you learn something like this."
- *Take your cues from the recipient.* Don't be surprised if people seem stoic or distant on hearing bad news, whereas others are tearful or even angry. It's hard for any of us to say how we will react in such circumstances. Patients typically say it is unhelpful when

someone attempts to impose a particular agenda or set of emotions on them (Maynard & Frankel, 2006). One patient Salander (2002) interviewed wondered: "Why did they have to be so dramatic? Suddenly, everybody looked so grave and became so low-voiced. It gave me a feeling of unreality" (p. 725).

- *Show genuine caring.* As one woman put it: "A hug or supportive word in passing worked miracles" (quoted by Salander, 2002, p. 727).
- *Be aware of personal and cultural preferences for bad news delivery.* Some people, such as members of traditional Native American cultures, prefer that bad news be delivered indirectly through metaphors and storytellings (T. L. Thompson & Gillotti, 2005). In some other cultures, speaking bad news aloud is considered unlucky.
- *Offer support.* Indicate your own support and offer other resources to help people learn, adjust, and cope.
- *Be ready with options and a plan of action.* Although some people may need time to take in the bad news before they make decisions, most say that having a specified next step helped them funnel their energy and emotion in positive ways and to feel less like helpless victims.
- *Schedule an information follow-up.* Keep in mind that few people can absorb and remember many details when they are feeling intense emotions. Written materials may help, as will a follow-up visit to talk about the details once the news has set in.

## Coping with Death

One positive aspect of death is that it draws people together. Loved ones who may not have seen each other in years unite again with a common concern. Death also provides an occasion for contemplating life and the purpose of living. A sense of insight and spirituality often surrounds death (McCormick & Conley, 1995). Moreover, by sharing in loved ones' deaths, people may become less fearful of death themselves. Joyce Dyer, who wrote *In a Tangled Wood* (1996) about her mother's 9-year experience with Alzheimer's disease, reflected after her death:

> I want to remember every moment I had with my mother, including every second of the last nine years. I want to remember her toothless grin, her screams, her growing fondness for sweets and then for nothing at all, the bouquets of uprooted flowers she picked for me from her unit's patio, the way she tried to fold her bib, the rare pats on my cheek that meant everything, her last words, her last party, her last dance. And I want to remember what I learned from aides and nurses, from volunteers and cleaning staff, from my mother's own sick friends. I don't want to forget a single thing. (Dyer, 1996, p. 136)

People may be surprised by the mixture of emotions they feel about death. Most of us are not sure what to expect, and consequently we are often uncertain how to act around dying individuals. Based on news reports and movies, people typically imagine death as violent and scary. However, the majority of deaths are nothing like that. Colin Parkes (1998) describes the typical death as a "quiet slipping away" without pain or horror.

One nurse described her initial discomfort when a young man in her care joked that he had to live quickly because he would not live long (Erdman, 1993). The nurse was eventually able to laugh with the young man when he quipped that he was watching movies on fast-forward and bathing his dog in the drive-through carwash to save time. Writes Erdman: "The nurse was at first caught off guard by the patient's comments, but the humor opened the door to further communication about death" (p. 59).

Three themes emerge in the narratives of older adults reflecting on the death of loved ones: loss, feelings, coping. The feelings are mixed, but not as negative as you might expect. In Caplan, Haslett, and Burleson's (2005) study of older-adult bereavement narratives, 36% of the feelings were negative (fear, loneliness, sadness), but 43% were positive (optimism, thankfulness for time spent together, and so on). Said one woman, whose husband died

in 1993: "I don't dwell on the sickness and problems of what happened then, but my thoughts and memories instead, think of all the good and wonderful life we had together with the six children" (p. 244).

As mentioned previously, health professionals may take a patient's death especially hard. Janice Rosenberg (1996) writes that a doctor is typically regarded as "super-scientist, able to confront death and beat it every time" (paragraph 3). Even physicians may expect themselves to be superhuman, and they may feel guilty and sad when they consider outcomes less than perfect. To make matters worse, doctors may consider it unprofessional to feel or show emotions (Haug, 1996).

Some researchers report success with end-of-life education for students and health professionals. In Hungary, fear of death diminished among participants in a course about medical care at the end of life (Hegedus, Zana, & Szabó, 2008). The researchers propose that the course was effective at easing fears because it emphasized that dying does not necessarily involve suffering and it presented a number of ways to preserve quality of life until the end.

Usually, whether a death is good or bad depends on the emotional coping resources of the people surrounding it. Supportive gestures are especially helpful, but insensitive actions are especially hurtful. McCue (1995) recommends assistance and social support for caregivers and loved ones. Often, he asserts, elderly individuals accept their own deaths as deeply personal and spiritual, but they are adversely affected by the fear and dread of well-meaning others. Supporting caregivers and families is important for their sake and for patients' sake.

In her book *On Death and Dying*, Elisabeth Kubler-Ross (1969) describes death as occurring in five stages: denial and isolation, anger, bargaining, depression, and acceptance. Not everyone experiences all five stages or in the order given, but dying individuals and the people around them are likely to experience many of these phases. Although with enough time and support many people eventually feel peaceful about death, they may at times refuse to believe what is told them, or they may feel angry, overwhelmed, sad, or hopeless. Often, people feel

## BOX 7.7 CAREER OPPORTUNITIES

# Social Services and Mental Health

Mental health counselor
Social worker
Psychologist
Social service manager
Hospice/palliative care provider
Home health aide
Senior citizen services providers

## Career Resources and Job Listings

American Mental Health Counselors Association:
www.amhca.org
Mental health counselor job profile:
www.jobprofiles.org/heacounselor.htm

American Psychological Association: www.apa.org
National Association of School Psychologists:
www.nasponline.org
American Board of Professional Psychology:
www.abpp.org
National Organization for Human Services:
www.nationalhumanservices.org
Hospice: www.hospicenet.org
Hospice careers: hospicechoices.com
Center for Hospice and Palliative Care:
www.centerforhospice.org/careers.cfm
National Association for Home Care and Hospice:
www.nahc.org
Senior citizen services provider job profile:
www.jobprofiles.org/heaelderlycaregiver.htm

*Also see social worker resources in Box 5.3.*

---

their God has let them down, and they react by showing anger or attempting to bargain for mercy. It may be reassuring to remember that these stages are common and legitimate components of the coping process.

## OVERSUPPORTING

Before closing this chapter on social support it is important to acknowledge that there can be too much of a good thing. Some attempts at social support hurt more than they help. Especially if "supportive" efforts are offered inappropriately or profusely, they can impair people's coping abilities. In this section we look at **oversupport,** defined as excessive and unnecessary help (Edwards & Noller, 1998). Following is a discussion of three types of oversupport: overhelping, overinforming, and overempathizing.

### Overhelping

**Overhelping** is providing too much instrumental assistance. This can make people feel like children or shield them from life experiences. People who

are overhelped may become needlessly dependent on others, feel left out of life activities, and begin to doubt their own abilities (Goldsmith, 1994).

Helen Edwards and Patricia Noller (1998) found that some women's take-charge attitude led them to be overly domineering in caring for their elderly husbands. Couples in this situation reported high conflict and low morale. Their relationships and their attitudes suffered.

### Overinforming

Forcing information on people when they are too distraught to understand it or accept it (**overinforming**) may only heighten their stress. Philip Muskin (1998) calls this "truth dumping" and warns people against it. Health-related information can be confusing and frightening. Facts change and outlooks vary. People may shy away from the truth, preferring to preserve hope or minimize their confusion.

### Overempathizing

Overempathizing is actually something of a misnomer, because it applies only to a particular type of empathy, called *emotional contagion*. In a general sense, **empathy** is the ability to show that you understand how someone else is feeling. Katherine Miller and colleagues (1995) have identified two components of empathy: **Empathic concern** is an intellectual appreciation of someone's feelings; **emotional contagion** involves actually feeling emotions similar to the other person's. Research shows that the second kind, emotional contagion, can be overdone.

One drawback of emotional contagion is that it can be exhausting. Miller and colleagues (1995) identified a link between emotional contagion and emotional exhaustion among people who work with homeless individuals. As you may recall from Chapter 4, emotional exhaustion is a component of burnout characterized by reduced motivation and compassion.

Taken to extremes, emotional contagion can also be detrimental to support receivers. Some of the literature on support groups warns that members sometimes empathize so much with each other that they perceive people outside the group to be ignorant and uncaring. Jeffrey Fisher and coauthors (1988) noted this effect among HIV/AIDS support group members. The perception that people outside the group are less empathic than those in it may discourage group members from developing social networks with diverse people.

Another danger is that people may hesitate to express themselves to listeners who are likely to become upset. In Eric Zook's (1993) case study, a man who cared for his dying partner at home remembers: "As long as I was kind of detached and logical about it, he would take it [his declining health] very well" (p. 117). The perceived need to seem unemotional and in control can make it seem that people do not need social support, when in fact they do.

Finally, some people find emotional empathy overwhelming or belittling. They may avoid scenes in which others seem to pity them. Wayne Beach (2002) describes the "stoic orientation" adopted by a father and son discussing the news that the mother was diagnosed with cancer. The son received the news calmly. Rather than reacting emotionally,

he initially responded with a series of "OK's" and technical questions such as "That's the one above her kidney?" (p. 279). Beach speculates that this factual, stoic orientation saved the father and son from immediately "flooding out." In this way, they were able both to maintain composure and to display that they were knowledgeable and capable of coping with the news.

## SUMMARY

A diverse number of behaviors make up social support. Support is useful in everyday life and in times of crisis. What is most supportive depends on the nature of the situation, the people involved, and their perception of health self-efficacy. Sometimes problem solving is the most effective coping strategy. In those instances, instrumental and informative support are likely to be appreciated. When the situation calls for emotional adjustment, nurturing support may be a useful way to help people feel better about themselves, express their emotions, and feel that others will stand by them in times of trouble.

Being normal sounds easy, but to members of society viewed as abnormal, achieving a sense of normalcy can seem as impossible as it is desirable. People do well to remember that individuals who have disabilities or are ill do not usually benefit from being treated as if they are childlike or helpless.

People usually cope more effectively when they can discuss sensitive topics than when they feel compelled to feign cheerfulness. Avoid assuming that individuals are coping well because are quiet or do not display much emotion. Research suggests these people often receive less support than others, although they probably need it just as much. Communication is most supportive when it allows distressed individuals to express themselves as they wish and to set the pace for talk and action. Supportive listeners are attentive, nonjudgmental, and able to help people understand their own emotions.

Information is often useful in coping, but as the theory of problematic integration points out, information sometimes creates as many uncertainties and contradictions as it does certainties. Sometimes it can be overwhelming.

Strong networks, including social support group membership, are often life-enhancing. Likewise, virtual communities and support groups expand the opportunities for communicating with people who have similar concerns and experiences. However, they can be limiting if people rely on online communities to the extent of avoiding face-to-face relationships.

What seems like a crisis is sometimes revealed as a valuable experience in which people learn and come into contact with things they may never have imagined. In transcendent experiences, people come to perceive an overarching meaning that makes sense of situations that initially seemed tragic or pointless.

As the need for lay caregivers has risen, the demands on lay caregivers' time have increased as well. Lay caregivers are an important source of social support, but they too need support. Support groups, skills-training programs, and the assistance of family and friends are promising sources of support for lay caregivers.

Medicine has traditionally considered death a failure, to be avoided at all costs, but groups such as hospice promote the philosophy that there is such a thing as a good death. For the most part, a good death unites people in a sense of peace and comfort. When people are able to cope effectively, death may bring people together and help them overcome their fears.

Sometimes efforts that are meant to be supportive hurt more than they help. Too much assistance can make people feel helpless and dependent. Too much information or ill-timed disclosures can tax people's coping ability, and emotional contagion can be exhausting and can discourage people from describing their feelings.

## KEY TERMS

social support
coping
problem solving
emotional adjustment
health self-efficacy
internal locus of control
external locus of control
crisis
normalcy
action-facilitating support
nurturing support
instrumental support
informational support
health information seeking
health information scanning
health information efficacy
theory of problematic integration
esteem support
emotional support
social network support
support groups
virtual communities
transcendent experiences
lay caregivers
Family and Medical Leave Act of 1993
hospice
palliative care
advance-care directives
physician-assisted suicide
euthanasia
oversupport
overhelping
overinforming
overempathizing
empathy
empathic concern
emotional contagion

## DISCUSSION QUESTIONS

1. What two efforts are usually involved in coping? Can you think of instances in which you did one or both of these? How effective would you rate your coping skills?
2. What does it mean to consider the body a "therapeutic landscape"?
3. How do an internal and an external locus of control differ? What impact does locus of

control having on coping and making health-related decisions?

4. Have you ever faced a crisis? Did you experience the sense that things might never be the same again? What coping strategies did you use? What types of support from others were most helpful?

5. How is a sense of normalcy related to social support?

6. What are two types of action-facilitating support? Give an example of each from your own experience.

7. In what circumstances might it be especially difficult to integrate problematic information? Why? Have you ever felt confused or overwhelmed by information? If so, how did you cope?

8. What are three types of nurturing support? Give an example of each from your own experience.

9. What are some communication strategies for supportive listening?

10. What are some tips for allowing emotional expression?

11. How are our social networks likely to change as we age? Why?

12. In what ways is social support linked to health and longevity?

13. What are some reasons and techniques for encouraging strong social network support?

14. In what ways is support group involvement typically beneficial? In what ways can it be harmful?

15. What are the advantages and disadvantages of virtual communities?

16. Compare the birth experiences of Carol Bishop Mills and her husband with those of Kate and Chris. What do you learn from these examples?

17. What does the term *transcendent experience* mean? Can you think of examples from movies or your own experiences?

18. What factors might convince (or discourage) you from registering as an organ donor?

19. Describe the typical lay caregiver for a frail older adult in terms of the caregiver's sex, health, and relationship to the older adult.

20. Describe provisions of the Family and Medical Leave Act of 1993.

21. What factors typically contribute to stress and burnout among lay caregivers?

22. Have you experienced the death of a loved one? How did it compare to the process described in "A Long Goodbye to Grandmother" (Box 7.5)?

23. In your opinion, is there such thing as a good death? If so, how would you describe it?

24. Why might caregivers adopt a life-at-all-costs perspective?

25. What are the potential disadvantages of a life-at-all-costs perspective?

26. What role does hospice play?

27. What is your opinion of the right-to-die issue (Box 7.6)? Why?

28. In what ways can people be oversupportive? What are the likely outcomes of different types of oversupport?

## ANSWERS TO *CAN YOU GUESS?*

1. Seven are daughters, three are sons (R. W. Johnson & Wiener, 2006).

2. Kidneys are overwhelmingly the most in-demand organs. They account for 76% of needed organs, followed at a distance by livers (17%) and hearts (3%) (Stevens, Lynm, & Glass, 2008).

# CHAPTER
# 8

# Cultural Conceptions of Health and Illness

*Unaware that the patient believes her soul will remain where she dies, the physician is frustrated by a woman's wish to leave the hospital when her condition is critical (Orr, 1996).*

*A patient unfamiliar with institutional medicine is disappointed when she is not cured by the X-rays her doctor orders (Uba, 1992).*

*Deeply committed to the healing power of positive thinking, a Navajo man becomes upset when his doctor describes the negative outcomes that may result from an upcoming surgery (Jecker, Carrese, & Pearlman, 1995).*

Diverse beliefs about health and illness profoundly affect health communication. Everyone is involved in making sense of health experiences. The way you talk about health, how you describe your aches and pains, the reasons you seek medical care or encourage others to—all these go beyond physical manifestations of illness. Joy Hart and Kandi Walker (2008) remind us that "we don't create a new slate each time we have a new experience" (p. 129). Instead, we base our current understanding on what we know from personal history, culture, and knowledge.

As the population becomes more diverse, it is especially important to appreciate culturally diverse ways of viewing health and illness. Misunderstandings can occur when people have different ideas about the nature of disease, how people are supposed to act in health care situations, and how illness reflects on people in the community.

For example, doctors who do not understand that Eastern cultures consider mental illness dishonorable may be frustrated when Asian patients seem depressed but vehemently deny it. If these patients refuse counseling, their caregivers may assume they are indifferent or obstinate. As a result patient–caregiver relationships may suffer, and these people may avoid medical care in the future. (For more on career opportunities in health care and diversity awareness, see Box 6.6.) In this chapter we examine evidence that cultural ideas influence well-being.

**Culture** refers to a set of beliefs, rules, and practices that are shared by a group of people. Cultural assumptions suggest how members should behave, what roles they are expected to play, and how various events and actions should be interpreted. In some cases one culture disdains what another reveres. For example, in some Russian cultures patients assume that doctors are incompetent if they do not wear lab coats and behave in a formal manner (Goode, 1993). Conversely, many Americans like doctors who seem casual and friendly.

We will explore the impact of culture on health and healing in this chapter, beginning with the question "Why consider culture?" and then profiling some major world cultures before surveying different ways of conceptualizing health and illness and the role sets that patients and caregivers play. Next is a cultural analysis of Viagra marketing, based primarily on Baglia's (2005) work on the subject. As you will see, the publicity surrounding this pharmaceutical product has had profound implications, not only for health, but for relationships and perceived social norms. The chapter concludes with communication strategies for intercultural health communication.

## WHY CONSIDER CULTURE?

Considering cultural differences is not merely an exercise in curiosity. It is an important prerequisite for working toward better health around the world. Consider the following statistics.

- Every day about 24,000 people around the world die from conditions that could have been cured with basic medical care. The yearly total is equal to the population of New York City (J. Donnelly, 2003).
- In India each year, an average of 10,700 children die of cancer, whereas about 350 children die of the same disease in the United Kingdom ("Children," 2003).
- In Tanzania, Africa, 2 of every 10 children will not live until age 5 (Spear, 2003).
- Around the world, about 11 million children die every year because of preventable conditions such as malnutrition and unsafe air and water ("About 11 Million," 2002).
- In developing countries, 1 in 16 women will die during childbirth, compared to 1 in 4,600 in the United Kingdom (Eaton & Dyer, 2003).
- Although the United States is the wealthiest country in the world, 28 countries outrank Americans in terms of life expectancy

(WHO Statistical Information, 2008). This is primarily because the gap between rich and poor is larger in the United States than in any other developed country.

Very often cultural barriers and perceived barriers limit our awareness. This occurs when people live across the world from each other and even when they are in the same country. Cultures different from our own may seem remote geographically and experientially. It's difficult to imagine that we could make a difference if we tried. But we all suffer the implications of that assumption. For one, we learn less about ourselves, life, and the world when we allow cultural barriers to separate us. Second, although we may perceive cultural and national boundaries, health threats do not. The outbreak of SARS, AIDS, and other communicable diseases makes it clear that health is a global phenomenon requiring global teamwork and interconnectedness. Achieving that will require a transcultural commitment to open communication, learning, and understanding.

Culture is also germane because cultural mores may make us more or less susceptible to health concerns. Consider sexual practices and the risk of HIV/AIDS. In many parts of Africa men's privilege to demand sex, even from women they do not know, contributes to an environment in which women can do little to protect themselves from AIDS. Gregory Kamwendo and Olex Kamowa (1999)—both of the University of Malawi in southern Africa—describe Malawian customs that put people at risk for sexually transmitted diseases. These customs include raids in which boys and men sneak into adolescent girls' huts during the night and have intercourse with them, ritual "sex education" in which *fisis* (anonymous male tutors) have sex with girls to test their readiness for marriage, exchanges in which men swap wives for sexual episodes, and spousal inherences in which a man "inherits" his brother's widow or his wife's sister. Underlying these customs is the belief that women cannot refuse sex or insist on condom use. Kamwendo and Kamowa write:

> In Malawi, women have no power to negotiate for safe sexual practices with their partners because sex

is a taboo subject even between husband and wife, and a woman who discusses sex openly is viewed as ill-mannered and promiscuous. (p. 172)

In Malawi, HIV/AIDS is more prevalent among married women than in any other demographic group.

In Mexico, men are often admired for having many sexual partners and for fathering many children (Pick, Givaudan, & Poortinga, 2003). Marital infidelity among men is as least implicitly tolerated. Women are expected to be chaste, but it is common practice for young women to use premarital sex to coax men to marry them (Pick et al.).

In India and China, girls and young women may be recruited to work as sex workers, or "hospitality girls" (Liao, Schensul, & Wolffers, 2003). Often, they do not have strong family backgrounds or economic means, so they have little opportunity to escape situations in which they are likely to be exposed to (and pass on) sexually transmitted diseases. But sex is such a taboo subject that the Indian government largely refuses to acknowledge explicitly the causes of AIDS. By some accounts, HIV/AIDS outreach workers are harassed by police officers (Chatterjee, 2003). The government has begun to take a stance against AIDS in recent years, recognizing that the number of people with HIV/AIDS in India is second only to the number in South Africa. However, much of the government rhetoric only hints at the causes of AIDS by decrying a "decline in national values"—presumably, but obliquely, the traditional values of monogamy and sexual restraint (de Souza, 2007, p. 261). In the same campaigns, impoverished women and children and middle-class women are typically cast as "innocent victims" (de Souza). Presumably, men who get HIV/AIDS are not worthy of the same sympathy. Indeed, they are more often viewed as immoral aggressors in spreading the infection. Although the Indian government has declared a "war on AIDS," de Souza says, in many ways it also minimizes the issue by playing down the overall numbers and stopping short of social reforms such as equal rights for women.

As interdependent citizens of the world it is imperative that we seek to understand the perspectives of people who are different from ourselves. In a lecture titled "The Small World of Global Health," physician and public health specialist J. P. Koplan (2002) makes the following point:

> We will have to recognize our interdependencies and look to each other for solutions. We know that a nipavirus outbreak in Malaysia has implications for hog farms in North Carolina. Effective tuberculosis control in India and Mexico affects TB rates in the United States, as does dengue fever control in Mexico and the Caribbean. Foodstuffs contaminated with pathogens or pesticides can originate abroad and appear on your kitchen counter. (p. 297)

Let's look at cultural ideas about health on a more fundamental level by investigating, next, how health and healing are defined in diverse cultures.

## A PROFILE OF CULTURES

> An Asian immigrant to the United States reports a perplexing set of symptoms, including a sense of heaviness and insomnia. Physical tests can detect nothing wrong. The patient attributes his illness to "too much wind" and "not enough blood," conditions resulting from his past immoral behavior. He is simultaneously being treated by a folk healer with meditation and herbal therapies. The American physicians eventually conclude that the man's condition exists "only in his head," although he vigorously denies any emotional upset (Kleinman, Eisenberg, & Good, 1978).

Examples such as this highlight the ways in which well-meaning people can trip over cultural gaps, sometimes with harmful consequences. There isn't room here to survey all the major cultures of the world, but I have done my best to integrate diverse information throughout the chapter and have chosen to spotlight three cultures here—Asian and Pacific Island, Hispanic, and Arab. These are highly populous cultures whose members have migrated around the world. Perhaps this introduction will pique your interest in learning more (see Box 8.1).

# More About Culture and Health

To learn more about cultural ideas concerning health, consult the book listed and visit the listed websites.

Dutta, M. J. (2008). *Communicating health: A culture-centered approach.* Cambridge, MA: Polity Press.

Transcultural Nursing Society and *Journal of Transcultural Nursing*: www.tcns.org

Ethnomed: www.ethnomed.org (includes multilingual health information)

Transcultural Nursing Society: www.tcns.org

Robert Wood Johnson Foundation on Vulnerable Populations: www.rwjf.org/vulnerablepopulations

*Journal of Multicultural Counseling and Development:* www.multiculturalcenter.org/jmcd

Guide to Choosing and Adapting Culturally and Linguistically Competent Health Promotion Materials: www11.georgetown.edu/research/gucchd/nccc/documents/Materials_Guide.pdf

## Asian and Pacific Island

More than half the world's population (56.4%) lives in Asia ("Global Population," 2004). Yet in many respects, the widest cultural gap in the world is between Eastern and Western cultures, making it particularly interesting and challenging for people in those cultures to understand one another (see Box 8.2).

Asians and Pacific Islanders typically do not perceive the mind/body dualism popular in Western thought. They tend to see mind and body as an interwoven whole. And because they have historically put great stock in traditional holistic healing methods, they often seek Western medical care only if other methods have not worked. At that point, they may expect a quick alleviation of symptoms, and they may be disappointed if the doctor doesn't prescribe something that offers instant relief ("Reducing Health Disparities," 2005).

Although Americans may consider caregivers friendly when they are energetic and nonverbally immediate, Asians and Pacific Islanders typically prefer a quiet, unhurried demeanor that begins with nonthreatening information and moves very slowly into the arena of personal concerns (Purnell, 2008). Following are some other insights about Asian and Pacific Island cultures.

- Most Asians and Pacific Islanders will not openly contradict or question another, especially not a high-status person such as a physician. They may use the word "yes" to signal that they understand the speaker, not as a sign that they agree. If they have questions, they may not ask them, for this might be seen as criticizing the speaker.

- Because of their high regard for status, patients may decline to take part in treatment decisions, preferring that doctors make decisions on their behalf ("Reducing Health Disparities," 2005).

- Physical touching and direct eye contact may be seen as overly personal and overly familiar.

- People from Asian cultures are typically not as emotionally expressive as Americans, and their nonverbal displays may mean different things. For example, in China it is common to smile when feeling sadness or discomfort ("Reducing Health Disparities," 2005).

- Asians and Pacific Islanders may be reluctant to say much about their health histories because this information feels private to them. Caregivers may do well to get one bit of information at a time ("Reducing Health Disparities," 2005).

- Members of many Asian cultures consider that the dead continue to have influence and relationships with the living (Lassiter, 1998). This often makes the ideas of autopsies and organ donation distasteful to them.

- Another frequent cause of confusion is that people in many countries, including some Asian nations, calculate age differently than in the West. For example, in Vietnam a person's age begins roughly when he or she is conceived and advances one year at every *Tet Nguyen Dan (Tet)*, the Vietnamese New Year.

BOX 8.2

# Eastern and Western Perspectives on Health

## West

From a Western perspective, illness is a foe and the body is largely a mysterious and unpredictable space. Juanne Nancarrow Clarke and Jeannine Binns (2006) bring these cultural ideas to the foreground in their analysis of heart disease coverage in popular magazines. They point out how subtle and not-so-subtle word choices depict the human body as being on the verge of war or disaster (think *heart attacks, asthma attacks, risk factors, warning signs*). As presented, the appropriate response to this danger is to be vigilant (*watch for warning signs*) and ready to engage in combat (*fight* disease). We often give someone a good prognosis because he or she is *strong* or *"a real fighter."* In so many words, attaining good health is portrayed as a battle against the forces within. One *fights for one's life* and, if victorious, *triumphs* over disease. Otherwise, people are said to *lose their battle* with heart disease (or cancer or any number of other diseases).

In this context, observe Clarke and Binns (2006), the body is depicted as "bad" and medicine as "good." If illness is a siege, medicine is the cavalry ready to come our defense. In Western media, medicine is described in such optimistic and glowing terms as *life-saving, state of the art,* and *tried, tested, and true.* Some medications (like Viagra) are even heralded as "miracle drugs" (Baglia, 2005, p. 28). All in all, the body is not to be trusted, but "the medical world is largely unquestioned and portrayed as if it is beyond criticism," conclude Clarke and Binns (p. 45).

## East

If you were raised in a Western culture, the idea of "being strong" and "fighting for your life" may make perfect sense. How else would you view disease? Actually, *quite* differently if you subscribe to an Eastern worldview. A classic intercultural exercise is to show people a picture of a snow-covered tree limb on the ground. People from Western cultures

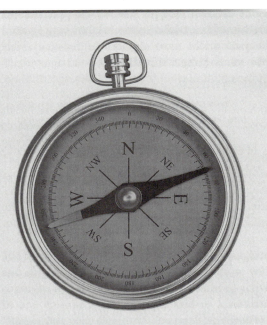

typically say the limb broke because it was too weak. Easterners usually say the opposite—that it broke because it was too strong, therefore too inflexible to bear the wind and weight. The Eastern idea of strength involves being supple and flowing. Think tai chi, qigong, karate, tae kwon do, and other methods of building spiritual and bodily awareness, flexibility, and fluid strength simultaneously.

Whereas Westerners are typically urged to take action at the first sign of illness, the Eastern way is to strive for health and balance all of the time. Rather than regarding the body suspiciously, Easterners are more likely to consider the body a natural place of harmony and well-being. They typically believe that the best way to maintain good health is to honor the body and follow its rhythms. Thus, rather than "fighting" an illness and using "strength" against it, people influenced by Eastern thought are more likely to focus on balance, harmony, and flexibility. Traditional Eastern medicine is based on awareness of subtle energy patterns. Interventions are typically mild and designed to enhance the body's natural functioning. Aggressive interventions such as surgery and strong drugs are viewed somewhat suspiciously because they may interfere with the body's natural rhythms. We might think of Eastern medicine as *health from within* rather than a *cure from without.*

That means that a child conceived shortly after Tet will be nearly 1 year old when born and will be considered 2 years old before the first anniversary of the birth (Purnell, 2008).

We will have a good deal more to say about Asian principles throughout the chapter, so let's turn now to health ideas in Hispanic cultures.

## Hispanic

*Hispanic* is a broad term encompassing people (most of them Spanish-speaking) whose heritage is associated with Latin America, South America, Spain, and some African nations. As you can imagine, this is a particularly diverse culture, but its members tend to honor several key principles, which we'll discuss here.

Among the highest of Hispanic values are the principles of *personalismo*—a preference for warm, friendly relationships rather than impersonal, institutional scenarios; *respeto*—embodied in respectful and deferential behavior toward people of greater age and social status; and *confianza*—the openness and trust among members of one's intimate circle (Añez, Silva, Paris, & Bedregal, 2008). These values translate to a preference for well-established, trusting relationships with caregivers, a general tendency to avoid conflict (especially with highly respected individuals), and sensitivity to displayed signs of respect. Understanding these cultural expectations, it is easy to imagine how offensive and foreign it may seem for a doctor to walk in, address a Hispanic patient by his or her first name, and then launch directly into medical talk without first working to build a close, friendly, trusting relationship.

Another belief held by members of some traditional Latino communities is *susto*, the conviction that a "shocking, unpleasant, or frightening experience" may cause physical illness (Willies-Jacobo, 2007, paragraph 18). Willies-Jacobo describes a patient visit during which a Latina mother said her 15-year-old son was sick because of *susto*. Although the boy disclosed that the *susto* involved something his father said, he and his mother refused to say anything more, leaving the doctor in a quandary, trying to decide if she should respect the family's desire for privacy or investigate to see if abuse was involved. To caregivers in similar situations, Willies-Jacobo recommends the following.

- *Conduct a cultural awareness assessment.* Learn as much as possible about the patient's culture, and incorporate that knowledge into assessment, diagnosis, and treatment considerations.
- *Assess family beliefs.* Keep in mind that overall culture does not tell the whole story. Every family has its own unique blend of beliefs and values.
- *Negotiate cultural conflicts.* Strive for ways to satisfy both patients' cultural expectations and the rigors of medical care. In this case the doctor met with the son individually and asked the mother what treatments she would consider helpful. Since there was no further reason to suspect abuse in this case, she resolved to keep an eye out for indications of maltreatment or emotional distress.

Cultural misunderstandings are one reason that Hispanic Americans tend to underutilize health services. Language and citizenship status are additional barriers for some. About 25% of Hispanic Americans are not insured, a number that has grown in recent years (Rutledge & McLaughlin, 2008). Hispanic residents who are not citizens of the United States are particularly unlikely to have health insurance or to seek care. Hispanic Americans may also find mainstream health messages culturally unappealing and/or assume that such messages do not pertain to them. Partly as a result, Mexican American women are more likely to die from breast cancer than members of any other ethnic group (Hubbell, 2006).

Following are some suggestions for communicating effectively with Hispanic individuals.

- Learn *un poquito de Español* (a little bit of Spanish). Warren Ferguson (2008) reminds us that "language is the currency of health care" and that learning even a small amount of the patient's language is a valuable investment (paragraph 1). As we saw in the last chapter, even *un poquito* makes a big difference.

- Begin with a warm and friendly greeting.
- Engage in friendly small talk and take time to build trusting relationships (*personalismo*).
- Show respect (*respeto*) through use of honorific titles such as Mr., Ms., Don, Señor, Señora, and Señorita. (It's okay to ask what title the person prefers.)
- Acknowledge and include family members and loved ones. Keep in mind that they are an important source of support and are often closely involved in making care decisions. "Family support is ever present," say Rick Zoucha and Barbara Broome (2008), adding that in Hispanic cultures, "family has meaning beyond blood or related connectedness.... Family may mean close friends of the family, known as 'compadres,' who may be present at times of health and illness" (p. 141). Health professionals should treat *compadres* with respect to avoid insulting the entire family.
- Keep in mind that religion is likely to be a source of great value and comfort to Hispanic individuals. It may also lead them to feel that health screenings and other measures are unnecessary because everything is in God's hands.
- If time matters, be specific. Time is typically a fluid concept in Hispanic cultures. Statements such as "Stop by after lunch" and "Take this medication first thing in the morning" may lead to misunderstandings.
- Traditional Hispanics may consult physicians only if care by a folk healer does not work. Be sensitive to this preference, and be aware that the patient may already be involved with folk treatments involving herbs, massage, prayer, and other remedies (Knoerl, 2007).

We turn now to a culture with origins in Africa and the Middle East.

### Arab

The interdependence between Western countries and the Arab world is unmistakable. Yet much of

---

what Westerners "know" about Arabs is based on stereotype and conjecture. Here we take an introductory look at Arab culture as it pertains to health and health care.

The Arab world includes 22 diverse countries in the Middle East and North Africa, including Egypt, Libya, Iraq, Iran, Kuwait, Saudi Arabia, Lebanon, Palestine, Yemen, and the United Arab Emirates, among others. These nations are united by proximity and their common use of the Arab language. Although some Arabs are of Christian or Jewish faith, Arabs are predominantly (92%) Muslim (Arab American Institute, 2000).

It's hard to judge the number of Arab Americans, because the U.S. census groups them in the larger category of white Americans. And because many Arab Americans fear discrimination, they often do not self-identify their ethnicity in other surveys (Ahmad, 2004). Most experts put the figure between 3.5 million and 7 million (Arab American Institute, 2000). Famous Arab Americans include Doug Flutie (Heisman Trophy winner), Tony Shalhoub (TV show *Monk*), Paula Abdul (TV show *American Idol*), Shakira (Grammy award–winning pop star); Donna Shalala (former U.S. Secretary of Health and Human Services and current president of the University of Miami), John Sununu (former White House Chief of Staff), and many more ("Arab Americans," 2006).

It is common for a traditional Arab household to include several generations as well as uncles, cousins, and others. Elders are deeply revered. Based on traditional gender roles, men are largely expected to provide for the family and women to raise the children and perform domestic tasks. Theirs is a collectivistic culture in which a dishonorable action by one member is considered to bring shame on the entire family. This means that some health conditions, such as mental illness and out-of-marriage pregnancies, may have powerful implications for the entire family. Health care professionals are encouraged to approach these matters delicately. Even when the issue is not a shameful one, many traditional Arabs prefer that doctors not tell the patient directly about a serious and terminal illness, but instead give the news to the nearest relative or the male head of the family, who will in turn share it with the others (Ahmad, 2004).

Many Arabs have migrated due to war and violence in their homelands. Because of this experience and because they often face social isolation and relatively few professional opportunities in their new communities, Arab Americans are especially susceptible to depression, anxiety, and suicide. However, mental illness is considered so shameful in their culture that they often deny they are in distress and avoid seeking help (Douki, Zineb, Nacef, & Halbreich, 2007).

Arab immigrants are likely to find the American health system alien and perplexing. Since most Arab countries have universal care, the concepts of managed care, copayments, insurance deductibles, and so on may be new to them. They may also be unaware of or reluctant to enroll in Medicare and Medicaid (Ahmad, 2004).

For the most part, Arabs are emotionally expressive and dedicated to being polite and agreeable (to such an extent that they may not disagree openly with their doctors). They enjoy getting to know health professionals and are typically put off by hurried transactions that do not involve a show of warmth and interest. They often show appreciation for health professionals with small gifts. To refuse these would be seen as a social rejection.

Because such a large percentage of Arabs are Islamic, let's turn now to the religious beliefs that influence the Arab culture and views of health.

Islam is the second largest religion in the world (behind Christianity), and its followers, Muslims, comprise about one-fifth of the world's population ("Major Religions," 2007). Muslims consider their religion to be a synthesis of Christianity and Judaism. They honor a number of prophets, many of whom overlap with the Christian faith, including Adam, Abraham, Moses, Solomon, and Jesus (Hammad, Kysia, Rabah, Hassoun, & Connelly, 1999). Muslims adhere to *Qur'an* (also spelled Koran), the scripture of Muhammad, whom they consider the final prophet. According to the Muslim faith, the angel Jibrīl (Gabriel) revealed the *Qur'an* to Muhammad as a set of universal, divine laws for human behavior. Thus, the *Qur'an* (Islam) is regarded as a way of life, including personal actions and spirituality as well as social structure, economy, politics, and so on (Hammad et al.). Muslim sects (e.g., Sunni, Shi'a, Sufism, Ahmadiyya) hold somewhat different beliefs, but most devout Muslims in every sect believe in Allah (God) and take part in ritualistic cleansing of the body, praying five times a day (preferably toward the east, the direction of the holy city Mecca, in Saudi Arabia), helping the poor, and fasting during daylight hours of Ramadan, an Islamic holy month. (Ramadan is based on the lunar calendar, so its dates differ from year to year.)

There are a number of implications relevant to health. For one, "Clinical staff should not be taken aback if a patient asks them, 'Which way is east?,'" say Adnan Hammad and colleagues (1999, p. 14). They should also be aware that Muslims' commitment to fasting—which they regard as a way to purify the body and maintain empathy for the poor and hungry—may at times dissuade them from taking oral and intravenous medications. They may even refuse critical, life-saving therapies during Ramadan. In such a case, say Hammad and colleagues, a health professional may appeal to a relative or family leader to convince the patient that it is permissible to take the medicine.

Health is important in the Muslim faith. Followers believe in free will, but they typically pray for good health, believing that Allah controls their ultimate destiny (Hamdan, 2007). Muslims may consider it presumptuous of a health professional to predict what will happen—be it death or a cure. They tend to perceive such predictions as overly bold and "as arrogant disrespect for God's will and an open invitation for disaster" (Hammad et al., 1999, p. 14). Adding the phrase "God willing" typically satisfies this concern.

Following are some other customs of which health professionals should be aware.

- In public, traditional Muslim women cover their bodies and sometimes their faces, as a show of modesty and in recognition that a man who looks on a woman with interest is committing "the spiritual equivalent of adultery" (Hammad et al., 1999, p. 15). By the same token, commenting on the appearance of a woman or child may be seen as improper. Instead, Muslims appreciate such comments as "What a nice child" or "You have a very nice wife" (Hammad et al., p. 21).
- Part of the Muslim creed is caring for people in need. Therefore Muslims may be present at the bedside of Muslim community members, even if they did not previously know them.
- *Halah*, the Muslim diet, forbids the consumption of pork or alcohol. This can make hospital food (including foods fried in animal lard) unacceptable and can be an issue with medications, such as some forms of insulin that are derived from pigs and cough syrup that includes alcohol.
- Traditional Muslims consider the left hand unsanitary (since it is presumably used for personal hygiene) and do not eat or drink with that hand. As a consequence, medical professionals should be careful not to put pills, drinking glasses, or food in the left hand.
- Muslim tradition largely dictates the separation of men and women, except in family interactions. This may mean a

preference for same-sex doctors and female-only labor and delivery experiences.

- Some Muslims are uncomfortable shaking hands with someone of the opposite sex, although this varies a great deal. Hammad and associates (1999) recommend that doctors extend a hand in greeting but not take offense if a Muslim person doesn't reach for it.
- Direct eye contact is often regarded as a sign of disrespect.
- The *Qur'an* is typically interpreted as defining a subordinate role for women, who are granted fewer rights and opportunities than men in Arab countries (Douki et al., 2007).
- Children are honored and celebrated.
- Fertility is revered to such an extent that the inability to bear children and even the onset of menopause can be seen as shameful (Douki et al., 2007).
- Premarital and extramarital sex are sources of profound disgrace, especially for females and their families. (Suicide over this disgrace is not uncommon in the Arab world [Douki et al., 2007].) Unmarried Muslim individuals may be insulted if physicians ask whether they are sexually active, believing this to be a judgment about their character.
- Muslims usually accept death without explanation as Allah's will, and custom dictates that they bury people very soon after death (on the same day, if possible). Autopsies are usually considered disrespectful and even horrifying, since traditional Muslims consider that the body feels pain until it is buried (Hammad et al., 1999).

Now lets turn to broader cultural perspectives about what it means to be healthy or ill.

## THE NATURE OF HEALTH AND ILLNESS

Cultures conceptualize health in various ways. Some consider that disease is manifested differently within each person. Others see disease as something objective and independent, outside patients' control and beyond their understanding. This section establishes two basic ways of viewing health—as an organic phenomenon and as a harmonious balance.

## Health as Organic

In many Western societies, germs or physical abnormalities are taken as signs of ill health. In the absence of these factors, a person is considered to be healthy. This perspective is consistent with the biomedical approach. The **organic perspective** assumes that health can be understood in terms of the presence (or absence) of physical indicators.

One strength of the organic perspective is its emphasis on scientific knowledge. Based on scientific principles, caregivers and researchers keep detailed patient records, conduct studies and experiments, identify risk factors, and link diseases to their causes (Marwick, 1997). This effort to learn and accumulate knowledge has led to remarkable advances in medicine, including pain remedies, diagnostic tests, vaccines, diverse treatment options, and numerous forms of medical technology.

Medical research has led to the development of **evidence-based medicine (EBM)**, the practice of making treatment decisions based on the results of scientific studies (Levin, 1998). EBM is used in many medical schools and hospitals as a strategy for avoiding medical waste and making effective decisions.

Physical evidence does not explain everything, however. A weakness of the organic model is its inability to account for conditions that cannot easily be verified. People who perceive illnesses that are not scientifically identifiable are often viewed with suspicion or labeled hypochondriacs. Patients with undetectable conditions such as chronic fatigue syndrome sometimes say the worst part is that so many people regard their condition as "not real" (Komaroff & Fagioli, 1996). Western society's faith in the observable survives despite evidence that science is imperfectly equipped to understand all aspects of the human body. Mental illnesses, long considered less real than physical illnesses, gained legitimacy in the 1950s as medicine began to recognize a chemical

basis for them (Byck, 1986). The difference is science's ability, not the illnesses themselves.

One downside of the organic approach is that its definition of health is fairly narrow, largely excluding social, spiritual, and psychological factors that are sometimes relevant to illness episodes. Partly as a result, Western doctors are typically reluctant to bring up spiritual concerns during medical visits (Todd, 1989). In fact, they are likely to avoid such issues, perhaps because it is time consuming to be so inclusive or because patients have such diverse beliefs it is difficult to understand or comment on them. But the organic approach can seem cold and impersonal, especially to people who are accustomed to a different style of care. African Americans have traditionally been dissatisfied with health care, partly because they feel snubbed by caregivers who seem disinterested in them as individuals (Levy, 1985; Spector, 1979). African American communities have traditionally placed great emphasis on community and religion. Compared to the personal concern of community members, clinical care can seem indifferent and unfeeling. Researchers led by Cheryl Holt (2008) found that African American women responded more favorably to breast cancer awareness booklets that featured spiritual beliefs and scripture than those that focused solely on medical information. The spiritual booklets portrayed the body as a temple, recognized God's role in preparing doctors, and stressed the value of balancing mind, body, and spirit. Both the spiritual and the strictly factual versions of the booklet included the same advice and tips for early detection, but African American women in the study thought more carefully about the information when it was grounded in spirituality (Holt, Lee, & Wright, 2008).

Furthermore, although classifying people as either healthy or sick satisfies the logic and precision of scientific thought, such simplicity may be at odds with human experience. As Charles Rossiter (1975) points out, *sick* and *healthy* are inadequate to describe all aspects of the human condition. There are varying levels of sickness and varying levels of health. Moreover, some people seem to be unhealthy although they do not have specific diseases.

Another drawback is that organic explanations can be confusing for patients. Some doctors work hard to overcome this. In their (2005) case study, Timothy Edgar and colleagues describe how one doctor, Dr. Price, explained type 2 diabetes to a teenager just diagnosed with it. Dr. Price compared the boy's condition to a logjam on a river, explaining that his body was able to convert food into energy (logs) but that the receptor sites in the body (where the logs/energy were to be unloaded) weren't working properly. Therefore, she explained, they needed to put fewer logs (less starch and carbohydrates) into his system and start an exercise program that would help "open" the receptor sites and help him feel more energetic.

Finally, based on either/or thinking, people may assume that if they are not sick, they are perfectly healthy. Not so, argue some theorists. They propose that true health is not only physical, but reflects a harmonious balance between many aspects of life, a perspective we turn to next.

### Health as Harmony

As you may recall from Chapter 1, the idea of health as harmony is supported by the World Health Organization, which defines health as "a state of complete physical, mental, and social well-being and not merely the absence of disease or infirmity" (WHO, 1948). From this perspective, health is cultivated through personal beliefs, contact with other people, physical strength, and other factors. From the **harmony perspective**, health is not simply the absence of physical signs of disease; rather, it is a pleasing sense of overall well-being. This perspective is in keeping with the biopsychosocial perspective.

Members of traditional Navajo cultures believe the best way to remain healthy is to maintain a balance between physical strength, social interactions, and spiritual beliefs (Bille, 1981). From their viewpoint, concentrating on only factor can upset the delicate balance. For example, striving for physical strength without also seeking spiritual growth is not healthy, and a person may become ill because of the imbalance. This is not to say that Navajo deny the existence of germs. They accept that germs cause

some diseases. But they also observe that some people are less vulnerable than others to germs. If several people are exposed to a contagious disease, some of them are likely to get sick, but others may not. Based on Navajo beliefs, people who live balanced lives are more likely to remain well, even when exposed to physical threats.

Members of the Odawa and Ojibway aboriginal communities in Canada believe that health is based on harmony with the environment, or Mother Earth (Wilson, 2003). As one member of the culture explained:

> She (Mother Earth) is something that heals you if you let it. You don't always feel it. You have to be thinking about it. You can't just go out for a walk and feel it. You have to be spiritually connected to feel her. (Wilson, third section, paragraph 8)

In this belief system it is therapeutic to live in harmony with the environment.

Members of some Asian cultures think of health in terms of balanced energy (Uba, 1992). According to the Chinese Tao, **yin and yang** are polar energies whose cyclical forces define all living things. *Yin* is associated with coolness and reflection, and *yang* with brightness and warmth. Cycles and combinations of yin and yang define human life and are a common element uniting all forms of existence. Within this belief, one's central life energy is called *Qi* (pronounced *chee*, sometimes spelled "chi"). Illness and even death may result if *Qi* is wasted or if yin and yang are not balanced. Life energy is sustained and balanced by awareness, rhythmic breathing, physical regimens, and meditation. The concept is often difficult to grasp and to study. "One reason *Qi* can so easily be left out of scientific descriptions of TCM [traditional Chinese medicine] is because of its invisibility," writes Evelyn Ho (2006, p. 425). *Qi* is sensed rather than measured or directly observed. And unlike Western medicine, in which the practitioner and the patient are treated as distinctly separate entities, *Qi* is a force that flows through them both. As one acupuncturist described it to Ho, an acupuncturist is "the conduit between the heavenly and the earthly *Qi* and it comes through you and through your hands and into the needle and the point" (p. 426). Some highly experienced people are said to see people's *Qi* and know what is wrong with them; others rely on touch. The importance of energy may lead members of some Asian cultures to resist undergoing surgery or receiving immunizations, believing these procedures will interfere with their life energy and the rhythms that define their well-being (Uba).

Across cultures, folk healing is typically oriented toward lifeworld concerns. Usually, a folk healer's role is to integrate social support with spiritual faith and physical treatment. The *curanderos* of Mexican American cultures and the hand-tremblers of some Native American cultures are good examples. These folk healers are usually well-known members of their communities (Bille, 1981). As such, they are familiar and accessible, without institutional boundaries or technical jargon. *Curanderos* and hand-tremblers take extensive personal interest in their patients and preside over rituals that bring members of the community together. In this way, healing involves a show of moral support and a sense of peace and belonging.

Health care that includes patients' lifeworld concerns has been praised as realistic and compassionate (Friedman & DiMatteo, 1979; C. B. Thompson, 1996). There is evidence that some people perceive more improvement when treated by folk practitioners than with conventional medicine (Kleinman et al., 1978). The discrepancy may amount to the distinction between healing and curing. McWhinney (1989, p. 29) calls *healing* a "restoration of wholeness," which includes spiritual and moral consideration, as opposed to purely physical *curing*, which he says may still leave a patient in "anguish of spirit" about the causes, effect, and fears associated with the illness.

One drawback of the harmony perspective is that it produces gradual and ambiguous results. Culturally speaking, people may be so concerned about maintaining harmony that they do not assert themselves. In Asian cultures particularly, people may avoid saying "no" or giving answers they think will displease the other person because they want to preserve interpersonal harmony (Purnell, 2008). Unlike organic medicine, which is devoted to analysis and comparison, attempts to establish harmony may be difficult to evaluate and measure (Cassedy, 1991). If immediate and measurable results are needed, the harmony perspective alone may seem insufficient. This is especially true for conditions such as cancer and broken bones, which have traditionally responded well to organic treatment. Harmony may help people resist disease and injury and recover more quickly, but most people agree that for some ailments nothing beats a trip to the ER or doctor's office.

A case in point is the rural community of Jharkhand, in eastern India, studied by Ambar Basu and Mohan Dutta (2007). After interviewing the impoverished residents of that region, Basu and Dutta noted that they live in a "twilight zone" between modernity and tradition. Many are no longer convinced of the power of traditional healers, *ojhas*, who may tell them that an illness is the result of someone's casting an "evil eye" on them, insufficient worship of the gods, or too few animal sacrifices. Residents say they often go to *ojhas* for minor illnesses because they are more affordable and accessible than doctors, who are often based in cities many miles from their village. However, most would prefer a doctor's care for serious illness, and they are acutely aware that distance and poverty preclude them from getting the care they want and feel they need (Basu & Dutta).

In closing this section, it's important to note that organic and harmony perspectives are not necessarily at odds with each other. As mentioned, physical health is a significant component of both perspectives. Moreover, each model may be appropriate in different situations, and sometimes they are both appropriate. Depending on the nature of the illness, a person might seek an organic remedy, a harmonizing one, or both. In some cases, conventional practitioners actively team up with folk healers. Amos Deinard, a pediatrician at the University of Minnesota Hospital, says, "Our attitude is, you bring your shaman and we'll bring our surgeon and let's see if we can work on this problem together" (quoted by Goode, 1993, paragraph 7).

## SOCIAL IMPLICATIONS OF DISEASE

One function of culture is to make sense of the world. Cultural assumptions act as guides to interpretation, indicating why things happen and what significance we should attach to various events (Garfinkel, 1967). For instance, death might be interpreted as a glorious ascension to the afterlife or as a tragic and regrettable occurrence. Illness may be regarded as an unfair or random affliction or as a valuable opportunity for renewed awareness. (See Box 8.4 for a description of the theory of health as expanded consciousness.)

Joy Hart and Kandi Walker (2008) describe their work with isolated villagers in Belize. One 16-year-old girl they met left the local clinic before having a pap smear because she was confused by a nursing student's description of the procedure. But she returned to the clinic after her mother told her "a pap smear was part of the journey of being a woman" (p. 130). The researchers reflect that the mother's explanation calmed the girl's fears because it was "more cultural and familial" than the nurse's explanation.

It is often difficult to make sense of disease. Some cultures honor scientific explanations. But even in those cultures, scientific accounts sometimes seem inadequate. At different times in history, epilepsy, cancer, tuberculosis, mental illness, AIDS, and other ailments have been viewed so negatively that people with these conditions were shunned or even imprisoned (Friedman & DiMatteo, 1979). Sick people may be regarded as a threat to the moral order because behaviors associated with their conditions are considered immoral or because their conditions seem contagious or frightening.

Many times, public reaction is not based on facts but on fears or cultural assumptions. Prior to 1950, people were so fearful of cancer they typically avoided telling anyone outside the family if a loved one was diagnosed with it (Holland & Zittoun, 1990). They often chose not to tell the patient either.

That has changed since the public has accepted that cancer is not contagious.

Social taboos have long surrounded the issue of mental illness as well. In sixteenth century and seventeenth century England, public horror over insanity was so great that the mentally ill were incarcerated as criminals, after which they were treated brutally and denied the right to marry or own property (MacDonald, 1981). Even today, in many areas of the world mental illness is considered God's punishment and people make great efforts to deny and conceal it (Purnell, 2008).

Even cultures steeped in organic definitions of disease may react with fear and loathing when confronted with certain disorders. It is common to blame ill persons for their conditions. This section considers the social effects of diseases regarded as threatening to the moral order. It surveys a variety of ideas about illness, including the notion of disease as a curse, the social stigma of some illnesses, moral issues of prevention, and the implications of referring to patients as victims. These ideas represent different (sometimes overlapping) ways of considering health and illness within the context of cultural beliefs.

### Disease as a Curse

Blaming someone is one way of making sense of frightening illnesses, write Dorothy Nelkin and Sander Gilman (1991) in a book about plagues. People may reason that disease is the result of curses inflicted by God or witches. It may be especially tempting to blame gods or witches when science and other explanatory models fail. White (1896/1925) proposes that as long as people cannot explain illness by natural law they attribute its cause and cure to the supernatural. As he puts it, "In those periods when man sees everywhere miracle and nowhere law...he naturally ascribes his diseases either to the wrath of a good being or to the malice of an evil being" (p. 1).

During the bubonic plague of the fourteenth century, more than one-third of the European population died (Slack, 1991). Struggling to make sense of this devastating epidemic, people killed tens of thousands

## BOX 8.4 THEORETICAL FOUNDATIONS

# Theory of Health as Expanded Consciousness

The majority of us spend our lives trying to stay healthy, and when we get sick we want nothing more than to be well again. We may be missing the point. According to Margaret Newman's **theory of health as expanded consciousness**, a health crisis is not necessarily negative or undesirable (Newman, 2000). Instead, health events are integral parts of life that provide opportunities for growth and change.

Newman is inspired by the David Bohm's (1980) concept that our everyday life is influenced by underlying patterns that characterize who we are and what we experience. Bohm conceived of two types of order—the **explicate order**, made up of the tangible elements of our existence, and the **implicate order,** comprising patterns beneath the surface. Although the tangible elements of our lives may seem like the "real thing" because we can see, hear, taste, and feel them, the meaning of what we do often lies within the underlying, implicate order. Bohm compares the dual nature of life to waves on the ocean. We can see the waves, but we will not really understand what causes them unless we explore the underwater currents that give rise to them.

Within this metaphor, a health event makes waves. It disrupts what might otherwise seem to be a peaceful, unremarkable existence. As nurse and nurse educator Newman (2000) observes:

> The thing that brings people to the attention of a nurse is a situation that they do not know how to handle. They are at a choice point. Each of us at some time in our lives is brought to a point when the "old rules" do not work anymore, when what we have considered progress does not work anymore. We have done everything "right" but things still do not work. (p. 99)

You might ask: And this is a *good* thing? According to Newman, yes. In her view, life is a process of attaining greater levels of understanding and awareness. When things stop working well, we experience a sense of chaos. But, she says, if we "hang in there," the uncertainty and ambiguity of a health crisis may become a means of seeing underlying patterns and transcending previous limitations. This can be a richly rewarding and liberating experience (Newman).

Imagine a person who has worked throughout her life to support others. She has devoted her energy and time to doing well at work, caring for her family, running errands, serving on committees, cleaning the house and yard, and so on. She is lauded with thanks and awards. Meanwhile, she appears less physically fit than she used to be. Her hair and clothing are not carefully groomed and tended. But this is nothing compared to what is happening within her. In fulfilling so many outward "obligations," she neglects her own spiritual and emotional growth. Although she interacts frequently with people, she does not share much of herself or appreciate the uniqueness of the people around her.

Suddenly (or what appears to be suddenly) the woman comes down with the flu and must cancel her commitments for several days. Faced with this prospect, she might put all her energy into fighting the illness, frustrated that it has interrupted her life. Or she might look for a deeper level of meaning. What does the illness (an outward manifestation) suggest about what is happening within her? And at an even deeper level, what does this disruption signal about the underlying pattern of her life? Perhaps this is an opportunity to reevaluate a pattern that appears virtuous on the surface but is harmful to her and others in the larger scheme of things. Perhaps understanding the pattern will allow her to restructure her life in a way that is more functional and adaptive, allowing her to develop her inner self as well as perform helpful tasks in the tangible world. Or perhaps she will ignore the underlying currents until they give rise to a much bigger, harder-to-ignore "wave," such as a stroke or a heart attack.

Seen this way, health events are opportunities for developing higher levels of understanding and more effective interactions with our environments. Greater

*(continued)*

**BOX 8.4** *(continued)*

harmony between inner and outer levels of existence provides the means for seeing beyond one's self and transcending old habits and assumptions. As Newman learned from her mentor, Martha Rogers, "health and illness should be viewed equally as expressions of the life process in its totality" (Newman, 2000, p. 7).

Newman (2000) coaches nurses to help people find the meanings and patterns revealed by their health experiences, whether or not their diseases are eradicated. She writes:

> Transcendence of the limitations of the disease does not necessarily mean more freedom from the disease; it does mean more meaningful relationships and greater freedom in a spiritual sense. These factors are considered an expansion of consciousness. (p. 65)

Furthermore, a health crisis is not merely a senseless or regrettable circumstance. Newman (1986) writes that, since she began to regard health as the expansion of consciousness,

> illness and disease have lost their demoralizing power....The expansion of consciousness never ends. In this way aging has lost its power. Death has lost its power. There is peace and meaning in suffering. We are free from the things we have feared—loss, death, dependency. We can let go of fear. (p. 3)

## What Do You Think?

1. Have you ever learned something valuable about yourself as the result of a health crisis?

2. What can caregivers and loved ones do to help people evaluate their life circumstances when an illness occurs?

3. In what ways are your health and outward, everyday life (explicate order) influenced by underlying factors (implicate order)?

## Suggested Sources

Bohm, D. (1980). *Wholeness and the implicate order.* London: Routledge & Kegan Paul.

Coward, D. D. (Fall 1990). The lived experience of self-transcendence in women with advanced breast cancer. *Nursing Science Quarterly, 3*(3), 162–169.

du Pré, A., & Ray, E. B. (2008). Comforting episodes: Transcendent experiences of cancer survivors. In L. Sparks, H. D. O'Hair, & G. L. Kreps (Eds.), *Cancer, communication and aging* (pp. 99–114). Cresskill, NJ: Hampton Press.

Malinski, V. M. (Ed.). (1986). *Explorations on Martha Rogers' science of unitary human beings.* Norwalk, CT: Appleton-Century-Crofts.

Newman, M. A. (1995). *A developing discipline: Selected works of Margaret Newman.* New York: National League for Nursing Press.

Newman, M. A. (2000). *Health as expanding consciousness* (2nd ed.). Boston: Jones & Bartlett.

Rogers, M. E. (1986). Science of unitary human beings. In V. M. Malinski (Ed.), *Explorations of Martha Rogers' science of unitary human beings* (pp. 3–14). Norwalk, CT: Appleton-Century-Crofts.

---

of women, accusing them of using witchcraft to make their neighbors ill (Nelkin & Gilman, 1991). Others attributed the plague to God's wrath over women's fashions, blasphemy, drunkenness, improper religious observances, and other behaviors (Slack, 1991).

Members of some African tribes attribute AIDS to the work of witches. Many of the Goba, who live in a rural area of Zambia, Africa, believe that death occurs naturally only in old age (Yamba, 1997). In all other cases, it is attributed to the work of witches in the community. (According to Goba beliefs, a person may be a witch and not know it.) The Goba use the same word (*ng'anga*) to refer to healers and to witch finders. When a young person dies, suffers an injury, or is unable to conceive children, the family is expected to hire a witch finder to identify and often to kill the witch believed to be responsible. Supposed witches are publicly challenged to survive impossible feats (such as drinking poison). If they do not survive, their guilt is assumed. Yamba reports that the tribe members maintain their belief in witches partly because they are unsatisfied with biomedical explanations of illness. If witchcraft is not involved in sexually transmitted diseases, then "why else, they argue, would two men be exposed to the same woman and yet one would become infected while the other would not?" (Yamba, paragraph 8).

All in all, people may suspect that supernatural forces are at work when rational explanations fail to make sense. One result of treating illness as a punishment or curse is that ill persons may be shunned and supposed witches accused and even killed. In light of this, people may not admit they are ill, and treatment may be withheld in the name of religion. In Europe in the 1700s some people refused the smallpox vaccination because it was regarded as interference with God's way (Nelkin & Gilman, 1991). For similar reasons, some Southeast Asians regard medical care as fruitless or a sign of weakness (Uba, 1992). Likewise, Kashmiri men in India, although at high risk for diabetes, frequently decline treatment or lifestyle changes because they feel that the disease is Allah's will and that they should enjoy life (including eating what they want) until it is their fate to die (Naeem, 2003).

## Stigma of Disease

Even when illness is not regarded as a supernatural curse, it may be culturally prescribed to consider people with certain diseases corrupt or immoral. As Erving Goffman (1963) uses the term, **stigma** refers to a type of social rejection in which the stigmatized person is treated as dishonorable or is ignored altogether.

Social theorists compare HIV and AIDS to a plague, in that infected persons are often avoided and seen as dangerous and unprincipled. Numerous studies tell of HIV and AIDS survivors who have been fired from their jobs and abandoned by

their families and friends (M. B. Adelman & Frey, 1997; Cawyer & Smith-du Pré, 1995). Stigmatized in this way, people with HIV or AIDS must often choose between two forms of isolation. Either they keep the diagnosis a secret (eschewing potential support) or they tell others and risk being shunned and avoided by them (Cline & Boyd, 1993).

One effect of social stigma is that people's individuality, even their humanity, is overshadowed by the discrediting characteristic. A participant in Rebecca Cline and M. Faye Boyd's (1993) study of HIV survivors says:

> I am finding it harder and harder to get away from AIDS....I am angry at people, society, for not looking at me as a normal person with a normal disease, putting labels on me and trying to isolate me, putting shame and guilt on me. (pp. 137, 139)

For those whose conditions stir society's fears and prejudices, disease is plainly more than a physical phenomenon. Some people die of embarrassment, too afraid or ashamed to seek care for medical conditions stigmatized by society. Others may keep their diagnoses secret for fear of retribution.

Sometimes people avoid medical evaluations because they are afraid of being stigmatized by the results. For example, although they are predisposed to breast cancer, highly religious Jewish women in Israel are less likely than others to seek genetic testing (Bowen, Singal, Eng, Crystal, & Burke, 2003). Given the history of persecution against Jewish people, these women are especially wary of being stigmatized as genetically "different" or "at risk" (Bowen et al.). As the following section shows, moral issues are often applied to illness, even when health is regarded as an organic phenomenon.

## The Morality of Prevention

It seemed for a time that reframing disease in scientific terms would shield sufferers from moral judgment. Ironically, Western society has attributed a moral quality to science, with the effect that people who get sick are often considered to be lazy or ignorant. The news is filled with health warnings and risk factors. Such information enables people to make healthy choices, enhancing their own well-being and assuring themselves of long, healthy lives. At least that is one implication: Take care of yourself and there is no reason you should become ill. Prevention information is enabling to an extent, but taken too far it may lead to prejudice against ill persons (Brody, 1987). One backlash of the prevention movement is that people may have so much confidence in prevention that they believe illness always results from laziness or indifference. The rationale is that, if illness can be prevented, ill people have not tried very hard to stay healthy.

"Why isn't it possible to just get sick without it also being your fault?" asks physician/essayist Paul Marantz (1990, p. 1186). Marantz describes the smug comments surrounding a young friend's unexpected death from heart failure. A medical resident minimized the man's death by dubbing him "a real couch potato" (Marantz, p. 1186). Marantz was angry that onlookers would judge his friend, even to the extent of making his premature death seem okay or deserved.

The fallacy that only the lazy or indifferent get sick compounds the hardship of being ill (Marantz, 1990). People do fall ill for reasons that are hard to explain, even though they have worked hard to stay healthy. Marantz and others propose that suffering is often made worse by the assumption that ill persons engineer their own misfortunes.

One alternative to blaming ill persons is to see them as victims of circumstances beyond their control. As you will see, however, there are social implications as well to playing the victim role.

### Victimization

As the average life span has increased, so has the duration of chronic diseases. Many people with serious diseases survive and lead relatively normal lives. This has created a semantic dilemma. These people are not accurately described as "patients." So what do you call a person with AIDS or cancer or emphysema? A common practice is to call them victims, as in "AIDS victims" or "cancer victims." However, many people so described resent the implications of that characterization.

A participant in Cline and Boyd's (1993) study declares: "I'm HIV positive but I'm not a victim! I'm a *survivor!*" (p. 144). Another participant in the same study concurs: "I hate that word. I'm not a victim because I'm not allowing AIDS to victimize me. The word 'victim' really ticks me off. And 'innocent victims' implies that there are 'guilty victims'" (p. 145). These people's reactions attest to the power of cultural metaphors. Words and images imply values and judgments, with serious implications for those involved.

The following section examines different ways of conceptualizing patients' and caregivers' roles.

## PATIENT AND CAREGIVER ROLES

Culturally speaking, there are right and wrong ways to "do" and to "treat" illness. That is, some behaviors are rewarded, whereas others bring social penalties. For example, members of Arab cultures expect women to cry out in pain during labor and delivery (Ahmad, 2004). But in some other cultures this is considered weak and unseemly, even a sign that the patient has been evil in the past. For example, members of traditional Hispanic cultures typically believe pain should be endured stoically because it is God's wish (Duggleby, 2003).

Likewise, people might be expected to remain "respectfully" quiet in medical encounters or to take a "responsible" role by sharing their thoughts. The rules for being a good patient and a good caregiver may be contradictory and confusing. Nevertheless, with people's health hanging in the balance, health care participants may fervently wish to behave correctly. (See Box 8.5 for more about Thai customs regarding family members' role as health advocates.)

This section examines different roles patients and caregivers are expected to play. A **role** is a set of expectations that applies to people performing various functions in the culture. For example, people may play the roles of patient, doctor, sister, friend, employee, and parent. Each role is guided by a set of culturally approved rules. Typically, one role exists in relation to another: patient–caregiver,

BOX 8.5 **PERSPECTIVES**

# Thai Customs and a Son's Duty

Absolutely nothing in Thai culture is as important as a son's duty to take care of his elderly parents. My paternal grandmother came to live with my family when I was 15 years old. She left Chonburi, a small city in the eastern part of Thailand, and moved to Bangkok after my grandfather died of a heart attack. Grandmother Kim had been paralyzed for 20 years because of a bad fall, so my father insisted she must come to live with us so we could take proper care of her and so she wouldn't be lonely.

Grandmother Kim was 91 years old then, but she still had a great memory, especially about finances. Even though she had no expenses of her own, she insisted that my father give her a monthly allowance. She kept perfect mental notes on the status of her money so that she could distribute it as she pleased. For example, every day before I left for school, Grandmother gave me some money to give to the monk she watched on television each day. She was looking after her future by buying merit enough to go to heaven when she died. Grandmother also gave me money for myself each morning, and she gave other people money as well.

Although she required a lot of care and assistance, Grandmother was not depressed. Instead, she seemed happy and content with her financial projects and with providing advice to our family. Still, my mother and I watched over her constantly and we hired a private nurse to help take care of her. My mother was a very skillful and competent caregiver, since she had taken classes at the hospital to prepare her to take care of Grandmother Kim.

After I graduated from high school, I pursued a bachelor's degree at a university far from home. I would go back every weekend, however. When she was 95, Grandmother began to get weak. The doctor said she might have lung cancer. I didn't think she had any diseases; instead, I believed it was her time to go to heaven. My father didn't think she had lung cancer, either. He was convinced her lungs were perfect because she had no symptoms of any lung problem. No matter how strongly my father opposed the doctor's opinion, the doctor insisted on a lung biopsy as soon as possible. We agreed not to tell my grandmother about any suspicion of cancer, since we thought it might be too hard for her to know. We agreed only to tell her she had suffered a stroke. As we waited during the surgery, my father confided in me that he was unsure he had made the right decision to let the doctor do a biopsy.

When the results came back, my grandmother didn't have cancer. After she came home, everyone expected her to feel better. Unfortunately, Grandmother got worse. We took her to another doctor, who said that, since a biopsy could make an elderly patient weaker, it had been inappropriate to do the procedure. My father asked the doctor how much time his mother had left in this world. He told us that Grandmother could not be expected to live longer than one year. She died within several weeks.

Although I was away at the university when Grandmother died, I quickly returned. It is Thai custom that kin and family have to see the dead person before the body is placed in the coffin. Therefore I had a chance to see her for the last time in the mortuary. As my mother and I got her dressed and cut her hair, I noticed that Grandmother's body was small and cold. I told my mother that Grandmother had kissed me and told me to be a good girl the last time I saw her. Up to this day, I still remember every single word she told me. I think she knew her time to go was close. However, she didn't show any signs that she was afraid of death.

My father blamed the first doctor for his mother's death, but he blamed himself most of all. He thought that, if he had insisted the doctor not perform the biopsy, she would have stayed with us longer. My mother and I both tried to comfort father. I thought the best way to relieve him of some of his sorrow was to tell him that it was time for Grandmother to go. She had stayed longer than most other people could; also she had suffered from a stroke and had been paralyzed for a long time. However, I do understand my father's feeling because he is a son, and his responsibility is to do everything to keep his mother alive and healthy.

—*Pem*

student–teacher, parent–child, and so on. A role may lose meaning without its counterpart (e.g., a teacher is not a teacher without students). Therefore, role-playing is a collaborative endeavor, and people usually adjust their performances to form meaningful combinations. This can be so compelling that people sometimes feel forced into roles they would rather not assume. For example, if your conversational partner adopts a parental role, you may feel like a child, and you may act that way even if you would rather not. To do otherwise might seem uncooperative and rude.

As you will see in this section, patients and caregivers often play complementary roles—as mechanics and machines, providers and consumers, parents and children, and so on. Keep in mind that these roles are collaborative achievements, supported by participants' mutual efforts. This does not mean that the participants always like the roles they assume. They may be motivated by a sense of cultural appropriateness or the perceived need to "play the scene" as the other person is playing it.

## Mechanics and Machines

From one perspective caregivers are similar to mechanics and patients to machines. The implication is that the patient is relatively passive and that the caregiver is expected to be analytical and capable of fixing the problems that are presented.

This perspective does not encourage emotional communication between patients and caregivers. The focus is more on identifying physical abnormalities and fixing them (Todd, 1989). When caregivers take on a mechanic role, they are typically more concerned with what they can observe and change than what the patient might be feeling.

Some people feel that scientific medicine is relatively mechanistic. That is, when caregivers take on the role of scientists, they are much like mechanics—concerned with the orderly physical functioning of the human body. As mechanics or scientists, caregivers are expected to be objective, value-neutral, and capable of collecting information, diagnosing the problem, and fixing it. From this perspective, it may seem inappropriate for caregivers to display

emotions or to call into play such intangible notions as faith and spirituality. Eric Cassell (1991) puts it this way: "Adjectives like warm, tall, swollen, or painful exist only for persons but, ideally, science deals only with measurable quantities like temperature, vertical dimensions, diameters" (p. 18).

One advantage of the mechanic/scientist role is that it reduces the emotional drain on caregivers. If patients are like machines who simply need fixing, emotions need not become part of the process (Bonsteel, 1997). At the same time, the confidence that people can be fixed may seem comforting and neat.

Of course, patients may not appreciate being treated like machines. Some argue that ignoring patients' descriptions and considering them passive in their own care amounts to a mechanized form of medicine in which the patient is treated as little more than a set of parts. Richard Swiderski's (1976) analysis of medicine through the ages concludes that doctors have often considered patients less relevant than their pulse rates, blood, and urine. This is an image the public has embraced as well, as evidenced by patients' disappointment when their physicians do not run tests or prescribe medications. One reason for overuse of antibiotics is patients' insistence that treatment be embodied in some physical form, even when pharmacology suggests it will have no effect (J. A. Fisher, 1994).

## Parents and Children

The popular expression "doctor's orders" suggests a relationship in which physicians issue directions that patients are expected to obey. This approach is referred to as **paternalism**, reflecting the idea that patients are like children and caregivers are like parents.

Members of some cultures carry this to an extreme. For instance, many South Africans (Herselman, 1996) and Asians (Uba, 1992) show respect for physicians' authority by outwardly agreeing with anything their doctors say, even when they do not understand the information or have reservations that will prevent them from following the medical advice.

## BOX 8.6 ETHICAL CONSIDERATIONS

# Physician as Parent or Partner?

Medical ethicist Robert Veatch (1983) reflects that physicians are often criticized as being "aloof and unconcerned" rather than concerned and attentive as people would like them to be. In short, physicians often act like strangers when patients wish they would act like friends or family members.

Paternalism (the idea that doctors are like parents) is a long-standing tradition. The Hippocratic oath, written approximately 2,500 years ago, beseeches physicians to use their best "ability and judgment" on each patient's behalf. This presumes that physicians are well acquainted with medicine *and* with the particular needs and preferences of each patient. Paternalism is also based on the belief that physicians are more capable of making medical decisions than patients are.

Some people feel paternalism is outdated. Veatch (1983) points out that it is difficult to know patients well in the current age of large patient loads, specialization, and emergency and outpatient care. These factors make it unlikely that doctors will understand the unique needs and preferences of each patient. The paternalistic model is also criticized as inconsistent with patient empowerment, which presumes that patients are knowledgeable and active agents in their own health care (Emanuel & Emanuel, 1995).

## What Do You Think?

1. Do you feel it is realistic or preferable for health caregivers to know their patients' feelings and values? If so, how might they accomplish this? If not, what alternatives would you suggest?
2. Can you think of circumstances in which you would want your physician to know your feelings and life circumstances?
3. Can you think of circumstances in which you would rather your physician did not know you well?
4. Do you feel patients are capable of making decisions about their own care?

## Suggested Sources

Emanuel, E. J., & Emanuel, L. L. (1995). Four models of the physician-patient relationship. In J. D. Arras & B. Steinbock (Eds.), *Ethical issues in modern medicine* (4th ed., pp. 67–76). Mountain View, CA: Mayfield.

Reilly, D. R. (2003, Winter). Not just a patient: The dangers of dual relationships. *Canadian Journal of Rural Medicine, 8*(1), np.

Veatch, R. M. (1983). The physician as stranger: The ethics of the anonymous patient–physician relationship. In E. E Shelp (Ed.), *The clinical encounter: The moral fabric of the patient–physician relationship* (pp. 187–207). Dordrecht, The Netherlands: D. Reidel.

---

David Hufford (1997) tells of a tragic case in which a 14-year-old Asian immigrant to the United States felt ashamed for complaining about abdominal pain after her doctor said it was normal menstrual cramping. She refused further medical care for a year, until the liver cancer that had gone undiagnosed was so advanced she died. Hufford points out the tragic consequences of stereotyping a young girl's condition, on the one hand, and adhering to cultural expectations that suffering be endured without complaint, on the other.

One implication of the paternalism model is that patients may be regarded as naive or incapable. There is a historical precedent for regarding patients as ineffectual, even as bungling intruders, in matters of their own health. In an 1871 commencement address at Bellevue Hospital College, the famous physician/poet/novelist Oliver Wendell Holmes (1891) warned graduates: "Your patient has no more right to all the truth you know than he has to all the medicine in your saddlebags.... He should only get so much as is good for him"

(p. 388). Holmes advised the graduates to adopt the habit of "shrewd old doctors" who keep a few stock phrases to quiet "patients who insist on knowing the pathology of their complaints without the slightest capacity of understanding their scientific explanation" (p. 389).

Another implication is that doctors may be expected to know what is best for their patients. Some theorists (e.g., Emanuel & Emanuel, 1995) feel this is a risky assumption because patients may have many feelings and desires unknown to their doctors. Expecting physicians to anticipate and act on patients' wishes may place an unrealistic burden on doctors and unfairly rob patients of opportunities to make their own decisions. (See Box 8.6 for more on this issue.)

## Spiritualists and Believers

Caregivers also may be cast as spiritualists who use their powers on behalf of faithful patients. The image of caregivers as spiritual figures (and even as gods) was established thousands of years ago. As discussed in Chapter 2, the Egyptian physician Imhotep was eventually granted the status of a god. Jesus has been called "the great physician" and is revered for legendary acts of curing the sick (L. G. Moore et al., 1987). Throughout history, physicians have been described as "little gods," a celestial metaphor that extends to nurses, often portrayed as "angels of mercy" (Moore et al., p. 232).

Anthropologists have compared the doctor's role to that of a priest, a powerful and somewhat mysterious authority figure. This awe-inspiring image may be strengthened by patients' reverence and physicians' displays of power. Pendleton and colleagues (1984) point to doctors' laboratory coats, specialized vocabulary, and honorific titles as supporting props in this image. They also suggest that the image is bolstered by an information imbalance that makes physicians' knowledge seem all the more marvelous. They write: "Powerful rituals, such as examining and prescribing, are the more charismatic in the absence of adequate explanations" (p. 9).

Among the most well-known healer/spiritualists are the shamans of traditional Native American cultures. A shaman is believed to coax a patient's disease into his or her own body and then expel it through strength of will (Swiderski, 1976). The assumption is that illness is an invasion of magical or supernatural forces. The faithful believe shamans can communicate with beings beyond the physical world, an ability that gives them magical abilities and healing powers.

The success of a spiritual ceremony is often said to rely on the patient's faith in the healer and the greater spiritual force that has accepted the healer as a medium. One result of this assumption is that failure to recover may be construed as an indication of the patient's insufficient faith (Kearney, 1978). For this reason, patients may be particularly trusting and may benefit from the power of positive thinking. However, if their conditions do not improve, they may be loath to admit it.

Another spiritualist group is the Christian Science Church, whose members believe that conventional medicine is anti-Christian. "They are taught that 'illness is an illusion' and can be cured only through prayer," explains Andrew Skolnick (1990, paragraph 5). Christian Scientists believe that orthodox medical care makes illnesses worse. Thus, they do not use drugs or surgery, and they refuse even simple home treatments like heating pads, ice packs, and back rubs. Christian Scientists' refusal to allow medical care has raised controversy across the nation, especially when children's lives are involved (Skolnick). Some believe that it is child abuse to deny children the medical care that might save their lives. For example, a Massachusetts couple, David and Ginger Twitchell, was convicted of involuntary manslaughter in 1990 after their 2-year-old son died from an obstructed bowel (Margolick, 1990). The couple had refused to allow doctors to treat the toddler, and he died what medical experts considered a preventable death. Others feel that requiring medical care violates Christian Scientists' right to worship as they choose. The Twitchells were acquitted of the charges in 1993 on the grounds that a state law exempted people from child neglect charges if they were acting in accordance with their religious beliefs. Not long afterwards, Massachusetts became the fifth state to revoke that law (Sanghavi, 2008).

A belief in the supernatural also characterizes the health beliefs of some southern Appalachians (Bille, 1981). In that culture, spiritual ceremonies involving faith healing and glossolalia (speaking in tongues) are believed to restore health. **Faith healers** are expected to channel the curative power of the Holy Spirit, which they pass to believers through ceremonies known as the laying on of hands. **Glossolalia** involves a trancelike state during which a worshiper seems to speak in a foreign language. It is believed that the language is known only to God or that it is a foreign tongue known to some but unknown to the worshiper except through divine inspiration (Lippy & Williams, 1988).

Even scientists acknowledge the power of faith, although they are not likely to regard it as the central focus of their work. Evidence supports that people who expect to be cured sometimes are, even when the "treatment" is an inactive **placebo** such as flavored water or sugar. Placebo effects are so common that medical researchers routinely give some research participants an actual treatment and give other people a placebo. If the treatment group does not experience greater effects than the placebo group, the researchers cannot be sure they are measuring anything more than the power of suggestion. Sometimes placebo effects are unintentional. When thermometers were introduced in a British hospital in the 1800s, some patients assumed they were curative and seemed to recover spontaneously before the treatment could be administered (White, 1896/1925). The reverse is sometimes true as well. People who have no confidence in a treatment may be unaffected by it. These examples do not prove that all disease can be reduced to the effects of faith and emotions. However, they do demonstrate that there is more to disease than meets the (microscopic) eye.

A religious-like faith in caregivers serves multiple goals. It inspires confidence (on the part of patient and caregiver), which may be an important part of healing. It also honors the extraordinary role caregivers play in managing life and health.

There is a downside, though, in dashed hopes and exorbitant malpractice claims. With the expectation that medicine can work miracles if done correctly, people may feel particularly angry when things do not go well, and they may rightly or wrongly charge that their caregivers are incompetent (Kreps, 1990).

## Providers and Consumers

It has become popular to describe health care in terms of consumerism. Patients are regarded as shoppers or clients who pay doctors primarily to provide information and carry out the patients' wishes (Roter, Stewart, et al., 1997). Consumerism is fueled in part by Internet resources. People can now look up extensive health information for themselves. What's more, websites such as ConsumerReportsHealth.org, DoctorScorecard.com, and AngiesList.com now offer reviews of hospitals, treatments, products, and doctors (including consumer reviews of doctors' bedside manner, perceived quality of care, price, the cleanliness of their offices, the courteousness of their staff members, and more).

Some theorists predict that competitiveness will make caregivers especially mindful of patient satisfaction (Lombardo, 1997). However, some caregivers who see themselves as serving a higher purpose than profit margins find the marketplace metaphors disturbing. Physicians also warn that consumer websites can have a backlash. For one, since anyone can file comments about a doctor online but most people won't, the comments that appear may not represent most patients' opinions. For another, physicians who are worried about their stats may be dissuaded from taking high-risk cases, which are more likely than others to result in lawsuits and disappointing outcomes. Thus, consumer reviews can inadvertently punish doctors for going out on a limb for patients with critical or rare conditions.

Howard Friedman and M. Robin DiMatteo (1979) caution that consumerism may be a risky conceptualization for all involved. If the customer is always right, they wonder, will medical centers that respect patients' treatment decisions later be held liable if adverse outcomes result? Friedman and DiMatteo also worry that pleasing patients may sometimes be at odds with helping them. Considering that the most effective medical options are sometimes the most unpleasant, how far will caregivers go to avoid upsetting their patients?

Similarly, consumerism seems to place cost as a top priority. Richard Glass (1996) is concerned that physicians may choose less aggressive treatment options if they are forced to be more mindful of cost than care. A physician himself, Glass maintains that patients "rightly expect something different from their doctors than from consumer goods salespersons" (p. 148). He argues that a marketplace mentality may have "perverse effects" on medical care, and he beseeches health care management not to interfere unduly in medical decision making.

There is some evidence that people who rely on health information do not view their doctors in quite the same way as before. Unlike generations past, they are unlikely to believe that doctors have all the answers (Lowrey & Anderson, 2006). This may diminish physicians' professional status. Or it may simply fuel a different kind of relationship, such as the one we'll discuss next.

## Partners

Only as partners do patients and caregivers assume roughly the same role. Of course, they each bring something different to the encounter in terms of experiences and expertise. But as partners, they are directed toward the same goals and they act as peers. The partner role is consistent with collaborative medical talk.

As partners, patients and caregivers ideally use a vocabulary they both understand and make decisions together. The success of health care managed in this way hinges largely on the quality of patient–caregiver relationships. In 1996, the *Journal of the American Medical Association* introduced a column called "The Patient–Physician Relationship." In an article launching the new feature, Glass (1996, p. 148) proclaimed the doctor–patient link to be

the "center of medicine," a covenant not to be compromised by impersonal reliance on technology or profit-oriented decisions. This emphasis underscores the importance of trusting communication between patients and caregivers.

Retired physician Francis Lombardo (1997) writes that he earned patients' trust and partnership by being a respectful listener. As he describes it: "Once a patient has sized you up as someone who won't hassle or ridicule him, he'll feel much freer to bring up those touchy topics himself, like the fact that he thinks he might be gay" (p. 121).

Some people find the partnership model appealing because it allows both patients and caregivers to have influence over medical decisions, as opposed to being strictly patient-centered or doctor-centered (Beck, Ragan, & du Pré, 1997; R. C. Smith & Hoppe, 1991). Hufford (1997) attests that patients have important and relevant statements to make about their own health. "Sick people, it turns out, often do know exactly what has been happening to them, what it feels like, and when it happens, and there is nothing fictional about it" (Hufford, p. 118).

One way to encourage patients' active participation is to follow the lead of Myra Skluth (2007) and create patient to-do lists. She and patients negotiate the terms of the to-do lists; then each keeps a copy. "This approach works very well," she says (p. 16). Because the to-do lists are in patients' charts, then "if they call with questions, the nurses know exactly what I told them. I can also review the items with them at the beginning of the next visit—what they accomplished, and what they didn't and why. I find my patients really appreciate this."

Few people criticize the idea of patients and caregivers as partners. However, this may be a difficult transition to make. Patients and caregivers have traditionally upheld the expectation that doctors will guide medical discussions and patients will be relatively quiet and passive in their doctors' presence (see Chapter 3 for a review of this literature.) A shift is possible, but it will require change and cooperation on both sides.

## Implications

These interaction models characterize various aspects of medical discourse, yet they are not as simple as they appear. Transactions often, perhaps always, involve elements of several models, even if one is dominant. Evelyn Ho and Carma Bylund (2008) make the point that holistic medicine such as acupuncture typically transcends and blends these models to such an extent that none of them provide an accurate description. One acupuncture intern in their study described holistic medicine this way: "It's about connecting yourself and your patients to the greater whole (the Tao, the yin-yang circle), and by doing so you both can rise to your highest potential" (p. 511). As Ho and Bylund observed, practitioners oriented to this goal were sometimes paternalistic, sometimes consensual, sometimes mechanistic. Mostly they invoked a blend of all the models. (We'll talk more about holistic medicine in Chapter 9.)

Now let's transition to a particular medical product with profound cultural implications.

## VIAGRA: CASE STUDY IN HEALTH–CULTURE OVERLAP

You know the commercials. In one, a man and woman sit disinterestedly at opposite ends of a sofa. He's watching a sports update and channel surfing and she's reading women's magazines. (Nothing sexist about that, right?) Then he gives her a meaningful look and tosses the remote control out onto the lawn. She follows with the magazines and telephone, he with a golf club. Then they tango their way into the bedroom to the tune of *Vivaaaa Viagra!*

Another commercial opens with a rather awkward man taking dance lessons with a Latina instructor. Then the scene shifts to a wedding reception at which the man, now confident and in control, whirls a diamond-bejeweled blonde woman around the dance floor as a voice-over intones: "Whatever steps you're taking to impress your partner, don't let erectile dysfunction get in the way." Soon the snappy *Vivaaaa Viagra!* tune accompanies the joyful couple's rush for the hotel elevator.

One thing is for sure: Viagra has captured people's attention. It's second only to Coca-Cola in terms of brand-name fame. It has been the subject of more than 54,000 news stories and 900-plus jokes on the *Tonight Show* (Parker-Pope, 2002). In *The Viagra Ad Venture*, Jay Baglia (2005) explores the cultural impact of the Pfizer product that at least one reporter has dubbed "the national drug of choice." Baglia's analysis reveals a carefully constructed deep-pockets campaign to define (in the most lucrative terms possible) what it means to be a man, supported by an adoring media and health officials' willingness to consider the male erection a medical necessity, thus covered by insurance and military benefits even when it threatens to break the bank. Let's look at a few of the most potent implications of the hype about the little blue pill.

## Implication 1: To Be a Man You Have to Get It Up

The Viagra commercials mentioned are similar to many Pfizer has released since launching the product in 1998 except that, as Baglia (2005) points out, the actors have gotten noticeably younger through the years. If you believe what you see, the difference between a boring, emotionally and physically remote relationship (in which you sit on opposite ends of the sofa) and joyous dancing toward the bedroom is an erect penis. Likewise, no matter what else a man does, an erection is a crucial element in "impressing" his partner. In fact, in the Viagra world, an erection seems to be the *most* important, maybe the *only* important, element in relational bliss (Baglia). No matter how lackluster things are between the man and the woman, women in the commercials seem to find the men in their lives instantly and irresistibly attractive when the pill takes effect.

The message is clear, says Baglia (2005): "Nothing tells a man he is masculine—not muscles, earning potential, an attractive partner, or even height—so much as his erection does" (p. 9). And if that is not reductive and insecure-making enough, Pfizer has raised the bar on acceptable "male sexual performance" so high that men are nearly certain to feel inadequate. (A man who scores 21 points or fewer on Pfizer's 25-point Sexual Health Inventory for Men is instructed to ask his doctor for help.) In the tricky game of measuring up to social expectations, it seems Pfizer has defined *normal* and *masculine* to suit its own ends. Judging by the 25 million males who have secured a Viagra prescription so far (Viva Viagra, 2008), men are buying it—literally and figuratively.

## Implication 2: To a Physical Ailment Let There Be a Physical Remedy

Following closely on the heels of a well-designed sucker punch to the ego, Pfizer offers this reassurance: Don't feel bad, men. It's not under your control. It's under *ours*. What used to be considered "male impotence"—a term that suggests no specific cause but conveys an "unmasculine" sense of powerlessness—is now referred to as *erectile dysfunction* (ED), a less emotional term that connotes a physical disorder (Baglia, 2005). Certainly there are physical conditions associated with some cases of impotence. But experts have long maintained that stress, emotions, relational health, and state of mind often play a part as well. The Viagra promise brushes those factors aside. If the commercials are to be believed, all it takes instantly to reignite a man's sexual interest and rekindle intimacy with his (female) partner is a pill (Baglia, 2005). (As we will soon discuss, gay men, although they are as likely as any other man to experience ED, are not part of the image Pfizer has created.)

You may have noticed the double standard. On one hand, a man is defined by his erectile function. On the other, ED is outside a man's control (Baglia, 2005). That's the conundrum that makes Viagra seem indispensible, even to many men who have no erectile dysfunction. Although ED is most common among men 65 and older, the fastest-growing segment of Viagra users comprises men ages 18 to 55 (Delate, Simmons, & Motheral, 2004).

Viagra ads have a *Take a chance! Live a little!* flavor that obscures evidence that the drug can be dangerous, even deadly. The early estimates of Viagra-related deaths range from 130 to 564 (U.S. FDA, 2001; Mitka, 2000), and there are at least 29 documented cases of sudden hearing loss and 38 cases of vision loss among men taking Viagra, Levitra, Cialis, or Revatio (U.S. FDA, 2007). Also worrisome is evidence that the key ingredient, sildenafil citrate, causes a 33% reduction in fertilization among mice injected with the drug (Glenn et al., in press). Early evidence suggests that it significantly reduces the chances of conception in humans as well (Glenn, McVicar, McClure, & Lewis, 2007). And even if Viagra doesn't cause health problems of its own, it may mask them. Some health experts urge men to address underlying factors that may contribute to ED, such as depression, stress, diabetes, kidney disease, hypertension, obesity, prostate cancer, and cardiovascular disease, rather than risk their health even more with a pharmaceutical work-around. (At one point, Pfizer boasted that underlying health concerns were coming to light in record numbers when men who wouldn't usually see their doctors made appointments to get Viagra. The prevalence of online subscription opportunities that don't require a medical exam seems to short-circuit that benefit, however.)

## Implication 3: Women Are Passive but Grateful Recipients of Male Attention

In influencing cultural ideas about masculinity, Pfizer simultaneously implicates women's identity. In Viagra ads it's the man's job to instigate intimacy and romance. He gives the meaningful look, takes dance lessons, presents the woman with flowers, buys a motorcycle, and so forth. Women seldom play a role except to respond, quite enthusiastically, to their men's sudden sexual interest. Women in the ads tend to embody passive, traditional roles. For example, Baglia (2005, p. 84) describes an article in *LifeDrive* (a Pfizer magazine dedicated to Viagra-related stories) that encourages men to demonstrate their "Casanova" potential by washing the dishes, explaining: "This is a gift she will truly love. Do some of *her* chores" (emphasis added).

In the five Viva Viagra commercials airing at the time of this writing, three women (all of them white) are shown in pre-Viagra situations. Two of them are sitting quietly, one reading magazines, the other writing on a greeting card. Each woman becomes animated (smiling and dancing) only when a man (also white) shows interest in her. The third woman is shown in a series of driveway shots in which she carries, at different times, a laptop bag, a cell phone, mail, dry cleaning, and groceries. In each case, she waves to a self-effacing, balding neighbor who drives by in a nondescript sedan. In all of these shots, the woman's hair, a common symbol of sexuality, is pulled back tightly and she is dressed conservatively. But this all changes when the man roars up one day in leather on a motorcycle, suddenly confident and assertive, and wordlessly hands the woman a helmet. She drops her groceries to the ground and rushes to press her body against his, throwing her head back in laughter (a classic vulnerable, flirtatious pose) as he wears a satisfied grin. The announcer promises: "Change it up a bit, and you're sure to get a reaction." *React* she does. In the next shot the woman is riding (as passenger) on the back of the man's bike, her blonde hair finally blowing in the wind as they roar down the highway on their way to share a room in a romantic Southwestern-style lodge. Once again, Viagra—the supposedly magic key to *his* sexuality—unlocks hers as well.

In these ads, there is no suggestion that the women might initiate romantic interactions themselves or that they might consider the men's sudden come-ons in any way resistible. It's more: *Got an erection? I'm yours!* If we infuse a bit of reality, it's probably more likely that women (and men) who respond enthusiastically are encouraged by factors extraneous to Viagra. Certainly, the men and women I know who are attracted to men say it's not men's erections but their confidence, consideration, and attentiveness that make them appealing. One woman in my Gender & Communication class quipped, "You want to talk about male enhancement? Make their *ears* bigger." There's no doubt members of both sexes could increase their sex appeal by becoming better listeners. But Pfizer has zeroed in on the male ego, hitting below the belt, if you will. The goal seems to be to undercut

men's self-confidence by making them doubt their sexual abilities and then promising to restore their confidence (at a price) by buying what Pfizer is selling.

As implied in the motorcycle commercial, Pfizer presents a world in which a man isn't a real man without, ahem, something big and powerful between his legs. In other ads, lest we miss the point, phallic images abound in masts, columns, buildings, and, in the Rafael Palmeiro commercial, "a dozen baseball bats' mushroom-capped handles pointing skyward" (Baglia, 2005, p. 78). Overall, the message is that, until a man can live up to these stiff images, his role as a sexual instigator is on hold; and because women are passive recipients waiting for the green light, theirs is too.

### Implication 4: There *Will* Be Dancing . . . If You're White and Straight

Viagra's first slogan was "Let the Dance Begin," and dancing has been a feature of most Viagra commercials ever since (Ovalle, 2008). So far, the dancing *always* involves heterosexual couples and is *nearly* always limited to white people.

"The equation dance = sex has long existed in film and media culture," observes Priscilla Peña Ovalle (2008, paragraph 2). The typical formula is that white characters learn to dance as a sign of their awakening sexuality. But nonwhite characters naturally have the moves and the rhythm. Translation: White people learn how to be sensual. People of color are innately "hypersexual" (Ovalle). It's a stereotype that confines ethnic minorities' identity and typically renders them subordinate to people who are portrayed as more "whole," "wholesome," or "mainstream." Even the Spanish term *viva* and the Latin music behind the Viva Viagra commercials connote an "ethnic sexuality," even though the main characters are white. In the "Tango" and "Surprise! [Dance Lesson]" commercials, all characters are white except the Latina dance instructor and (if you look *really* close) members of the Latin band playing at the wedding reception. " 'Viva Viagra' reminds me that, as a thirty-something Chicana, I am not the target demographic," Ovalle concludes (final paragraph). "I am forced to recognize my status as a temporary partner on the floor."

It's a rub with which women are all too familiar. Exploitive sales pitches that depict feminine attractiveness in Anglo terms spare women of color to some extent. For example, eating disorders have traditionally been less prevalent among black women than among white women. However, being typecast as other, subordinate, or outright nonexistent is no better. In many ways, it's worse. Baglia (2005) concludes that, in the pervasive images Pfizer presents, masculinity is portrayed in mostly white, relentlessly heterosexual ways. In this context, "other ways of being a socio/sexual human being don't exist" (p. 98).

## Implication 5: Intimacy Equals Vaginal Penetration

The suggestion that Viagra yields sexual excitement and intimacy is so palpable that many men are surprised when they don't automatically feel aroused. "What happens when a man first takes a Viagra pill? Absolutely nothing," writes Tara Parker-Pope (2002, paragraph 10). She explains that the drug isn't an aphrodisiac (although, I might add, it plays one on TV). "Among several men interviewed who have used the drug, not one of them experienced any feeling or sensation after taking the pill," Parker-Pope says. "The nothingness is so intense that the most common reaction is a slight panic that the drug isn't going to work" (paragraph 11).

Just as Viagra doesn't produce sexual feelings in men, neither does it create instant intimacy between people. True intimacy, Baglia (2005) reminds us, doesn't come in a pill but through communication, closeness, trust, and mutual respect. And sex comes in many forms that do not require a rigid member.

R. V. Scheide—who despite having no actual ED symptoms conned his doctor into giving him a Viagra prescription but, to his credit, feels a little bad about it—asks with at least a modicum of sarcasm:

In today's fast-paced life, who has *time* for true intimacy? Scheide (2006) invokes George Ritzer's idea of the McDonaldization of society to suggest that we treat sex the same way (Ballantine, Roberts, & Ritzer, 2008; Ritzer, 1993). McSex, we might call it, is served up quickly, without much wait and with very little effort or forethought—à la Viagra. Or least that's the sales pitch.

Is that what we want—a "Viagra utopia" of fast-food sex in which masculinity and intimacy are reduced to the likelihood of a penile erection? Are erections so essential to intimacy and happiness that it's worth risking men's health and sometimes their lives to attain them? These are important questions. But they are often lost in the hype. Most media accounts, far from challenging the shaky presumptions of Pfizer's campaign, have endorsed Viagra as "the new miracle drug," "the potency wonder drug," and "the new national drug of choice" (quoted by Baglia, 2005, p. 28). Granted, some writers *have* taken issue with the dangers and fallacies of the Viagra promise. Baglia quotes a *Newsweek* reporter who made the point that "a poor lover plus Viagra does not make a good lover, but merely a poor lover with an erection" (p. 37). But the risks of Viagra are typically downplayed, and most media professionals are not stepping up to include marginalized populations in the conversation. Of 52 Viagra-related news stories Baglia studied, none of them mentioned gay men in reference to erectile dysfunction.

With an advertising budget of about $100 million a year, Viagra is unlikely to disappear from the media or the public conscience (Stephens, 2004). And the introduction of similar drugs with similar advertisements is likely to compound the effect. Maybe, despite ourselves, we'll find the nearly ubiquitous *"Vivaaaa Viagra"* tune stuck in our heads. But there is one thing we *can* do, says Baglia (2005). We can stop to consider the implications and think for ourselves. Recognizing that culture doesn't affect only health communication—that sometimes it's the other way around—we can be skeptical consumers of health information. We can recognize the marginalizing effects of narrow

## BOX 8.7 RESOURCES

## More About Viagra, Health, and Culture

Baglia, J. (2005). *The Viagra Ad Venture*. New York: Peter Lang.

Friedman, D. M. (2003). *A mind of its own: A cultural history of the penis*. New York: Penguin.

Loe, M. (2004). *The rise of Viagra: How the little blue pill changed sex in America*. New York: New York University Press.

definitions of masculinity, femininity, intimacy, sex, race, ethnicity, gender, health, and so, and we can reject exclusionary images that cast some among us as less vital or important than others. (There is a great deal more to say about the Viagra phenomenon. For information about Baglia's book and other resources, see Box 8.7.)

### COMMUNICATION SKILL BUILDERS: DEVELOPING CULTURAL COMPETENCE

Although it is useful to be aware of overall cultural differences, be careful about assuming cultural beliefs based on people's appearance or ancestry. For example, Hispanic Americans may have roots in Central America, South America, or the Caribbean—all of which have different customs (Murquia, Peterson, & Zea, 2003). To recognize cultural and individual differences, Betty Pierce Dennis and Ernestine Small (2003) suggest that caregivers consider the following questions when getting to know people from other cultures.

- How do the client and family members identify themselves? For example, do they call themselves American, Jamaican, Puerto Rican, Russian American, or Ghanaian?
- Are the caregivers' questions answered by the client or by another family member?

- Is there a family member who always speaks first? Who makes decisions?
- Do the family members speak with the caregiver in English and to each other in another language?
- Will you need an interpreter? Is so, select one that fits the family structure. For example, if only men respond to interview questions, a child or a female would not be an appropriate interpreter.
- Determine how respect is shown. Ask what titles should be used. First names may be regarded as disrespectful.
- Here in the United States, maintaining eye contact shows interest and involvement. Is it the same or different in the client's culture?
- Food is very cultural. What are the food choices of the client? Are ethnic dishes preferred? Can arrangements be made with the family based on the medical needs of the client?

### SUMMARY

Social desirability and cultural modes of expression influence the way people think about health and illness. As we strive to become better communicators it is important to understand cultural diversity, for a number of reasons: Cultural beliefs and customs influence health-related behavior; in today's global environment, health concerns in one country or ethnic group have repercussions for everyone; and surmounting cultural barriers enhances our ability to learn and to work together for better outcomes.

People from traditionally Asian and Pacific Island, Hispanic, and Arab cultures are similar in that they tend to value trusting relationships and to prefer health care encounters in which caregivers take time to know the patient. They are also sensitive to status differences, sometimes to the extent of masking their disagreement or confusion so as not to offend the caregiver or create disharmony. People from Asian cultures may seem reserved to Westerners because they often avoid direct eye contact and emotional expressiveness except in close relationships. Traditionally Hispanic individuals place a high value on warm, trusting relationships and respect. They typically consider that close friends and family members are integral in coping with hardship. Caregivers who do not realize this can cause offense and interfere with social support. Traditional Arabs may be alarmed if their physicians make predictions, believing that only Allah controls the future and that humans invite disaster by making bold forecasts about what will happen. Like Asians, they are likely to consider mental illness shameful and to deny that they are in emotional distress. Islamic diet and customs can seem alien to Westerners, but they are understandable with a little effort. Finally, learning even a bit of a patient's native language can help caregivers be more effective.

From one perspective, disease is an organic phenomenon and what shows up under a microscope may be more to the point than a patient's subjective experiences. Consistent with the biomedical model, this perspective considers undetectable conditions less real than physically verifiable ones. From another perspective, some people believe health is affected by harmony among such factors as relationships, spiritual forces, the environment, behavior, and energy fields within the body. The organic perspective lends itself to scientific and statistical analysis, whereas the harmony perspective recognizes illness as a phenomenon that occurs for different reasons in different people. Health is believed to reflect harmony among all aspects of a person's life. From this perspective, personal viewpoints, habits, and social networks are considered integral parts of the health equation.

The premises that underlie diverse beliefs may be more similar than they seem. Even staunch supporters of the organic approach admit that stress and attitude affect healing. And people in many cultures acknowledge an organic element as well as a spiritual element to disease. The theory of health as expanded consciousness proposes that a health disruption can be a valuable opportunity for reflection and change.

Diseases and their implications are open to cultural interpretation. Particularly when great uncertainty surrounds a disease or when medicine can do little to help, people are likely to assume that supernatural forces are at work. Society may also stigmatize people who have dread diseases as being menacing and contemptible. At the other extreme, people may regard ill individuals as helpless victims.

Cultural values and assumptions are embodied in the roles patients and caregivers play. How one interprets illness has an effect on the type of healing process preferred. If disease is regarded as a physical phenomenon, patients may be like passive machines and caregivers like mechanics or scientists. Patients may be considered incapable if they are cast as children seeking the guidance of parent-like caregivers who know what is best.

Caregivers have been deified to varying extents. Even orthodox practitioners who pride themselves on science-based care are regarded with awe for their extraordinary ability to understand and treat illness. In some cultures, healers are spiritual leaders, expected to channel supernatural powers for the benefit of faithful patients. Considering patients and caregivers to be consumers and providers is more enabling for patients, but some people worry that medical care may suffer if it is forced to uphold the rules of the marketplace. Finally, as partners, patients and caregivers work to build mutually satisfying relationships and care plans.

Sometimes health-related products and the way they are marketed have profound effects on cultural ideals. Viagra is one such product. Some analysts question marketing strategies that seem to downplay the risks of Viagra while exaggerating men's need for it. Especially worrisome is the degree to which Pfizer and some other advertisers create and escalate social insecurities in the name of making money.

By becoming more culturally competent we increase our understanding of ourselves and others. The next chapter expands the discussion of diversity to organizational culture and diverse types of health-related professionals.

## KEY TERMS

culture
*personalismo*
*respeto*
*confianza*
*susto*
*halah*
organic perspective
evidence-based medicine (EBM)
harmony perspective
yin and yang
*Qi*
theory of health as expanded consciousness
explicate order
implicate order
stigma
role
paternalism
faith healers
glossolalia
placebo

## DISCUSSION QUESTIONS

1. In what ways does diverse cultural knowledge help us to be more effective concerning health communication?

2. Do you have experience interacting with people from diverse cultures? If so, what are the most important things you have learned?

3. Describe some of the cultural beliefs and practices of Asians and Pacific Islanders. How might these influence health communication?

4. How do Easterners and Westerners typically regard health and wellness? What elements of each perspective appeal to you? Why?

5. Discuss the importance of *personalismo, respeto,* and *confianza* in traditional Hispanic cultures. How might these ideas influence health communication?

6. What is a *compadre*? What should health professionals know about Hispanic culture in regard to *compadres*?

7. Describe some of the cultural beliefs and practices of Arabs and Muslims. How might these influence health communication?

8. Have you ever experienced health care in a different culture? If so, what was your experience like? How was it similar to the health care you experience at home? How was it different?

9. What are the strengths and weaknesses of the organic approach?

10. What are the strengths and weaknesses of the harmony approach?

11. Can you think of times when your health was affected by organic factors? By issues of harmony? By both?

12. Describe the idea of yin, yang, and *Qi* and how they influence traditional Chinese ideas about health and health care.

13. Describe the principles of the theory of health as expanded consciousness. What is the role of the explicate order? The implicate order? What role do nurses (and other caregivers) play in helping people cope with health episodes?

14. What are the implications of regarding illness as a curse?

15. Why might members of a society stigmatize ill individuals? Some people feel that smoking has become a stigma in the United States. Do you agree or disagree? Why?

16. How can an emphasis on prevention lead to prejudice against ill people?

17. What are some of the expectations regarding care for family members in Thai culture?

18. Name and describe some of the role sets that patients and caregivers play.

19. Which of these roles have you played as either a patient or a caregiver? Which roles appeal to you most? Why?

20. How is each role set you described likely to affect health communication?

21. Do you feel that Pfizer exploits men in the way it markets Viagra? Why or why not?

22. Do you think companies that advertise medical products should be sensitive to the ways they influence cultural ideas about masculinity, femininity, sex, and race? Why or why not?

*are you more paternalist, consumerist, collaborative?*

*for class discussion* ✗ *any other examples?*

## ANSWERS TO *CAN YOU GUESS?*

1. In order, from the largest number of speakers to the least: Mandarin Chinese, Hindi (India), English, Spanish, and Bengali (India and Bangladesh) (R. G. Gordon, 2005).

2. The number 168 is the luckiest of those listed because it involves the lucky number 8; and when said in Chinese, 168 sounds like "the success is rolling in" (Tse, 1999). The number 74 is unluckiest because it sounds similar to "will die" (Tse).

# PART IV

# COMMUNICATION IN HEALTH ORGANIZATIONS

# CHAPTER 9

# Culture and Diversity in Health Organizations

*About 150 years ago, a father received a letter from his daughter, saying she wished to become a physician. He replied: "If you were a young man I could not find words in which to express my satisfaction and pride…but you are a woman, a weak woman; and all I can do for you now is to grieve and to weep. O my daughter! Return from this unhappy path. (Bonner, 1992, p. 11)*

Well into the 1900s, many people believed that women lacked physical strength and intelligence and were too emotionally unstable to practice medicine (Bonner, 1992). Furthermore, it was considered scandalously immodest of women to touch and see portions of other people's bodies.

There was not much room in medicine for minorities either. Until the 1960s, African Americans were refused entrance to U.S. clinics and hospitals. Black doctors were forced to open their own hospitals because they were not allowed to practice alongside white practitioners (Cassedy, 1991). As you will see, health organizations are much more diverse than in the past, but they still do not reflect the diversity in the overall population.

This chapter describes the role of culture and diversity in health organizations. **Health care organizations** provide products, services, and information to help people maintain health and manage illness and injuries. Health organizations include pharmacies, doctors' offices, clinics, diagnostic centers, long-term care facilities, managed care

organizations, fitness and wellness centers, counseling services, home health agencies, insurance companies, nonprofit agencies such as the American Heart Association, and more.

Health care organizations have a powerful impact on health communication. Organizational members create the environments in which health care is provided and are largely responsible for the tone, quality, and timing of health care transactions. We would all like to think of health care organizations as centers of excellence in which members are professional, compassionate, and devoted to their work. Whether this is the case or not depends largely on the culture of the organization—what is expected, how members define their roles, and what actions and attitudes they value.

As you will see, organizational members and clients differ most visibly in terms of race and sex. But even more importantly, they differ in terms of job duties, occupations, skills, and experiences. You will read about health care organizations that top the charts in patient and employee satisfaction. You will also learn more about efforts to bring additional women and minorities into medicine. The chapter showcases professional diversity by spotlighting communication issues that influence nurses, nurse practitioners, physician assistants, hospitalists, allied care personnel, and holistic care providers. You will read about the advantages of diversity in terms of personal growth and innovation and the challenges of working with people with different visions and ideals. Making the most of diversity requires skillful handling of the conflicts that arise naturally from our differences. We will look at various kinds of conflict common in health organizations and at tips for successful conflict management.

BOX 9.1

## Can You Guess?

1. How much do female physicians make as compared to male physicians?
2. What's the average salary of a registered nurse in the United States?

*Answers appear at the end of the chapter.*

## ORGANIZATIONAL CULTURE

During the Industrial Revolution, it was popular to think of organizations as smooth-running machines (Hawkins et al., 1997). However, a general shift in ideology has occurred since the 1970s. Now people are more likely to view organizations as cultures. As defined by Edgar Schein (1986), an **organizational culture** is made up of members' basic beliefs and assumptions about the organization and its place in the larger environment. In Schein's view, organizational culture has a taken-for-granted quality. That is, members accept established ways of thinking and acting so thoroughly that they rarely question them.

Organizational culture is important because it represents a common set of assumptions that help guide people's actions and interpretations. For example, people in medical organizations (and society overall) commonly address physicians as "Doctor." However, nurses are not usually addressed as "Nurse." If Maria Brown is a doctor, she is probably called Dr. Brown. If she is a nurse, she is probably called Maria. Scholars of organizational culture examine conventions such as these to see what values they imply.

To illustrate, Campbell-Heider and Hart (1993) propose that doctors' expertise is emphasized by addressing them in terms of their medical degrees. They are treated as distinctly different from other people. (For many years, nurses were taught to stand when doctors entered the room.) By contrast, calling nurses by their first names, with no honorific title, suggests they are "everyday people" not much different from patients, clerks, or others who also go by first names. This may put patients at ease because nurses seem more casual and friendly, less intimidating, than doctors. At the same time, however, it may make nurses seem significantly less powerful and educated in the eyes of patients, doctors, and supervisors. Nurses may even buy into the low-status image themselves, displaying meek subordination even when it is in patients' interest and their own to speak up (Campbell-Heider & Hart, 1993). In Schein's (1986) view of culture, people do not intentionally address doctors and nurses differently. They have simply come to accept "normal" ways of behaving and may not be fully aware that their actions support cultural values.

### Cultural Integration and Transformation

The significance of viewing organizations as cultures is that people are not regarded as mere cogs in a machine, as in the industrial metaphor. Instead, they are individuals whose thoughts and values help define the organization and shape its activities. Organizational cultures are accomplished through communication. As Charles Conrad (1994) writes: "Cultures are communicative creations. They emerge through communication, are maintained through communication, and change through the communicative acts of their members" (p. 31).

Schein (1986) suggests it is important to consider how the organization's philosophy is embodied in rules, goals, and the physical environment. It is also important to consider whether people in the organization share the same philosophy about their work, what customs they observe, how their personal expectations mesh with the organization's, how they communicate with each other, and what motivates them (Schein, 1986).

When Linda Deering assumed the role of chief nurse executive at Delnor-Community Hospital in Geneva, Illinois, she had a few ideas. "Being the new whippersnapper, I was frequently in the president's office telling him what was right and wrong with his organization," she told me during an interview. "Bless his courage, he listened. He challenged me that, if I thought I could do something about it, go to it." Deering was inspired by research evidence that caregiver relationships influence patient outcomes. "That grabbed me," Deering recalls. "Before we were forever spending our time on clinical skills and education. Those are important, but this was something that changed how I was going to do my job as a leader. If *disharmony* on a medical unit puts patients at risk, then my top job has to be *harmony*." Deering began to focus on communication, relationships, and organizational culture.

Deering took the bold stance that, if done right, work is a joy. She and other Delnor leaders began to look for opportunities to praise employees. They also implemented a peer-recognition program called BOB (Best of the Best) Awards. Employees created BOB Award coupons to give coworkers when they did something exceptional. People who received BOB awards could cash them in for $5 gift certificates. "It was a little rough at first," Deering acknowledges. "We gave a lot of undeserved gift certificates for things like bringing cookies to work. But we had to look at it a year later and say, 'You know what? They're more joyful than before.'" As staff morale improved, employees began to raise their expectations and their achievement levels. Now Delnor staff members give out about 400 BOB Awards per month. Deering says they are well worth the expense.

Organizational cultures are influenced by the broader cultures in which they operate and by members' personal preferences. People within an organization have preexisting assumptions about the community, the world, and their place in it. These may be more or less consistent with their coworkers' beliefs and with the organizational culture. A **culturally integrated organization** is one in which members share a common language and set of assumptions (Schein, 1986).

Sometimes people seek intentionally to alter an organization's culture. When the staff of Delnor-Community Hospital decided to redesign the corporate culture, they began at the top. "We knew the leaders had to display a passion for excellence or other people wouldn't pick up on it," says Brian Griffin, director of marketing and public relations. Then they focused on employee satisfaction, reasoning that patients would not get top-quality care if staff members were discontent or uninvolved. In 2002, Delnor was number 1 in the nation in terms of employee satisfaction in hospitals its size. In 2007, Delnor was honored as the 4th Best Place to Work in Illinois, based on employee perceptions of communication, teamwork, and benefits ("Best Places," 2007).

Before the cultural transformation, Delnor had a 25% annual turnover of nursing staff. "That's horrible," Deering says. "It wasn't horrible for our region at the time. But it's horrible. Think about it. That's one-fourth of our nurses changing each year." Now Delnor enjoys an extraordinarily low turnover rate of 8%. (The national average is 20%.) Deering estimates that the lower turnover rate saves the hospital about $1.5 million a year. Patient satisfaction at Delnor has also improved—from a respectable 70th percentile ranking in the 1990s to scores that are consistently in the 90th percentile and above now.

Following are some lessons the Delnor staff has learned about orchestrating a cultural transformation.

- *Train leaders, and keep training them.* "Of those who have arrived in positions of management and leadership, very few of us have really had training on how to lead people effectively," Deering says. Delnor sponsors a two-day leadership retreat four times a year. Participants learn new skills and set goals for the next quarter.

- *Don't underestimate the importance of leadership.* "When you have an effective team, you have an effective leader," Deering attests. "When you have a team that's struggling, you have a leader who's struggling." The Delnor staff learned to model the behaviors they wanted others to adopt. "As a leader you can't ask your staff to engage in these behaviors unless you're doing them yourselves. And we weren't," Deering says. "I had to change too. I had to change the way I walked to meetings. I'm a marcher. I like to walk quickly, with purpose. I like to read on the way to meetings. I had my head down. I wasn't engaging people. I had to change." The changes had an effect. "When 75 leaders started acting a little nicer a little softer, everyone noticed," Deering says.

- *Establish clear expectations, and don't set the bar too low.* "In health care we haven't always been effectively run businesses," Deering says. "I think it's born out of 24/7 shifting. We tolerated very bad behaviors. I mean, I could tolerate a bad nurse on the night shift, because if I confront her what might happen? I might lose her. And if I lose her, who might have to take the night shift?" To turn things around, Delnor leaders asked employees to set standards for everyday behaviors such as answering the phone and greeting people in the hallway. "When you take the time to put the right behaviors down on paper and get everyone in the organization to commit to it in writing, you can enforce it throughout the organization," Deering explains.

- *Hold people accountable.* "I happened to be the first manager who fired someone for not following behavior standards," Deering says. "That changed the organization overnight. The word was out that if you don't follow the rules you might lose your job!" Another

benefit of accountability is seeing clear results. "There is nothing more satisfying that seeing those results," Deering says. "And it will radically change the way I'm going to spend my time in the next quarter when I see results that aren't moving."

- *Don't hide behind excuses.* Previously, Delnor employees assumed nurse turnover was sustained by the high number of affluent nurses who could afford to leave their jobs and by competition from doctors willing to pay top dollar for staff nurses. Now that turnover rates have dropped, they are forced to admit those were excuses. "Are we still in an affluent community?" Deering asks. "Of course we are. Has the competition changed? No! *We* changed. The truth is every system is perfectly designed to produce the results it is producing. I didn't like that because it meant I had to change my behavior. But when we changed as leaders, good things started happening."

- *Involve everyone.* Another step was to get everyone involved. Deering and her colleagues instituted a system of shared governance, allowing the people who carry out decisions to make the decisions. "We started putting decision making at the lowest level possible," Deering explains. "They know because they're doing the work. Decisions can't rest in the hands of a few leaders. It's got to be permeated in the organization."

- *Praise lavishly.* "We learned that criticism doesn't work," Deering says. "I think because we're scientists, by nature we're highly trained to see what's wrong. That's a good skill, but it doesn't work very well in raising the human spirit. Praise and recognition work. Take it down to a simple thing: 'You look good in lavender.' Oh yeah? I'm going to start wearing a lot more lavender!"

- *Strive for excellence, and profits will follow.* Deering recalls when "the number one topic on the table was money." Organizational leaders met to discuss how they could increase the bottom line. "Now you know what the topic is? It's quality, patient satisfaction, or employee morale. When you focus on service, people, and quality, you're going to get volume and financials. Put your attention where it ought to be, and the rest will take care of itself."

## Advantages of Diversity

It may be tempting to hire people whose ideas conform to organizational beliefs and to develop highly unified beliefs among employees. It is certainly advantageous when organizational members commit to pursuing the same vision and mission. However, taken to extremes, members' like-mindedness can cause organizations to become stagnant and unimaginative. In a rapidly changing industry such as health care, stability is a risky illusion that numbs members to the need for continued evolution. From the perspective of complexity theory, the greatest risk to a complex system is a continued state of equilibrium (Pascale, 1999). Threats to the system—if not too overwhelming or explosive—stimulate change and improvement. A good example is Baptist Health Care in Pensacola, Florida. In the mid-1990s, in an attempt to save the hospital, organizational members launched a full-scale cultural overhaul. "We were in trouble," recalls Pam Bilbrey, now senior vice president of corporate development. With a "nothing to lose" philosophy, they began bold and innovative changes that catapulted the once-hobbling medical center to the top of the charts in patient satisfaction (du Pré, 2005).

Organizational theorists agree that diversity is valuable because it enhances the potential for creative problem solving. Research is consistent—innovative thinking is enhanced when diverse people bring different viewpoints to bear on a problem (Milliken & Martins, 1996).

Another advantage is that diverse employees are well suited to serve diverse consumers, possibly expanding the organization's clientele (Gardenswartz & Rowe, 1998). Employers who consider diverse applicants also have a wider selection and thus a better chance of finding outstanding

employees (Gardenswartz & Rowe, 1998). Overall, diversity is a catalyst for growth and expansion—both for the organization and for individuals within in it.

Diversity does present challenges, however. A diverse workforce can seem fragmented, with different members working toward different goals. And research shows that employees are often less satisfied and less likely to remain in highly diverse workplaces (Milliken & Martins, 1996). One reason is that members of minority cultures often feel undervalued, as if their contributions and ideas are not considered important. Perceived discrimination is a major contributor to employee dissatisfaction. Among Americans workers who feel their employers are not invested in workplace place diversity, only 21% say they are "extremely satisfied" with their jobs. But 61% of people in diversity-friendly organizations are "extremely satisfied" (Leonard, 2006).

Research shows that people are likely to be stereotyped on the basis of their most visible differences—skin color, age, and sex (Milliken & Martins, 1996). Before they even open their mouths to share ideas, members of minority cultures may find that others have made judgments about their intelligence and importance. Ironically, visible differences usually say far less about a person than "invisible" variables such as education level, length of employment, personality, and so on (Milliken & Martins, 1996). Sometimes organizations present the appearance of diversity on the surface, but actual differences are discouraged. (See Box 9.2 for more on this.)

The first step in encouraging diversity is to allow diverse people into the organization. The next section describes how women and minorities have slowly gained acceptance in medicine.

## HISTORICAL PATTERNS OF ACCEPTANCE

This section examines historical patterns that have regulated the number of women and minorities in medicine. As you will see, the numbers have improved somewhat, but women and minorities still strive for equal treatment.

## BOX 9.2 THEORETICAL FOUNDATIONS

# Model of Multiculturalism

Having established that health care is becoming more diverse and that there are advantages and challenges to diversity, the question is how to maximize the rewards and minimize the potential drawbacks. Evidence suggests that most health organizations have a way to go before they honor diversity in its fullest sense.

The process of integrating diverse viewpoints in an organization is typically gradual. Taylor Cox Jr. (1991) suggests that organizations develop along a continuum from **monolithic organizations** that recognize only one culture, with few minority members, to **plural organizations** with more minority members but continued pressure to conform, to **multicultural organizations** that integrate many diverse cultures and ideas.

Although organizations may hire people who are diverse, they often squelch diversity as soon as new employees walk in the door. Cox (2001) calls these "diversity-toxic cultures." As he puts it:

> Due to the pressure to conform, members who have high cultural distance from prevailing norms of the work culture tend to either leave the organization or modify their thinking—and their behavior—to achieve acceptance. The result is that apparent differences of cultural groups, such as an increasing presence of women, may represent only small differences in worldviews. (pp. 12–13)

Health care, overall, is in a state of pluralism. About 12.9% of members in the American College of Health Care Executives are from minority racial and ethnic groups (Kirchheimer, 2008). This is an increase from years past, but it's still less than half their representation in the overall community, and leadership training is still not adequate to give them a leg up, says Andrés Tapia, chief diversity officer for a national health care consulting firm. As Tapia puts it, "Diversity is the mix. Inclusion is making the mix work" (quoted by Kirchheimer, 2008, p. 6). In other words, diversity is increasing but full-scale acceptance is yet to come. Linda Larkey (1996) points out that discrimination operates beneath the surface in plural organizations. These "pseudoprogressive" organizations purport to honor diversity, and members may even believe they are doing so. But subtle prejudices keep some people from excelling or advancing.

A **glass ceiling** exists when women and minorities are excluded from management positions or are denied equal compensation for similar work. A study by the American College of Health Care Executives (2002) shows that African Americans in health care management make about 13% less money than white managers who have the same education and experience. Women do not fare any better. Female health care executives make about 19% less than their male counterparts—a gap that has grown rather than diminished in recent years (Tieman, 2002).

## What Do You Think?

1. Have you ever been judged by your appearance before you had a chance to prove yourself?
2. In what ways do the organizations to which you belong honor diversity? In what ways do they squelch diversity?
3. Are you surprised by the salary disparities described here? Why or why not?
4. What are the implications for health communication if people in health care organizations do not value diversity?

---

### Female Physicians

In the book *Woman as Healer*, Jeanne Achterberg (1991) describes women's place in medicine and society from ancient times to the modern day. Achterberg describes ancient cultures that honored women as skillful and intuitive healers, primarily because of their "cosmic link" to the earth and the birth of new life. The healing image of an Earth Mother was largely abandoned during the Middle Ages, however. Christianity depicted women as the embodiment of original sin and decreed that church positions be restricted to men. Women who continued to practice healing arts were often regarded as heretics and witches. Women were tortured and burned by the thousands when plagues ravaged Europe and women were accused of using witchcraft to spread the disease (Achterberg, 1991, p. 85). Women were further excluded from medicine during the sixteenth century with the advent of scientific medicine. Largely prohibited from academic pursuits, women were not seen as qualified caregivers because they lacked scientific knowledge (p. 99). Not until the 1900s were women allowed to adopt professional caregiver roles. Even then, they were mostly restricted to holistic medicine.

The first woman known to receive a medical degree was Elizabeth Blackwell, who graduated in 1849 from the Geneva Medical School of Western New York (Duffy, 1979). Ironically, she had to leave America to find a hospital willing to host her clinical training. When she returned, she was forced to open her own clinic because no hospital would allow her privileges.

By the middle of the nineteenth century a few medical schools had begun accepting women applicants, and by 1859 about 300 women physicians had begun medical practices in America (Bonner, 1992). But all of them were denied privileges in established hospitals, and they were forced to open their own clinics and hospitals, specializing mostly in homeopathic and herbal medicine.

By necessity, women physicians were allowed to practice during times of war. About 55 female doctors served in the U.S. Army during World War I (Bonner, 1992). However, they lost professional ground during the Great Depression of the 1930s, when female doctors were strongly discouraged from filling jobs men wanted.

In 1970 the Women's Equity League filed a class action suit against all U.S. medical schools, accusing them of unfair discrimination. At the time, only about 9% of medical students in the United States were women (Waalen, 1997). Continued efforts by women's groups and civil rights leaders led to affirmative action laws requiring schools and businesses to accept qualified minority applicants. By 2002, 44% of medical students in the United States were women ("Educational Programs," 2002). And in 2005, for the first time there were as many female as male medical students in the United States ("Minorities in Medical," 2005). Similar trends are occurring in many places around the world. In 2003, officials in Singapore abolished a long-standing policy that two-thirds of the seats in medical schools be reserved for men. Now nearly half of the medical students in that country are female (Chieh & Tan, 2007).

*Building Equity*  In the last 30 years women have gained significant entrance into medical communities. However, female physicians still make only 63% as much money as their male counterparts ("Investigating," 2008). This is partly because women usually choose lower-paying specialties such as pediatrics and family medicine and are vastly underrepresented in high-paying specialties such as neurosurgery, oncology, and cardiology. Female physicians are half as likely as males to be surgeons and twice as likely to be pediatricians (Magrane, Lang, Alexander, Leadley, & Bongiovanni, 2007, Table 2). Research suggests that this is primarily because women have few role models in highly specialized fields and because they still encounter unfair discrimination on the way there (Benzil et al., 2008). One study found that, although female medical students performed as well as their male counterparts, the women consistently underestimated their abilities, possibly because they received less encouragement and endured more discrimination (Blanch, Hall, Roter, & Frankel, 2008).

Gender inequities persist in medical schools as well, where male professors are more likely than women to advance in the ranks. In U.S. medical schools, women hold about 39% of entry-level professor positions but only 17% of the highest-ranking teaching positions (Magrane et al., 2007, Table 3). Furthermore, male department chairs outnumber female chairs 7 to 1 in U.S. Medical schools (Magrane et al., Table 9). Female medical professors earn about 11% less than men in comparable positions, even adjusting for rank, specialty, and years in field (A. L. Wright et al., 2003). More than 30% of female medical faculty members have felt discriminated against, compared to only 5% of men (Wright et al., 2003). In the right atmosphere, however, the numbers can change. The staff of Johns Hopkins University School of Medicine was able to increase the number of female associate professors (the second-highest faculty rank) from 4 to 26 within 5 years (Fried et al., 1996). The school increased women's participation in leadership, implemented equitable pay scales, increased awareness of gender-related stereotypes, and rescheduled meetings to conflict less with family life. The results benefited both male and female faculty. More convenient meeting times boosted attendance across the board. Women *and* men perceived their treatment to be more equitable than before, were more satisfied with their opportunities for advancement, and rated themselves significantly more optimistic about their careers.

*Communication Styles*  Overall, research does not show dramatic differences between the way male and female caregivers communicate with patients. There are often slight differences, however. Women tend to display more interest in patients' life contexts and feelings, possibly because they are often trained to be primary caregivers (Christen, Alder, & Bitzer, 2008). Female physicians are more likely than men to attend medical school so that they can treat people who are poor or underserved and to maintain that commitment until graduation and beyond (Crandall, Volk, & Loemker, 1993; Shannon, 2006).

Patients' preferences for male and female caregivers are mixed. Adult patients are typically amenable to a variety of communication styles—when the physician is male. But female patients seeing female physicians are most satisfied when the doctor communicates in a caring and compassionate manner (Schmid Mast, Hall, & Roter, 2007). Other studies show that verbal aggressiveness is often considered appropriate for male, but not female, physicians. Female physicians who behave contrary to cultural expectations (as in being verbally aggressive) are often viewed negatively by patients, who consequently are less likely to follow the doctor's advice (Burgoon & Burgoon, 1990; Conlee, Amabisca & Vagim, 1995). Overall, it seems that patient expectations are often framed in terms of gender, particularly when the provider is female, and even more so when the provider *and* the patient are female.

Children's gender preferences may differ from their parents'. When researchers asked 200 children being seen in an emergency department if they would prefer a male or a female doctor, 78% of the boys and 80% of the girls expressed a preference for a female doctor (Waseem & Ryan, 2005). Their parents had different ideas. Some 60% of the parents preferred a male doctor. Among both children and parents, the physician's sex was a more important criterion than the physician's professional standing. None of the children and only 21% of the parents said they would like "the best" physician regardless of gender (Waseem & Ryan).

These findings may be based more on cultural expectations than on actual communication differences, however. Medical socialization, professional constraints, and personal style may mitigate some of the differences between male and female speech. Patients are sometimes surprised to find that there is actually less difference than they expect between the communication styles of male and female caregivers (Gorter, Bleeker, & Freeman, 2006).

## Minorities in Medicine

The racial and ethnic diversity of America is underrepresented in the health professions. Although African Americans, Hispanics, and Native Americans together make up 29% of the U.S. population, only 14.6% of the country's physicians and 10.7% of registered nurses (RNs) are from these groups (American Association of Medical Colleges, 2007; "Minorities," 2005; "Registered Nurse," 2007). In some areas, the disparity is even more striking. In the Boston area, only 3.2% of physicians are African American or Hispanic American, although those groups comprise 13% of the state's population (Powell, 2003). And the numbers are not improving. Only 37 of 600 physicians who graduated from

Massachusetts medical schools in 2000 were black or Hispanic (Peter, 2003). This is not to say that white doctors intentionally let people of color die. A more reasonable explanation is that the social conditions and discrimination that make minorities at risk for health concerns also create disadvantages in medical settings and limit their opportunities to become medical professionals. It's a regrettable imbalance because, as you will see here, caregivers from underrepresented groups are often more willing to serve, and more capable of serving, people in those communities.

*History* A history of racial discrimination has affected patients as well as caregivers. Well into the 1960s African Americans were barred from most hospitals in the United States (Cassedy, 1991). They could neither be treated nor practice medicine alongside white citizens. Members of other minorities were also discouraged from becoming doctors and often had little in common with the physicians they were allowed to consult.

Of necessity, African Americans formed their own medical societies and hospitals. By 1910 the United States was home to nearly 100 hospitals and 7 medical schools catering to African American citizens (Duffy, 1979). Denied membership in the AMA and other medical societies, African American doctors formed their own. In 1895 they founded the National Medical Association. (The organization remains active, with a current membership of 30,000).

African American hospitals and universities suffered from meager funding and harsh criticism. Not until the 1960s did the United States implement affirmative action laws and ban segregation in federally funded hospitals. No longer would federal money be used to build "separate but equal" facilities (Duffy, 1979). (See Box 9.3 for more on affirmative action.)

*Current Representation* There have been some signs of increased acceptance. In the 1990s, Jocelyn Elders became the first African American U.S. Surgeon General, and her successor, David A. Satcher,

became the second. In the same decade the American Medical Association (AMA) inaugurated its first woman president, Nancy W. Dickey. But even then, following decades of racist policies, less than one-third of minority doctors in the United States were AMA members (Foubister, 1997).

In 2008, the AMA issued a formal apology for its history of racial discrimination. Ronald Davis (2008) wrote on behalf of the association, remarking that "the AMA failed, across the span of a century, to live up to the high standards that define the noble profession of medicine" (p. 323). He concluded:

> The medical profession must have diversity in the physician workforce—equivalent to that in the general population—and equity in health care delivery for all persons....
>
> To some, whether looking back or looking forward, attaining equality of opportunity in medicine may seem an audacious goal, but it is not optional for the medical profession. It is within reach, and the nation will celebrate the day when racial harmony is achieved in health care for the benefit of patients, communities, and the medical profession. (p. 325)

*Communication Effects* Physicians from underserved groups are usually well qualified to care for minority patients and more willing than their peers to provide such care. About 48.7% of minority medical students say they will provide care for the underserved, compared to 18.8% of white students, and 16.2% of students from nonwhite minority groups who are already well represented in medicine (mostly Asian Americans and Americans with ancestry from India, Pakistan, and the Pacific Islands) (Saha, Guiton, Wimmers, & Wilkerson, 2008). And contact with diverse classmates seems to help others become more sensitive to cultural differences as well. Medical students whose classmates are highly diverse are 33% more likely than others to feel confident in their ability to care for minority patients and 44.2% more likely to advocate for equitable care for everyone (Saha et al.).

## BOX 9.3 ETHICAL CONSIDERATIONS

# Is Affirmative Action Justified or Not?

Everyone wants the best doctor possible. The question is whether race and ethnicity have a place in that equation. Based on civil rights legislation passed in the 1960s, state **affirmative action** laws require publicly funded universities to give preference to minority applicants who meet admission requirements. Contrary to what many believe, affirmative action does not require acceptance of unqualified persons, nor does it set quotas requiring a certain number or percentage of minority members. Institutions are under no obligation to accept individuals who do not meet qualifications. However, if minority applicants meet the established criteria for admittance, they may be chosen even if nonminority applicants also meet or exceed the criteria. Affirmative action is meant to offset historic patterns of discrimination that have limited opportunities for women and minorities and have resulted in their being significantly underrepresented in professional positions.

Controversy over affirmative action escalated when nonminority applicants who met (or exceeded) the minimum requirements for medical school admission were passed over in favor of minority candidates. In 2003, after three white students sued because they were not accepted into the University of Michigan, the U.S. Supreme Court ruled that the university can give minority applicants special consideration, but it cannot continue its policy of granting minority candidates a portion of the points needed for a favorable admission review (Newbart & Grossman, 2003).

Opponents of affirmative action argue that prospective doctors should be chosen only on the basis of their qualifications. In 1996 the California Board of Regents banned state schools from considering the race and ethnicity of university applicants. Courts in Texas did the same after white students sued because they were denied admission to the University of Texas Law School. In 1999 Florida governor Jeb Bush removed race from consideration in state university admission programs, effectively ending affirmative action in that state's higher education system. Mississippi, Washington, and Louisiana have followed suit. The number of minority applicants to medical schools in those states has dropped 17%, compared to a 7% drop in other states (AMA Minority, 2008).

People who favor affirmative action argue that the public is poorly served by physicians who do not reflect the diversity of the overall population. Research shows that exposure to diverse classmates helps doctors become more open-minded and aware of cultural differences. For example, medical students at Harvard and the University of California overwhelmingly agreed that sharing classes with diverse students helped them become better doctors (Whitla et al., 2003). And minority caregivers are especially willing and able to serve minority patients who are currently least served by medicine and most at risk for health problems (Mitka, 1996).

## What Do You Think?

1. Do you feel medical schools should consider sex, race, and ethnicity when reviewing applicants? Why or why not?
2. How do you respond to the argument that affirmative action sometimes allows people to be accepted into medical school although others' credentials are higher?
3. How do you respond to the argument that affirmative action is needed to help the medical profession more closely reflect the concerns and backgrounds of patients?

As it stands, patients from minority races and ethnic groups in the United States are likely to be treated by doctors whose backgrounds are different from their own. Levy (1985) observes that physicians may be more critical of, and less comfortable with, patients of another race. Or they may be overly paternal or condescending. Caregivers may also under- or overestimate cultural differences (Daly, Jennings, Beckett, & Leashore, 1995). As a result, they may consider behavior abnormal because it does not conform to their expectations or may perceive unhealthy irregularities as mere cultural differences. Caregivers may not be aware that they are acting differently or offensively. However, members of minority groups may be especially sensitive to communication that seems disrespectful or dismissive, and they usually fear discrimination or humiliation more than most patients (Levy, 1985).

## DIVERSE TYPES OF HEALTH CARE

Members of health organizations are diverse not only in terms of sex and race. They differ by profession as well. Many people think of medicine in terms of doctors. But doctors cannot meet every health care need. In fact, the expectation that they *should* do it all places an enormous burden on their shoulders. One solution is to expand people's notion of caregiving to include a wider range of providers. This section offers a brief overview of diverse professional roles in health care.

### Nurses

Nursing is unique, in that it provides ongoing support for patients through periods of recovery and adjustment. Nurses typically spend more time with patients than doctors do and devote themselves more to patients' personal concerns.

RNs are the largest segment of health professionals, and 59% of nurses work in hospitals (U.S. Bureau of Labor Statistics, 2003). And the career outlook is promising. The number of jobs for RNs is expected to grow more quickly than for any other profession (in or out of health care) over the next decade (U.S. Bureau of Labor Statistics, 2007b).

Traditionally, nurses have been rewarded with personal satisfaction but not much else. For much of the nation's history, nurses had little power or status in the health industry. They were often treated more as maids than as professional caregivers. And, although nurses worked long and unusual hours, their salaries were notoriously low. That has changed in some ways.

*Nursing Shortage*  A nationwide nursing shortage has been the most obvious impetus for recent changes. By 1989 there were at least 200,000 unfilled nursing jobs in the United States. Three-quarters of the nation's hospitals were short-staffed (Kleinmann, 1989). In an effort to attract nurses, health care leaders raised salaries, improved working hours, and gave nurses more opportunities for advancement.

The nursing shortage of the 1980s and 1990s reflected the culmination of many factors. One was the women's movement, which had begun to expand career opportunities. Women began to pursue a variety of professions, including medicine. Between 1974 and 1986, the number of first-year college students aspiring to become nurses dropped by 75% (K. C. Green, 1988). The nursing shortage abated somewhat in the 1990s. Relief was short-lived, however. Numbers started to slide again, and by 2008 the United States was short-staffed by 116,000 RNs. That number is expected to reach a staggering 1 million by 2020 (AHA, 2008).

In addition to the factors already described, a number of other conditions aggravate the current nursing shortage. One is insufficient funding for colleges and universities. At a rally in Olympia, Washington, 600 nurses and nursing students protested to raise awareness that nursing schools turn away would-be nursing students every year because they do not have the budgets or facilities necessary to accept more students ("Nursing Lobby," 2003). In one typical year (2007), U.S. nursing schools turned away 40,283 qualified applicants because they didn't have enough faculty, classrooms, clinical hosts, or money to train them (American Association of Colleges of Nursing, 2008). Meanwhile, the need for more nurses is urgent and unmistakable. Among 400 hospital CEOs surveyed, 99% urged the country to train more RNs (Council on Physician and Nurse Supply, 2007).

Another factor is that men have not entered nursing at the rate once expected. Although some men were attracted to the field in the 1980s and 1990s, their numbers never got very high. Only about 5.4% of nurses in the United States are male (U.S. DHHS, 2006).

A third additional factor involves population shifts. At the same time nursing school enrollment has plummeted, a growing elderly population is increasing demands on the health care system. The number of people over age 85 will triple between 2008 and 2050, reaching an unprecedented 19 million, increasing the overall need for health services by at least 40% (U.S. Census Bureau News, 2008).

Most alarming is evidence that—although health care needs are increasing—the number of nurses (which is already insufficient) is expected to *decrease*. This is partly because nurses themselves will retire (U.S. Department of Health and Human Services [DHHS], 2002). About 41% of RNs in the United States are already 50 or older ("Registered Nurse," 2007). At the same time, other nurses are leaving the profession midcareer. Nearly one in five RNs in the United States is not employed as a nurse. That equates to about 490,000 qualified people who have opted out of the nursing workforce (U.S. DHHS, 2006). Many say they burned out working in understaffed units. Because of the nursing shortage and to save money, many hospitals and residential care facilities have fewer staff members than before. This includes nurses, nurse aids, technicians, and housekeeping staff. Nurses are often called on to fill the gaps (Apker, 2001). Stress is also elevated by the demands of caring for sicker patients. Reimbursement limits provide financial incentive to keep patient visits to a minimum and perform minor services on an outpatient basis. As a result, hospital patients today are "quicker and sicker" than in the past. Rather than a patient load in which some patients are quietly recovering and others are really sick, *everyone* is really sick. Hospital nurses in

Hendrich and colleagues' (2008) study walked an average of 3 miles per 10-hour shift. The researchers conclude: "A picture emerges of the professional nurse who is constantly moving from patient room to room, nurse station to supply closet and back to room, spending a minority of time on patient care activities" (p. 31). The researchers note that it is no surprise that nurses leave the profession. Hendrich and colleagues urge health care leaders to consider ways to make nurses' jobs more efficient and less demanding.

The nursing shortage not only affects health care professionals. It also hurts patients. An extensive study of 799 hospitals by the U.S. Department of Health and Human Services revealed that patients in understaffed units are significantly more likely than others to have urinary tract infections, pneumonia, shock, and upper gastrointestinal bleeding—all conditions that can often be averted or minimized with careful attention ("HHS Study Finds," 2001). Patients in understaffed units were also more likely to have extended hospital stays and less likely to be successfully resuscitated after cardiac arrest. The researchers found that understaffing doesn't save money or lives. Researchers conducting a more recent study came to the same conclusion. Jack Needleman and associates (2006) found that hospitals can actually save money by hiring more RNs because nurses in well-staffed units have fewer emergencies, patient deaths, and mistakes to manage.

Many analysts feel that, to navigate the health challenges ahead, we must help health care professionals do their jobs without burning out. This will mean giving them the freedom to create pleasant work environments that foster teamwork and relieve stress, resisting the temptation to overwork staff members, and providing frequent breaks and replenishment.

## Hospitalists

There is not only a nursing shortage. Experts predicts that the United States will also be short-staffed by 96,000 physicians by 2020 ("Physician Workforce," 2005). Hospitalists may help make the most of doctors' time. **Hospitalists** are physicians who work directly for hospitals, helping to monitor and care for patients while they are receiving around-the-clock care. Hospitalists positions were created in the United States beginning in the late 1990s in an effort to reduce costs and improve care.

Based on the traditional model, a physician sees patients in his or her office most of the day and visits patients in the hospital once or twice a day. This provides rather limited opportunities to confer with patients and their families and to make treatment and discharge decisions. By contrast, hospitalists are always on duty. The idea is that hospitalists can save physicians from traveling back and forth and hospitalists can more quickly review test results, make decisions, and meet patients' needs. Sometimes this means patients get to go home a day or two earlier than they would have. And because hospitalists know the hospital even better than other doctors do, they may be better able to help patients understand and navigate the system (Volpintesta & Kanterman, 2008). The potential downsides are that hospitalists are less familiar with patients and their conditions than their regular doctors, they are sometimes stretched quite thin caring for a wide range of patient needs, and patients don't have the comfort of dealing with a doctor they have come to know and trust (B. Fisher, 2008).

In a study of 45 hospitals, Peter Lindenauer and associates (2007) found that the length of patient stays was slightly shorter at facilities that employed hospitalists. But overall costs were about the same across all the hospitals. The researchers speculate that hospitalists' salaries and their tendency to rely too much on diagnostic tests (probably because they are less familiar with patients' health histories) tend to counterbalance the savings of sending patients home sooner.

## Midlevel Providers

Many patients who visit their doctors for minor concerns or routine checkups are now likely to be seen by midlevel providers instead. Two types of midlevel providers are nurse practitioners (NPs) and physician assistants (PAs), both of whom are specially trained and state licensed. (Another acronym associated with NPs is ACNP, which stands for *acute care nurse practitioner*.)

In the hierarchy of most medical enterprises, NPs and PAs are of equal status, about midway between that of doctors and nurses. The main difference is that PAs are trained in medical schools and NPs in nursing schools.

Restrictions limit what midlevel providers can prescribe and diagnose and require them to practice under the supervision of physicians. For minor health concerns, however, NPs and PAs function very much like doctors and are often employed in doctors' offices. They perform routines exams, do minor biopsies, suture cuts, and handle other minor concerns (Freeborn & Hooker, 1995).

Research indicates that patients are typically satisfied with midlevel practitioners. NPs and PAs are usually able to spend more time with patients than doctors can, and they tend to focus on social and personal concerns in addition to biomedical matters (Charlton, Dearing, Berry, & Johnson, 2008; Cipher, Hooker, & Sekscenski, 2006; Laurant et al., 2008). (See Box 9.4 for more about careers in nursing and midlevel care.)

## Allied Health Personnel

Allied health encompasses a broad array of careers involving (to name just a few) speech pathology, physical and occupational therapy, massage therapy, chiropractics, nutrition, athletic training, pharmacology, radiology and ultrasound, respiratory therapy, and dental assistance. Allied health personnel are already crucial to health care, and many people predict they will become increasingly visible members of interdisciplinary care teams in the years ahead. Researchers in New Zealand found that the average hospital patient is seen by 17.8 health professionals, even more (26.6 professionals) if they have surgery (Whitt, Harvey, McLeod, & Child, 2007). The majority of these are allied health professionals, and numbers are similar in the United States. There is not yet a large body of research about communication and allied health personnel, but their contributions to patient care are noteworthy.

## BOX 9.4 CAREER OPPORTUNITIES

# Nursing and Midlevel Care

Licensed practical nurse
Registered nurse
Clinical nurse specialist
Nurse practitioner
Case manager
Nurse manager/director
Health care administrator
Physician assistant
Educator/professor

## Settings

Home health pratices
Private practices
Assisted living centers
Schools
Acute care facilities
Health department
Outpatient care centers
Hospice
Hospitals
Medical office

Insurance companies
Retail clinics

## Career Resources and Job Listings

U.S. Department of Labor: www.careervoyages.
    gov/healthcare-nursing.cfm
DiscoverNursing.com
National Student Nurses Association: www.nsna.org
U.S. Bureau of Labor Statistics: www.bls.gov/oco/
    ocos083.htm
National League for Nursing: wwwnln.org
American Association of Colleges of Nursing:
    www.aacn.nche.edu
American Nurses Association: nursingworld.org
Bureau of Health Professions: bhpr.hrsa.gov
National Association of Clinical Nurse Specialists:
    www.nacns.org
American Academy of Nurse Practitioners:
    www.aapn.org
American Society of Registered Nurses: www.asrn.
    org
American Academy of Physician Assistants:
    www.aapa.org

---

- Community-based health educators represent an effective way to help reduce the knowledge gap among ethnically diverse members of the community (States, Susman, Riquelme, Godwin, & Greer, 2006).
- Paramedics and other emergency management personnel are often the first to respond in a crisis, be it a personal emergency or a widespread disaster (Heideman & Hawley, 2007).
- Social workers have been successful at creating diverse teams to help people with cancer improve their quality of life. Such teams might include experts in nursing, physical therapy, legal issues, financial mattes, community resources, and more (C. H. Miller et al., 2007).

- Multidisciplinary teams that include physical and occupational therapists, psychologists, and others can help people cope with chronic pain and resume many life activities (Breton, Miller, & Fisher, 2008; Stanos & Houle, 2006).
- Because dental assistants usually greet and welcome patients and spend more time with them than dentists do, assistants are helpful in easing people's fears and letting them know what to expect (Abbe et al., 2007).
- Massage therapists and others can help the parents of children with disabilities provide at-home care for them (Cullen & Barlow, 2004).
- Professionals in London are experimenting with the use of perioperative specialist

## BOX 9.5 CAREER OPPORTUNITIES

## Allied Health

About 60% of medical personnel are in allied health. This list is a fraction of the more than 100 careers in allied health.

Medical transcriptionist
Medical billing and coding specialist
Medical librarian
Anesthesiology assistant
Physical therapy assistant
Occupational therapy assistant
Recreational therapy assistant
Respiratory therapy assistant
Medical laboratory technician
Pharmacy technician
Ultrasound technician
Medical assistant
Phlebotomy technician
Radiology technician
Dental assistant
Athletic trainer
Audiologist
Dental hygienist
Nutritionist/dietician
Massage therapist

Speech pathologist
Medical sonographer
Medical illustrator
Surgical assistant
Physical therapist
Occupational therapist
Recreational therapist
Respiratory therapist
Emergency medical technician/paramedic

### Career Resources and Job Listings

Association of Schools of Allied Health Professions: www.asahp.org
Journal of Allied Health: www.asahp.org/journal_ah.htm
U.S. Department of Labor: www.careervoyages.gov/healthcare-alliedhealth.cfm
American Health Information Management Association: HealthInformationCareers.com
AMA Health Professions Career and Education Directory: www.ama-assn.org/ama/pub/category/14598.html
U.S. Bureau of Labor Statistics Occupational Handbook: www.bls.gov/OCO

---

practitioners (PSPs), who help people prepare for surgery and educate them about postoperative procedures. So far, PSPs are proving to be a cost-effective way to avoid medical errors and make sure patients are well informed (Kneebone et al., 2006).

This is just a brief overview of allied health. Other examples are incorporated throughout the book. For more about careers in allied health, see Box 9.5.

### Retail Clinics

Another effort to make health care more afford-able and accessible involves the recent creation of

retail clinics such as those at some CVS, Walgreens, Wal-Mart, and Target locations. The first retail clinics in the United States opened in 2000. There are now more 1,000 of them located in 37 states, and the number is expected to top 6,000 in the next few years (Laws & Scott, 2008). Most are staffed by NPs or PAs who provide immunizations, give advice on minor health concerns such as pink eye and ear infections, and provide health monitoring services such as blood pressure checks (Mehrotra, Wang, Lave, Adams, & McGlyn, 2008).

The U.S. Food and Drug Administration now allows pharmacists to prescribe some drugs that used to require a doctor's order. These drugs are referred to as behind-the-counter (BTC) drugs, in comparison to over-the-counter drugs (which require no prescription) and prescription drugs (which require a physician's approval). Ten other countries, including the United Kingdom, France, Germany, Canada, and Australia, also allow pharmacists to prescribe BTC drugs. Some people think that expanding pharmacists' authority in this way will ease demands on physicians, reduce the costly use of emergency departments, and help make medical care available to the underserved (Laws & Scott, 2008). But many, including the AMA, are opposed to the idea, on the grounds that pharmacists don't have the ability to examine patients properly or review their medical records. And because pharmacies don't typically share their databases with each other or with doctors, patients possibly could visit multiple pharmacies and receive inappropriate amounts of prescription drugs or drugs that interact with one another. It is also unclear how medical malpractice laws (which vary from state to state) would apply to pharmacists and midlevel providers. (Check the FDA website at www.fda.gov for updates on this issue.)

## HOLISTIC CARE

Medical options such as acupuncture, meditation, and chiropractic, once derided as quackery, are gaining acceptance. As you will see, there are a number of reasons for this newfound acceptance. One is that the culture of medical professionalism is quickly becoming more diverse. The following section describes holistic forms of medicine, factors fueling recent interest in them, and their advantages and drawbacks.

### Definitions

The term *alternative medicine* has traditionally been applied to therapies that have not been scientifically researched and consequently approved by professional associations such as the AMA. However, "alternative" is not a particularly accurate description of these therapies. As Lisa Schreiber (2005) points out, it's not an either/or proposition.

Many people use "alternative" therapies in conjunction with other treatments. For example, meditation, prayer, and yoga are not biomedical means of treating cancer, but most oncologists agree that, if they are useful in promoting emotional well-being, they are valuable components of a treatment regimen.

Some have adopted the term *complementary medicine* or *alternative and complementary medicine (CAM)*. But these are problematic as well, in that they define these therapies not by what they *are* but simply in terms of their (implicitly peripheral) relation to biomedicine. Another semantic alternative is the term *traditional medicine,* used in parts of the world such as Africa, Asia, and Latin America. However, this term seems to exclude recent innovations. At a preconference meeting on alternative and complementary medicine at the National Communication Association some years ago, I was part of an extended conversation on this issue. In the end, I think none of the delegates were entirely satisfied with the vocabulary available so far. For lack of a better term, I take Schreiber's suggestion and use the term *holistic medicine* here rather than alternative and/or complementary medicine. Some make a good point that not all methods that fall within this rubric are holistic; but, for the most part, their approach is more holistic than biomedical therapies, which are grounded to a large extent in identifying specific causes and cures of illness. A brief glossary that explains the wide variety of holistic therapies is available in Box 9.6.

### Popularity

There are several reasons for the recent popularity of holistic medicine. First, Americans are receptive to the idea. About 38% report that they use holistic therapies such as acupuncture, chiropractic, aruveyda, meditation, and hypnosis ("National Health," 2007). Holistic care is particularly popular among women and those with chronic health concerns such as back pain (Astin, 1998). Acceptance is even greater in some areas of the world. The World Health Organization (WHO) (2003, Update 83) reports the following.

BOX 9.6

# Holistic Medicine at a Glance

**Acupuncture** is believed to stimulate and balance the body's energy flow (Qi) through the use of tiny needles inserted in the skin.

**Aruveyda** is based on ancient Indian practices, including yoga, diet, and meditation.

**Biofeedback** involves learning to recognize the body's physiological states (such as tension) and to control them.

**Chiropractic medicine** focuses on the physical alignment of the spine, muscles, and nerves.

**Herbal therapies** use plant extracts such as chamomile, licorice, and St.-John's-wort to treat ailments ranging from skin conditions to asthma and depression.

**Holistic care** emphasizes overall well-being (physical and emotional), with an emphasis on maintaining health, not just curing ailments.

**Integrative medicine** combines biomedical and naturopathic therapies.

**Homeopathic medicine** uses very small doses to escalate symptoms in an effort to stimulate the body's immune system. (By contrast, most mainstream medical care is *allopathic*, relying on remedies that counteract symptoms.) *Homeo* is derived from the Greek word meaning "same," and *allo* comes from the Greek word for "other."

**Naturopathic medicine** focuses on diet and the use of herbal therapies to help people maintain good health.

**Oriental medicine** includes therapies such as herbal remedies, acupuncture, and massage. It is based on establishing a healthy flow of energy through the body and achieving harmony between mind, body, spirit, and surroundings.

**Osteopathic medicine** is taught in traditional medical schools. This branch of medicine focuses on the muscular and skeletal system, treating the body as an integrated unit.

**Reiki** (pronounced RAY-kee) is based on the Japanese tradition of channeling energy through the healer's hands to increase the patient's spiritual strength, leading to better physical health.

---

- Herbs represent 30% to 50% of medicines consumed in China.
- In San Francisco, London, and South Africa, 75% of people with AIDS use complementary medicine.
- Worldwide, herbal medicines are a $60 billion-a-year market that continues to grow.

Second, well-trained caregivers are becoming more plentiful. In the United States, chiropractic is one of the fastest-growing occupations, expected to increase 14% between 2006 and 2016 (U.S. Bureau of Labor Statistics, 2007a). More than 50 colleges in the United States are devoted to chiropractic, oriental medicine, and/or naturopathic medicine (Cooper & Stoflet, 1996).

Third, research dollars are more available than in the past. In 1997, the U.S. Congress voted to fund an Office of Alternative Medicine as part of the National Institutes of Health (NIH). This new NIH office offers funding for researchers interested in testing the efficacy of diverse therapies. For example, it has funded research on the effects of Chinese herbal therapies, biofeedback, and music in the treatment of people with head injuries and the effects of substances, such as shark cartilage, that some believe diminish cancerous tumors.

Finally, many insurance companies and physicians are now giving the go-ahead to nonbiomedical treatments. About 64% of physicians surveyed have recommended holistic therapies to their patients ("Physicians Divided," 2005), and Medicare and workers' compensation plans in all 50 states reimburse chiropractic care.

## Advantages

There are several reasons for the growing popularity of holistic care. For one, such care typically involves low-cost and low-technology methods. If these are useful, they stand to reduce health care costs. This is good news for insurance companies. It is also good for managed care organizations if people simultaneously maintain their involvement in conventional care (which they seem inclined to do). WHO is supporting research to see if low-cost herbal remedies can effectively treat malaria, AIDS, diabetes, and other conditions in impoverished areas of the world (WHO, 2003, Update 83).

Second, complementary methods are usually based on simple principles that may be more understandable and less frightening to patients than conventional medicine (H. Brown, Cassileth, Lewis, & Renner, 1994). Patients often feel they better understand and can even manage their own holistic care. Astin (1998) found that people who use holistic therapies often choose them because they reflect their personal philosophy about health. For the most part, these people are not dissatisfied with biomedicine, which suggests they will continue to see both physicians and holistic care specialists.

Third, holistic therapies are usually more directed to health maintenance than is biomedicine, which has traditionally focused on curing and treating. The new imperative to conserve health care resources and money makes prevention appealing.

Fourth, holistic practitioners often spend more time with their patients and develop closer relationships with them than do biomedical practitioners. This may suit people who feel that most medical settings are too impersonal.

Finally, people may turn to holistic therapies if other methods offer little or no help. Symptoms of anxiety, for instance, which aren't cured by medication, may sometimes be managed by relaxation and biofeedback.

## Drawbacks

Many holistic therapies are nonthreatening. Energy work, relaxation, and minute traces of natural substances (as in homeopathy) are unlikely to hurt anyone. However, some therapies involve the use of herbs and other naturalistic products. Because these products are considered dietary supplements rather than drugs, the U.S. Food and Drug Administration does not require manufacturers to register them or prove their safety before they go on the market. Consequently, many supplements are not thoroughly researched. This is worrisome, first, because significant health risks are associated with some natural therapies. Taken by the wrong person or in the wrong amount, they can be deadly. Some natural remedies have caused lead poisoning, hepatitis, or renal failure (H. Brown et al., 1994). The herb germander, often included in herbal teas and tablets, has been linked to acute nonviral hepatitis. The herb ephedra, sold as a natural enhancement for bodybuilding, affects the heart and blood vessels and can cause dangerously high blood pressure. It has been linked to at least 17 deaths (Capriotti, 1999; WHO, 2003, Update 83).

Another concern is that people may be swindled into buying useless products. Cancer patients, for instance, are vulnerable to advertisers who claim to provide the latest life-saving serum. Shark cartilage sells for as much as $115 per bottle, although there is no convincing evidence that it diminishes cancer.

Third, WHO (2003, Update 83) warns that endangered plant species may be wiped out in the zeal to provide health benefits (and reap the financial awards) associated with high-demand herbal remedies. Already, harvesters have endangered rain forests in Malaysia, Africa, and the Amazon. Environmentalists urge world citizens to consider regulations, herbal farming, and ocean-based cultivation to protect the planet's wildlife.

A final drawback is principally an issue of perception. People who use holistic medicine may be inclined not to tell their doctors about it, which can lead to dangerous drug interactions. Only about one-third of Americans who use holistic therapies

# Curricula on Holistic Medicine

The Association of American Medical Colleges provides guiding principles and an annotated bibliography for faculty who wish to integrate information about holistic therapies. See Gaster, Unterborn, Scott, and Schneeweiss's article "What Should Students Learn About Complementary and Alternative Medicine?" in the October 2007 issue of the *Journal of the Association of American Medical Colleges* (volume 82, pp. 934–938).

tell their physicians about them (Kennedy, Chi-Chuan, & Wu, 2007). A study of 80 people with cancer in the United Kingdom revealed that, when doctors were dismissive or critical of holistic therapies, people were more likely either to abandon them or to avoid mentioning them to the doctor (Tovey & Broom, 2007). One woman interviewed for the study described her doctors' reaction to acupuncture: "They didn't actually ridicule it, but they said, hmmm [frowns]. I felt like they didn't really want to talk about it" (p. 2556). In another study, physicians were more likely to suggest acupuncture and chiropractic if they knew the practitioner and felt confident that he or she was well trained (Hsiao et al., 2006). However, they were unlikely to know holistic practitioners unless they were part of the same practice, as when physician/acupuncturists or physician/chiropractors were on staff.

The next section examines the conflict that can sometimes result when people have diverse goals and diverse ways of thinking and behaving.

## MANAGING CONFLICT

As you have seen, diversity comes in many forms. People are diverse in terms of gender, race, culture, and profession. Even people who grow up in the same community may have different views and goals. Diversity is a driving force behind innovation and growth. It is also a source of conflict. **Conflict** results when people perceive that some goals are incompatible with others.

Conflict is not necessarily negative, nor is it avoidable. To some extent, conflict is a natural product of diversity. One of the reasons diversity gives rise to new ideas is that people's ideas are different. Conflict is also inevitable in times of change, when new ideas conflict with established ways of doing things. Even people in relatively homogeneous organizations experience conflict.

Conflict is a natural component of health care, with its mix of professions and people. However, it is especially important to manage health-related conflict well because the goals of health care are so important and because the emotional intensity of medical settings can cause conflict to escalate out of control. This section looks at three types of conflict common to health organizations: conflict of interest, violent conflict, and role conflict.

### Definitions

**Conflict of interest** is internal and occurs when a person wishes to meet multiple objectives but meeting one objective means sacrificing another. In this section, you will see how doctors are being called on to provide quality care but, at the same time, cut costs. Some people fear that meeting one objective will mean sacrificing the other.

Conflict can also be interpersonal, as when some people's goals and objectives are different than other people's. As Linda Putnam and Marshall Scott Poole (1987) define it, **interpersonal conflict** occurs when people who depend on each other have conflicting goals, aims, and values that seem to stand in the way of accomplishing their objectives. This conflict can turn violent. In this section, you will see why health organizations are sometimes dangerous places to be.

At another level, people may experience role conflict. A **role** is the way a person is expected to behave when performing certain functions within the culture. People often play multiple roles at the same time (e.g., friend, doctor, boss, subordinate). **Role conflict** occurs when a person is playing more than one role but the expectations for those roles conflict. For example, nursing home residents often regard their caregivers as surrogate family members (Hullett, McMillan, & Rogan, 2000). However, although caregivers typically consider emotional support to be the one of the most important parts of their job, emotional support is not often part of their official duties, and some facilities discourage caregivers from becoming too friendly with residents. Thus there is a conflict between what caregivers and residents feel is important and what the caregivers are rewarded for doing as employees (Hullett et al., 2000). In this section you will see how nurses struggle to be patient advocates at the same time as they serve as subordinates to doctors and supervisors. The following discussion examines how each of these forms of conflict is actualized in health settings.

## Conflict of Interest

Despite pressure to cut health care costs, physicians have a particular duty to tell the truth and to be as helpful as they can. In this regard, they are in a different position than most business people. To illustrate, if a sign in a restaurant windows says, "Best coffee in the world," you can easily judge for yourself whether the claim has merit. And it does not matter much either way. But claims made about more important services—such as medical care and financial advice—*do* matter. The stakes are higher, and it is difficult to know if providers' claims are true. In those situations, it is important to know you can trust the source.

The legal term **fiduciary** refers to people such as doctors, attorneys, and bankers who are expected to uphold the public's trust. As Marc Rodwin (1995) explains it:

> Fiduciaries advise and represent others and manage their affairs. Usually they have specialized knowledge or expertise. Their work requires judgment and discretion. Often the party that the fiduciary serves cannot effectively monitor the fiduciary's performance. The fiduciary relationship is based on dependence, reliance, and trust. (paragraph 11)

Rodwin worries that doctors cannot truly be fiduciaries (trustworthy) while they are being pressured to make financial decisions that may not be in patients' best interest (also see Morreim, 1989). For example, imagine that physicians work for an organization that withholds a portion of their pay unless the care they prescribe for patients comes in under budget (a common practice in managed care organizations). Or imagine that physicians are paid on a capitation basis (a set amount per patient regardless of the care provided). When a doctor says treatment is not needed, is it the truth or a cost-cutting fiction? Patients who are aware of the pressure to cut costs may wonder.

Rodwin (1995) worries what will become of the patient–physician relationship if people cease to believe they can trust their doctors' advice. If public trust in medical decisions erodes, the quality of health communication will suffer. Distrustful patients may not take medical advice seriously, may feel it is not worth seeking care, and may blame caregivers for adverse outcomes even when the caregivers acted in good faith. Furthermore, if people receive substandard care because their doctors are pressured to save money, can patients sue the managed care organization rather than the doctor? Not according to the U.S. Supreme Court, which ruled in 2004 that managed care organizations cannot be sued for malpractice (Ramstack, 2004). This puts doctors in the rather precarious position of being personally and financially liable for decisions that may be strongly influenced by others, including their employers.

## Violent Conflict

One reason communication in health organizations is so important—and so difficult—is that health care takes place in a high-pressure atmosphere. It is characterized by emotional highs and lows. This is true for employees as well as for patients and their loved ones.

In some instances, working together in high-pressure situations can foster a sense of camaraderie and mutual support. Former nursing student Frank Kelly (1996) remembers a particularly demanding shift during which he and a staff nurse were kept busy changing soiled bedclothes and attending to seizure patients. He recalls being inspired by the calm compassion of the other nurse:

> She had a quiet manner tending to the philosophical, and I found myself drawn to her astonishing patience....[She] never gave the slightest hint of annoyance...."If she can do it then so can I," was my thought. (p. 28)

Kelly was surprised at the end of the shift, when the nurse turned to him and said, "Your patience is wonderful....I couldn't keep going if it weren't for you" (p. 28). Without realizing it, they had been role models for each other.

Sometimes stressful situations turn ugly, however. Frustration can boil over, leading to hurt feelings and even violence. In a study of 6,300 nurses, 13% said they had been physically assaulted in the last year, and 38% had been threatened, verbally abused, or sexually harassed (Nachreiner, Gerberich, Ryan, & McGovern, 2007). In another study of nurses and other personnel in two Veterans Administration (VA) health centers, nearly 73% said they had experienced nonphysical violence in the previous year, and 21% had experienced physical violence (Lanza, Zeiss, & Rierdan, 2006). Most of the perpetrators (70%) were patients.

More violent assaults occur in health care settings than in any other type of workplace. Indeed, nearly half of all nonfatal workplace assaults in the United States occur in health care and social service settings (Occupational Safety & Health Administration [OSHA], 2004). One reason is that people are worried and anxious. Another is that violence often culminates in a trip to the hospital. Emergency personnel and others are called on to treat people who are violently out of control, are on drugs, or are victims of violence. Gang members and substance abusers may frequent health care facilities, either for treatment, to visit patients, or because they hope to steal drugs ("Guidelines for Preventing," 1997).

Security is a challenge in health care settings. Most facilities are open to the public, some of them 24 hours a day. As a result, workers come and go at all hours, and so do visitors. This makes it difficult to know who is on the premises, if they are carrying weapons, and how agitated they may be.

***Communication Skill Builders: Defusing Violent Situations*** Skillful communication can sometimes defuse violent situations. Communication specialists help people learn to spot the warning signs that individuals may become violent, such as agitated movements and unusually loud or quiet speech. They can also help people develop communication strategies for conflict situations. Following are some communication techniques recommended by OSHA (2004) to reduce violent conflict.

- *Keep people well informed so that they do not wait anxiously.*
- *Listen patiently to people's concerns.*
- *Establish ground rules for discussions (such as no loud voices).*
- *Avoid making statements that might be interpreted as defensive or demeaning.*
- *Make it a point to be aware of your surroundings, and keep an eye out for coworkers who may be in danger.*
- *Develop secret distress signals to summon help when you need it.*
- *Avoid being alone with agitated individuals.*

### Nurses' Role Conflict

Nurses serve as patient advocates, meaning they seek to protect patients' interests and speak out for them when necessary. Because nurses often spend a great deal of time with patients, they are in a good position to monitor their overall health. At the same time, however, nurses play a subordinate role, obligated to follow instructions given by physicians and supervisors. The roles of patient advocate and subordinate are sometimes at odds. Consider the following scenario.

> The nurse takes a deep breath and walks into the hospital room. It should be a happy time—the patient is going home today. Instead, the patient looks worried and upset. He still feels ill and is scared to leave the hospital. Although his vital signs are

strong, the nurse agrees. This patient is not ready to go home. The patient turns to her with tears in his eyes and asks, "Why are they sending me home?" The nurse doesn't know what to say.

In situations such as this, nurses are in a difficult position. They are not at liberty to criticize the doctor's decision in front of the patient. To do so would undermine the doctor–patient relationship, anger the doctor, and perhaps cause the nurse to be fired for insubordination (Begany, 1995; Marin, Sherblom, & Shipps, 1994). And physicians are under pressure themselves to keep costs down. All the same, it is difficult for nurses to carry out orders when they believe patients' health is at risk. The dilemma is especially difficult to manage because patients often feel comfortable talking to their nurses, and nurses work hard to earn their patients' trust. In a study of 1,900 nurses, Mark Orbe and Granville King III (2000) found that many nurses were distressed by role conflict when they felt colleagues' actions were putting patients at risk but they feared they would be ignored or punished if they reported the bad behavior.

One option is for nurses (and other personnel) to participate more in clinical decision making. In Orbe and King's (2000) study, nurses who felt they were supported by peers and supervisors were likely to report wrongdoing, which may save lives and protect the organization from lawsuits. By contrast, nurses who feel excluded are more apt to feel emotionally exhausted and to leave their jobs (Ellis & Miller, 1993). Some people believe that empowering nurses to make more routine decisions may relieve some of the strain on doctors (Beebe, 1995). However, others worry that it is risky for nurses to make decisions about patient care because they are less educated than doctors and because doctors are ultimately responsible for patients' well-being.

By long-standing convention, nurses do not challenge doctors' authority, and most doctors are not in the habit of asking nurses' opinions. This may stem partly from sex-role differences (historically, most doctors were men and most nurses were women), partly from educational differences, and partly from authority roles instilled in doctors as medical students (Sharf, 1984). But sex roles among health professionals are changing, and many nurses are now highly educated. The number of RNs with master's and doctorate degrees rose by 37% between 2000 and 2004, when the latest national survey was conducted ("Registered Nurse," 2007). Based on traditional patterns of deference, however, doctors may still be insulted when other caregivers seem to question their authority. The following section provides suggestions for dealing effectively with multiple viewpoints in health organizations.

## COMMUNICATION SKILL BUILDERS: INTEGRATING DIVERSE EMPLOYEES

Here are some suggestions for better integrating diverse employees into health care organizations.

- *Analyze your own biases.* At all levels of the organization, people should take honest stock of their ideas and prejudices. Even unconscious assumptions can affect people's behavior and minimize the degree to which diverse members are accepted in the organization (Law, 1994).
- *Learn about other cultures.* Members of other cultures may have different accents, languages, and styles of dress. It is helpful to understand that they are different, not purposefully defiant (Law, 1994). It is also useful to remember that people in other cultures may have different concepts of time. Be explicit about your expectations.
- *Set a good example.* It is especially important for managers and supervisors to show that they honor diversity (Blank & Slipp, 1998). Not only does this contribute to job satisfaction and commitment, it also sets an example for people who may be unsure of how to act around diverse coworkers and clients.
- *Create flexible hiring criteria.* Look for "talent and potential" rather than focusing solely on previous experience (Rubenstein, 2008).

- *Make assumptions cautiously.* People sometimes misunderstand each other because they assume everyone thinks as they do. Blank and Slipp (1998) use the example of an Asian American employee who works late and seems very satisfied with his job. Supervisors are unaware that this employee considers it unacceptable to refuse to work late or to show signs of discontent, so they are surprised when he leaves for another job. Members of some cultures may also consider it improper to make their accomplishments known or suggest themselves for raises or promotions (Blank & Slipp). Smart supervisors reward efforts, even when employees do not call attention to them.
- *Know the law.* It is illegal to discriminate on the basis of age, race, gender, or national origin. Become familiar with laws governing hiring procedures, job interviews, and employment termination.
- *Help people develop their skills.* The entire organization benefits when its members are equipped to do their jobs well and to communicate effectively with others. Help all employees develop the skills necessary to succeed. Do not overlook basic communication skills, which may differ from culture to culture.
- *Make diversity a priority.* Odette Pollar (1998) suggests a communication audit to identify the organization's level of diversity and its strengths, limitations, and goals. Task forces and diversity awareness programs can be used to establish diversity as a primary objective, help people learn to behave respectfully, and exchange ideas in a cooperative and innovative way.
- *Implement a mentorship program.* To welcome new and marginalized employees into the organization, Max Messmer (1998) suggests the creation of mentoring programs, in which long-standing employees team up with newer ones to show them the ropes and help them see that their input is important.

Messmer says the program reduces training time, opens new lines of communication, establishes trusting relationships, and helps people become established in the organization when they might otherwise feel left out.
- *Groom future leaders.* "Identify our leaders of tomorrow and cultivate their development and education," suggests health care consultant Gail Donovan (2008).
- *Do not be too sensitive.* When people make culturally insensitive remarks in your presence, explain why the statement is hurtful and show that there are no hard feelings (Grensing-Pophal, 1997). Most people do not mean to be offensive.
- *Celebrate diversity.* The true benefits of diversity occur when people consider it not simply a difficulty to be managed or tolerated but a rich asset to enjoy (Pollar, 1998).

## SUMMARY

Organizational culture influences how people behave in health organizations. Culture comprises values and assumptions so familiar that most people are no longer conscious of them. Nevertheless, the implications of culture are profound. Treating organizations as cultures means considering the viewpoints of organizational members, not simply assuming people will perform tasks as if they are cogs in a machine. Cultural assumptions are embodied in written guidelines and in unspoken rules of interaction, all of which imply certain values and assumptions. Personal preferences also play a role, especially as people with diverse ideas come together to solve problems and establish goals.

Members of organizations (and the people they serve) are diverse in terms of race, gender, national origin, ethnicity, ability, and other factors. Diverse coworkers are likely to come up with new ideas, but they may initially feel uncomfortable together and must overcome their prejudices if everyone is to participate fully and feel valued within the organization.

Health care is influenced by the social climate surrounding it. Civil rights advancements since the 1960s have brought unprecedented diversity to medicine. Women doctors are now present in numbers nearly equal to their portion of the population, but the proportion of minority doctors is still only half that of the population overall, and women and minorities still experience the lingering effects of discrimination. Affirmative action laws are active in some states but not others.

Nurses have long played a significant role in health care, and they make up the largest segment of caregivers. The nursing shortage has led health care leaders to increase nurses' pay and status, although many nurses still feel excluded from medical decisions. Nurses' communication is typically characterized by extended contact with patients and a concern with biopsychosocial issues. Stress and staffing issues make it imperative that we consider how to help nurses function at top levels and feel that their efforts are valuable and well rewarded.

The emerging emphasis on staying healthy may place patients in contact with diverse caregivers, including hospitalists, midlevel providers, allied health personnel, and holistic practitioners. These caregivers are typically able to devote time to talking about patients' lifeworld concerns. Moreover, their contributions may lighten doctors' loads. New medical settings are emerging as well, in the form of retail clinics.

Holistic care specialists focus primarily on lifestyle changes and natural remedies. These diverse therapies are gaining popularity based on public interest, an increase in trained care providers, new research, and increased acceptance by health plans and biomedical practitioners. Holistic care is appealing to many people because it is relatively inexpensive, easy to understand, prevention-oriented, and personal. Some people seek holistic care when they are not satisfied with the results or nature of biomedicine. In the majority of cases, however, people continue to see physicians and other practitioners as well. The downsides are that some products are not well researched before they go on the market,

people may be tricked into buying useless products, and large-scale harvest of natural remedies threatens the environment. Although individuals may assume that natural products are not harmful, they can be deadly. All in all, it is a good idea to become knowledgeable about herbs and supplements before trying them.

Whether diversity results from different ideas, different types of people, or changing environments, it is likely to result in some degree of conflict. For example, there is a potential conflict of interest between providing quality patient care and cutting costs. Even if physicians manage the conflict successfully, patients' trust may be damaged if they perceive that their doctors are not acting in their best interests. The intense emotions inherent in health settings can escalate to violence if people are already prone to violence or if they believe they (or their loved ones) are being neglected or mistreated. Finally, role conflict results when people are expected to speak on patients' behalf but also to follow orders without question. Health care employees of all types are exposed to higher-than-normal amounts of violent conflict. Communication can be a valuable tool in assessing and managing violent situations.

Experts suggest that health organizations can become truly multicultural if they make diversity a priority, honestly assess personal and organizational barriers to cultural acceptance, develop knowledge and skills to communicate effectively, and work together to avoid hurt feelings and enjoy the benefits of diversity.

In closing, it is important to acknowledge that there is far more diversity than can be covered in one chapter or book. White males, who make up the largest contingent of physicians, differ from each other in personal preferences, family background, beliefs, and more. For the most part, personal differences are too numerous to describe on paper, and research about the communication behavior of different types of caregivers is still relatively scarce. However, an awareness of the diversity in health care may help put available health communication research into perspective.

## KEY TERMS

health care organizations
organizational culture
culturally integrated organization
monolithic organizations
plural organizations
multicultural organizations
glass ceiling
affirmative action
hospitalists
conflict
conflict of interest
interpersonal conflict
role
role conflict
fiduciary

## DISCUSSION QUESTIONS

1. What is the significance of regarding organizations as cultures rather than as machines?
2. Would you like your boss to be more like Linda Deering? Why or why not?
3. In your experience, what factors are most likely to make employees feel unappreciated? Valued? Inspired?
4. What are some advantages and challenges of diversity within an organization?
5. Have you ever felt that you were prejudged by others before your ideas got a fair hearing? If so, on what qualities or assumptions did people judge you?
6. How do monolithic, plural, and multicultural organizations compare?
7. What do you make of Kirchheimer's (2008) proposition: "Diversity is the mix. Inclusion is making the mix work" (p. 64)?
8. What is meant by the term *glass ceiling*? Have you seen evidence of glass ceilings yourself? Think of specific schools, businesses, and government organizations. Are top-level leaders as diverse as the overall population? Why or why not?
9. What historical factors have influenced women's acceptance as doctors?
10. Do you perceive a difference in the way female and male caregivers communicate? If so, do you have a preference between them? Why or why not?
11. Describe the history of African American doctors in the United States.
12. How does affirmative action differ from the quota system?
13. Do you favor affirmative action policies when choosing medical students? Why or why not?
14. What are the risks involved when caregivers are culturally different from the people they serve? In your opinion, how can these risks best be minimized?
15. What historical factors have influenced nursing today?
16. What factors have led to the nursing shortage?
17. What are the effects of the nursing shortage?
18. In your opinion, what are some things organizational leaders can do to make sure nurses do not burn out?
19. What is a hospitalist? What are some advantages and disadvantages of using hospitalists? Would you like to be cared for by a hospitalist if you were a patient? Why or why not?
20. What are two types of midlevel providers? How are they alike and how are they different?
21. What are some ways that allied health personnel can (and do) make a difference?
22. What are the pros and cons of retail clinics? Have you ever seen a practitioner at a retail clinic? Would you if you had the chance? Why or why not?
23. What factors contribute to the popularity of holistic medicine? What are the potential advantages? Disadvantages?
24. Have you ever taken part in holistic treatment (e.g., meditation, herbal supplements, acupuncture, chiropractic)? If so, what was your experience? Did you tell your doctor about it? Why or why not?
25. What does it mean to say physicians are fiduciaries? How might the pressure to cut medical costs affect their fiduciary role? In your opinion, how can we avoid this?

26. Why is violence relatively common in health settings?

27. What are some tips useful in avoiding violent situations?

28. In what way do health care professionals experience role conflict?

29. According to Cox, what are the three levels of diversity in organizations?

30. What are some tips for managing diversity effectively?

## ANSWERS TO *CAN YOU GUESS?*

1. In the United States, female doctors make about 63 cents on the dollar as compared to male physicians, largely because women typically engage in lower-paying medical specialties ("Investigating," 2008).

2. The median salary for registered nurses in the United States is $57,280 (U.S. Bureau of Labor Statistics, 2007b).

# CHAPTER
## 10

# Leadership and Teamwork

*A critically ill patient was admitted to Mayo's hospital in Phoenix shortly before her daughter was to be married, and she was unlikely to live to see the wedding. The bride told the hospital chaplain how much she wanted her mother to see her get married, and he conveyed this to the critical care manager. Within hours, the hospital atrium was transformed for a wedding service, complete with flowers, balloons, and confetti. Staff members provided a cake and a pianist, and nurses arranged the patient's hair and makeup, dressed her, and wheeled her bed to the atrium. The chaplain performed the service. On every floor, hospital staff members, other patients, and visiting family and friends ringed the atrium balconies "like angels from above" to quote the bride. The wedding scene provided not only evidence of caring to the patient and her family but also a strong reminder to the staff that the patient's needs come first. The event reflects the clinic's spirit of volunteerism at its best. (Berry & Seltman, 2008, p. 57)*

This moving story is evidence of Mayo Clinic's simple vision, known to every employee and used as the basis for all decisions: *The needs of the patient come first* (Berry & Seltman, p. 24). Volunteerism refers to employees' willingness to do more than they have to do because they want to make a difference and they know organizational leaders will back them up. The Mayo vision dates back to 1863, when William Morrall Mayo opened a medical practice on an unpaved street in Rochester, Minnesota. The War Between the States was just ending. Patients drove to the clinic on horses and buggies, and Dr. Mayo's front walk was bordered by hitching posts rather than parking spots. He eventually passed the practice and his guiding philosophy along to his sons Will and Charlie, who also become physicians and oversaw the creation of what we now know as Mayo Clinic, one of the

largest and most respected medical centers in the world.

We'll talk more about Mayo Clinic and other centers of health care excellence throughout this chapter, which focuses on the influence of organizational leadership, teamwork, and satisfaction. But before we begin, let's consider whether such factors actually matter. Health care is in a period of rapid change and intense competition. Funding agencies, rather than providers, establish the going price for medical procedures. And although health needs are escalating, there are personnel shortages in many professions, such as nursing and primary care. It's tempting to push leadership development, teamwork, and satisfaction to the bottom of the priority list and focus mostly on the bottom line. But that's a mistake according to many analysts, including health care leadership consultant Quint Studer, who has twice been named one of the top 100 Most Powerful People in Healthcare by *Modern Healthcare* magazine ("100 Most," 2002, 2008). Studer recalls a 1998 survey in which health care executives outlined their strategies for organizational change. The executives listed technology, provider networks, and new services. "What didn't make the list?" Studer asks. "Not patient or employee satisfaction, nor leadership development. As a result, these goals did not receive attention or resources" (Studer, 2002, p. 7). Studer says these executives were missing the mark. He advocates a different approach—creating cultures of excellence in which employee and client satisfaction are paramount and, although goals are clearly defined, leadership is dispersed throughout the organization.

Studer and others argue that organizational culture and shared leadership are especially important *because* health care is in a state of transition. Change is difficult to manage in isolation, but when people are actively involved in facing challenges as a team, they can often transform them into opportunities for innovation and transformation. The trick, say experts, is to establish guiding principles that point the way even when the landscape changes. A case in point is Mayo Clinic, which has remained cutting edge for more than 145 years, all the while maintaining a simple, timeless, nonnegotiable commitment to put patients' needs first.

This chapter describes the conditions that make it necessary for health care organizations to break free of the traditional, slow-moving bureaucratic model in favor of more innovative leadership and teamwork. Communication skills are crucial as people from many disciplines come together to share ideas and establish new policies. Experts share tips for working in teams, training new leaders, collaborating on creative solutions, developing a shared vision, evaluating existing rules, and managing crises.

## CURRENT ISSUES

Health care has changed dramatically in the last few decades, primarily because of efforts to control costs. As you may recall from Chapter 2, in the 1970s insurance and governmental agencies began to limit the amounts they would pay for medical services. Health organizations were subsequently faced with deficits unless they cut their own costs. Organizations unable to adapt quickly or efficiently enough closed their doors. Some 949 U.S. hospitals closed between 1980 and 1993 (American Hospital Association [AHA], 1994). Hospitals in minority neighborhoods were especially hard hit. Between 1990 and 1997, 70% of hospitals in predominantly African American or Hispanic neighborhoods closed (Robert Wood Johnson Foundation, 2001). Closures have tapered off since 2000, but a 12% drop in the number of hospital emergency departments has officials worried about the country's ability to respond to disasters ("Advance Data," 2006; Kaji, Koenig, & Lewis, 2007). And many existing facilities, especially in rural areas, face uncertain futures. Based on the latest numbers, one-third of the nation's hospitals are losing money (AHA, 2008). Let's review a few of the most influential market conditions.

## Consolidation

Health organizations that once operated independently are now likely to be part of corporate enterprises. By the mid-1990s, more than half the hospitals in the United States had been bought by large corporations (Shortell, Gillies, & Devers, 1995). Many others merged with competitors or formed alliances with other health organizations. **Integrated health systems** are formed when care providers collaborate to offer a spectrum of health services (Jennings & O'Leary, 1995). An integrated health system may include hospitals, outpatient surgery centers, doctors' offices, fitness centers, nursing homes, rehabilitation centers, hospices, and more (Slusarz, 1996).

The idea is that, by sharing resources, consolidated organizations can reduce their operating costs and be more competitive. That's not easy to accomplish, however. Takeovers, mergers, and alliances present immense communication challenges. For one, long-standing competitors may suddenly find themselves working together. Health care executive Eleanor McGee recalls a consolidation the late 1990s this way: "We went from 2,000 employees to 5,000 employees in 2 years. We didn't know each other. We didn't like each other. We didn't have a common vision. We didn't even have a common mission" (quoted by du Pré, 2005, p. 312). In circumstances like that, organizational members may struggle to form new relationships and find ways to integrate their ideas, or they may do as many health systems have done and continue to operate as separate entities under one (rather invisible) umbrella. Partitioning is understandable, but it hampers organizations' ability to share resources and coordinate patient care. Later in the chapter we'll examine how Mayo Clinic has managed to fully integrate a comprehensive array of services.

Another challenge of integration is that, as organizations become more complex, it's difficult to manage them by the old rules. In *Good to Great,* Jim Collins (2001) summarizes the challenge:

> Entrepreneurial success is fueled by creativity, imagination, bold moves into unchartered waters, and visionary zeal. As a company grows and becomes more complex, it begins to trip over its own success—too many new people, too many new customers, too many new orders, too many new products. What was once great becomes an unwieldy ball of disorganized stuff. (p. 121)

It's hard to maintain clarity as an organization grows. Rapid change can feel disorienting and overwhelming. And whereas people in a small organization often perceive themselves to be one cohesive team, factions and division are common in larger organizations. Leaders often react to these forces by establishing hierarchies and chains of command (in short, bureaucracies) to impose order and control. This may help organizational members feel more organized, but it also suppresses creativity and makes it clear that upper-level leaders, not employees, are in charge of the organization's design and destiny. In Collins' terms, an "executive class" with most of the power and perks begins to emerge, distinctly separate from others in the organization. As

this happens, "the creative magic begins to wane as some of the most innovative people leave, disgusted by the burgeoning bureaucracy and hierarchy" (Collins, p. 121). In short, centralized, bureaucratic decision making is an effort to keep everyone marching in the same direction, but it can be sluggish and inhibiting. We'll talk more about these challenges and opportunities throughout the chapter.

## Controversy Over Specialty Hospitals

With health care dollars limited, people in health organizations have a clear incentive to allocate resources wisely. Because their income is limited to capitated fees and set reimbursements, organizational members try to anticipate as accurately as possible what health services people are likely to need (Azevedo, 1996). Some people wonder why medical centers don't specialize more—perhaps agreeing that one hospital will offer cardiac care, another neurological care, and so on. This has happened to some extent. In fact, entrepreneurs in some states, such as Louisiana, have gone so far as to open what are called "boutique hospitals" that offer acute-care services such as cardiac care and orthopedic surgery. These hospitals often advertise highly personalized care and luxurious amenities. Many of them cater to people who can afford to top off what their insurance pays with additional out-of-pocket payments.

The downside of boutique hospitals—and, to some extent, specialization overall—is that some procedures (traditionally including cardiac and orthopedic care) are more generously reimbursed than others. Without income from these comparatively lucrative services, comprehensive hospitals are less able to make up the difference on services that, although in high demand, don't have high reimbursement rates. Hospitals routinely lose money on some services, such as emergency and trauma care and care for the uninsured. Thus, specialty hospitals may run comprehensive hospitals out of business or at least cause them to scale back on staff and technology and/or to close particular departments. This is worrisome because people who cannot afford boutique hospitals may lose access to high-quality care; and if comprehensive-care hospitals close, everyone in the community may lose access to services not offered by medical boutiques.

Another argument against specialized hospitals is that medical concerns are often complex. For example, complications from heart surgery may require the immediate attention of a neurologist. Scattering specialized services across a geographic region makes it more difficult to respond quickly to patients' complex and emergent needs.

The issue of boutique hospitals is controversial and is likely to get more attention in the years to come. Some states already have (or are considering) certificate-of-need laws that require start-up hospitals to demonstrate that they will not be duplicating existing services and laws requiring physicians to tell patients upfront if they have a financial investment (such as being an owner or stockholder) in a boutique hospital at which they treat patients.

## Efficiency

Another strategy is eliminating waste and maximizing efficiency. People in some health organizations are using techniques such as Six Sigma to analyze the efficiency of everyday procedures such as ordering lab tests, delivering meal trays, dispensing medication, and responding to patient requests. **Six Sigma** is a process in which analysts chart each step in a workplace process, time how long each step takes (computing averages, ranges, and standard deviations), and chart the various outcomes. The goal is to determine which actions add value and which contribute to waste and errors. These considerations are particularly important in health care because of the high costs involved and because even a small error can have drastic consequences. Carolyn Pexton (nd) explains:

> In terms of impact to the patient, a defect in the delivery of health care can range from relatively minor, such as food on a tray that doesn't match the doctor's orders, to significant, such as operating on the wrong limb. In a worst-case scenario, the defect can be fatal, as when a medication error results in the patient's death. (paragraph 5)

Even errors that don't harm the patient's health, such as waiting an extra day in the hospital for lab results, are costly. Experts estimate that avoidable errors account for 30% to 60% of U.S. health care costs (Panchak, 2003), and medication errors alone cause more than 1.5 million patient injuries per year ("Medication Errors," 2006).

As you might expect, analysts often find that existing procedures don't always work according to their original design, so people adapt various work-arounds. Over time, coworkers may adopt so many work-arounds that immense variations and holes in the system develop. For example, Chuck DeBusk and Art Rangel Jr. (nd) studied discharge procedures in a hospital nursing unit. They found that it took an average of 3 hours to discharge a patient, with an enormous standard deviation of 128.7 minutes. That means it might take 1 hour or it might as easily take 5 hours. The analysts soon realized that every nurse on the unit followed a slightly different procedure. For example, after getting the physician's signature on discharge paperwork, the second step was getting patients to sign. Some nurses placed paperwork awaiting patient signatures in a bin for other nurses to pick up (usually about 73 minutes later). Other nurses didn't use the bin but went directly to patients for their signatures (which usually required only 9 minutes). Because no one could estimate how long it would take to get signatures, the nurses typically waited until all signatures were in to call a social worker to educate the patient about aftercare procedures (another 120- to 160-minute wait). And even once all discharge procedures were final, there wasn't a standard way to alert the unit secretary, so patients sometimes waited around until someone noticed and called for transport. All the while, other personnel were tied up trying to get incoming patients into the beds being vacated. The Six Sigma analysts were able to work with the nurses to create what they call a "lean process map," a streamlined procedure that shaved more than 2 hours off the discharge process, with very little variation. The new process reduced patients' average wait to 47.8 minutes, made everyone's job easier, and minimized the chances of error and oversight.

BOX 10.1 **RESOURCES**

## Six Sigma and Other Efficiency Process Models

deBusk, C., & Rangle, A., Jr. (nd). Creating a lean Six Sigma hospital discharge process. An iSixSigma case study. iSix Sigma Healthcare. Retrieved October 16, 2008, from http://healthcare.isixsigma.com/library/content/c040915a.asp

Panchak, P. (2003, November 1). Lean health care? It works! *Industry Week.* Retrieved October 16, 2008, from http://www.industryweek.com/ReadArticle.aspx?ArticleID=1331

Pexton, C. (nd). Framing the need to improve health care using Six Sigma methodologies. iSixSigma. Retrieved October 16, 2008, from http://healthcare.isixsigma.com/library/content/c030513a.asp

Rooney, J. J., & Vanden Heuvel, L. N. (2004, July). Root cause analysis for beginners. *Quality Progress, 37*(7), 45.

Vanden Heuvel, L., & Robinson, C. (2005, Summer). How many causes should you pursue? *Journal for Quality and Participation, 28*(2), 22–23.

(For more about Six Sigma and similar techniques, see Box 10.1.)

## Marketing and Advertising

Health organizations have traditionally relied on word-of-mouth promotion, but competition has led to more diverse marketing strategies. The AMA, which banned physician advertising in 1914, lifted the ban in 1975 under pressure from the U.S. Supreme Court, which felt that the ban restricted public information and physicians' livelihood (Kotler & Clarke, 1987). Although doctors have been somewhat reluctant to advertise aggressively themselves, many insurance companies and managed care organizations are avid advertisers, as are pharmaceutical companies, which spend more than $2 billion a year to advertise prescription drugs (Kane, 2003). (You will read more about this in Chapter 11.) Although competition is fierce,

"selling" medical services remains a controversial subject. For a discussion of the ethical issues involved, see Box 10.2.

## Consumerism

Patients have choices in the health care marketplace. Choice is underlined not only by advertising and marketing efforts but also by an unprecedented amount of health information available in the news media and on the Internet. In this context, patients are well-informed consumers asked to choose between different health services vying for their business.

As a result of these factors, people in health organizations must strive for consumer satisfaction. This is a challenge because, as Berry and Seltman (2008) point out, "being a patient is about the least amount of fun anyone can have as a consumer" (p. 167). And the stakes are high. Every patient wants and deserves to be treated as an individual with unique needs and perceptions. Ignoring or inconveniencing patients is not a good way to keep their business. Consequently, many medical centers have eliminated the paperwork that used to make hospital admissions a lengthy and frustrating process. Instead, personnel now obtain information over the phone in advance so that people feel less hassled when they arrive for treatment. Some others have authorized employees to reimburse patients for lost items (e.g., dentures, eyeglasses, pillows, or clothing) and to award gift certificates and coupons when they see fit. A nurse once told me, "It's amazing how much goodwill you can inspire with a free lunch!" After employees at the hospital where she worked were given cafeteria coupons to pass along to others, patient satisfaction increased considerably. Says the nurse:

> Now, when we see a patient's family that has been waiting around for results or a procedure, we can say, "I'm sorry you have had to wait so long. Please have lunch on us. We'll have everything ready by the time you get back." There's no amount of advertising that can outmatch a free meal when you are hungry, tired, and frustrated! And it makes us feel good to help. We're not the bad guys. We're the ones who

## BOX 10.2 ETHICAL CONSIDERATIONS

# Should Health Organizations Advertise?

Members of the American Medical Association long believed that it was unethical to promote medical services for the purpose of making money (Walt, 1997). They have since lifted the ban on advertising, but although many types of health care organizations (e.g., hospitals, managed care organizations, nursing homes) do advertise, physicians have typically limited themselves to simple ads, such as those that announce the opening of a new practice.

Some people object to advertising medical services and products. Robert Boyd (1997), for one, argues that "media hype" has no place in health. He warns that it is confusing enough to keep up with medical research without being bombarded by sales pitches promoting various health products and services.

A related worry is that claims made by health organizations (such as "Best cancer care") are hard to evaluate and patients do not typically have the expertise to know when advertisers are making exaggerated or inaccurate claims. Moreover, seriously ill patients and their loved ones may be particularly vulnerable to advertising claims because they so badly want to believe a cure is possible (Irvine, 1991).

Others fear that health advertisements will alarm people and make them needlessly preoccupied with health issues. Alison Bass (1990) describes a hospital advertisement that shows a woman examining her breasts for lumps. The headline reads: "This woman just missed the cancer that will kill her" (p. 1). Bass concludes: "People who provide health care have begun playing on the very fears and anxieties they are supposed to alleviate" (p. 1).

There is also concern that advertising will damage the professional image of caregivers. Critics cringe at sales ploys that make health professionals seem silly or greedy. For example, some clinics have offered money-back guarantees if patients are not satisfied with the care they receive. Health ethicist John La Puma (1998) wonders if free toasters will be the next marketing strategy.

People who support health advertising have a simple but compelling case as well. They feel that advertising is a useful way to let the public know about service providers and services (Bass, 1990). Proponents of health-related advertisements maintain that consumers are wise enough to be skeptical about advertisers' claims and to avoid being taken in by misleading promises.

### What Do You Think?

1. Should doctors advertise their services? Why or why not?
2. Some physicians feel that lawyers' professional image has been tarnished since they have begun to advertise on television. Do you agree? Why or why not? Do you think it would be the same for physicians?
3. Should other providers (e.g., hospitals, drug companies, rehabilitation centers, managed care organizations) advertise? Why or why not?
4. If advertising is allowed, should there be any restrictions on what the ads may (or must) contain?

---

understand and help—not just the patients, but their families too.

### Staffing Shortages

In the midst of other challenges, people in health care organizations are struggling to attract and keep qualified personnel. As you may remember from Chapter 9, experts estimate that U.S. health care organizations will be short-staffed by 1 million registered nurses by 2020, and 116,000 positions are already vacant (AHA, 2008). This makes it imperative for leaders to do whatever they can to attract and keep qualified personnel. This includes

## BOX 10.3 CAREER OPPORTUNITIES

## Health Care Leadership

President or CEO
Chief operating officer
Chief financial officer
Health information manager
Director of human resources
Strategic planning director
Medical director
Nursing director
Departmental director (e.g., Department of
  Nursing, Surgery, Medical Records, Human
  Resources, Marketing, Public Relations, Education,
  Information Technology, Billing, Risk Management)

Medical office manager

## Career Resources and Job Listings

U. S. Bureau of Labor Statistics: www.bls.gov/oco/
  ocos014.htm
Association of University Programs in Health
  Administration: www.aupha.org
American College of Health Care Administrators:
  www.achca.org
American College of Health Care Executives:
  www.healthmanagementcareers.org
Medical Group Management Association: www.
  mgma.org

---

listening more closely to employees' needs, responding to their ideas, and involving them in collaborative efforts to create satisfying environments. We'll talk about these more throughout the chapter.

All in all, people in health care are reacting to a new set of challenges—to conserve resources, to develop a clearer understanding of community health needs, and to attract and satisfy clients and employees. One of the most notable changes is a shift from bureaucratic management to an emphasis on human resources. (See Box 10.3 for more on career opportunities related to health care leadership.)

### CHALLENGING THE BUREAUCRACY

Like most businesses that developed during the Industrial Revolution, U.S. health organizations (especially large ones) adopted a bureaucratic model. A **bureaucracy** is a highly structured organization with a clear chain of command, centralized power, specialized tasks, and established rules for operation (Weber, 1946).

Over the years, the bureaucratic model has strengthened health care organizations in some ways and weakened them in others. The principle

weakness—top-down leadership that is often insulated and slow moving—has become a liability few organizations can afford. A case in point is the U.S. Veterans Administration (VA). Although the VA is the second-largest bureaucracy in the American government, leaders in VA health systems have launched an extensive effort to become less bureaucratic. Describing the VA's planned transformation, Vestal, Fralicx, and Spreier (1997) explain:

> The rigid, functionally focused, command-and-control culture that has long been a hallmark of VA must be replaced by one that values speed, flexibility, and the processes for delivering high-quality, cost-effective patient care. (p. 339)

An effort is under way to restructure the VA health system so that employees are empowered to respond to consumers' needs, not simply to the dictates of the bureaucracy. Employees are increasingly encouraged to think of ways to please customers, solve problems, work together in teams, and come up with innovative methods to improve care and conserve resources.

As in the VA, members of many health care organizations are considering new options. A few of those options are presented here. As you will see, future trends are still more easily defined by questions than by answers, which means leaders and teams have a particularly challenging and exciting task ahead of them.

## Hierarchies or Partnerships?

In a classic bureaucracy, a strict hierarchy establishes who the bosses are. The organizational chart is vertical, meaning there are many layers of management, and managers at each level supervise a relatively small number of people (Hamilton & Parker, 1997). The old saying "It's lonely at the top" is especially true in a vertical organization. Few people make it that far. Although top-level managers make most of the decisions, employees are encouraged to communicate, mostly with those directly above and below them, meaning that high-level administrators typically have little contact with the majority of organizational members.

*Advantages*  There are some advantages to a vertical hierarchy.

- Centralized authority provides stability and a common sense of purpose. This is important in health care organizations, which may have dozens of departments and different types of employees. Particularly with mergers and consolidations, it may be difficult to maintain a common vision without strong leadership at the core.
- A strict hierarchy reduces ambiguity. It is clear who has decision-making power. This is useful when making quick or important decisions. In emergencies, for example, paramedics know exactly which procedures they are authorized to begin and which procedures require the approval of a supervisor or physician. This clarity can save time and prevent mistakes inexperienced personnel might make.
- Appointed decision makers can help with decisions about marketing, new service

lines, staffing, and other issues that cross departmental lines.

*Disadvantages*  Centralized authority also has drawbacks. Nurse executive Ann L. Hendrich strongly urges that people in vertical health care organizations consider a change of format. As she puts it: "In the new market there will be two kinds of organizations—quick and dead" (quoted by Porter-O'Grady, Bradley, Crow, & Hendrich, 1997, paragraph 10).

- Centralized decision making is *not* usually quick. Opportunities for change are often lost or delayed, which can be fatal in today's fast-moving market.
- High-level decision makers typically do not have direct contact with clients or frontline personnel.
- Employees don't usually have the authority to make exceptions for special circumstances or to customize services for individual customers. (In plenty of organizations the wedding in the story that began this chapter would be discouraged or outright forbidden.)
- When service breakdowns occur, frontline employees usually have to wait for authorization from "higher-ups" before they can resolve the issues. The result is often a frustrating delay on top of an already-disappointing situation.
- Hierarchies inhibit trust and open communication. Employees may be reluctant to suggest ideas or to be honest with people in positions of higher power, particularly since there is typically little opportunity to get to know and trust them. For example, employees in the billing department may be reluctant to admit that the new computerized billing system they requested is not working well.

Consultant Fred Lee (2004) offers a good example of how frustrating centralized decision making can be. He arrived at a hospital early one morning to conduct a training session, only to find that the classroom was locked. A security officer arrived, but, although he had a key, he had to get his supervisors' permission to open the door, and they were not available. After waiting in the hall for a while (along with the workshop participants), Lee suggested that hospital administrators might be in the office by then. "That won't do any good," said the officer. "I don't take orders from administration. I have to call my dispatch office, which is located across town.... Until they tell me to open the classroom, I can't. I'm really sorry" (p. 86). The officer finally did get permission and opened the classroom, but Lee reflects on the absurdity of the policy. He wonders: "How could central dispatch, 20 miles away, have a better understanding of the situation than the officer at the scene? Any information about the problem would be coming from the officer anyway" (p. 86). Lee sympathizes with the employee who was rendered powerless (and was no doubt embarrassed) because supervisors did not trust employees enough to give them authority to act on their own judgment.

*Opportunities for Change* Faced with the need to adapt more quickly than a bureaucratic framework allows, members of some health care organizations have taken steps to minimize the hierarchy. Following are some ideas from the experts.

*Give Employees the Power to Say Yes on the Spot* In *Customer Satisfaction Is Worthless, Customer Loyalty Is Everything,* Jeffrey Gitomer (1998) proclaims that "policy" is the "single most annoying word a customer hears besides 'no'" (p. 68). He points out that customers don't want to hear about policies—they want solutions to their problems. Gitomer imagines a scenario in which a employee is able to say: "Hey, you're in luck!—I just looked it up in the policy book and it says right here I can do everything you want, just the way you want it" (p. 68). He acknowledges that this fantastic scenario is unlikely to come true and that *some* policies are necessary. But Gitomer forbids people from using the p-word with customers. Instead of telling customers or patients that you can't do something

because of a policy, he suggests, say "yes" to a different way of solving their problems.

To try this out, I challenged students in an advanced leadership class to say "yes" for one week to customer requests whenever possible in their jobs. The students, who were employed in a range of careers, from health to banking to student services, all reported the same thing a week later. "Customers were shocked," they said. "They weren't expecting to hear yes." Many of the customers asked some version of "Really?!" or "Are you sure?" Clearly, there aren't a lot of organizational cultures in which people are empowered to tell customers yes!

*Go Horizontal* Giving team members the authority and resources to manage themselves enables vertical organizations to eliminate some layers of middle management and to disperse leadership throughout the organization. When done effectively, empowerment allows teams to create systems and work environments that are tailor-made for success. If they have adequate training, authority, and resources, teams usually don't need much supervision, particularly if everyone is responsible for meeting clear goals. For example, as the staff at Baptist Hospital in Pensacola, Florida ushered in a new age of empowerment, they began posting patient satisfaction scores on hallway bulletin boards, challenging units to maximize their scores. The satisfaction scores, which are updated regularly, are visible to patients and employees. And easy-to-read charts make it clear how department scores compare to each other. Lynn Pierce was a nurse manager in a low-scoring unit when this tradition began back in the late 1990s. Although she frequently made excuses for her unit's scores when they were kept private, having them posted changed her point of view. "I started thinking, 'My [patient satisfaction] numbers are going to come up! I won't be left behind,'" she says (quoted by du Pré, 2005, p. 317). Pierce says she began seeing patient requests, not as time-consuming chores, but as opportunities. She laughs, "'You want a Coke?' I'd call Dietary and say, 'Send 'em a six-pack!'" (p. 317).

*Create Participative Decision-Making Structures* Empowerment should extend beyond departmental boundaries. Employees are usually more satisfied with their jobs and more committed to staying with the organization when they have input on overarching decisions as well (Bucknall & Thomas, 1996; McNeese-Smith, 1996). **Participative decision making (PDM)** means people are involved in making the decisions that affect the organization (Goldhaber, 1993). PDM is typically good for morale and effective at yielding high-quality decisions. It puts everyone in a position of leadership. But keep in mind that many people need help adjusting to such a role. Bob Murphy, a former hospital administrator and now a coach with the Studer Group, puts it this way: "There's an old saying: 'What's the difference between a nurse on Friday and a nurse leader on Monday?' . . . A weekend to think about it!" The same is often true of personnel in other areas. Following are some tips for increasing the communication effectiveness of people throughout the organization.

*Train for Leadership* The Leadership Institute at Baptist Hospital in Pensacola has become so popular that people travel from around the country to take part in workshops and benchmarking sessions there. Here are some of the leadership lessons the Baptist staff shares with others.

- *Provide ongoing leadership training.* Involve midlevel and upper-level managers in day-long leadership training programs at least four times a year, and invite people throughout the organization to take part in series of briefer workshops. Also help people develop leadership experience by involving them in self governance.
- *Keep no secrets.* If people are to be accountable as leaders, they must know where they stand and how the organization is performing. Make current financial records and satisfaction survey reports available to all employees so that they can chart their success

**BOX 10.4**

## Can You Guess?

1. What percentage of health care administrators work in hospitals? What percentage work in physician offices and nursing homes?
2. What is the outlook for future health care administrators?

*Answers appear at the end of the chapter.*

and receive immediate market feedback on what works well and what does not.

- *Make organizational leaders accessible.* Avoid placing administrative officers in far-off or segregated areas. Encourage leaders to interact freely throughout the organization and to share conversations, praise, and ideas.
- *Reward people for sharing ideas.* Develop a program that invites employees' suggestions and rewards them for submitting workable ideas that improve services, save money, and increase employee morale.
- *Respond to ideas.* Even when the ideas cannot be implemented, people want to know they have been heard. Designate committees to review ideas, respond to them all, and initiate implementation whenever possible.
- *Celebrate successes.* Send handwritten thank-you letters to employees and their families and post thank-you letters from patients. Hold celebrations when the organization reaches key goals. Informally praise people who do good work, and develop formal recognition programs to honor heroic efforts.

### Authority Rule or Multilevel Input?

In bureaucratic language, **rational-legal authority** is based on "rationality, expertise, norms, and rules" (K. I. Miller, 1999, p. 13). In health care this translates to a reverence for those who are most educated, have the most up-to-date knowledge, and have earned the most impressive titles and credentials (Cadogan, Franzi, Osterweil, & Hill, 1999). Health care employees typically advertise their credentials right upfront. Their name badges list their job titles and, very often their degrees and accreditations. For example, the initials CRNA behind a person's name stand for Certified Registered Nurse Anesthetist. Patients may not fully grasp the difference among credentials, but professionals probably do.

*Advantages* Most people agree that health care is not a job for amateurs.

- The emphasis on education and experience is justified by the immense knowledge and responsibilities associated with providing top-quality care.
- Attention to norms and rules helps ensure that treatment is given in time-honored and consistent ways by people who are well qualified to provide it.

*Disadvantages* Status differences can cause rifts and intolerance. Health care is often characterized by what Kreps (1990) calls **professional prejudice**. Some professionals are considered more prestigious than others based on their training, their authority, or their place in the organization. For example, critical care nurses may be given higher status than maternal-child or psychiatric nurses (M. Smith, Droppleman, & Thomas, 1996). This presents a number of disadvantages.

- People without impressive titles (including patients) may be excluded from discussions even though they have valuable information and ideas to share.
- Low-ranking and nonclinical personnel may be treated with less respect than doctors and nurses, and nurses may be treated as subservient to doctors.
- Status differences can provoke animosity between coworkers and lead to turf battles in which one department or profession asserts that it is more important than another, thus more deserving of new equipment, pay raises, additional staff, or the like (Albrecht, 1982).

Unfortunately, efforts to cut expenses and limit resources have aggravated this long-standing competitiveness in many institutions (P. S. Forte, 1997).

- Authority rule stifles creativity. Mayer and Cates (2004) propose that "Do it because the boss says so!" is a flawed argument (p. xvii). Simply following orders isn't very fulfilling and doesn't lend itself to service excellence.

*Opportunities for Change* From a communication standpoint, there is value in education and seniority, but overlooking low-ranking employees is a mistake. Often, frontline employees are more familiar than anyone about clients' wishes and the organization's daily routines. Steve Miller, a worldwide manager at Shell Oil Company, emphasizes the need to treat members throughout the organization as intelligent change agents:

> In the past, the leader was the guy with the answers. Today if you're going to have a successful company, you have to recognize that no leader can possibly have all the answers. The leader may have a vision. But the actual solutions about how best to meet the challenges of the moment have to be made by the people closest to the action. (quoted by Pascale, 1999, p. 210)

With a similar belief, Mayo Clinic staff members attribute a great deal of their success to team spirit and their respect for each other. "I know by name the custodians that work in the emergency department, and I appreciate them as much as I appreciate my physician colleagues," says Anne Sadosty, an emergency care physician with Mayo Clinic (quoted by Berry & Seltman, 2008, p. 58).

Minimizing status differences doesn't make leaders obsolete. As James Pepicello and Emmett Murphy (1996) put it, empowering organizational members "does not relieve leadership of its responsibility to lead" (paragraph 17). It does means that leaders' role is different. No longer is leadership defined by one's position or title; instead it is characterized by interpersonal skills, including the ability to inspire, recognize, and reward others (Jobes & Steinbinder, 1996, paragraph 23). Leaders in horizontal organizations are responsible for communicating the organization's overall goals, enabling team members to participate fully, and rewarding them for contributions. Otherwise, employees may feel adrift and overwhelmed, particularly if they are accustomed to the close supervision provided within a vertical hierarchy (Porter-O'Grady et al., 1997). Research shows that employees are typically dissatisfied and unmotivated if they are unsure what is expected of them, if they lack the skills to perform new duties, or if they are discouraged by managers who do not seem to support organizational changes (Northouse & Northouse, 1985).

In their article "The View from the Middle," two midlevel managers in health care organizations suggest the following communication strategies for leaders in participative environments (Bachenheimer & DeKoven, 2003).

- *Be a leader <u>and</u> a team member.* Organizational leaders are responsible for providing direction, but they should also be team members who listen to and work alongside others.
- *Choose your words—and your medium— carefully.* Do not use e-mail to communicate praise, advice, criticism, or critical information. Discuss sensitive and important information face to face or over the telephone.
- *Make the most of meetings.* Plan meetings carefully, invite everyone to participate, listen actively, and follow up afterwards.
- *Invite ideas and follow up on them.* Bachenheimer and DeKoven urge leaders to follow up on everything—every promise, every conversation.
- *Invite solutions.* Create an environment in which people are encouraged to present solutions, not just describe problems.
- *Think and act positively.* Acknowledge challenges, but present the organization in a positive light.
- *Praise people for their efforts.* Recognize those who try hard even if things do not go exactly as planned.

## Specialized Jobs or Mission-Centered Expectations?

A **division of labor** means that workers have specific tasks to perform. No one person takes a project from beginning to end. This is the idea behind assembly lines. The assumption is that workers operate at maximum efficiency performing simple, repetitive tasks.

Of course, health organizations did not take medicine to the extreme of assembly line production. But they did adopt a division of labor. Whereas rural physicians traditionally performed the gamut of activities—from delivering babies, to keeping medical records, to performing surgeries, to collecting fees—health organizations during the Industrial Revolution began to separate these tasks (Reiser, 1978). Nurses were assigned specific duties, such as giving injections, taking health history information, and so on. Bookkeeping and scheduling were taken over by staff members trained to perform those tasks. Physicians also began to specialize. Although almost all doctors in the 1800s were general practitioners, one in four doctors specialized in a particular type of medicine by 1929, and three out of four doctors were specialists by 1969 (Reiser, 1978).

*Advantages* There is something to be gained from specialization.

- As medical knowledge and the business of providing health care have become more complex, specialization helps people stay abreast of facets that would be overwhelming for any one person.
- A division of labor also helps maintain the image of caregivers as public servants rather than as businesspeople. As health organizations evolved, doctors usually did not discuss fees with patients. Specially trained staff members took charge of financial details, leaving caregivers to (presumably) ignore monetary concerns in single-minded pursuit of better health for their patients.

*Disadvantages* A division of labor enabled health care professionals to become highly focused experts, but to a large extent it also created boundaries between them.

- Members of one department or specialization are unlikely to communicate or collaborate with professionals in another, leading to duplicated efforts, treatment complications and overlaps, and lost opportunities for collaborative decision making.
- Caregivers are largely excluded from health care management. Gradually, hospitals and clinics ceased to be run by doctors and were instead managed by people with backgrounds in business, management, and finance. This trend was supported by the complexity of new tax laws and business regulations, which made managing health care organizations more complicated. Although business expertise was welcome, many caregivers began to feel disconnected from policy decisions.
- People with specialized job duties are not likely to go beyond them. For example, any number of employees may walk past a spill in the hallway because it is not their job to clean it up. By contrast, consider the story of Ryan Miller, a van driver for Creighton University Medical Center in Omaha, Nebraska. When Miller noticed that the rubber tips on a patient's walker were worn out, he went to a medical supply store on his own time, got new tips, and gave them to the patient. This kind gesture went far beyond his official job duties (*What's Right in Health Care*, 2007, p. 592).
- Specialization is not designed to address the reality that top-quality care transcends the efforts of any one person or department.

*Opportunities for Change* Members of some organizations are realizing that it is as important to work *together* as it is to work hard. For example, during a rather lengthy wait to see the doctor recently, a nurse assistant hurrying by noticed me in the waiting room. She stopped to apologize for the delay and to explain that an emergency had disrupted the doctor's schedule. This simple gesture dispelled my irritation. I am sure it was not part of her job description to do this, but by making the extra effort, she improved my estimation of the entire experience. This sort of gesture is most likely in organizations in which leaders establish overarching goals and reward employees for taking the initiative to satisfy clients' needs.

*Promote a shared vision.* Studer (2003) compares an effective health care leader to the conductor of an orchestra, whose job is to achieve the following:

- *Establish goals for the performance.*
- *Keep everyone on the same page.*
- *Define the contribution of each individual.*

In other words, a good organizational leader recognizes that harmony results from clear expectations and the coordinated performance of individuals. Although each person will make unique contributions, everyone must be in sync to be successful.

At Missouri Baptist Medical Center, employees are encouraged to "make their patients' day," even when that requires going beyond their job descriptions. Therefore, when nurse assistant Leo Carter was caring for an elderly patient who was agitated and near death, Carter sought a means of soothing the man without restraining him. A fellow nurse remembered that the patient had been a symphony conductor. Leo ran to his car to get a clarinet, which he played quietly in the man's room. Stephen Lundin and colleagues (2002) describe what happened:

> As the soft, mellow notes drifted through the room, something happened. The old man stopped thrashing. He closed his eyes and smiled. Lying on his back, he raised his arms and began to wave them back and forth. Perhaps, deep in his mind, he was standing in a great concert hall once again, wearing coat and tails, with a baton in his strong hands, leading *his* orchestra. After a few minutes the old man's arms dropped slowly to his sides and he slept quietly through the night. (p. 93)

In short, when people are united by a strong mission but encouraged to go beyond traditional boundaries, unforeseeable circumstances become opportunities to make a difference.

### Strictly by the Rules . . . or Not?

Ask people to define bureaucracy and they are apt to mention red tape. Bureaucracies are known for their paperwork. Nearly any task requires that a form filled out, signed, and submitted to the appropriate people. Ask why, and an employee is likely to pull out more paper in the form of written rules and procedures.

*Advantages*  In some ways, paperwork and guidelines are well suited to health care.

- Careful records allow health care organizations (and oversight boards) to review care procedures and evaluate their efficacy and cost effectiveness.
- Written records keep teams members informed about patient care. Standardized forms help ensure that information is recorded in a form others can quickly read and understand. This is crucial for managing medical emergencies and around-the-clock shift changes.
- Established policies reduce ambiguity and may give people a sense of security and predictability (Vestal et al., 1997). For example, clear rules for employee evaluation and advancement discourage favoritism and provide performance guidelines (Eisenberg & Goodall, 2004).
- People are less likely to overlook important information (or to skip crucial steps) if they are following established procedures. Missing even a small detail can have tragic consequences when people's lives are at stake.

*Disadvantages*  Adherence to written guidelines presents some disadvantages, however.

- People may be frustrated by what they see as needless amounts of paperwork. As you may recall from Chapter 2, hospital nurses today spend twice as much time completing paperwork as they spend providing direct patient care.
- Established policies can jeopardize customer service. Because few people have the authority to override policies, when an unforeseen problem arises, the best an employee can do is to request that a policy be reconsidered (which may take weeks or months) or to refer the situation to someone higher on the ladder, hoping it will eventually reach someone with authority to grant an exception (Hamilton & Parker, 1997). In the meantime, clients are likely to feel mistreated, to share their grievances with others, and to look for other organizations more responsive to their needs.
- The emphasis on following written policies, asking specific questions, and filling out forms can also discourage open communication. Patients' input may be largely limited to the information requested on forms, where there is often little room to add comments not specifically requested (C. B. Thompson, 1996; Wyatt, 1995).
- Professionals may rely on written communication more than face-to-face discussions. Although notes and charts are informative, they are a meager substitute for interactive discussions when it comes to making collaborative judgments.
- Overly restrictive rules limit team members' ability to be creative, to go beyond the norm, or to make unique contributions.

*Opportunities for Change*  Jim Collins (2001) argues against strict rules, saying that "the purpose of bureaucracy is to compensate for incompetence and lack of discipline—a problem that largely goes away if you have the right people in the first place" (p. 121). In place of bureaucratic rules, Collins advocates organizational cultures that nurture talented people with similarly high values and that allow them to be creative and entrepreneurial in the pursuit of a common vision. The result, he says, is a far cry from the boring, stodgy atmosphere of a bureaucracy. Instead, "you get a magic alchemy of superior performance and sustained results" (pp. 121–122). Collins' prediction isn't pie-in-the-sky management advice. He and a team of researchers consistently found this quality in America's top 22 companies, each of which had outperformed its competitors for at least 15 consecutive years.

The same idea is echoed by James F. Nordstrom, former cochair of Nordstrom Department Store, which is world famous for outstanding customer service. Nordstrom proclaims, "We hate the rules." He proposes that "the minute you come up with a rule you give an employee a reason to say no to a customer" (quoted by Spector & McCarthy, 2005, p. 141). Nordstrom has only one rule: *Use good judgment in all situations.* Consequently, when a Nordstrom associate at the Washington, DC, store learned about a woman who had arrived in the area in the midst of a medical crisis (her husband was about to have emergency brain surgery) and who didn't have a car or clothing appropriate for the climate, the associate personally picked the woman up at the hospital, brought her to the store, helped her select clothing, and drove her back to the hospital. The associate knew that in extending this kindness she would be fulfilling Nordstrom's mission of serving customers, and she wouldn't be breaking any rules to do it. The Nordstrom culture abounds with similar stories of service excellence.

Irwin Press (2002), a well-known patient satisfaction expert, recommends that health care leaders take the following steps to eliminate unnecessary rules and to make sure the remaining ones make sense.

- *Ask employees to identify "really stupid rules."* "This is fun and focuses analytical attention on the often arbitrary nature of regulations" (Press, p. 42). By identifying what does not make sense, organizations can get rid of rules that impede performance.
- *Next, examine rules that make sense but do not work well.* For example, Press asks, is it necessary that nurses deliver meal trays? Could other staff members perform this task and free nurses to respond more quickly to patients' requests?
- *Remember that patients don't much care about the paperwork.* "No matter how firmly we argue that paperwork is a necessary part of care, patients don't see it this way. Paperwork is not the hands-on care that patients want or that they base their evaluations on" (Press, p. 39).
- *If the rules and paperwork are important, allow time and space to complete them.* Press urges leaders to analyze employees' job duties to make sure they are compatible. For example, it is unrealistic to expect an employee to answer the phone, file reports, and simultaneously respond to others' needs. Frustration—and poor service—are likely to result. Instead, provide adequate time and space to complete necessary procedures and paperwork. If the regulations are important, make fulfilling them part of the job.

## TEAMWORK

Simply defined, a *team* is "a set of individuals who work together to achieve common objectives" (Unsworth, 1996, p. 483). Teamwork is nothing new to health care. Doctors, nurses, technicians, clerks, and others have long relied on each other to reach common objectives. But the rules and reasons for teamwork are changing.

To apply the terminology of management guru Peter Drucker, health care teams used to function like baseball teams, but now they must act like doubles tennis partners. Drucker (1993) writes that (managerially speaking) a doubles tennis game is different than a baseball game. In baseball each player is assigned a position with a specific set of tasks to perform. The pitcher pitches, the catcher catches, the batter bats, and so on. The game is specialized and precise. Doubles tennis is different—faster, less precise. Players have basic positions but must always be poised to help each other, and there is scarcely time to stand still.

To flourish today, health care teams must function like tennis partners, argues Mary Fanning (1997). They must be ready for the unexpected and be prepared to help each other. Caregivers used to play their positions with little overlap (like baseball players). A patient might see a physical therapist, a nurse, a doctor, and a laboratory technician—but one at a time, never all together (Zimmermann, 1994). Technically, the caregivers were working toward the same goal, but they contributed in specialized ways, independently. The problem is that team members who do not communicate with each other are likely to drop the ball. Lack of communication can lead to duplicated efforts, costly (and sometimes life-threatening) delays, frustration, and wasted time. Teamwork can minimize the waste and frustration. However, like leadership, teamwork is not always easy to accomplish.

There is a saying at Mayo Clinic that "teamwork is not an option" (Berry & Seltman, 2008, p. 51). The medical center is unusual in that, although it is one of the largest in the world, it is truly integrated. To appreciate how, let's consider a patient care scenario somewhere else. Typically, a patient with a serious health concern schedules an appointment with a primary care physician, who refers her to a separate facility for diagnostic tests, where the staff sends her back to the doctor for results, who refers her to a specialist in a different location, who might recommend surgery at still a different place, and so on. The patient probably has to make appointments with each provider separately, supply her health history and insurance information at each office, and perhaps wait weeks or months between appointments. The physicians involved with the patient's care probably do not work directly for the hospital, nor are they likely to have an easy or quick way to communicate with each other or review an overall medical chart for the patient. (In most cases there is no overall patient chart. Instead, each doctor maintains a separate chart detailing his or her work with the patient.)

By contrast, Mayo Clinic is a fully integrated system of doctors, specialists, therapists, hospitals, laboratories, and everything else needed to provide comprehensive medical care. Everyone involved—including the physicians—works for the clinic. They are all linked via sophisticated communication technology and, very often, proximity close enough to allow face-to-face conversations about patients. The Mayo Clinic team practices what they call *destination medicine*. When patients go to Mayo for serious health concerns, they should be prepared to stay in town for a few days. In that time they are likely to be seen by several specialists, have diagnostic tests done, and undergo treatment—all on the same campus. Even surgeries are typically scheduled on a next-day basis. The whole process—from the initial consultation, through visits with specialists, diagnostic tests, and even surgery and recovery—might take 3 to 5 days, compared to weeks or months elsewhere.

Mayo's streamlined efficiency is supported by an organizational culture that values and rewards teamwork and a carefully designed infrastructure. All appointments are made through one centralized system. This saves time and energy and allows the staff to coordinate the timing and sequence of tests and treatments properly. Pathologists and radiologists immediately evaluate diagnostic test data, usually before the patient leaves the office, in case more data is required. The results are immediately posted in the patient's electronic medical record. Every caregiver has a computer and instant, online access to the patient's comprehensive medical record, including all test results and other physicians' notes. This makes it feasible for everyone to get the full picture, to avoid delays or duplications, and to work effectively as a team. All the while, physicians are free to collaborate and to refer patients to each other without loss of income because they are all on salaries and are all part of the same team. "It's like you are working in an organism; you are not a single cell out there practicing," says Mayo physician Nina Schwenk. "I have access to the best minds on any topic, any disease or problem I come up with and they're one phone call away" (quoted by Berry & Seltman, 2008, p. 53).

## BOX 10.5 THEORETICAL FOUNDATIONS

# A Model for Innovative Leadership

When writers for the *Harvard Business Review* interviewed 100 innovative business leaders, they identified some common characteristics among them (Davenport, Prusak, & Wilson, 2003). For one, innovators are *idea scouts*, always looking for new ideas within the organization and outside it. They talk to people and really listen. They are also *tailors* who modify new ideas to suit the organization's needs, all the while inviting frequent and candid input from others. As the process continues, the best innovators are *promoters* who sell their ideas to people throughout the organization, communicating effectively and enthusiastically with top and middle management as well as frontline employees and clients. Finally, innovators are *experimenters*. They pilot and test new ideas on a small scale to prepare them for wider adoption. Importantly, innovators are *not* do-it-all-myself types. When an innovation has been tested and refined,

they "get out of the way and let others execute" (Davenport et al., 2003, p. 58). The implications for communication are clear: Observe, listen, invite feedback, sell your ideas, experiment, and enable others.

## What Do You Think?

1. In what ways are you an idea scout? Think of the best idea scout you know. How does he or she do it?
2. What steps might you follow to tailor ideas to a particular organization or group of people?
3. What skills are needed to promote new ideas?
4. Have you ever been part of (or coordinated) a pilot study or experimental program? Did you feel it was worthwhile? What did you learn during the process?
5. Why are skillful innovators not "do-it-yourself" types when it comes to implementing widespread changes?

## Advantages

One advantage of teamwork is that members are able to apply multiple perspectives to a problem, enhancing innovation and creativity. This applies to overarching issues, such as new cost-cutting measures and service lines, and to everyday dilemmas. Cathy Smith of St. Joseph Hospital in Orange, California, remembers trying to prepare Katie, a frightened 13-year-old girl with autism, for surgery. A child life therapist at the hospital offered a doodle board, and Katie was amused as long as her father drew pictures on it with her. But when it was time to leave his side, the girl was frightened and resisted caregivers' efforts to prepare for her surgery. "The question for the nurses became 'How do we get our artist into the operating room with the least amount of struggle?'" says Smith. After conferring with each other, one nurse crawled onto the patient's bed to draw with her while the other wheeled them into

pre-op. "The anesthesiologist was surprised to see two people instead of just one, but the nurse kept talking and drawing. The doctor was able to mask the patient to sleep while she and the nurse next to her continued to draw," Smith says. "The patient was then moved to the OR and the surgery ensued smoothly" (*What's Right in Health Care*, 2007, pp. 469–470). Such creative teamwork is no doubt rewarding for professionals and for patients. (See Box 10.5 for more about encouraging innovation in health care organizations.)

Another advantage is that interdisciplinary teamwork blurs the line between departments and presents new opportunities for diverse employees to take part in decision making (R. Green, 1994). One result is that doctors and nurses are again playing a major role in health care management (Pepicello & Murphy, 1996).

Third, teamwork reduces costly oversights that may occur when people are devoted to highly specialized tasks. Health care organizations can no longer afford (if ever they could) the oversights that result when team members do not communicate with each other. Ask any hospital employee about patients who have gotten "lost in the system." Usually the story is that the patient is scheduled for a series of treatments or tests, but somewhere along the way everyone assumes the patient is with someone else—until they realize the poor soul has spent hours lying on a gurney in the hallway. (I am told of a case, years ago, when a patient went up and down in the staff elevator for hours, with everyone assuming an escort was waiting at the next stop.)

Bureaucracies are especially vulnerable to these kinds of oversights because many tasks do not fall squarely within the boundaries of any job description. Workers who concentrate on specialized tasks may not take the initiative to go beyond their borders. They may not even realize they should. Teamwork encourages people to look at the larger picture and to pitch in, even with tasks that are not specifically assigned to them. For example, nurses who notice that lab results have not arrived on time may take the initiative to find out if tests were run and why results are delayed. This extra effort can save time and money in the long run (Sullivan & Wolfe, 1996).

Fourth, teamwork is well suited to biopsychosocial care. Members of some organizations have concluded that the best way to keep patients healthy is to pay attention to their broad range of concerns. As physician Alan R. Zwerner advises:

> The dog ate a 100-year-old patient's glasses, and she's not eligible for a covered pair for another year? Give her a pair. Free. It could prevent a fall that would break her hip. There is a reward for quality care, patient satisfaction, and doing the right thing at the right time. (quoted by Azevedo, 1996, paragraph 22)

Teams can help provide care that simultaneously addresses a variety of issues, such as patients' personal resources, nutrition, exercise, psychological well-being, and more. The object is not to replace physicians with teams, but to help physicians provide broader care than they can provide alone.

Interdisciplinary care teams can provide more complex biopsychosocial care than could any one caregiver (Frasier, Savard-Fenton, & Kotthopp, 1983).

Finally, team members may benefit from their involvement with coworkers. Teamwork allows professionals to share the immense responsibilities of health care, provide mutual support, and learn from each other (Abramson & Mizrahi, 1996). For example, an ethics committee can help guide caregivers and family members and relieve some of the pressure that an individual making a difficult decision alone might face (Harding, 1994). This support may be especially important as health care employees deal with the stress and uncertainty of providing care while adjusting to industry changes.

## Difficulties and Drawbacks

None of this means teamwork is easy. Although teamwork presents many advantages, there are potential disadvantages as well. For one thing, teamwork takes time. If a quick decision is needed, an individual may be better qualified to make it. Some nurses in Julie Apker's (2001) study appreciated opportunities to be part of shared-governance teams. Others said that there was not enough time for it. Said one nurse: "I don't feel it's fair to give someone a project if they don't have time" (quoted by Apker, 2001, p. 125). Furthermore, especially if they are rushed or intimidated, team members may resort to **groupthink**, that is, going along with ideas they would not normally support (Janis, 1972).

Teamwork can be particularly difficult in health care organizations. Professionals from different disciplines often have very different ideas about health, which creates the potential for competition and conflict (Abramson & Mizrahi, 1996). A study of 320 doctors and nurses revealed that 73% of the physicians felt they collaborated well with nurses, but only 33% of the nurses agreed (E. B. Thomas, Sexton, & Helmreich, 2003). The discrepancy may lie in their different expectations. Whereas physicians were mostly satisfied with the communication, nurses reported feeling left out and intimated about expressing themselves freely with doctors. Busy schedules make it hard to arrange meetings, especially if the organization is not supportive in allowing time for teamwork. There is also a question of leadership. Doctors have traditionally been accustomed to calling the shots, but dominating group interactions may defeat the purpose of teamwork (Sharf, 1984).

## Communication Skill Builders: Working on Teams

True teamwork means appreciating the contributions of everyone on the team. Few organizations honor this ideal more than Mayo Clinic. Denis Cortese remembers his early experiences as a physician at the clinic (related by Berry & Seltman, 2008, p. 44). "I was unaccustomed to have a desk attendant tell me, a physician, that I needed to adjust my schedule to see a patient right away," Cortese says. But then another physician pulled him aside. "He explained that at Mayo Clinic, the focus is always on the patient. And whichever member of the staff is interacting with the patient deserves our full support," Cortese recalls. He says he quickly learned to trust the desk attendants and to respond to their requests:

> The one who asked me to change my schedule had years of experience and she knew how to listen to patients.... It was my job to help her.... I've never forgotten that lesson.... It's still my job—it's all of our jobs—to serve patients directly, or provide service for those who are serving patients. After 35 years, it is still a privilege. (p. 44)

Cortese is now CEO of Mayo Clinic.

Considering the advantages and difficulties of effective teamwork, experts present the following suggestions to help team members communicate effectively.

- *During meetings, minimize distractions and sit so that all members can easily see each other* (Sharf, 1984).
- *Establish ground rules for attendance, discussions, and decision making* (Farley & Stoner, 1989).
- *Before trying to solve a problem, make sure group members agree on the nature, importance, and cause of the problem.*

- *Make an effort to understand each group member's background and expertise.* Often, one group of professionals is not clear on what another group is trained to do. For example, doctors surveyed were not able to describe accurately the duties of social workers (Abramson & Mizrahi, 1996).
- *Be aware that conflict is a natural part of group work.* Group members who remain committed to the task often work through the conflict to achieve a mutual sense of accomplishment (Northouse & Northouse, 1985).
- *Encourage all group members to contribute ideas* (Sharf, 1984).
- *Be willing to compromise* (Sharf, 1984).
- *Summarize group discussions out loud to clarify the group's viewpoints and perspectives* (Sharf, 1984).

We now turn to a particularly challenging arena for leadership, communicating effectively in crisis situations.

## CRISIS MANAGEMENT

By their very nature, health organizations are likely to be part of crises. As Kathleen Fearn-Banks (1996) defines it, from an organizational perspective, a *crisis* is "a major occurrence with a potentially negative outcome affecting an organization, company, or industry, as well as its publics, products, services, or good name" (p. 1). In health care, the crisis usually has an external origin: a natural disaster, an accident, or an outbreak of contagious disease. In such cases, health care organizations (especially hospitals and health departments) may be called on to explain the crisis and to keep the public informed about it. In some cases the crisis originates within the organization—a fire, a baby kidnapped from the nursery, charges of extortion. In any case, it is important to have a well-developed plan for handling crises, collecting information, and making information available to members of the organization, the media, and the public.

## BOX 10.6 CAREER OPPORTUNITIES

# Health Care Marketing and Public Relations

Public relations professional
Strategic planning manager
Marketing professional
Advertising designer
Physician marketing coordinator
Community services director
In-house communication director
Pharmaceutical sales representative

## Career Resources and Job Listings

Society for Healthcare Strategy & Market Development: www.shsmd.org/shsmd_app/index.jsp

International Association of Business Communicators: www.iabc.com
Public Relations Society of America: www.prsa.org
Public Relations Society of America Health Academy: www.healthacademy.prsa.org
American Association of Advertising Agencies: www.aaaa.org
American Advertising Federation: www.aaf.org
Strategic Health Care Communication (job listings): www.strategichealthcare.com/career
U.S. Bureau of Labor Statistics: www.bls.gov/oco/ocos020.htm
PharmaceuticalSales.com

---

In Chapter 12 we talk extensively about handling public health crises, so we'll keep this overview brief. But it's worth mentioning that crises have implications not just for the public. There is an organizational component as well. Crisis management is a job for communication specialists, especially those in public relations. Here are some helpful tips for preparing a crisis plan and managing publicity during a crisis, based on Fearn-Banks' (1996) book *Crisis Communication*.

- Let people within the organization know what constitutes a crisis and whom to contact at the first sign of crisis.
- Designate a primary spokesperson for the organization (usually the CEO), and help that person decide what information to release and how.
- Develop good relationships with media professionals before a crisis occurs, and do not play favorites during a crisis.
- Educate people in the organization about how to handle a crisis and how to get information.

- Keep up-to-date contact information for designated spokespersons, media professionals, stakeholders, and emergency management professionals.
- Maintain supplies that will be necessary if electricity or Web access is unavailable.
- Plan ahead how you will accommodate members of the media.

See Box 10.6 for more on career opportunities related to community relations and crisis management.

## AIMING FOR SERVICE EXCELLENCE

Many of the ideas in this chapter are oriented to service excellence. Based on decades of experience conducting patient satisfaction surveys, Press (2002) presents five reasons to focus on patient satisfaction: (1) High satisfaction is linked to patient cooperation with treatment protocols, even when they are frightening or uncomfortable, (2) satisfied patients experience less stress than others, (3) highly satisfied patients actually *feel* better than others and recover more quickly, (4) patients who have positive experiences become "apostles" for the organization, promoting it to others, and (5) there is a high correlation between satisfied patients and satisfied employees. All of these add up to competitive strength and bottom-line gains. As much as a 30% of profits are based on patient satisfaction (Press). But there's one more reason not to be overlooked. In their book *Leadership for Great Customer Service,* physicians Thom Mayer and Robert Cates (2004) suggest that the number-one reason "to get customer service right in healthcare is...it makes the job easier" (p. xx). They observe that team members *like* coming to work when they feel they are making a difference rather than swimming upstream, when they enjoy the work they do and are able to have creative input, and when they feel valued and supported by coworkers and supervisors. As a way to wrap up this discussion of organizational structure, culture, and values, here are 10 tips from the experts on building cultures that sustain these ideals. You'll see that much of the emphasis is on employee satisfaction. As many have observed, it's unlikely that dissatisfied employees will lead to happy customers, but happy employees will go far beyond the job description to do a good job.

***1. Flip the pyramid.*** In a classic bureaucratic pyramid, the people at the top make most of the decisions, get the biggest perks, reap the greatest financial rewards—and seldom see or talk to service-line employees or clients. Everyone in the organization tries to please the bosses. And patients and customers aren't even on the chart.

Some theorists advocate turning the pyramid upside down. In an inverted pyramid, the largest and highest tier is devoted to patients and customers. Everyone in the organization is oriented to pleasing *them.* The next-highest tier is made up of frontline service providers—a diverse assortment of all those who have direct contact with the people you serve (e.g., nurses, volunteers, physicians, cafeteria staff, housekeeping, valets, and so on). Subsequent layers are devoted to supervisors. In true servant-leadership style, CEOs and presidents are on the bottom. From this perspective, their job is to listen, encourage, support and remove barriers so people can do what they do best. Leaders should help team members define a mission for the organization and make sure the mission is clear and well supported. The staff at Nordstrom Department Store embraces the inverted-pyramid style (Spector & McCarthy, 2005), as do CEOs in many top-performing organizations (J. Collins, 2001).

A classic example of a servant leader was Ken Iverson, former CEO of Nucor Steel. Iverson eliminated executive perks, cut his own salary to be in line with others', reduced the staff at corporate headquarters to 25 people (in a company with 7,000 employees), and put frontline employees' needs first. Nucor, which was nearly bankrupt when Iverson assumed leadership, became a $3.5 billion Fortune 500 company. In his book *Plain Talk,* Iverson (1997) summarizes his philosophy this way:

> The people at the top of the corporate hierarchy grant themselves privilege after privilege, flaunt those privileges before the men and women who do the real work, then wonder why employees are unmoved by management's invocations to cut costs and boost profitability....When I think of the millions of dollars spent by people at the top of the management hierarchy on efforts to motivate people who are continually put down *by* that hierarchy, I can only shake my head in wonder. (pp. 58–59)

Lest this sound too critical of presidents and CEOs, who usually *do* work very hard and try their best, it's important to note that an inverted pyramid serves them well, too. They are spared the immense pressure of being responsible for decisions at all levels. Instead, accountability is dispersed throughout the organization (see Tip 5). Leaders in a supportive role are more a part of the overall team, and what they lose in authority they typically gain in genuine appreciation and loyalty from the people they serve.

***2. Hire carefully, and continually recruit internal talent.*** The biggest drain on employees isn't usually serving demanding clients, it's putting up with negative coworkers. Collins (2001) identifies getting the "right people on the bus" as the first tenet of effective leadership. Mayer and Cates (2004) whole-heartedly concur. They ask: "Are there days when you come to work and see the people you are working with and think to yourself, 'Bring it on! Whatever we've got to do today, this team of people can make it happen!'?" (p. 7). If so, they say, you are surrounded by A-team players, the type who love a challenge, have a positive attitude, and inspire everyone around them. But if you said no, you understand the concept of B-team players. They inspire a different internal dialogue on the way to work, one that sounds more like, "Shoot me, shoot me, shoot me! I can't work with him—I worked with him yesterday!" (p. 7). Mayer and Cates describe B-team players as negative, lazy, late, confused, and always surprised by the demands of the job. B-team players are "fundamentally toxic," in that it just takes one to poison things for everyone. A major part of a leader's job, maintain Mayer and Cates, is getting B-team members either to reform (which may mean moving to a different position more in line with their talents and passions) or to leave. Even better, whenever possible, is hiring the right people for the right jobs in the first place.

Disney restaurant manager George Miliotes says that experience has taught him to look for two basic qualities in potential team members: "Is this person happy and is this person smart? If you are smart, we can teach you anything. If you are happy, I know you will make the customers happy" (quoted by F. Lee, 2004, p. 121).

Linda Minton of Parkwest Medical Center in Knoxville, Tennessee, describes how she knew that a new nurse, Paul, would be an A-team member. A woman in her 80s with Alzheimer's was admitted for a blood transfusion under Paul's supervision. When the woman became afraid and pulled out her IVs, her daughter was tearful and distraught. The patient repeatedly requested to be left alone and allowed to go home, but Paul knew she needed the life-saving treatment. Minton recalls:

Paul again quietly explained that she could not go home, but he also asked if there were anything else she might like to do. Quickly she responded, with a big smile on her face, "I would like to dance." Paul, who is not a dancer, said, "You will have to lead." She agreed, and so—they danced. What a wonderful sight, seeing this lovely lady calmed by the impromptu dance. It was at that moment that we all knew Paul had a place at Parkwest Medical Center. (*What's Right in Health Care*, 2007, p. 666)

In line with this attitude is nurturing team members and giving them ample opportunities to use their talents. Continual recruitment and hiring from within (at least part of the time) allow leaders to cultivate A-team members they are sure about. In a way, point out Berry and Seltman (2008), employment is a job interview "that lasts for years" (p. 29).

**3. *Teach the culture.*** Mayo employees hear the clinic motto, "The needs of the patient come first," within the first 5 minutes of new-employee orientation and several times a day thereafter. As one employee said, "Mayo becomes part of your DNA" (quoted by Berry & Seltman, 2008, p. 26). Having a strong, clear purpose provides unity even among diverse people and departments. Everyone contributes it different ways, but they all know and agree on what they are trying to achieve.

**4. *Empower the front line.*** Mayer and Cates (2004) advise: "Make no decision at a higher level than can be made at a lower level" (p. 58). They point out that health care is a personal service offered at an individual level, therefore "the people responsible for the service delivery must be entrusted with the power to make service meaningful" (p. 58). This chapter is filled with remarkable stories that result from empowering committed people to do their best.

**5. *Hold people accountable.*** A key component of empowerment is holding people at every level of the organization accountable for pursuing goals they help to set. Setting goals helps people make sure their efforts are aligned. And regularly measuring progress toward the goal (e.g., satisfaction scores, reduced employee turnover, higher profits, more business) helps team members gauge what's working and what isn't. Measurement also provides opportunities to recognize and celebrate success. To make the process effective, experts suggest that measurement not be used to punish team members. If so, they will have an incentive to set goals too low or to enhance the results artificially. Instead, measures should be based on what team members *themselves* want to know so that they can continually improve. In Mayer and Cates' (2004) terms, measurement should be a tool, not a club.

**6. "Blow their minds."** This is Nordstrom's philosophy. The Nordstrom team realizes that doing the job right isn't enough. People expect that. Inspiring customer loyalty requires giving people *more* than they expect. Mayer and Cates (2004) put it this way:

> How much credit do we give airlines for getting us from point A to point B and not killing us? How about *none*—we expect that. Your patients expect excellent clinical care (the destination). But they also expect excellence service (the journey). (p. 26)

Nordstrom aims for "fabled service"—the type you talk about around the dinner table that night. By most estimates, customers who indicate they are "satisfied" (4 on a 5-point scale) may or may not come back to the organization. People expect to be satisfied. Only those who rate themselves "very satisfied" (5 on a 5-point scale) are likely to be loyal customers. Some organizations miss this distinction when they combine scores and conclude that, say, "95% of our customers are satisfied or very satisfied." Cognizant of the immense difference between "satisfied" and "very satisfied," Disney considers anything less than a 5 to be a failing score (F. Lee, 2004).

**7. Use service failures as a springboard.** A few years ago I conducted a series of service-excellence workshops for the staff of a large hospital. Over several days' time, as each new group of participants came through, I asked them to think of times they had received excellent customer service. Their answers were inspiring.

One woman ordered a dress from a department store to attend her niece's wedding out of town. First, the store's tailor made a mistake with the alterations. Then the dress wasn't ready when it was promised. Eventually it was the day before she was to fly out for the wedding and the woman still did not have her dress. She was frustrated and ready to buy something off the rack at another store and never do business with the original store again. But then a very gracious sales associate called her to apologize and say that she would personally drive to the tailor's, retrieve the dress, and deliver it to the woman's home that evening. The associate arrived on her doorstep with the dress as promised, and the woman was so touched by her apologies and extra effort that she has been a loyal customer ever since.

Another workshop participant said she bought a new Saturn automobile, but two days later it died on her way to work. Frustrated and fearing that she had just invested in a lemon, the woman called the dealership. An associate answered immediately, apologized, and said he would be there (on the roadside where she was stranded) in 10 minutes. To her astonishment he arrived even sooner, handed her the keys to a new loaner car, and encouraged her to be on her way. The Saturn representative waited for the tow truck, had the woman's car fixed (a minor adjustment to the computer), and delivered it to her driveway a few days later. She proclaims herself a lifelong Saturn customer.

As I listened to these stories and many more like them, it occurred to me that they were all service-recovery stories. Things certainly did not go perfectly. Indeed, in nearly every instance the customer was ready to walk away forever—frustrated and inclined to tell everyone he or she knew about the poor treatment. But in each case, an associate (who was often not to blame for the service failure) turned the situation around by apologizing and giving far-better-than-expected service. The moral is that service recovery is often an opportunity to turn a customer into a loyal fan.

Mayer and Cates (2004) offer the following tips for service recovery.

- *Address the issue immediately.* Denying or ignoring a complaint is the worst thing you can do.
- *Listen without interrupting, acknowledge the problem or mistake, and apologize for it.*
- *Ask for another chance to get it right.*
- *Ask how you can fix the problem, and tell the customer what to expect next.*
- *Fix it—and then some!*
- *Follow up, and let the person know what you have done to ensure that such mistakes don't happen in the future.*

**8. Recognize and create moments of truth.** Jan Carlzon, the highly successful CEO of Scandinavian Airlines, titled his 1987 memoir *Moments of Truth*. In the book Carlzon advances the idea that satisfaction and loyalty are made or broken during 50,000 moments of truth every day. These moments occur any time people develop an impression of the organization based on how they are treated. The Mayo Clinic staff encountered a moment of truth when a woman seeking care in the emergency department declined to be admitted, although she was quite ill. In encouraging her to share her concerns, the staff learned that she was from out of town and had left her dog in her truck, parked in the hospital lot. The staff might have discharged her as she requested. Instead, a nurse volunteered to take care of the woman's truck and her dog. The nurse wasn't even dissuaded when he realized the truck was an 18-wheeler! He got to work, arranging with the local shopping mall to park the truck in their lot for a few days, and recruited a fellow nurse with a commercial license and truck-driving experience to move it there. Then he looked after the dog until the patient was well enough to leave the hospital.

**9. Round for excellence.** Studer (2003) maintains that feedback is as crucial as oxygen. As a health care administrator, he borrowed a technique from physicians and began "rounding" everyday—visiting units through the hospital to talk to patients, families, and employees. He typically introduced himself this way: "Hi, I'm Quint Studer. I work for you." After a few questions about the person's experiences and the positive things going on in his or her unit, Studer made it a point to ask, "Do you have the tools and equipment to do your job?" or "What can I do to make your job easier?" And, even more remarkably, he followed through. At one hospital, stories are still told, years after Studer left, about the changes he made happen. He got reliable hot water in the ICU after more than a decade of doing without, he put up lights in the parking lot, built fences, and delivered new equipment and supplies—usually the very next day!

**10. Tell stories and honor heroes.** Stories such as the ones in this chapter become guiding principles for others. They portray what is best and most noble in the things we do. One of the most effective ways to support a culture is to encourage its stories. Good leaders appreciate their value and share them often. Here's one more, from Lafayette General Hospital, where I used to work. This true story was told every Christmas, in departments all across the hospital.

> An ambulance arrived late in the evening on Christmas Eve with a woman and her two young children, who had been involved in an automobile accident. The children were okay, but the woman died soon after arriving at the hospital. Her husband was working on an offshore oilrig, and police were unable to reach him. The emergency department staff was devastated for these two children who had just lost their mother and were stranded in a hospital with no family on Christmas Eve. The nurses, doctors, and unit receptionist tried to comfort and entertain the children as best they could until their shift change. The stores were closed, so they took turns driving to their homes to get supplies and gifts to create a makeshift holiday for the children. Sacrificing time they might have spent relaxing with their own families, the nurses worked into the night so that, when the children awoke on Christmas morning, the room was decorated with a tree surrounded by presents. Many staff members had brought their families to the hospital to share Christmas morning with the children. "The employees' kids were amazing," remembers one nurse. "Here they were, in a hospital on Christmas

morning, watching children they didn't know open gifts that had been under *their* trees with *their* names on them the day before. And they were just so happy to share. There wasn't a dry eye in the place, I can tell you!"

## SUMMARY

Bureaucratic elements are still evident in most health organizations, and it's doubtful that they can or should be completely abandoned. However, the need to contain costs, respond to changing consumer demands, and diversify services has led some health organizations to change their patterns of leadership and teamwork. Many are reshaping their bureaucratic structures to become more adaptive and innovative. The new emphasis is on participative decision making, employee and patient satisfaction, and interdisciplinary teamwork.

Heath care has traditionally been offered via a pod approach, in which groups of specialists provide care in separate departments or locations. But it is increasingly important to operate, instead, as interdisciplinary teams whose members support each other and avoid wasteful duplications. With this approach, what might otherwise take weeks or months to accomplish can occur within a few days.

Interdisciplinary teams help organizations bridge communication gaps between people in different departments and professions. Teamwork reduces the oversights that occur when workers focus on only one aspect of a job. Interdisciplinary teams are well qualified to provide biopsychosocial care and to develop services that combine cost efficiency and quality care. Team members may find comfort and support in working together. However, they will be challenged to overcome time constraints, professional differences, and the tendency simply to go along with what other members want.

Processes such as Six Sigma are designed to analyze workplace procedures carefully so that people can avoid wasting time and money. Well-designed systems can also reduce stress and minimize errors.

Satisfaction and service excellence are particularly important, considering that people are health care consumers who make deliberate choices about the care and services they are willing to pay for. There is a strong incentive for health care organizations to create appealing work environments and to strive to retain and develop the talent they have.

## KEY TERMS

integrated health systems
Six Sigma
bureaucracy
participative decision making (PDM)
rational-legal authority
professional prejudice
division of labor
groupthink

## DISCUSSION QUESTIONS

1. What are some communication challenges in newly integrated health systems?
2. Have you ever felt that work was fun? That it was boring and restrictive? What made the difference?
3. Why are people in some states opening boutique hospitals? Are you in favor of these organizations? Why or why not?
4. What is involved in a Six Sigma analysis?
5. In your opinion, should physicians advertise? If not, why not? If so, should their ads adhere to particular regulations or ethical guidelines?
6. In your experience, if being a patient is "the least amount of fun someone can have as a consumer," what are some factors that can make it a positive experience overall?
7. What are advantages and disadvantages of a vertical hierarchy? What are some opportunities for change?
8. Do you agree with Jeffrey Gitomer that policy "is the "single most annoying word a customer hears besides 'no'" (p. 68)? Do you have experience with this as a customer? As an employee?

9. What are some communication challenges involved in creating a horizontal organization? How can we best meet those challenges?

10. What does participative decision making (PDM) mean? What are the advantages of PDM? The challenges?

11. What suggestions do experts offer for training organizational leaders?

12. In what ways is rational-legal authority advantageous in health care organizations? In what ways is it limiting? What are some opportunities for improvement?

13. How can professional prejudice affect communication between health workers?

14. What communication skills are involved in collaborative leadership?

15. How can a division of labor make people more productive? In what ways does it interfere with communication? What are some ways to unite people in pursuit of a common vision?

16. What are the advantages and disadvantages of relying on rules? Why do some customer service experts hate the rules? Following Irwin's advice, how might you evaluate the rules in a health care organization?

17. What are some stupid rules you encounter regularly as a student, a consumer, an employee, or in some other role? Why don't these rules work? How would you change them?

18. How is the staff of Mayo Clinic able to accomplish in several days what usually takes weeks or months elsewhere? Would you like being a patient in such an integrated system? Why or why not? Would you like being a professional in such a system? Why or why not?

19. What are the qualities exhibited by innovative leaders in Davenport and colleagues' (2003) study (Box 10.5)?

20. What are the advantages of teamwork in today's health care organizations? What factors make teamwork difficult to achieve?

21. What are some tips for making teamwork productive?

22. What are some suggestions for improving service excellence? Which are your favorites among the ones listed in this chapter?

## ANSWERS TO *CAN YOU GUESS?*

1. There are about 262,000 health care administrators in the United States. Some 37% work in hospitals, and another 22% work in medical offices and nursing homes (U.S. Department of Labor, 2007).

2. Employment prospects are expected to increase 16% between 2006 and 2016, faster than the overall average (U.S. Department of Labor, 2007).

# PART V

# PUBLIC HEALTH: MEDIA, CRISIS, POLICY REFORM, AND HEALTH PROMOTION

# CHAPTER
# 11

# Health Images in the Media

---

*Do What Hubby Tells You?*

*When a group of British researchers found that submissive women were slightly less likely to have heart attacks than other women, they prepared a media release they felt was accurate, interesting, and readable. Many media organizations ran the release or suitable portions of it. However, others misconstrued the study to mean that women should return to being housewives. Headlines about the study admonished, "Put Down That Rolling Pin Darling, It's Bad For Your Heart" and "Do What Hubby Says and You'll Live Longer. Professor's Shock Advice to Women." The researchers were discouraged by journalists' handling of the story, calling the supposed link between submissiveness and housewifery "bewildering" (Deary, Whiteman, & Fowkes, 1998).*

The researchers in this example say they learned a valuable lesson: Where health is concerned, the mass media is both friend and foe. The publicity helped the scientists share valuable knowledge and promote their work. However, inaccuracies and exaggerations made them wonder if some of the stories did more harm than good.

In this chapter we examine health's presence in mass communication. **Mass communication** is the dissemination of messages from one person (or one group of persons) to large numbers of people via media, including television, radio, computers, newspapers, magazines, billboards, video games, and other means of sharing information with large audiences (Biagi, 1999). As you will see, there is evidence that media messages encourage people to overeat, doubt their attractiveness, drink alcohol,

smoke, and neglect physical activity. However, mass communication is also irreplaceable for getting health information to large numbers of people. Such information may enable them to better understand their own health and experience more control over their lives. People who watch a range of TV news programs, documentaries, talk shows, and even soap operas are typically better informed about health than nonveiwers (Dutta, 2007).

As we further explore the way that mass media messages shape our ideas about health, we will first examine health images in advertising, news, and entertainment. As you will see, research often shows a link between media use and various behaviors, such as overeating and drinking. Remember that this does not prove that the media, or the media alone, *cause* these behaviors. Mass-mediated messages are only one of many influences on health. Their effects are likely to be lessened or exaggerated by a range of other factors, including personal preferences, culture, social networks, and health status. The chapter concludes with information about media literacy—a systematic process of becoming more skeptical and more informed mass media consumers so that we do not unwittingly buy into harmful and unrealistic ideas.

## ADVERTISING

Most of us feel that we are not personally susceptible to persuasive messages in the media, but we think other people are. W. Phillips Davison (1983) coined the term **third-person effect** to describe this perception. For example, teens often believe their peers will be more likely to smoke if they see pro-smoking messages in the media, but they tend to feel immune from media effects themselves (Gunther, Bolt, Borzekowski, Liebhart, & Dillard, 2006). Most research suggests that we are all influenced more profoundly than we think.

### Direct-to-Consumer Advertising

*"This product may cause headaches, drowsiness, stomach upset, liver problems, heartbeat irregularities…"*

In 1985, the U.S. Food and Drug Administration (FDA) ruled that pharmaceutical companies could advertise product categories to the public. But the most dramatic change came later, in 1997, when the FDA relaxed the rules even more to make the United States one of only two countries (the other is New Zealand) to allow brand-name prescription drug advertising. Selling prescription drugs in public venues such as the mass media is called **direct-to-consumer advertising (DTCA)**, as compared to *physician marketing*, in which drugs are marketed to doctors, who, in turn, make patients aware of them as they perceive a need to do so.

Since 1997 names such as Claritin, Zyrtec, and Lunesta have become as familiar as Coca-Cola and Tic Tacs. And along with the ads have come a now-familiar list of disclaimers—so familiar that one guest on an online medical site asked the doctor: "Do *all* prescription drugs cause diarrhea and dry mouth?" These *are* common side effects, but you hear about them so much because of a rather nebulous FDA guideline known as "fair balance," which states that, if advertisers present the potential benefits of a drug, they must also report potentially harmful side effects. In the name of fairness (sort of), for every promise of relief you are likely to hear a list of disagreeable outcomes you might also experience. The "sort of" means that the guideline is only loosely and rather lopsidedly upheld. For quick evidence of this, compare the lengthy information in a magazine pharmaceutical ad to the brief disclaimer you hear on a TV or radio commercial for the same drug!

The "fair balance" guideline also explains why some prescription drug ads make no claims at all. The announcer might just say, "Ask your doctor about Zertec." Per FDA guidelines, an ad that doesn't make a *positive* claim doesn't have to provide cautionary information either. In the case of no-claim ads, sponsors apparently believe that you will recognize the drug and its purpose by name, that the disclaimers, if mentioned, would scare you away, or that you will be curious enough to ask about or research the drug. In reality, about 3 in 10 Americans say they have sought additional information after seeing a drug advertisement (whether it made a specific claim or not), and 5 in 10 report talking to a friend, relative or physician about the drug (DeLorne, Huh, & Reid, 2006).

*Advantages of DTCA* From one standpoint, advertisements for needed products are beneficial. Without advertising, consumers might not know that treatment options exist for indigestion, asthma, allergies, depression, restless legs, and the like (Calfee, 2002). But it's hard to say how many people actually "ask their doctor" about advertised drugs. Soontae An (2007) found that people were mostly likely to bring up advertised medicines when they considered themselves to be knowledgeable about health matters. This may be a small percentage of the public. In one U.S. study, only 1 in 10 people reported making drug-specific requests at the doctor's office (DeLorne et al., 2006). And patient surveys in New Zealand yield similarly low numbers (Dens, Eagle, & De Pelsmacker, 2008). But doctors tend to report a higher frequency of requests. In a *Consumer Reports* study of American physicians, 78% said patients occasionally ask them for drugs they have seen advertised on TV ("Finally," 2007). The discrepancy may arise because doctors perceive implied requests even when patients don't ask for advertised drugs outright.

Another advantage of DTCA is that active competition can inspire product development. The public presumably benefits when drug companies strive to offer the most appealing and useful products. For example, high interest in cholesterol-reducing drugs spurred research and development efforts in the 1990s (Calfee, 2002). By targeting people at moderate risk for heart attacks, drug companies expanded their markets and motivated consumers to visit their doctors for preventive treatment before their conditions worsened. Marketplace stimulation has not lived up to its full potential, however. A substantial number of "new" drugs are actually what Marcia Angell (2004) calls "me too" drugs—close copycats of already-existing products.

*Disadvantages of DTCA* Although health information is beneficial within limits, it also has drawbacks. For one, expensive advertising drives up the price of health products. Prescription drugs are one of the fastest-growing health costs in the United States, topping $216.7 billion in 2006, which is five times higher than in 1990 ("Prescription Drug," 2008). Part of the price goes to advertising, which went from zero two decades ago to $10.4 billion in 2007 ("Prescription Drug"), this at a time when 70% of Americans feel that drug companies value profits more than people ("Americans Value," 2005).

Second, physicians worry that—based on the dazzling scenarios in prescription drug commercials—people may believe that high-priced designer drugs are better than others and that drugs will not only cure anything that ails them, but yield increased

happiness and excitement as well. Consider a few examples from Rebecca Cline and Henry Young's (2004) content analysis of pharmaceutical ads:

- 93% of the models in arthritis drug ads were shown engaging in physical activity,
- 100% of the models in ads for HIV treatments appeared healthy, and
- 85.7% of models in cancer-related ads appeared healthy.

"The message is obvious," the researchers conclude. "With treatment by prescription drugs, the consumer with the associated condition can be attractively healthy looking and lively" (Cline & Young, p. 151). As a result of unrealistic expectations, consumers may squander money on unnecessary medications, seek prescriptions for the wrong reasons, feel disappointed when their doctors do not prescribe the drugs they see in the media, or feel disappointed when the results are less dramatic than advertisers led them to believe.

Concerns about DTCA have intensified as advertisers have become bolder, promoting not only drugs but devices used in complex medical procedures. For example, the makers of a stent involved in coronary angioplasty launched their "Life Wide Open" advertising series in 2007. The ads show models enjoying a range of sporting and outdoor activities, presumably after having their clogged arteries cleared by angioplasty. However, there is little mention of how dangerous angioplasty actually is. And critics worry that ads promising "quick and easy" cures will dissuade people from taking care of themselves in the first place. The authors of an article in the *New England Journal of Medicine* write:

> A specialized medical device such as a stent can be selected and implanted only by someone with a very sophisticated medical understanding that no member of the lay public could realistically expect to gain from a DTCA campaign. (Boden & Diamond, 2008, p. 2197)

Boden and Diamond (both physicians) wonder: Is it responsible to "sell" a specialized and risky medical procedure in a 60-second time slot?

That question becomes even more significant when we consider evidence that drug companies sometimes downplay their products' risks. When Wendy Macias and colleagues studied 106 pharmaceutical TV commercials, they found that 2 violated the FDA's "fair balance" requirement and another 10 were borderline. The rest gave customary but minimal amounts of information about potential side effects (Macias, Pashupati, & Lewis, 2007). Even more frightening is that the side effects drug companies are (under)reporting often come from research they have funded and overseen themselves. The FDA requires research evidence that drugs are safe and useful before they are put on the market. The problem is that drug companies pay for most of this research themselves, and they have an interest in seeing the drugs released as quickly as possible, with as few documented side effects as possible. There are reports of drug company executives firing researchers, refusing to release adverse research findings, denying research funding when methods are not expected to yield the desired results, and so on. Sergio Sismondo (2008) concluded that pharmaceutical companies "not only fund clinical trials but also routinely design and shape them" (paragraph 5). He reports that drug companies often have their staff statisticians perform data analyses and then hire people to write the research reports and corral them through the publication process.

A tragic example is the Merck Pharmaceutical Vioxx case. After years of denying that its top-selling pain medication (Vioxx) posed significant health risks, Merck officials finally withdrew the drug in 2004. By that time, between 27,000 and 60,000 people had died from the drug's side effects (Lyon, 2007). In studying Merck documents and communiqués, researcher Alexander Lyon found that a pervasive "market mentality" led Merck decision makers to suppress and minimize information about Vioxx's harmful side effects. Lyon recommends that pharmaceutical companies be kept separate from research about the products they sell.

Third, some experts worry that Americans are developing an unhealthy preoccupation with their own health, based largely on the amount of health care products and information now surrounding them. "We're not exactly a nation of hypochondriacs. But we're close," writes Jennifer Harper (1997, p. 40).

Finally, while some people are overrepresented in DTCA images, others are left out of the picture, reinforcing health disparities. Here are some examples.

- Although heart disease is the leading cause of death among men *and* women, nearly two in three ads show only men (Cline & Young, 2004).
- Although black Americans are more likely to die from heart disease than their white counterparts, models in cardiovascular treatment ads are almost always white (Cline & Young, 2004).
- Only 5% of drug advertisements in general-readership magazines show black models without white models also present (Mastin, Andsager, Choi, & Lee, 2007).
- Hispanic American models are rarely pictured; when they are, the ads are mostly for HIV/AIDS treatments (Cline & Young, 2004).

There are exceptions to the mostly-white rule, but you have to look in black-oriented publications to find most of them. According to Teresa Mastin and colleagues (2007), about 75% of the pharmaceutical ads in black-oriented magazines feature only black models. But even these ads present a distorted picture of what African Americans need. For example, heart-care ads in general-audience women's magazines outnumber similar ads in black women's magazines 4 to 1. And 80% of the ads directed to black females are for birth control pills, a bias that is not present in general-readership women's magazines. Mastin and colleagues conclude that direct-to-consumer ads are not educating *all* consumers about health risks and treatment options (Mastin et al., 2007).

***Communication Skill Builders: Evaluating Medical Claims*** As you have seen, consumers who rely on advertisements for health information do not always (or even often) get a clear picture. Here are some tips for evaluating the claims in medication ads.

- *Don't put too much stock in the wording.* Joel Davis (2007) found that people were most optimistic about drugs when the side effects were presented in language that downplayed their severity, such as "Side effects were mild and might include…" "Side effects tend to be mild and often go away," and "Few people were bothered enough to stop taking the drug." Keep in mind that reassuring word choices don't necessarily mean these drugs are safer than others.
- *Look to print sources for detailed information.* Broadcast commercials mention potential side effects only briefly. Magazine ads include a great deal more information (Boden & Diamond, 2008).
- *"Newer" doesn't necessarily mean better.* Pharmaceutical companies vie for the public's attention by advertising "newest" and "latest" therapies. But the rush to the marketplace doesn't actually mean the medication is "improved" or even that it is safe (Lyon, 2007).

Even advertisements that seem unrelated to health care often affect people's health by influencing social expectations about how they should behave, what they should eat and drink, and how they should appear. The remainder of this section discusses advertising's impact on nutrition, alcohol, and body image.

## Nutrition

It's been called the "coach potato physique," characterized by soft bulges where muscle ought to be. Heavy television viewing is consistently linked to obesity, partly because TV offers a triple punch to good nutrition. People usually burn few calories while watching, they have a tendency to snack while viewing, and the commercials usually encourage consumption of non-nutritious foods (Dennison,

Erb, & Jenkins, 2002; Signorielli & Staples, 1997). As you will see, commercials sometimes handicap people's knowledge of nutrition and influence their food preferences for the worse. As the researchers in one study concluded, in the content of television commercials, "fruits and vegetables are virtually nonexistent" (Kotz & Story, 1994, paragraph 11).

*Obesity* The prevalence of TV commercials for fatty and sugary foods may have serious implications for health, considering that overweight people are at elevated risk for heart disease, cancer, diabetes, and sudden death. African American women are at especially high risk for obesity and related concerns. This may be partly because of advertisements. When Linda Godbold Kean and Laura Prividera (2007) compared ads in *Essence* (aimed mostly at female African Americans) and *Cosmopolitan* (targeted to women in general), they found that 13% of the ads in *Essence* were for fast food, compared to 1% of the ads in *Cosmopolitan*. Furthermore, *Cosmopolitan* readers were exposed to more weight-loss products and claims (mentioned in 41% of the ads) than were *Essence* readers (12% of ads). (While these messages may be helpful to *Cosmopolitan* readers trying to maintain a healthy weight, it should also be noted that many of the weight-loss claims—such as those for low-carbohydrate whiskey—were not exactly health conscious.)

The editorial content in magazines is not making up the difference. Articles in general-audience women's magazines such as *Ladies Home Journal* and *Good Housekeeping* offer twice as many recommendations to cut back on fast food as the articles in *Ebony, Essence,* and *Jet* (Campo & Mastin, 2007). The general-audience magazines placed more emphasis on small portions and whole-grain and high-protein foods. By contrast, the African American magazines were more likely to present fad diets and to encourage women to rely on God and religious faith to help them lose weight (Campo & Mastin).

Another media distortion, in the United States and abroad, is that media messages often cast obesity as a beauty issue rather than a serious health concern. Swedish researcher Helena Sandberg (2007) argues that this trivializes weight's importance and leads people to think that a healthy size is more important for women than for men. Indeed, males are typically less concerned about their weight than females, even though male obesity rates are nearly equivalent to women's ("New CDC Study," 2007). And when overweight men do want to lose a few pounds, the majority do not aim low enough. Researchers report that about 59% of overweight men envisioned an ideal weight for themselves that was still overweight by medical standards (Neighbors & Sobal, 2007).

As the next section shows, weight and nutrition issues begin in childhood.

*Effects on Children* Since 1988 the incidence of childhood obesity in the United States has doubled among children ages 6 to 11 and tripled among 12- to 19-year-olds ("Childhood," 2008). These youth are at risk for heart disease, diabetes, sleep apnea, joint problems, and high blood pressure.

Part of the problem is that children are exposed to an average of 5,500 televised food commercials pear year (Desrochers & Holt, 2007), and the commercials often misrepresent what healthy food is all about. For example, no matter how much TV they watched at home, first- through third-graders in Kristin Harrison's (2005) study were roughly equivalent in their nutritional knowledge of products,

such as fruit and dairy, that are not heavily advertised. But when Harrison asked children to choose the more nutritional option between cottage cheese and fat-free ice cream and between orange juice and Diet Coke®, those who watched a lot of television were more likely to consider (incorrectly) that the highly advertised diet products were better for them. The chances are high, Harrison concluded, that children exposed to a lot of commercials will assume that diet products are, by nature, more nutritious than other foods.

The distortion continues in the supermarket. A Canadian study of 367 products marketed to children revealed that 89% of them were unhealthy (C. Elliott, 2007). Fruits and vegetables constituted less than 1% of the products aimed at kids, and 62% of unhealthy products—despite having high levels of sugar, fat, and sodium—came in packages that touted their "nutritional value."

*Activity Levels* It should be noted that advertising is not entirely to blame for the obesity linked to TV viewing. Some researchers suggest that the sedentary nature of heavy viewing is as unhealthy as the content. Children who watch 4 or more hours of TV a day have significantly higher body fat and body weight than children who engage in more vigorous pastimes, even when their calorie intake is similar (Andersen, Crespo, Bartlett, Cheskin, & Pratt, 1998). And heavy television viewing may lead to other unhealthy behaviors. For example, youngsters who watch a lot of television are more likely than others to smoke (Gidwani, Sobol, DeJong, Perrin, & Gortmaker, 2002). Researchers speculate that extensive viewing substitutes for physical activities and social development that might otherwise help teens avoid peer pressure.

High media use is also linked to sleep deprivation. Children today sleep an average of 2 hours less per night than children in the early 1980s (Zimmerman, 2008). Authorities blame TV, video, the Internet, and computer games. They say these activities sometimes cut into sleep time and leave children too excited to sleep when the lights do go out. Children may also feel less sleepy because they aren't getting much exercise and because the glow from TV and computer screens inhibits melatonin secretion, an important chemical in sleep functioning (Zimmerman).

## Alcohol

If media messages influence the way people eat, they are also likely to influence the way they drink. Particularly worrisome is the industry's apparent agenda to recruit drinkers when they are still underage. When market researchers asked teens to name their favorite TV commercials, Bud Light came in first and Budweiser was fourth ("Television," 2006). Young people may remember and like these commercials so much because the spots are designed for them. Consider the following.

- More alcoholic beverage commercials air before 9 p.m.—when you might expect young viewers to be watching—than later in the evening. Additionally, there is a spike in commercials on weekdays from 3 to 5 p.m. Researchers speculate that these commercials are intentionally aimed at school children since "it would be a reasonable assumption that most people in employment will not have returned home until after 5 p.m." (Alcohol Concern, 2007, p. 13).
- Based on their content, 1 in 6 magazine ads and 1 in 14 commercials for alcoholic beverages are apparently aimed at teens (Austin & Hust, 2005).
- Compared to adults of legal drinking age, underage radio listeners hear 8% more ads for beer, 11.6% more ads for malt liquor, and 14.5% more ads for distilled alcoholic beverages such as whiskey, vodka, and tequila (S. Elliott, 2003).
- The number of alcohol advertisements to which children are exposed increased 38% between 2001 and 2007 ("Youth Exposure," 2008). More than 40% of those ads appeared in specifically youth-oriented programs.
- African American youth see about 66% more beer and ale magazine advertisements and 81% more ads for distilled beverages than other people their age (S. Elliott, 2003).

Alcoholic beverage companies buy heavily in magazines aimed at young, minority audiences and employ rappers and youthful-appearing spokespersons designed to catch the attention of young people. Says the director of an alcohol and drug recovery center in San Francisco: "The models they use in the ads have to be 21, but they're the youngest 21-year-olds you'll ever see" (quoted by F. Green, 2003, p. 1C). And this early exposure seems to make a significant difference. The odds that a seventh- or eighth-grader will drink wine or beer are 44% greater if he or she is exposed to a large number of alcohol advertisements (Stacy, Zogg, Unger, & Dent, 2004).

*Source of Knowledge* As early as age 9, children typically know a lot about alcoholic beverages based on what they have seen advertised (Austin & Nach-Ferguson, 1995). And children with brand-name knowledge (the ability to link brand names with certain types of alcohol) are more likely than others to try alcohol (Mastro & Atkin, 2002). The implication is that advertising has an influence on what children know and sometimes on what they do. Children and adolescents may be especially susceptible to the ideas cultivated by persuasive media messages. (See Box 11.2 for a theoretical exploration of media effects on children.)

*Glamorized Images* Beer commercials often show drinkers surrounded by beautiful women, fun-loving friends, and exotic locales. But the reality is not nearly so glamorous. Alcohol-related accidents kill 5,000 underage drinkers per year in the United States, and the risk of drinking problems later in life is five times greater for people who begin drinking before age 15 than for those who wait until they are 21 (U.S. Department of Health and Human Services, 2007). What's more, heavy drinkers risk liver damage, hypertension, and strokes and are more likely than their peers to hurt others (and to be hurt) in accidents and acts of violence (Nestle, 1997). Considering these risks, beer companies are sometimes criticized for portraying drinking episodes as fun and sexy.

## BOX 11.2 THEORETICAL FOUNDATIONS

# Cultivation Theory and Social Comparison Theory

In a video about sexist images in advertising, *Killing Us Softly 3*, Jean Kilbourne (2000) observes that people frequently tell her they are not affected by the media. "Of course, they are usually standing there in their Gap t-shirt while they say this," she laughs.

The fact is that we are all affected by the media to varying extents. The two theories described here—cultivation theory and social comparison theory—consider how media messages influence our attitudes and expectations about the world.

Cultivation theory helps explain why children may be especially vulnerable to advertising messages. According to **cultivation theory**, people develop beliefs about the world based on a complex array of influences, including the media. Media's influence is not uniform or automatic, but it is likely to be most profound if (a) media images are highly consistent, (b) people are exposed to large amounts of media, and (c) these people have a limited basis for evaluating what they see and hear (Gerbner, Gross, Morgan, & Signorielli, 1994). To clarify, consider that children have fewer experiences and less knowledge than adults. Because of this, they are less able to perceive that media images may be wrong or unrealistic. The same principle would hold true if you watched a documentary about a faraway land about which you knew very little. People familiar with that land might see inaccuracies in the documentary that you would be unable to identify.

The effect is compounded among high media users because not only is their exposure high, but the more

time they spend tuned into mass media, they less opportunity they have to experience activities that might provide a basis for comparison. Researchers in Thailand found that children who watched TV more than their peers were more likely to think television portrayals were realistic and to want to be part of TV families (Jantarakolica, Komolsevin, & Speece, 2002). Children in the United States spend an average of 1,023 hours a year watching TV, which is more than the time they spend engaged in any other activity except sleep ("By the Numbers," 2007).

Social comparison theory helps explain why people yearn to emulate the models they see in the media. Proposed by Leon Festinger (1957), **social comparison theory** suggests that people judge themselves largely in comparison to others. Want to know if you are attractive, popular, healthy, or smart? The only answer may lie in how you stack up to the people around you. Social comparisons can be useful when they enhance self-esteem or serve as the basis for reasonable self-improvement. However, they become dysfunctional when the comparison establishes an unrealistic standard (like being supermodel thin or weight-lifter strong).

## What Do You Think?

1. In what ways are you influenced by media messages?
2. If you are around children, what reactions do you observe as they are exposed to messages in the media?
3. How do you think we can minimize the effects of media images that establish unrealistic standards of attractiveness?

Some people worry that beer ads showing "the good life" will affect young people's views about drinking. Research supports that lifestyle-oriented beer advertisements are more appealing to adolescents than ads focusing on product qualities like taste. Adolescents surveyed by Kathleen Kelly and

Ruth Edwards (1998) preferred beer ads showing fun lifestyles, but this preference was not linked to the youths' intention to drink. But sizeable research suggests that young people (especially boys) *may* be more likely to drink if they find beer commercials appealing (Chen, Grube, Bersamin, Waiters, &

Keefe, 2005; Grube & Wallack, 1994; Slater et al., 1997). When Betty Parker (1998) studied college students' reactions to beer commercials she found that some students considered the commercials unrealistic based on their own experiences, but others regarded them as fairly accurate and even as instructional guides for how to enjoy drinking.

Health warnings all but drown in the ocean of pro-alcohol messages. Alcoholic beverage ads outnumber responsible drinking PSAs at least 20 to 1 ("Youth Exposure," 2008). The good news is that, despite the odds, responsible drinking messages may have some influence. Itzhak Yanovitzky and Jo Stryker (2001) observed that, over time, binge drinking among youth decreased in the midst of news coverage about its harmful effects. The downturn is not likely to continue, however, unless media professionals can keep the dangers of binge drinking on the public agenda.

## Body Images

Consumers are repeatedly warned that their skin, weight, hair, breath, clothing, and teeth are "problem areas" requiring vigorous and immediate attention—at a price. Theorists call this **pathologizing the human body**, making natural functions seem weird and unnatural (Wood, 1999). In short, advertisers are accused of making people feel bad about themselves so that they will be willing to pay for "needed" changes.

Adolescents are particularly susceptible to these messages (Kowalski, 1997). With the physical and social changes of adolescence comes a heightened self-consciousness that makes it easy to escalate (and capitalize on) teens' insecurity. Advertisers often encourage an obsessive concern with physical appearance, sometimes to the detriment of people's health and self-esteem. "Advertisers realize that having your period is the grossest thing in the world, and they want to help," quips Ann Hodgman (1998, p. 38), adding: "As long as Procter & Gamble can scare a teen into thinking that [a boy] can see her bulky maxi through her dress, she'll buy Always.... If a teen wasn't obsessing about it before, Tampax wants her to start."

Advertisements aimed at teens are working, judging by sales figures and the number of products on the market. Teenagers spend an average of $70 billion annually on clothes (C. Williams, 2003). Additionally, they are encouraged to buy (or convince their parents to buy) skin care creams, lotions, powders, perfume, makeup, shaving cream, shampoo, bath oil, mouthwash, toothpaste, and more. Bardbard (1993) points out that—aside from making teens feel unattractive without them—these products can be health risks when they cause rashes, hives, eye irritation, or other reactions.

One problem is that media images are inherently unrealistic. Whether these images are fashion spreads in Singapore and Taiwan that focus mostly on facial beauty or American images that emphasize sex appeal, clothing, and the body, fashion designers and other advertisers establish alluring but unattainable standards and then rake in profits as people strive to measure up (Frith, Shaw, & Cheng, 2005). For example, researchers calculate that, to attain the proportions of a Barbie doll, a woman would have to be more than 7 feet tall, with a bust 5 inches larger than normal and a waist 6 inches smaller (Duewald, 2003). The same contrast is evident between the average-size woman, who wears a size 12 to 14 ("plus" sizes by fashion-industry standards) and fashion models, who typically wear size 0 or 2 (Betts, 2002). Model Coca Rocha remembers fashion moguls' advice when she began modeling at age 15. "They said, 'You need to lose more weight. The look this year is anorexia. We don't want you to be anorexic, but that's what you need to look like'" (quoted by Scott, 2008, paragraph 12).

After a number of fashion models died from malnutrition, fashion industries in some countries begun to crack down. The Council of Fashion Designers of America has urged designers to inch up the average size of models in their show. So far, the increase is barely perceptible—models who wear sizes 2 and 4 rather than 0 (Scott, 2008). In bolder efforts, fashion leaders in Spain now deny runway jobs to models with a body mass index below 18 (the recommended range is 18.5 to 25), and fashion leaders in London require models to show doctors' certificates that they are healthy or, if they have eating disorders, that they are being treated for them (Cartner-Morley, 2007).

*Health Effects* Unrealistic standards can have serious health consequences. About 90% of American women within a normal weight range wish they were thinner, and more than 50% of underweight women either like their weight or wish they were thinner (Neighbors & Sobal, 2007). Men typically express less dissatisfaction with their bodies, but 20% of men in Neighbors and Sobal's study wanted to gain weight, and 48% wanted to lose.

Although obesity is a serious health threat, extreme efforts to change one's body can be dangerous or even deadly. About 9 million Americans (the majority of them female) suffer from eating disorders, which may damage their hearts and livers, make their bones brittle, and even kill them ("Eating Disorder," 2007). Although eating disorders often start in adolescence, they do not end there. In fact children are likely to feel their bodies are inferior partly because their parents are preoccupied about their own weight and appearance (C. Maynard, 1998).

Anabolic steroid abuse is another problem among people hoping to become more muscular. More than 1 million Americans have abused steroids (National Institute on Drug Abuse [NIDA], 2007). The risks of steroid abuse include cardiovascular disease, liver damage, hair loss, sterility, aggressiveness, and depression. Nearly 30% of teenagers in the United States say illegal steroids are readily available to them (NIDA, 2007), but the profile of the average steroid abuser will probably surprise you. He is 30 years old, Caucasian, highly educated, and well employed and, though not active in sports, is interested in developing a more muscular appearance (Cohen, Collins, Darkes, & Gwartney, 2007). Researchers observe that for most steroid users, the goal is to measure up to Western ideals of masculine attractiveness rather than to excel at sports.

*Eternal Hope* Why do people keep buying into what the media sells? There is some evidence that people are hopeful when they see idealized models and are optimistic that they can attain the same look. Philip Myers and Frank Biocca (1992) were surprised when female college students in their study reacted favorably to television programs and commercials featuring slender women. Immediately after viewing these images, most viewers were more elated than depressed, and they tended to consider *themselves* to be thinner than usual. The researchers concluded that media images make idealized body shapes seem attainable, causing an optimism that may later turn to disappointment because it is infeasible for most people to look like that.

## NEWS COVERAGE

When America's Health Network announced it would show a live Internet broadcast of a woman giving birth in June 1998, more than 50,000 curious viewers logged on to witness the event (Charski, 1998). Now live births can be viewed most days on cable TV, as can plastic surgeries and a host of other medical procedures. Additionally, health is the topic of special-interest television channels, magazines, books, and radio advice programs. Americans have access to more health information than ever before, in the form of websites and news, entertainment, and educational programming.

Madge Kaplan, a health news reporter on the public radio program *Marketplace,* says covering health issues is "a rich, exciting and suspenseful journey" (Kaplan, 2003, paragraph 4). "My hope is that health care reporting stay closely tied to the central purpose of health care—service to patients.... This means we need to do a better job illustrating our story subjects' multidimensional character" (paragraph 13).

The main criticism of health news is that, in the rush to provide the latest information, media professionals sometimes oversell scientific findings and overlook ongoing, everyday concerns. This section examines health news in terms of accuracy and sensationalism and discusses the advantages of media coverage. It concludes with a discussion of interactive technology, which is revolutionizing the way people get health information.

## Accuracy and Fairness

Although many media professionals do an admirable job informing the public about health issues, a sizable number of health stories are misleading and exaggerated. When researchers compared 25 scientific studies to 60 newspaper and magazine articles about them, they found numerous inaccuracies and did not consider any of the stories to be excellent reflections of the research (Motl, Timpe, & Eichner, 2005). The most common errors occurred when writers overgeneralized the results of medical studies. For instance, a study of older women might be reported simply as a study about women or older adults, although the heath concerns of these populations may be significantly different. Such inaccuracies are particularly troubling since it is often difficult for readers to verify scientific information for themselves.

One worry is that overly optimistic news about medical research will give people false hope. As early as 1997, headlines in major publications suggested an imminent cure for AIDS ("When AIDS Ends" in the *New York Times Magazine* and the "The End of AIDS?" in *Newsweek*). Jon Cohen (1997) cautioned: "If treatments don't live up to unrealistic expectations, researchers fear a public backlash against medical science" (paragraph 2). Premature reports about cures for cancer raise the same fear (Arnst, 1998).

Sometimes news reporters seem to cater to commercial interests. In a study of magazines written for African American women, researchers found 1,500 tobacco advertisements but only 9 articles about smoking as a cause of cancer (Hoffman-Goetz, Gerlach, Marino, & Mills, 1997). Considering that cancer is the leading cause of death among elderly African American women, the researchers suggest that editorial decisions were made in advertisers' interest rather than readers'. (See Box 11.3 for more on the accuracy of health news sources.)

---

**BOX 11.3 RESOURCES**

# Health News Ratings

Go to healthnewsreview.org to see how experts rate the accuracy of health news in specific TV programs, networks, magazines, and newspapers. You can also access there a list of 5-star health stories selected by experts on the basis of their accuracy and usefulness.

---

Sometimes the concept of "accuracy" is problematic in itself. For example, Raul Reis (2008) reports that Brazilian and U.S. newspapers cover the issue of stem cell research differently. Brazilian papers tend to focus on it as a scientific matter, whereas American journalists more often focus on the ethical implications. Where health is concerned, there are more than two sides to any coin.

## Sensationalism

Media professionals are also criticized for favoring sensational health news rather than useful information about everyday concerns. For example, SARS and West Nile virus (characterized in such terms as "mysterious" and "deadly") get far more coverage than heart disease, which is the world's leading cause of death (T. R. Berry, Wharf-Higgins, & Naylor, 2007). And reporters forecasting a potential bird flu pandemic rely largely on sensational stories that do not provide enough information for the public to feel prepared and confident if the crisis arises (Dudo, Dahlstrom, & Broussard, 2007).

In some instances, snappy headlines have little to do with scientific evidence. A study conducted for *Consumer Research Magazine* revealed that women's magazines such as *Redbook*, *Mademoiselle*, *McCall's*, and *Better Homes and Gardens* published frightening health stories without documentation to back them up (Zipperer, 1997). Menacing headlines included "Will Pollution Ruin Your Chance of Having a Baby?" and "Is Your Lawn Making You Sick?," although there is little or no scientific evidence that the implied risks actually exist.

## Advantages of Health News

Despite the criticisms, health news does offer several advantages. Media organizations are credited with increasing people's awareness about health. And even when medical news is not what scientists would wish, its presence keeps health on the public agenda and (hopefully) garners support for medical science (Deary et al., 1998). For example, coverage of breast cancer has substantially increased since the 1970s and has focused mostly on new treatment methods and scientific breakthroughs (S. Cho, 2006). That's good, except that some other forms of cancer receive only minimal coverage (T. R. Berry et al., 2007).

It should also be said that news writers are not entirely to blame for misleading health coverage. The fault lies partly with the nature of news and the nature of science. It is the nature of news to be unusual and recent (Taubes, 1998). The public is hungry for current and interesting information, and media organizations strive to provide it. However, it is the nature of science to be meticulous and cautious, weighing diverse evidence over long periods of time (Taubes). Consequently, news writers are at a disadvantage trying to cover scientific news accurately. The latest study may reach different conclusions than the study before it or after it. Science is full of reliable accounts that, for one reason or another, arrive at different conclusions, so even the experts don't agree (Vardeman & Aldoory, 2008). For example, gastroenterologist Tadataka Yamada (2008) owns up to being in the "Acid Mafia," his humorous term for physicians who initially refused to believe evidence that gastric ulcers are caused by bacteria rather than stress. Finally, to convince the skeptics, one of the medical researchers actually drank a solution containing the bacterium and became ill because of it. Yamada eventually came around, and the researchers he had doubted won a 2005 Nobel Prize. "New ideas should not have to fight so hard for oxygen," Yamada (p. 1324) now preaches. Even if that does happen, health news writers trying to report up-to-date information are likely to find themselves with considerable ambiguity on their hands.

Furthermore, reporters may be ill prepared to meet the extraordinary challenges health coverage presents. Medical terminology and statistical analyses make medical science difficult to understand and interpret, and comparatively few reporters are trained to do so (Tanner, 2004a, 2004b). On the bright side, with many sources of health news available, the chances are greater that people can evaluate and compare information, judging for themselves what is credible and useful (Eng et al., 1998).

## Communication Skill Builders: Presenting Health News

Here are some suggestions Melissa Ludtke and Cathy Trost (1998) offer to help media news writers present fair coverage.

- *Favor the factual over the sensational and trendy.*
- *Do not allow ongoing issues to fade from coverage.* "Put a fresh face on coverage of long-standing health issues like asthma, lead poisoning and infant mortality" (paragraph 20).
- *Never rely on just one source.* Consult a number of experts; read a variety of reliable literature.
- *Set the record straight.* If a health news item is revealed to be untrue or misleading, update the public.

Also see Box 11.4 for career opportunities in health journalism.

In the next section we consider a relatively new medium in mass dissemination of health messages—the computer.

## Communication Technology: Interactive Health Information

The interactive nature of computer-based communication allows a more customized approach to sharing health information. Rather than simply receiving mass-mediated messages, users can respond to them, ask questions, request more information, and choose how and when they wish to receive information (Street, 1997). As the options

## BOX 11.4 CAREER OPPORTUNITIES

# Health Journalism

Print or broadcast health news reporter
Health news editor
Media relations specialist
Nonprofit organization publicity manager
Health publication editor
Journal or magazine editor

## Career Resources and Job Listings

Association of Health Care Journalists: www.
healthjournalism.org/prof-dev-jobs.php
Association for Education in Journalism and Mass
Communication (includes job listings): aejmc.org

Broadcast Education Association (includes job
listings): www.beaweb.org
Foundation for American Communications: www.
facsnet.org
Henry J. Kaiser Media Fellowships for Health: kff.
org/mediafellows/index.cfm
Knight Center for Specialized Journalism
Fellowships: knightcenter.umd.
edu/?q=fellowships
National Association of Broadcasters (includes job
listings): www.nab.org
National Press Foundation: www.nationalpress.
org
U.S. Department of Labor Occupational
Outlook for News Analysts, Reporters, and
Correspondents: www.bls.gov/oco/ocos088.htm

---

become more sophisticated, people can also go online to review case studies and experiment with computer simulations of various treatments, such as radiation and chemotherapy (Rains, 2007).

*Advantages* Computerized communication has several advantages, according to the authors of *Health Promotion and Interactive Technology* (Street, Gold, & Manning, 1997).

- The opportunity for feedback and response improves the chances for effective communication.
- The interactive nature of computerized information makes it highly memorable and engaging. Children with asthma who took part in an interactive computer program about asthma subsequently displayed fewer symptoms, needed less medication, and required fewer visits to the emergency room than children exposed to printed materials (Krishna et al., 2003).
- Information is quickly available when consumers need or want it, accommodating different needs and schedules.

- Graphics, color, and print size can be tailored to meet the needs of people with special needs and preferences.
- People have more control over the information they receive as compared to radio or TV, which can overwhelm people with information they do not consider relevant.
- Computer users can easily store information, replay items of interest, and forward information to others.

These advantages signal an empowerment on the part of media users that may affect their health knowledge and behaviors.

*Drawbacks* Computer-mediated communication is not without disadvantages, however.

- Although format changes are available, access for people with visual disabilities is still discouragingly limited. For example, not all health-related websites offer automated screen readers that allow people to hear a voice that reads the contents of the webpage and describes the graphics.

- Information is not always complete or reliable. Among 36 websites designed to educate teenagers about sexually transmitted diseases, only 2 provided information on how to negotiate with partners for safer sex practices (Keller, Labelle, Karimi, & Gupta, 2002). Another team of researchers found 41 inaccuracies in 18 cancer information websites (Bernstam, Walji, Sagaram, Sagaram, Johnson, & Meric-Bernstam, 2008).
- Online communication typically occurs without touching or watching other human beings, which limits nonverbal feedback and may add to people's sense of isolation (Quittner, 1995).
- Access is limited to people who have computers and know how to use them. Most researchers agree that using computers has become a fairly simple process. However, underprivileged populations are usually the most in need of health information but the last to get information technology (Eng et al., 1998).
- Important messages may be lost in the vast amount of information available. A recent Google search for "breast cancer" yielded more than 43.5 million hits.
- Technology specialist Tony Gorry points out that more information and quicker access is not always beneficial. For some people, multimedia is "confusing, disturbing, and may in fact not be understood" (quoted in "Reflections," 1997, p. 224).
- Fraud is hard to police online. Consumers must be vigilant about double-checking advice and product claims.

### Communication Skill Builders: Using the Internet

Because there is reliable and unreliable health information on the Internet, experts offer the following suggestions.

- Do not trust information if there is no author or sponsor or if the source given is not well known.

- Visit HealthNewsReview.org to see how experts rate the quality of information from various sources and to access a list of 5-star health news stories.
- Look for another source if the sponsors are trying to sell a product rather than offer free information. Plenty of websites make reliable health information available free.
- Do not rely on information if it is dated, references are missing, or references do not seem legitimate.
- Keep in mind that legitimate health practitioners do not speak in terms of "secret formulas" or "miraculous cures." Only con artists use such language (Kowalski, 1997). Other red-flag claims include such wording as "Treats all forms of cancer," "Cancer disappears," and "Nontoxic" ("Beware of Online," 2008, np).
- Don't be convinced by case studies of "actual" satisfied customers. An isolated case does not prove a product's effectiveness, and this may not be an actual customer (Kowalski, 1997).
- Do your own research. Read medical journal articles. Ask health professionals.
- Read the fine print very carefully. Look for disclaimers and vague wording.
- Report suspicious claims to the Federal Trade Commission, Better Business Bureau, or state attorney general's office.

## ENTERTAINMENT

Medical settings have long been popular for entertainment programs. Shows such as *Marcus Welby* and *General Hospital* were forerunners of today's popular medical dramas. This section examines how medical care and health issues are portrayed in entertainment programming. As Webb and colleagues (2007) point out: "In today's media-saturated world, education has become indistinguishable from entertainment and…popular films have an impact on beliefs, behaviors, attitudes, and knowledge" (p. e1226). Even programs designed entirely to entertain can have important implications for health.

## Portrayals of Health-Related Behaviors

*The mad scientists cackles as he prepares his next victim. The music rises, the lights dim...*

Characterizations like this are fun, but they are also suggestive. People base their perceptions of mental illness and other health concerns partly on fictional portrayals. In this section we examine the implications of media portrayals of mental illness, disabilities, sex, and violence.

*Mental Illness and Dementia* One media distortion is the traditional portrayal of mentally ill persons as violent and dangerous. That characterization never reflected reality. Only about 11% of people with mental illnesses are violent, which is roughly equal to the proportion of violent people in the overall population. James Willwerth (1993) attests: "In reality, most mentally ill patients are withdrawn, frightened and passive" (paragraph 6).

The incidence of violence among characters with mental illness has decreased in recent years. And for better or worse, some forms of mental illness have become popular topics in entertainment programming. One example is *Monk*, a USA Network program about a quirky, brilliant detective with obsessive-compulsive disorder. The series has won an Emmy and a Grammy—and it has been honored by the U.S. Substance Abuse and Mental Health Services Administration (SAMHSA) and the Anxiety Disorders Association of America. In the show, Monk is fond of saying that his obsessive attention to detail is "a blessing—and a curse." In some ways, it makes him extraordinarily good at what he does. In other ways, it limits and frightens him. A viewer poll on the *Monk* website asks guests to vote for Monk's weirdest phobia from a list that includes puppets, slime, driving, milk, monkeys, and more. However eccentric, such generally likeable media portrayals make a difference, according to SAMHSA administrator Charles G Curie. "The entertainment industry is a powerful vehicle for helping shape public opinion," says Curie. "Positive portrayals show the nation that people with mental health problems do live, learn, work, and fully participate in the American community" (SAMSHA, 2005, paragraph 5). Some applaud *Monk* for showing an appealing character who, although affected by a serious mental illness, is a brilliant and much-admired professional. Others are less comfortable with the show, pointing out that Adrian Monk is portrayed simultaneously as "needy, emotional, and plagued by self-doubts" (D. A. Johnson, 2008, paragraph 8).

*Disabilities* Television tends to perpetuate unrealistic stereotypes about people with physical disabilities. "The one-dimensional victim often portrayed in popular media accounts bears little resemblance to the actual lives of individuals with intellectual disabilities," writes researcher Carol Pardun (2005), who studied 3,900 media portrayals and newspaper articles about people with disabilities. Pardun found that 50% of media depictions show people with disabilities working in careers, whereas only about 32% of people with disabilities are actually employed, and 60% live in poverty, a condition not usually reflected in media portrayals. Pardun found that people with disabilities are disproportionately depicted as victims to be pitied and that persons with intellectual disabilities are nearly invisible in the media.

One effort to give people with disabilities a voice is *Ouch,* a website sponsored by the British Broadcasting Corporation (BBC). *Ouch* is an open forum in which people with disabilities can share views and read columns, calendars, and news items of interest. The largest number of features (29%) are about entertainment (movies, music, comedy, and so on), followed by health (15%) and travel and society (tied at 8%) (Thoreau, 2006). The website provides a safe place for readers to talk about episodes others might not understand. For example, Thoreau describes a funny and revealing article, "Holiday Diary: A White Man Abroad," in which a man with albinism reflects on a vacation with his friends. He wonders if he should color his hair before the trip to look a "wee bit more 'normal' " and worries about too much sun exposure, quipping, "I'm a white cap, for crissakes, and I'm gonna fry like a sausage in the sun" (quoted by Thoreau, p. 458). He also describes his relief that, once the vacation begins, he seems to "be topping the score" in terms of attracting women (p. 458). Thoreau reflects that the man's witty self-commentary finds an appreciative audience on the website but that an underlying theme of the article is the writer's sense of being, in many ways, isolated from and different than his friends.

*Sex* You're likely to see a lot of sex on TV, but exactly how much depends on when you watch. Sex in primetime programs has steadily but modestly decreased since 1975 (Hetsroni, 2007b). But other programs—such as soap operas and reality shows—have made up the difference. Overall, the proportion of programs that depict or imply sexual intercourse has doubled (from 7% to 14%) since 1997/1998 (Kunkel, Eyal, Donnerstein, Farrar, Biely, & Rideout, 2007). In programs that include sexual references, characters *talk* about sex about 4.6 times per hour and *have* sex (usually implied rather than shown explicitly) about 2 times per hour (Kunkel, Eyal, Finnerty, Biely, & Donnerstein, 2005). Kunkel and associates (2005) write: "If the topic of sex on television was frequent in the past, it is now nearly ubiquitous" (Conclusion, paragraph 8).

A few other trends are notable as well.

- More homosexual couples than ever before are having sex on the small screen (Hetsroni, 2007b). Whereas TV references to homosexual sex were virtually nonexistent in 1975, the topic is now raised once every 3 or 4 viewing hours during primetime (Hetsroni).
- There has been a dramatic decrease in the amount of teen sex portrayed on TV (Kunkel et al., 2005). TV sex is more likely to occur between married partners (Hetsroni, 2007b).
- There are slightly fewer acts of sexual aggression on TV than in the past (Hetsroni, 2007b).

In terms of safer-sex references, the numbers are higher than they used to be but still quite low. About 1 in 25 TV sex scenes includes verbal or visual reference to safer-sex methods (Kunkel et al., 2005). But such references are far more scarce (about 1 in 200 episodes) when you figure in music, magazines, and movies aimed at teen audiences (Hust, Brown, & L'Engle, 2008). Stacey Hust and colleagues surveyed more than 3,000 middle school students about their favorite programs, magazines, songs, and recording artists and then content-analyzed the most popular choices. They found that, across formats aimed at teen audiences, safer sex is still depicted as "humiliating and humorous" (p. 14), boys are portrayed as sexually ravenous, and sexual protection is considered girls' responsibility. The researchers report: "In the rare instances when condoms were discussed or depicted, boys had condoms as a kind of toy, whereas girls were more knowledgeable and more likely to have a condom when it was needed" (p. 17). Even when condoms were present, they were usually treated comically rather than as topics of serious discussion with health consequences.

There is evidence that adolescents exposed to large amounts of sex in the media are more likely than others to have sex at a young age. In one study, researchers compared 12- to 17-year-olds in the 90th percentile of TV-sex viewing with same-age peers in the 10th percentile or lower. Heavy viewers were significantly more likely to have sex within a year of the study (R. L. Collins et al., 2004). Other research suggests it's not just how *much* sex adolescents view, but how realistic they consider it to be. In a study of Dutch teens, Peter & Valkenburg (2006) found that adolescents (particularly boys) who viewed what they considered to be realistic online sex typically considered it instructional about how to have sex in real life. They were subsequently more likely than their peers to consider having sex in the near future and to approve of sex in casual relationships.

Of course, we can't assume that media sex causes interest in real-life sex. It may be the other way around—that people who are already interested in sex more readily seek out media depictions of it. Either way, the issue is important, considering that sexually active adolescents are at higher risk than adults for contracting sexually transmitted infections (STIs), including HIV ("Sexual Health," 2008). Nearly 46,000 adolescents in the United States have already contracted HIV, and about 9.1 million are stricken with other STIs every year. Additionally, about 42 in 1,000 female teens give birth in the United States each year ("Sexual Health").

*Violence* Contrary to popular opinion, primetime television is not more violent than ever before. Based on Amir Hetsroni's (2007a) meta-analysis of 40 years of related research, the incidence of primetime violence peaked in the late 1970s and the mid-1990s, when viewers were likely to see between 5.5 and 7.3 assaults per hour. By 2002, murders in primetime television were half as numerous as in 1997. Violence may be down, but there's still a lot of it. No matter what time you watch TV, you are likely to see violence in two out of three programs (S. L. Smith, Nathanson, & Wilson, 2002). And the movies are no better. Even the previews are violent. About 75.7% of movie previews include violence, and 56% show sexuality (Oliver & Kalyanaraman, 2002).

One criticism of media violence is that the effects are so unrealistic. People run through machine gun fire unscathed. They are shot or stabbed but continue to perform like athletes. Evil characters die, but heroes seldom do. George Gerbner (1996) calls it happy violence: "'Happy violence' is cool, swift, painless, and always leads to a happy ending, so as to deliver the audience to the next commercial in a receptive mood" (paragraph 10). In a study of PG-13 movies, Theresa Webb and colleagues (2007) report that, although violence was prevalent, enduring harm to victims was "either nonexistent or largely unrealistic" (p. e1226). In the fast-paced world of entertainment, it seems violence is popular but lengthy recoveries are boring. The result is an on-screen world in which violence lacks serious consequences.

Most researchers agree that there is an association between violence in the media and violence in real life. As the first generations to grow up with television have reached adulthood, the evidence is convincing that children exposed to media violence are more likely than others to engage in violent behavior themselves (Huesmann, Moise-Titus, Podolski,

& Eron, 2003; Wartella, 1996). Graphic violence in video games has also been linked to aggression among children (Eastin & Griffiths, 2006; Pesky & Blascovich, 2007). In one study, youth who played a video game with "blood on" (an option that displays gory depictions of characters' wounds) were slightly but significantly more likely than "blood-off" players to indicate feelings of anger and to say they would react violently if someone ran into them on the sidewalk (Farrar, Krcmar, & Nowak, 2006).

Of course, not everyone reacts to media violence in the same way, and it is difficult to isolate media effects among the many factors that influence people (Haridakis, 2006). Women tend to use the media to moderate their mood when they feel angry, whereas males studied were more likely to choose programs that mirrored their anger (Knobloch-Westerwick & Alter, 2006). For some people, violence in the media is a substitute for acting out. For others, media images tend to escalate their sense of aggression. One prevalent effect of media violence, even when people do not feel more aggressive themselves, is that high media users tend to feel afraid and to overestimate the threat of violence in their environment (Nabi & Sullivan, 2001; Romer, Jamieson, & Aday, 2003).

## Portrayals of Health Care Situations

Medical dramas seem to offer a backstage pass to medicine. What most people "know" about the interior of a surgery unit or a doctor's lounge they learned from television. Areas usually off limits to the public are open for inspection, or at least it seems that way. In some ways, medical dramas are likely to give people mistaken impressions about the way medical work is done.

*Medical Miracles* Based on television portrayals, it may seem that heroic rescues and miraculous recoveries are the norm. Kimberly A. Neuendorf (1990) dubbed the tendency to portray doctors as "all-powerful and all-good" the "Marcus Welby syndrome." Health crises arise and are resolved on TV in 30-minute or 1-hour segments, compared to the weeks or months often required to resolve real-life medical conditions.

One group of researchers (Diem, Lantos, & Tulsky, 1996) studied instances of CPR (cardiopulmonary resuscitation) in TV episodes. On television, CPR was usually administered to children and young adults, and most of them recovered fully and quickly. Some even regained full health in a matter of minutes. In everyday life, however, CPR is most often used to help older adults having heart attacks, and it only saves 2% to 30% of actual patients, many of whom suffer lasting disabilities. Susan Diem and coauthors conclude that television medical dramas encourage people to believe in miracles that are not likely to occur.

Entertainment programming also perpetuates myths about organ donation. In their study of network television programs, Susan Morgan and colleagues (2007) found numerous storylines about organs sold illegally, people murdered for their organs, doctors giving preferential treatment to their favorite organ recipients, and people allowed to die prematurely so that others could have their organs. The researchers also found fictional accounts of organ recipients who behave criminally or irresponsibly, squandering the life-sustaining gift they have received. On television, donors are often depicted as "good people," but a corrupt system sometimes treats them as nothing more than "spare parts" (Morgan et al., p. 148). All of these depictions—though the stuff of exciting drama—are grossly unrealistic. "We often wonder where members of the public get 'crazy ideas' about organ donation like the existence of the black market, the corruption of the organ allocation system, and the untrustworthiness of doctors," the authors reflect. "The answer may have been quite literally in front of us for years" (Morgan, Harrison, Chewning, Davis, & DiCorcia, 2007, p. 149).

## Entertainment and Commercialism

It is usually easy to tell the difference between a commercial and a television program or movie. But what if a commercial looks like entertainment or commercial messages are subtly embedded in entertainment programming?

*Entertainomercials*   Journalists have coined the term **entertainomercials** to characterize sales pitches that resemble entertainment programming ("Entertainomercials," 1996). A classic example involved Joe Camel, the former cartoonlike mascot of Camel cigarettes. R. J. Reynolds Tobacco Company introduced the colorful, sunglass-wearing camel in 1988 advertising. Although company officials insisted the animated character was not meant to capture children's interest, it had that effect. Sales of Camel cigarettes to children rose from $6 million per year to $476 million per year (DiFranza et al., 1991). Within a few years, children were as familiar with Joe Camel as with Mickey Mouse (Fischer, Schwartz, Richards, & Goldstein, 1991). Under public and legal pressure, Reynolds ceased using images of Joe Camel in 1997, after a 10-year run (Vest, 1997).

*Product Placement*   The tobacco industry is also involved in another type of commercial/entertainment blend called product placement. *Product placement* means that a sponsor pays (with cash, props, services, or so on) to have a product or brand name included in a movie, a television program, a video game, or some other form of entertainment (Babin & Carder, 1996). Subtle product placements (sometimes called *stealth ads*) can be considered a form of subliminal advertising, in that the viewer may not be consciously aware of seeing items displayed but may develop an impression about them based on their association with other elements of the drama (Erdelyi & Zizak, 2004). At the very least, critics argue, when viewers suspend disbelief to enjoy the reality of an entertainment program they shouldn't have to worry that they are being exposed to embedded commercial messages all the while.

For a time, the Federal Communication Commission (FCC) forbade paid product placements within television programs. The rule was only loosely enforced, however, and it went out the window in a culture filled with online pop-up ads anyway. The Nielsen Company, famous for establishing viewership ratings, now has its own product placement division. Company officials report that 204,919 brand-name references or images appeared in U.S. TV shows in the first six months of 2008 (Moss, 2008). The leader of the pack was *American Idol,* which included 4,636 of those product placements (N. Anderson, 2008). A number of reality shows, such as *Survivor* and *Big Brother,* also make the top 10. As this book went to press, the FCC was considering new guidelines—not to ban product placements (that's probably a lost cause)—but to make viewers more aware of them. Although some watchdog groups have called for the word ADVERTISEMENT to appear on the screen each time a product is shown, the reality will probably be closer to a listing of product sponsors in programs' opening and/or closing credits.

Product placements have always been allowed in movies, and the numbers are increasing. Steven Spielberg earned $25 million for placing 15 brand-name products in the movie *Minority Report,* leading at least one reviewer to comment on the irony of the characters' on-screen resistance to a mind-controlling regime (King, 2002). Other notable examples include Reese's Pieces in *E.T.,* the Dr. Pepper can that Peter Parker uses for target practice in *Spider-Man,* the FedEx trucks and planes in *Castaway* (not to mention the FedEx box that is with Tom Hanks' character for most of the movie), AOL logos and the famous AOL line "You've Got Mail" in the movie titled with that line, and the sports cars showcased in James Bond movies.

Product placements become health communication when they concern the way people think or behave concerning health issues. This may range from an emphasis on fast food and cigarettes to athletic gear. A particular concern arises when product placements are used to dodge restrictions on conventional advertising. Tobacco industry documents obtained in the 1990s suggest companies secretly reward actors and producers to display their cigarettes prominently in the movies (Basil, 1997). Stars, including Sean Connery, Sylvester Stallone, Paul Newman, and Clint Eastwood, have allegedly accepted expensive cars and jewelry in return for smoking brand-name cigarettes on the big screen. Promoting cigarettes in this way violates several restrictions: (1) the prohibition on advertising tobacco on radio, TV, or in the movies, (2) the ban on celebrity endorsements, and (3) federal law requiring health warnings on all tobacco packages and advertisements (Basil, 1997). These restrictions, initiated in the 1960s, are based on medical evidence that tobacco products are serious health hazards (Jacobson, Wasserman, & Anderson, 1997).

As the next section shows, some people have decided to fight fire with fire, using the product placement strategy to promote recommended health behaviors. See Box 11.5 for ethical issues related to health images in entertainment programs.

### Entertainment-Education Programming

Producers may embed subtle messages in programs, not to sell products but to educate or persuade people regarding health matters. Efforts to benefit the public using an entertainment format are known as **entertainment-education** or pro-social programming. The idea, say Piotrow and colleagues, is that "no one enjoys being lectured to but everyone enjoys and often learns from entertainment, whether broadcast through radio or television, or performed in person" (Piotrow, Rimon, Merritt, & Saffitz, 2003, p. 5).

Entertainment producers today are likely to be lobbied by health advocates urging them to incorporate health messages in their scripts, props, and story lines. The Hollywood, Health & Society program helps entertainment writers portray health issues in accurate and informative ways. Medical experts and Hollywood insiders provide tip sheets about health issues and offer story ideas and scripts to incorporate health information in entertainment programming. On the website (www.learcenter.org/html/projects/?cm=hhs), entertainment writers can find information about topics ranging from AIDS, to bat bites, to car seats, to suicide, and West Nile fever.

The Entertainment Industries Council sponsors a similar program as well as a website (eiconline.

## BOX 11.5 ETHICAL CONSIDERATIONS

# Is the Entertainment Industry Responsible for Health Images?

Does the entertainment industry have a responsibility to promote healthy behaviors? Some claim that entertainment writers and producers behave irresponsibly when they consistently portray unhealthy and unrealistic images of life and health.

One way the media distorts reality is by showing unhealthy and violent behaviors without the natural consequences (Gerbner, 1996). People are shot with guns but continue to run and fight. Others overeat but appear to be slender and healthy nevertheless (J. D. Brown & Walsh-Childers, 1994). Another way media messages often misrepresent health is by depicting ill (especially mentally ill) individuals as dangerous, corrupt, and antisocial (Signorielli, 1993).

Taking the concept of reality TV to new extremes, some programs have begun staging medical tests as public forms of entertainment. For example, on a television program in the United Kingdom, fathers were invited to air their suspicions about their partners' infidelity. The results of paternity tests on the men's children were announced on the air (V. English, Critchley-Romano, Sheather, & Sommerville, 2002). Medical ethicists observe that the United States has set a precedent for this type of reality-shock programs. Whereas documentaries about giving birth and undergoing plastic surgery may be educational, programs like the one just described are meant only to shock and entertain. Some question the ethics of using medical procedures as entertainment and violating the privacy of nonconsenting participants (such as the men's children).

Some people argue that the entertainment industry need not offer such a shocking or distorted view of reality. They challenge Hollywood to create engrossing yet realistic programming. Going one step further, some people advocate pro-social programming to educate people while they are entertained.

On the other side of the issue, people argue that entertainment programming should not be harnessed to a social agenda. They feel that artistic creativity is compromised when writers and producers must adhere to social guidelines. Moreover, they say, it is difficult to know whose agenda should prevail. When health professionals disagree about specific guidelines for healthy living, is it entertainers' job to decide which viewpoint should be represented? If the industry is held to a standard of realism, they wonder what will become of fantasy themes and movies made famous by earlier generations, when different social expectations prevailed.

## What Do You Think?

1. Does entertainment programming influence people's behavior? For instance, would people be more likely to use condoms if they saw their favorite characters talking about them in television programs or movies?

2. Should entertainers consider how their programs might influence audience members?

3. Do you think it is irresponsible of the entertainment industry to misrepresent the natural consequences of violent or otherwise-unhealthy behavior?

4. Do you think it would diminish the entertainment value of your favorite movies and TV shows if they showed healthy behaviors or realistic consequences?

5. Do you believe programs designed specifically to promote healthy behaviors would be popular in the United States? Do you think such programs should be created? Why or why not?

org) and a guidebook useful in depicting health and social issues in entertainment programming. Council sponsors suggest terminology to convey accurately the dangers of high-risk behaviors. For example, they caution against using the term *hard drugs* because it implies incorrectly that drugs that are not "hard" are relatively harmless. The council also recommends that characters be shown using seat belts and other safety devices.

In some countries, entire programs have been created to promote healthy behaviors. After *Nunl Dhuhyo!* (Open Your Eyes!) segments began airing on Korean television, the number of people who signed cornea donation cards increased from 1,239 to 13,733 (Bae & Kang, 2008). In the show, celebrity hosts conduct moving interviews with people who are hoping for cornea transplants to restore their sight.

A radio drama in Ethiopia, *Journal of Life,* depicted a main character who contracted HIV during an isolated sexual indiscretion and then unknowingly infected his wife. A random survey of the radio audience revealed that most listeners became emotionally involved in the storyline and that their resolve to engage in safer-sex practices increased the more episodes they heard (R. A. Smith, Downs, & Witte, 2007).

Sponsors of a multimedia entertainment-education campaign in North India broadcast a variety of PSAs and entertainment-education programs about HIV and AIDS (Sood, Shefner-Rogers, & Sengupta, 2006). In one program, *Jasoos Vijay,* radio and television audiences followed the actions of a detective with HIV played by a popular Bollywood actor. As the storylines progressed, audiences learned more about the discrimination, the medical care, and the diverse abilities and contributions of people with HIV/AIDS, and they were invited to get personally involved by writing in each week to share their views on who-done-it before Vijay solved the crimes. Another component of the campaign was a year-long reality TV show in which the show's producers traveled to communities throughout North India to engage young people in lively challenges that tested their knowledge of HIV/AIDS. Suruchi Sood and colleagues (2006) report that people exposed to the

---

### BOX 11.6 **RESOURCES**

# More About Product Placement and Entertainment-Education

Greene, M. C., Strange, J. J., & Brock, T. C. (Eds.). (2002). *Narrative impact: Social and cognitive foundations.* Mahwah, NJ: Lawrence Erlbaum.

Shurn, L. J. (Ed.) (2004). *The psychology of entertainment media: Blurring the lines between entertainment and persuasion.* Mahwah, NJ: Lawrence Erlbaum.

Zillmann, D., & Vorderer, P. (Eds.) (2000). *Media entertainment: The psychology of its appeal.* Mahwah, NJ: Lawrence Erlbaum.

---

campaign were more knowledgeable than others about HIV transmission and more likely to talk to others about the issue.

Other forms of influential education—which may or may not be created intentionally for the purpose—are the narratives in books, movies, plays, TV shows, and even the stories people share with each other personally. When people identify with the people portrayed and feel emotionally involved with them, they can be transported to worlds beyond their personal experience (M. C. Greene, 2006). Such narratives can be culturally sensitive and eye-opening (Petraglia, 2007). People may model the actions (good or bad) of the characters and allow themselves, through the story, to consider new ideas and perspectives. Evocative narratives can create what Melanie Greene (2006) calls a "mental simulation" of situations that are new or frightening. A particularly promising use of narratives is their value in helping people cope with health challenges such as cancer. Noted theorist Melanie Greene (2006) proposes that "narratives have the potential to both change cancer-related beliefs and motivate health behaviors" (p. S178).

For more on product placement and entertainment education, see Box 11.6.

## Impact of Persuasive Entertainment

Before you become too optimistic (or perturbed) about the prospects for incorporating messages within entertainment, it is important to ask: Beyond the effects already mentioned, do messages in entertainment programs make much difference?

Some theorists believe media images affect the way people view society, but not necessarily the way they view themselves personally. **Social adaptation theory** suggests that people evaluate messages by considering how useful the information is likely to be in their lives (Perse, Nathanson, & McLeod, 1996). In this regard, entertainment may have an edge over news. Leslie Snyder and Ruby Rouse (1995) found that people perceived entertainment portrayals to be more relevant to their lives than news items, probably because entertainment episodes tend to be more intimate and vivid. Snyder and Rouse's study revealed that movies and television programs increased people's perception of personal AIDS risk, while news coverage decreased their sense of being personally vulnerable. The researchers concluded that the dramatic nature of entertainment programming often makes it seem up-close and personal, whereas news seems to depict what happens to "other people."

Concerning product placement, there are a few (but not many) striking success stories. After a character on *The Young & the Restless* saved a child using CPR techniques he "learned at the Red Cross," the Red Cross received thousands of calls from interested people (Drum, 1997). When a product placement deal put James Bond behind the wheel of a BMW Z3 roadster in *Goldeneye*, the car maker had to put anxious buyers on waiting lists ("Let Us Put," 1996). Likewise, the sales of Reese's Pieces rose 65% after the release of *E.T.*, which depicted them as the favorite snack of a lovable outer space creature (Babin & Carder, 1996).

Success stories aside, most product placements seem to do no more than increase brand-name recognition. College students who watched movie clips that included product placements were more inclined than others to say they would choose the brand from a range of similar alternatives (Moonhee & Roskos-Ewoldsen, 2007). But this depended largely on how prominently the product figured in the movie. Background depictions did not have much effect, but audiences were influenced by products that characters (especially likeable characters) used actively, especially if they were integral to the plot.

One cause for concern is the underlying power dynamic of some education-entertainment programs. From a critical-cultural perspective, Dutta (2006) argues that education entertainment programs are typically designed to serve the goals, values, and priorities of the funding entity rather than those of the target community. The result can be a form of cultural hegemony in which the values of the dominant culture are imposed on members of the marginalized community, without respect for (or even awareness of) the community's own values, culture, and circumstances. Another danger is that sponsors will focus on individual aspects of a problem—as in having fewer children per family—rather than tackling larger and more systemic issues such as the need to allocate resources fairly to all people (Dutta). These efforts tend to hurt more than they help, particularly considering that the philanthropic goal of a funding entity is often based on a deeper, more self-serving desire to create stable markets for its good and services, ensure tranquility in regions rich with natural resources, and so on. The tendency to impose the agenda of the powerful can be offset by involving community members in open dialogue and participation before, during, and after campaigns. But Dutta warns that many "participatory" efforts actually involve choosing between options preselected by campaign designers. In his view, only when social programming is created with an open and rich appreciation for the circumstances, culture, and needs of the focus community can we expect it to foster real and meaningful change. (We'll talk more about the critical-cultural perspective in Chapter 14.)

## MEDIA LITERACY

This chapter concludes where it began, with the reminder that the media's influence is by no means uniform. People are affected differently and to varying extents. Perhaps the best defense against excessive or negative media influence is the ability to analyze messages logically (Austin & Meili, 1994). This is a central tenet of media literacy.

**Media literacy** is defined as awareness and skills that allow a person to evaluate media content in terms of what is realistic and useful (adapted from Potter, 1998). According to Dorothy Singer and Jerome Singer's (1998) seminal overview, media-literate individuals are aware that advertisers are apt to highlight (and even exaggerate) the attractive aspects of their products and to downplay the disadvantages. They evaluate the creators' intent and try to figure out what is not being said and why. Media-literate individuals are also skillful at identifying portrayals that are unrealistic or have been enhanced by special effects. Overall, media-literate individuals tend to evaluate messages in terms of fairness and appropriateness, weighing ideas for themselves.

## Teaching Media Literacy

Media literacy instruction usually involves an informative, an analytic, and an experiential stage. Arli Quesada and Sue Summers (1998) have described these stages well, and the discussion here is based on their work.

In the **informative stage,** participants in media literacy programs learn to identify different types of messages (persuasive, informative, and entertaining) and different types of media (television, radio, newspapers, and so on). They learn about the strengths and limitations of various media. For example, Internet resources are vast and accessible, but some sources are not trustworthy. Participants also learn about production techniques and special effects.

In the **analytic stage,** participants discuss their perceptions of media in general and of specific media messages. In this stage they typically deconstruct messages with guidance from a trained leader. **Deconstructing** a message means breaking it down into specific components, such as key points, purpose, implied messages, production techniques, and

---

**BOX 11.7 RESOURCES**

## Tobacco and Media Literacy

Real Parents. Real Answers: www.realparentsrealanswers.com

Teens, Tobacco & The Media resource guide: depts.washington.edu/thmedia/view.cgi?section=tobacco&page=teenprojects

Center for Media Literacy: www.medialit.org/reading_room/article420.html

American Legacy Foundation: www.americanlegacy.org

---

goals. For instance, beer commercials often present a social reality in which drinking is fun and sexy. In deconstructing a beer commercial (or any other media message), participants try to identify the message's purpose, what information is missing from it, and how it compares to their own social reality. They might conclude that beer companies make drinking look fun to sell their products, but the reality is something more than or different from what the commercials show. Finally, in the **experiential stage**, media literacy programs challenge participants to write their own news stories, design ads, perform skits, and participate in other creative efforts to help them understand the process and demystify the way media messages are created. Adolescents who have taken part in tobacco-related media literacy programs are more likely than others to think carefully about tobacco commercials and to decide not to smoke (Pinkleton, Austin, Cohen, Miller, & Fitzgerald, 2007). A particularly useful technique is to have them create their own antismoking messages (Banerjee & Greene, 2006). (See Box 11.7 for resources about tobacco media literacy.)

Media literacy skills have been taught successfully to people of different ages. In one project, third-graders watched a 28-minute video about advertising techniques and took part in guided discussions (Austin & Johnson, 1997). Following this brief exercise, they were more likely than other children to identify commercials as sales pitches, to see them as unrealistic, and to judge for themselves whether the behaviors depicted were appropriate and desirable.

A similar project helped college students critique fashion advertisements, noting how extremely thin or muscular the models were (Rabak-Wagener, Eickhoff-Shemek, & Kelly-Vance, 1998). The students were challenged to redesign the ads using models of different body sizes, ages, ethnicities, and physical abilities. They were consequently less likely to believe people should look like supermodels and were more satisfied with their own bodies.

Media literacy can be taught at home when parents help children understand aspects of the media messages they encounter. This is known as **parental mediation**. Adults are often able to make children aware of inaccuracies and discrepancies in media messages. For example, "Why does this program show thin people eating fattening foods?" (Austin, 1995) or "Is the violence shown in this program realistic?" (Nathanson & Yang, 2003). Research suggests that children get maximum benefits from media (while minimizing unfavorable influences) when their parents (1) limit media exposure, (2) choose programs with care, (3) watch, listen, or read alongside them, and (4) discuss program content with them (Austin, 1993; Austin, Roberts, & Nass, 1990; Singer & Singer, 1998).

Although the research about media literacy is encouraging overall, it does not suggest a cure-all. Some stereotypes persist, even when people have explicitly been told they are not valid. College students who watched a movie about a mentally ill murderer were more negative in their assessment of mentally ill persons than students who viewed an unrelated film (Wahl & Lefkowits, 1989). This was true even when the students saw a message stating that violence is not a characteristic of mental illness. The authors conclude that awareness and information campaigns will not be entirely successful at counteracting negative media portrayals.

## SUMMARY

Whether you regard the media as friend or foe, mass-mediated messages are an important component of health communication. The distinction in this chapter between advertising, news, and entertainment is useful for explanatory purposes, but do not forget that actual media exposure involves a great deal of blending and juxtaposing. For instance, a news story about eating disorders may be followed by an advertisement featuring unnaturally thin models. Such clashes are common, and contradictions of this nature may mitigate the effects of health-conscious messages.

Although it is difficult to say to what degree people's actions are affected by advertising, significant influence is suggested by the number of people who eat the unhealthy food advertisers promote, drink the beverages they sell, and strive to emulate supermodels. As Timothy Gibson (2007) puts it, "Our physical health depends, at least in part, upon the health of our media environment" (p. 125). Based on cultivation theory, children and adolescents may be especially susceptible to advertising messages because their frame of reference is limited. Social comparison theory suggests people strive to measure up to "idealized" characters in the media, even when the ideals are far from attainable. Sometimes advertisers make natural conditions seem bad or unnatural (pathological) so that people will pay money to change them. Although advertising offers many advantages, it can be harmful if it encourages poor nutrition, drug and alcohol abuse, or an unhealthy reliance on cosmetics and fad diets.

As one of only two countries to allow direct-to-consumer advertising, the United States is navigating relatively uncharted ground. DTCA offers a few advantages but presents a number of challenges and ethical dilemmas related to social justice, research objectivity, full disclosure, and market agendas versus altruism.

News coverage of health issues is important for sharing valuable knowledge. However, news audiences should remember that scientific findings are usually tentative, news stories tend to focus on unusual concerns, and coverage may be influenced by the desire to please advertisers or attract new audiences.

Interactive technology combines elements of mass media with interpersonal communication. Participants are able to access information written for mass audiences, but they have the option of responding, asking questions, making requests, and choosing what information they wish to receive. The challenge now becomes securing computer access and discriminating between reliable and unreliable information.

Entertainment portrayals may influence what people believe about medical care, risky behavior, and people with disabilities. Sex and violence are shown mostly for entertainment value, not as serious subjects with health consequences. In reality, medical miracles are less common than as shown on television, and people are more diverse.

Do not be surprised if the food, drinks, cigarettes, vehicles, and props in your favorite programs and movies were put in purposefully to please advertisers. Although product placements may not look like commercials, advertisers go to great expense hoping that they will function like commercials. Health advocates use the same tactic to insert health messages into some entertainment programs, a practice known as education-entertainment programming.

Finally, media literacy allows people some control over how media messages affect them. Wise consumers learn to distinguish between reliable and unreliable information by critiquing media messages to determine their purposes, strengths, and limitations.

## KEY TERMS

mass communication
third-person effect
direct-to-consumer advertising (DTCA)
cultivation theory
social comparison theory
pathologizing the human body
entertainomercials
product placement
entertainment-education
social adaptation theory
media literacy
informative stage
analytic stage
deconstructing
experiential stage
parental mediation

## DISCUSSION QUESTIONS

1. What is the third-person effect, and does it ring true with you? Do you assume that other people are influenced more by media messages than you are? Why or why not?

2. In what ways are pharmaceutical drug advertisements beneficial? In what ways can they be harmful?

3. Have you ever become interested in a drug because you saw it advertised? If so, why? Did you do more research or ask your doctor about it? Why or why not?

4. Do you think it matters that some types of people aren't depicted in pharmaceutical ads as often as others? Why or why not?

5. What are some tips for being an effective consumer relevant to pharmaceutical advertisements?

6. How does television viewing seem to affect children's eating habits and knowledge of nutrition?

7. What evidence suggests that alcoholic beverage makers target underage youth? Have you seen experience of this yourself? If so, how? Did it have any effect?

8. Based on cultivation theory, why do you think children are particularly susceptible to media messages?

9. In what ways do advertisers pathologize the human body? What are the health implications?

10. In what ways are health news items frequently distorted in the mass media? What are some reasons for this?

11. What are the advantages and disadvantages of health news coverage in the mass media?

12. What are some suggestions for reporters covering health topics?

13. What are some advantages and drawbacks of using interactive computer technology to educate people about health?

14. Name some tips for avoiding health scams and for using the Internet wisely.

15. If you have seen the TV show *Monk,* do you regard the portrayal of mental illness as mostly favorable or unfavorable? Why?

16. What are some recent trends in how sex is portrayed in entertainment programming?

17. Based on what you have read, is it reasonable to conclude that viewing a lot of sex on TV or online will lead adolescents to have sex at a younger age? Why or why not?

18. What did Gerbner mean by the term *happy violence*? Can you give some examples from your own media experience?

19. How might people be misled by media images of health care situations?

20. Do you favor FTC guidelines that require producers to make it clear that they have accepted money for product placement? Why or why not? What method of disclosure do you think would be most effective?

21. How does promoting cigarettes in the movies violate advertising regulations?

22. Name some examples of education-entertainment programming. Have you noticed product placements before? Do they influence your buying preferences?

23. Describe some examples of entertainment-education programming.

24. When is entertainment-education most effective? What ethical considerations should be involved?

25. Describe the steps in teaching media literacy.

## ANSWERS TO *CAN YOU GUESS?*

1. On average, broadcast and cable TV stations devote less than one-third of a minute (17 seconds) per hour to PSAs. That is less than one-half of 1% of airtime. And 46% of PSAs run between midnight and 6 a.m. ("Study Finds," 2008).

2. In 65 years, the average person will spend a total of 11.3 years in front of a TV set ("Nielsen Reports," 2008).

# CHAPTER 12

# Public Health Crises and Health Care Reform

In 1986, a strange malady began afflicting cattle in Great Britain. Affected animals stumbled and staggered, unable to walk normally. Some of them became paralyzed. All died within a year of displaying symptoms, their brains partially eaten away by a disease that came to be called *bovine spongiform encephalopathy (BSE)*, or, more commonly, mad cow disease.

Scientists were unable to explain how the cattle got the disease, but it was similar in some respects to a neurological disease, scrapie, that had long affected sheep. Affected sheep would compulsively scratch themselves on fence posts and other materials. They, too, would inevitably wither and die, their brains full of spongy holes.

The similarity between scrapie and BSE was apparent, but scientists and public health experts lacked definitive answers to some important questions: (1) Through what means was the disease being transmitted from sheep to cattle, if that was indeed the source? (2) Could the disease jump to humans next?

The stakes were high. On the one hand there was no evidence, only conjecture, that the disease could be communicated to humans. Alerting the public might cause widespread fear. And there were economic concerns. Short of exterminating all the cattle in Great Britain, authorities were unsure how to stop BSE. On the other hand, silence would rob people of the opportunity to avoid exposure to what was, potentially, a deadly, incurable disease. British officials reassured the public that there was no known risk.

All the while, following a procedure common at the time, many of the deceased animals were being ground up and their bones and tissue (which are potent and inexpensive sources of protein) incorporated into feed for livestock, including other cows. In the early 1980s, to cut costs, farmers had altered the process to allow fatty and nerve tissue to remain in the mixture. By the time researchers realized that the disease was spread through contact with infected brain and nerve tissue, it was too late. Farmers had literally fed the disease to surviving members of their herds and perhaps to humans as well.

In 1988, officials banned the use of animal products in livestock feed, but the ban was not strictly enforced for several more years (Henahan, 1996). They also called for the slaughter of infected cattle and those behaving suspiciously. But because the government initially compensated farmers at only about 50% of market value for sacrificed animals, farmers had little economic incentive to be vigilant (Dora, 2006).

In the meantime, British officials continued to insist there was no cause for alarm. In 1990, the Minster of Agriculture, John Gummer, staged a public photo opportunity during which he fed his 4-year-old daughter a hamburger (Lyall, 2000).

The public was not reassured. By 1993 more than 1,000 cases of BSE were surfacing every week (Henahan, 1996). To make matters worse, it emerged that the incubation period was as long as 7 years. Cattle are typically slaughtered when they are 3 to 5 years old, meaning that untold numbers of infected (but as yet asymptomatic) animals were being allowed into the animal and human food supply.

British authorities were still telling people not to worry. But the numbers kept escalating. Ultimately 200,000 cattle in Great Britain were diagnosed with BSE, and 3.7 million were destroyed in precautionary efforts, causing the "near destruction of Great Britain's cattle industry" (M. O. Adams & Osho, nd, p. 1).

In 1995 and 1996, two teenagers died in Great Britain from a variant of Creutzfeldt-Jakob disease (vCJD), a fatal neurological disorder that causes brain damage similar to that of BSE. Researchers speculated that BSE might be involved. Other cases followed, and vCJD was definitively linked to beef consumption.

Finally, 10 years after they became aware of BSE, British officials publicly admitted the risk to humans. In the book *Mad Cows and Mothers' Milk,* Leiss, Powell, and Whitfield (2004) lament that it took so long. They say officials' eagerness to downplay the issue resulted in "years of mismanagement, political bravado, and a gross underestimation of the public's capacity to deal with risk" (pp. 3–4).

Investigators for national and worldwide agencies have reviewed the mad cow disease saga, seeking lessons and identifying factors that led British officials to suppress this public health threat even as evidence of its severity mounted. They speculate that the following factors played a role.

- In Great Britain, as in many countries, agency boundaries made it unclear who had ultimate jurisdiction and whose interests should prevail. Involved were agencies in charge of food safety, agriculture, public health, international commerce, and more.

- Economic concerns discouraged aggressive action. Alarming the public might mean a drop in beef consumption; bankruptcy for farmers, meat packers, and others; food shortages; and so on. (Ultimately inaction proved more costly. Not only did domestic consumption plummet, but at one point British beef was banned worldwide).

- Officials were wary of creating panic.

- Decision makers were hesitant to make judgment calls without scientific data.

- Officials were overwhelmed when the public and media urgently desired information, but the information available was changing and incomplete. Spokespersons often deemed it preferable to deliver words of comfort than to admit how much they didn't know.

- Because vCJD mimicked some of the symptoms of other neurological disorders, it was difficult to know exactly when, or if, BSE had affected humans.

- Officials were reassured by patterns of the past. Scrapie had been plaguing sheep for about 200 years with no known transmission to humans. It was tempting to assume BSE would be the same (Ashraf, 2000).

- National leaders assumed that precautionary measures (e.g., changing livestock food and slaughtering infected herds) would be enough to halt the disease trajectory.

These factors underscore the complexity of public health and risk communication. It is easy to judge harshly from a distance and with the advantage of hindsight, and certainly we all want public health professionals to be honest with the public. But perhaps the greatest lesson is that handling a public health crisis is anything but easy. Dissecting past experiences is not meant to condemn the perpetrators so much as to help us avoid making the same mistakes again.

The BSE saga has calmed somewhat in recent years. Because researchers were able to ascertain how the disease was spread and regulators took action (albeit slowly), about 95% of BSE cases have been confined to Great Britain, and the numbers have decreased dramatically. However, boundaries are porous in our world economy. Cattle have been diagnosed with BSE in 24 countries (World Organisation for Animal Health, 2008). As of this writing, isolated cases were still being reported.

The greatest failure was one of communication. The public was kept in the dark about a lethal health threat. If people had been warned earlier of a danger—even a danger about which little was known—they could have chosen for themselves whether to eat beef. To date, 164 people have died from vCJD (Creutzfeldt-Jakob Disease Statistics, 2008). The numbers have tapered off since 2004, but one fact has scientists worried: The disease can take more than 25 years to incubate in humans. It's possible that people are infected and don't know it yet.

The complexity and importance of public health require us to be especially vigilant, principled, and well prepared. This chapter focuses on the overlap of a number of perspectives—public health, risk communication, crisis communication, and health care reform. We could spend an entire book on any one of these topics, and I encourage you to pursue them in more depth. Resource boxes throughout the chapter will get you started. But for now, there is an advantage in focusing on the overlap. It gives us an opportunity to look at real-life episodes with a rich appreciation for the complexities that confront the people who experience them. Although public health, risk, and crisis communication are not synonymous, it is often difficult within any one experience to say where one stops and the other starts. Likewise, an emphatic lesson of public health communication is that it does no good, it fact it often does harm, to encourage healthy behaviors when people lack the support and resources to carry them out. Consequently, we'll conclude this chapter with a discussion of reform ideas meant to make good health a more built-in feature of everyday life.

## WHAT IS PUBLIC HEALTH?

As the mad cow disease saga illustrates, public health involves the well-being of entire communities. Mary-Jane Schneider (2006) puts it this way:

Just as a doctor monitors the health of a patient by taking vital signs—blood pressure, heart rate, and so forth—public health workers monitor the health of a community by collecting and analyzing health data. (p. 121)

And public health doesn't stop there. In the same way that a physician is devoted to keeping people well, public health professionals are concerned with maintaining the good health of the entire population (Schneider, 2006). They seek to accomplish this through education, community partnerships, health campaigns, immunizations, and other medical care by maintaining healthy standards in restaurants, day care centers, schools, and much more. There are approximately 3,000 local health departments in the United States (Gursky, Inglesby, & O'Toole, 2003). (See Box 12.1 for more on career opportunities in public health.)

In the classic definition presented by Charles-Edward A. Winslow (1923), **public health** is

the science and art of preventing disease, prolonging life, and promoting physical health and efficiency through organized community efforts for the sanitation of the environment, the control of community infections, the education of the individual in principles of personal hygiene, the organization of medical and nursing service for the early diagnosis and preventive treatment of disease, and the development of the social machinery which will ensure to every individual in the community a standard of living adequate for the maintenance of health. (originally published in Winslow's *The Evolution and Significance of the Modern Public Health Campaign*, 1923, reprinted in the "History of Public Health," 2002, np)

This definition prescribes that public health professionals be both proactive—seeking to avoid unhealthy conditions, illnesses, and injuries—and diligent about monitoring and responding to health needs that arise.

Modern thinking about public health recognizes that one-way communication hasn't worked very well. As Piotrow and colleagues (2003) put it,

## BOX 12.1   CAREER OPPORTUNITIES

### Public Health

- Epidemiologist
- Health educator
- Health researcher
- Communication specialist
- Media relations professional
- Health campaign designer
- Environmentalist
- Health inspector
- Nutritionist
- Nurse
- Physician
- Risk/crisis communication specialist
- Nonprofit organization director
- Fundraiser
- Professor/educator
- Public policy advisor
- Health department administrator
- Business or billing manager
- Patient advocate or navigator
- Social worker
- Emergency management director

### Career Resources and Job Listings

- Pfizer Guide to Careers in Public Health: www.whatispublichealth.org/careers/index.html
- American Public Health Association CareerMart: www.apha.org/about/careers
- Partners in Information Access for the Public Health Workforce: phpartners.org/jobs.html
- Public Health Jobs Worldwide: www.jobspublichealth.com
- U.S. Department of Health & Human Services Careers: www.hhs.gov/careers/
- Association of Schools in Public Health: www.asph.org
- World Health Organization: www.who.int/employment/vacancies/en
- Centers for Disease Control and Prevention (CDC): www.cdc.gov/about/opportunities.htm

Also check the websites of your local hospitals and health departments.

---

health communication is "no longer simply repeating untested slogans like 'A small family is a happy family'" (p. 2) or distributing how-to guides on contraceptive methods. Instead, professionals are oriented more toward **social mobilization**, large-scale efforts in which community members and professionals work interactively to define goals, raise awareness, and create hospitable environments for healthy behaviors. Social mobilization relies on teamwork, diversity, shared leadership, and active involvement (Patel, 2005). For example, in an effort to stop the spread of leprosy in Bihar, India, World Health Organization (WHO) officials met with experts and citizens in the region. They realized that it was uncommon for local residents to check themselves for early signs of leprosy because

they had very few full-length mirrors, they typically showered outdoors while partly clothed, and even married couples did not often see each other naked (Renganathan et al., 2005). More than a catchy slogan would be needed for people to establish the habit of checking their skin for subtle changes. Community members would willingly have to alter their lifestyles and customs. Changes of this sort are usually most successful when they are promoted by community opinion leaders rather than outsiders.

Public health involves an array of health concerns. Traditionally, ongoing concerns such as diabetes, cancer, and heart disease fall within the rubric of *health promotion*, a topic we will cover more thoroughly in Chapters 13 and 14. *Risk communication* usually refers to health concerns that occur in a particular time and place, such as exposure to harmful substances, workplace dangers, and so on (Glik, 2007).

## RISK AND CRISIS COMMUNICATION

The National Research Council (1989, p. 21) defines **risk communication** as an ongoing process that involves not just one message but many diverse messages about risk factors as well as interactive discussions about how people perceive these factors and judge the risks and how they feel about the risk messages themselves.

With mad cow disease, the officials chose largely to downplay the risk and to discourage open discussion about the danger BSE might pose to humans. That decision was, and has continued to be, widely criticized. A full 6 years before officials went public about the risk, the British journal *Nature* chided authorities for keeping people in the dark:

> Never say that there is not danger (risk). Instead, say that there is always a danger (risk), and that the problem is to calculate what it is. And never say that the risk is negligible unless you are sure that your listeners share your own philosophy of life. ("Mad Cows and the Minister," 1990, p. 278)

The article stressed that that the Minister of Agriculture "should be obliged to tell it like it is" (p. 278) and admonished that the cost of false reassurance was fear, distrust, and economic instability. "The British will not eat beef for fear that it will kill them, and the price has fallen ever further" (p. 278).

Downplaying the risk of eating beef ultimately created a sense of public distrust that made it difficult to believe anything the government said. Although risk communication professionals are sometimes in the business of soothing fears, in this case health officials violated an important tenet of risk and crisis communication: *Be open about what you know, even if you don't have all the answers.* False reassurance—what Peter Sandman (2006a) calls "optimism masquerading as information" (paragraph 9)—can actually heighten fears and mistrust. This is supported by a second lesson that

belies conventional wisdom: *Citizens rarely panic when they are well informed.* Reporting on 50 years of research about people's behavior during disasters, Lee Clarke (2002) observes that, despite the "panic myth," people rarely act irrationally or selfishly in crisis situations. Instead emergencies usually bring out the best in people. "When danger arises, the rule—as in normal situations—is for people to help those next to them before they help themselves" (Clarke, p. 24).

Sandman (2006b) describes three "risk communication traditions": (1) helping people who are *insufficiently concerned* appreciate that a serious risk exists, (2) reassuring and calming people who are *excessively concerned*, and (3) working with people who are *appropriately concerned* (those who are "genuinely endangered and rightly upset") to help them cope and function effectively (p. 257). The dividing line between categories is sometimes hard to define, but we may view them as a continuum along which the first category is typical of risk communication and the last of crisis communication.

In its broadest sense, crisis communication can involve any number of events—a natural disaster, a scandal that rocks a political campaign, an epidemic, a chemical spill, and so on. In this chapter, we will focus on communication about crises that involve public health. The CDC (2008) defines health-related **crisis communication** as:

> An approach used by scientists and public health professionals to provide information that allows an individual, stakeholders, or an entire community to make the best possible decisions about their well-being, under nearly impossible time constraints, while accepting the imperfect nature of their choices. (paragraph 2)

The definition is telling, in that it acknowledges "the nearly impossible" demands and the inherently "imperfect" nature of crisis management. Public health expert Deborah Glik (2007) observes that a crisis involves "unexpectedness, high levels of threat, an aroused and stressed population, and media looking for breaking news stories" (p. 35). Practitioners work hard to lay solid groundwork and learn everything they can, but overwhelming demands and emotions can challenge even the most experienced professionals.

## Managing Perceptions

In her review of risk communication research, Katherine McComas (2006) observes that people tend to perceive some risks, such as being attacked by a shark while swimming at the beach, to be greater than they actually are, whereas people tend to have "optimistic biases" or "illusions of invulnerability" about other, statistically more threatening, risks, such as smoking and sun exposure (p. 78). This is particularly true when the risky behavior has pleasant or socially rewarding implications. For example, despite warning messages we have heard, we may tell ourselves that we're too young to get skin cancer, that we'll put on sunscreen later, or that having a suntan is worth the risk.

Ratzan and Meltzer (2005) point out that consumers are not wrong when they see things differently than experts; they just have a different vantage point. "These two audiences receive different information, process it in unique ways, and respond to conclusions based on their own set of circumstances and concerns" (Ratzan & Meltzer, 2005, p. 324). It is complicated, of course, because members of the public are not uniform in their perceptions. For example, you may have felt your anxiety rise while reading about mad cow disease, perhaps because you have been to England, have seen news footage of infected cows struggling to walk, or know how devastating a debilitating disease can be. Meanwhile, some readers may feel insulated from the issue and wonder what all the fuss is about. There is no "right" way to feel. Instead we must remember as health communication practitioners that belittling or ignoring diverse perspectives is typically ineffective and even unethical.

## How Scared Is Scared Enough?

While interacting with the public about health risks and crises, it is sometimes difficult to judge how much fear is productive and how much is disabling. It sometimes seems that public health advocates

want people to be afraid of something nearly all of the time. As Dawn Hillier (2006) puts it, well-meaning health promoters sometimes feed the public "a steady diet of fearful programmes about impending calamities" (p. 30). After a while, people may be either too fearful to make effective choices or so weary of fear appeals that they discount them altogether. However, a *rational* fear of horrible outcomes is healthy and motivational. It's a fine line to walk. Sandman (2006b) captures the dilemma well when he writes:

> The Holy Grail of crisis communicators is to get people to take precautions without frightening them. This is like trying to write a novel without using the letter "e"; it may be possible, but it's certainly a handicap. (p. 258)

By way of example, Sandman quotes a *New York Times* headline that read "Fear Is Spreading Faster Than SARS." He retorts: "As if it weren't supposed to....If the purpose of fear is to motivate precautions, after all, then the fear must come before the precautions are needed" (p. 259). We'll talk more about fear appeals in Chapter 14.

## In the Heat of the Moment

An assortment of "lessons learned" appear in italics throughout this chapter. As I alluded to earlier, one of the lessons is that *crisis communication looks easier on paper than it feels in reality.* Vicki Freimuth (2006) recalls the challenges that health communication specialists at the Centers for Disease Control and Prevention (CDC) faced after the 2001 anthrax attacks:

> Health communicators have a particularly difficult time with speed, as they are accustomed to conducting formative research, carefully segmenting audiences, planning messages, and pretesting before releasing them. [In a crisis] all of these activities have to occur in hours, not days, weeks, or months. Theory and research are still critical, but must be internalized by the communicators so they are available to use on the spot. (p. 144)

And a cool-headed commitment to safety can be even more difficult at the actual site of an emergency.

Dave Johnson (2006) recalls the chaos at the World Trade Centers when they were attacked in 2001:

A violent explosion rips through your office complex. Multiple fires are burning. An ominous plume of heat, fire, dust, debris and an unknowable mixture of perhaps asbestos, silica, lead and other metals floats into the atmosphere.... Firefighters and police and EMTs, over which you have no authority, arrive on the scene. The fire chief says "Get out of our way." His guys, and the police, don't wear proper protection.... Your own workforce is shocked. Some rush past the fires and debris, into the plume, searching for comrades.... It's chaotic. You're operating in a fog of disaster.... What do you say to your own workforce? To those outside your control, such as the firefighters? To the crowd of reporters? To threatened residents and business owners? And to your CEO, who won't wear a hard hat or respirator or safety glasses because, "We don't want to scare people"? (p. 58)

Johnson, who is editor of *Industrial Safety & Hygiene News*, presents some of the lessons learned about risk communication at ground zero.

- *"Beware of overly optimistic risk assessments,"* as when an EPA administrator prematurely announced one week after the disaster that the air in New York City was "safe to breathe" (p. 58). False reassurance can undermine experts' credibility and put people in danger.
- *Understand the different information needs of various stakeholders.* The ground zero team found that, after workers heard officials reassure the public that the site was safe, supervisors had a hard time convincing workers to use proper safety gear and caution.
- *"Understand the emotions and fears you are dealing with"* (p. 60). People who are worried, anxious, angry, or grief-stricken are likely to brush aside safety concerns, then be sorry later.
- *"Expect resistance to your message"* and *don't give up* (p. 60). Use a range of methods if necessary. When even New York City

Mayor Rudy Giuliani balked about wearing a hardhat, the ground zero team presented him with one that said "VIP - Mayor" on the front. "It worked," said Stewart Burkhammer, an environmental safety and health consultant working at ground zero. At other times, Burkhammer said, bluntness worked better than subtlety. He once told the crew at a morning safety meeting, "I'm not going to be the one to tell the mayor we just killed somebody, so clean up your act" (quoted by Johnson, p. 62).

- *Foster relationships and open communication with partners (media, emergency personnel, and so on) before, during, and after a crisis.*
- *Be proactive rather than reactive.* "Communicate and instruct as much as possible in advance of an emergency," recommends Burkhammer. "We spent a lot of time being great reactors.... A lot of things were done by feel and guess. I think we were very poor proactors" (p. 62).

Box 12.2 presents a framework to help guide your efforts as you prepare for and manage a health crisis. With these lessons in mind, let's examine a few case studies involving risk and crisis communication around the globe.

## CASE STUDIES: A GLOBAL PERSPECTIVE

In the past it was largely feasible to contain contagious illnesses such as smallpox and yellow fever to geographic sectors. Now, because more than 2 billion people a day fly to locations it would have taken days, weeks, or months to reach in the past, "an outbreak or epidemic in any one part of the world is only a few hours away from becoming an imminent threat somewhere else" (World Health Report, 2007, p. x). (See Box 12.3 for a profile of famous disease carriers and some tough considerations about personal liberties and public welfare.)

What's more, diseases—and their resistance to known drugs—are multiplying. Margaret Chan, director-general of WHO, cautions that "new diseases

BOX 12.2 **THEORETICAL PERSPECTIVES**

# Risk Management/ Communication Framework

Imagine that, after eating lunch in their school cafeteria, 125 local children have become ill, with some of them then hospitalized. As the health education supervisor at the health department, you are expected to help manage the crisis. Your staff has received 25 calls from worried parents and 15 calls from media professionals, and the issue hasn't even hit the news yet. What do you do first?

You might start by refreshing your knowledge of Scott Ratzan and Wendy Meltzer's (2005) **risk management/communication framework** (RMCF). Drawing on extensive experience in crisis and risk communication,[1] Ratzan and Meltzer developed their model to be an elegant and useful synthesis of guidelines presented in the WHO Maxims for Effective Health and Risk Communication, the U.S. Food and Drug Administration (FDA) Model for Risk Management, Covello's (2003) Best Practices in Public Health Risks and Crisis Communication, and other trusted models.

## Establishing the Foundations

If you are wise, the first step in managing the crisis actually began long before it occurred. Experts recommend developing interactive and trusting relationships with stakeholders when things are calm. They also recommend creating teams and crisis management plans and practicing what to do when a crisis occurs. Another precaution is to collect information that will be helpful,

---

[1] Ratzan, MD, MPA, MA, is founding editor-in-chief of the *Journal of Health Communication: International Perspectives* and is Vice President of Government Affairs in Europe for Johnson & Johnson. He served on a WHO team that analyzed the mad cow disease saga and drafted Maxims for Effective Health and Risk Communication, and he has helped draft global health communication strategies working on teams associated with the U.S. Agency for International Development, the American Medical Association, the Institute of Medicine, and other groups.

Meltzer is managing editor of the *Journal of Health Communication* and has a master's degree in public health from the George Washington University School of Medicine and Health Sciences.

quick at hand, and tailored to different audiences. Ratzan and Meltzer (2005) point out that there isn't always time in a crisis to construct and pretest new messages carefully. In your case, having ready access to good information about food-borne illnesses will make your job a great deal easier.

## Partnering with Stakeholders

Stakeholders are important before, during, and after a crisis. Ratzan and Meltzer (2005) embrace a broad definition of *stakeholders* as "anyone and everyone touched by the event" (p. 325). In your case, this might mean parents, children, school employees, reporters, public officials, health professionals, food distribution and preparation personnel, state agencies, and more. Ratzan and Meltzer observe that there are several benefits of engaging stakeholders: (1) They give you valuable, diverse input, (2) they can be (should be) active partners in achieving shared goals, and (3) mutual trust will allow you to be honest and open with each other.

In the current crisis, you might not know all of the stakeholders personally, but if you have made it a point to interact with at least a few key people in each group, you will be more effective in this crisis. What's more, you can activate your network to extend outreach to stakeholder groups. For example, if the health department supplies local schools with nurses, you might enlist the nurses' help in communicating with stakeholders. In the same way, you might call on health inspectors, media relations staff, PTA presidents, and others. If you have laid good groundwork and are open and trustworthy with stakeholders, a crisis can renew and strengthen relationships rather than damage them (Ratzan & Meltzer, 2005; Ulmer, Seeger, & Sellnow, 2007).

## Communicating with the Public

The majority of what you want conveyed will be passed along through mass media. Understanding media professionals' goals will help you work as partners rather than as adversaries. Be mindful that reporters have a stake in presenting immediate, accurate, and interesting information to the public. They look as foolish as you do if they pass long inaccurate information. But this doesn't mean you should keep them waiting until you know everything. "Today's media have a need for constant information updates to fill 24-hour broadcasts," Ratzan and Meltzer (2005) advise, adding: "Crisis communicators need to be aware that if they do not supply information, the media will report what they have" (p. 328).

In communicating with the public (either in person or through media channels), Ratzan and Meltzer (2005) recommend, be "clear, honest and compassionate" (p. 330). Being clear requires that you consider the different needs and literacy levels of stakeholders. Information that might make sense to researchers and clinicians can bewilder and frighten members of the public. All the while, show that you care and are feeling emotions. "This is the exact reason Mayor Giuliani was so successful at managing a citywide crisis" after the 9/11 terrorist attacks, say Ratzan and Meltzer (p. 331). City residents believed that he genuinely cared. However, be sure that you don't allow your emotions to exaggerate or minimize the severity of the crisis. Your words and demeanor convey to the public how they should think and feel about the crisis. Always "think before you speak," urge Ratzan and Meltzer (p. 331).

## Internal Communication Strategies

In the general rush to meet public and media demands it is easy to neglect teamwork in a crisis. But this oversight can lead to devastating mistakes. Ratzan and Meltzer (2005) underscore the importance of communicating regularly with members of your team. Depending on the duration of the crisis, you might call daily or twice-a-day briefings at which everyone can compare notes and impressions.

With these principles in mind, RMCF presents five stages of risk management (quoted verbatim from Ratzan & Meltzer, 2005, p. 335):

1. *Risk assessment:* Estimation and evaluation of risk
2. *Risk confrontation:* Determining acceptable level of risk in a larger context
3. *Risk intervention:* Risk control action
4. *Risk communication:* Interactive process of exchanging risk information

5. *Risk management evaluation:* Measure and ensure effectiveness or risk management efforts

As indicated, each of these stages involves partnering with stakeholders (members of the public, experts, media professionals, and others), making decisions, creating messages and communication strategies, and continually monitoring and refining your strategies.

## What Do You Think?

With regard to the "sick schoolchildren" crisis described at the opening of this box:

1. Where would you begin? What would you do first?
2. What stakeholders might you involve, and why? What questions would you ask each stakeholder group?
3. How would you enlist the stakeholders as active partners in the process?
4. How will you get (and convey) answers to reporters' questions such as the following? How sick are the children? Could this be deadly? Can you arrange interviews with some of the children or parents? How likely is that other children will come down sick? Have you definitively linked the illness to food served at school? If so, what food was it? Who is responsible for food at school? Is there a chance that the tainted food was distributed to other schools as well? To restaurants? To grocery stores?
5. What will you do when your staff can't keep up with all the phone calls, much less research the issue and contact stakeholders?
6. When the crisis has passed, how will you evaluate the success or failure of your efforts?
7. What might you do to prepare for future risks and crises?

## Suggested Sources

Covello, V. (2003). Best practices in public health risk and crisis communication. *Journal of Health Communication, 8*(1S), 5–8.

Ratzan, S., & Meltzer, W. (2005). (2005). State of the art in crisis communication: Past lessons and

*(continued)*

---

**BOX 12.2** (*continued*)

---

principles of practice. In M. Haider (Ed.), *Global public health communication: Challenges, perspectives, and strategies* (pp. 321–347). Boston: Jones and Bartlett.

Sixth Futures Forum on Crisis Communication. (2004, May). Reykjavik, Iceland. World Health Organization. Available online at www.euro.who.int/document/E85056.pdf

---

## BOX 12.3 TYPHOID MARY AND TB ANDY

In 2007 Andrew Speaker, an Atlanta resident with drug-resistant tuberculosis (TB), traveled by plane to Europe and back, even though doctors say they told him not to fly because of the risk to others. Tuberculosis is dangerous and highly contagious, particularly in the recirculated air of an airplane cabin. Nearly 2 million people a year die from TB, mostly in developing countries (Global Health, 2008). The disease has made a deadly comeback in recent years because new strains have emerged that do not respond to drug therapy, and people with immune deficiencies such as HIV and AIDS are particularly susceptible to TB whether they have been immunized or not.

In Speaker's case, authorities in Italy were alerted to his health status, and they refused to allow him to board a flight back to the United States. So Speaker and his wife (they were on their honeymoon) flew to Canada instead, where his status went unnoticed, and they were able to fly back to Atlanta. Many fellow airline passengers, angry that Speaker knowingly exposed them to a dangerous disease, later filed charges against him ("Plane Passengers Sue," 2007).

Some journalists nicknamed Speaker "TB Andy," referencing another famous figure in history, Typhoid Mary. In the years preceding 1906, Mary Mallon was a cook for wealthy families in New York. Authorities began to notice that, in the homes where she worked, an extraordinary number of people contracted typhoid fever. At the time, about 10% of people who got typhoid died from it. Mallon resisted being tested or being taken into custody. Indeed, she "brandished a meat fork and threats" so vociferously that it took five police officers to bring her in ("TV Program," 2004, paragraph 6).

Tests showed that Mallon was a typhoid carrier, although she manifested no symptoms herself. She was forcibly quarantined in a hospital on an island in New York City's East River. Her distraught letters from the time relate that she felt like a kidnap victim and a "peep show" ("In Her Own Words," 2004, last paragraph) Mallon was released after about 6 years. But when she disobeyed orders and returned to cooking professionally, she was taken into custody for the rest of her life. Historians have mixed feelings about whether Mallon was treated fairly or not.

### What Do You Think?

1. Should the state take people into custody if they refuse to take actions (such as wearing gloves or face masks, agreeing not to fly, and so on) that would protect others from catching their illnesses? Does it matter what illness it is? Do colds and flu count? What about illnesses that are somewhat, but not highly, contagious?
2. Should airlines beef up their "no fly" lists so that people with highly contagious diseases are not permitted aboard? Why or why not?
3. If a person knowingly exposes others to a contagious disease, should the people who are exposed have the right to sue? Would you? Why or why not?
4. Historians have noted that Mary Mallon had little means of earning a living besides being a cook. If protecting others means changing careers, should the government help pay for new vocational training or education?

5. People whose immune systems are compromised by illness, chemotherapy, or other conditions are particularly susceptible to diseases that wouldn't endanger others. Should we exercise greater-than-usual precautions when we know that such people are in our communities? Why or why not? What precautions would you consider reasonable?

6. In some countries people who have colds wear disposable face masks (like surgical masks) in public to protect others. Should other countries adopt this practice as well? Why or why not? Would you wear a mask when you had a cold? Why or why not?

7. Many illnesses could be prevented if people washed their hands before eating. In Japan, even fast-food restaurants provide moist towelettes with every meal. Should other countries adopt this practice? Why or why not?

8. A common means of transmitting illness is shaking hands with others and then touching food. Some people suggest we would be healthier (and perhaps avert epidemics) if we bowed or waved in greeting instead of shaking hands. What do you think?

*For an excellent video about Mary Mallon, as well as discussion guides and ethical analyses, see www.pbs.org/wgbh/nova/typhoid.*

---

are emerging at the historically unprecedented rate of one per year"(World Health Report, 2007, p. vi). WHO identified more than 1,110 epidemics between 2002 and 2007 (World Health Report, 2007).

Contact with other people, especially a *lot* of other people, can be hazardous to your health. But health risks involve more than communicable diseases. They also encompass environmental issues, safety practices, intentional and accidental exposure to hazardous substances, contaminated food and water, natural disasters, and more. The good news is that globalization has also improved worldwide awareness of public health. After a catastrophic tsunami hit Southeast Asia in 2004, people around the world cooperated to send more than 50 medical aid teams and $4 billion to the region (Council on Foreign Relations, 2005).

We could fill volumes with descriptions of public health issues around the world. We won't do that. Instead, let's look at a few case studies that illustrate some key principles, challenges, and lessons. The following discussion focuses on AIDS, bioterrorism, SARS, and avian flu.

## AIDS

AIDS has been called the greatest public health challenge in the last half century. It has killed more than 25 million people since 1981, and about 33 million people are now living with HIV or AIDS (UNAIDS, 2008). The death rate is up to 2 million people per year. And the crisis is particularly bad in Africa, where about 75% of those deaths occur (UNAIDS).

One challenge of AIDS is that related behaviors are sometimes considered taboo, immoral, or too personal to be discussed. What's more, cultural rules about these behaviors vary widely from culture to culture. For example, although members of Western cultures mean well, their Judeo-Christian worldview can be baffling to others. Americans missed the mark when they designed public health messages urging people in Namibia, Africa, to prevent HIV by abstaining from premarital sex and by being faithful to their spouse. These concepts are not meaningful to most Namibian citizens, who are accustomed to polygamy and who tend to define marriage very loosely (Hillier, 2006). Hillier concludes: "Prevention campaigns have been silent about polygamous sexual cultures... [They have] elevated the Christian monogamous marriage to the most desirable norm but it is not the only or most common form of sexual union" (p. 18). As a result, many foreign efforts are culturally unacceptable, therefore ineffective at changing people's behavior.

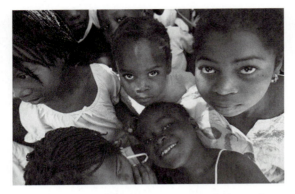

Children in sub-Saharan Africa can only hope for a brighter future than current conditions predict. That region now has the highest concentration of HIV infection in the world.

*Source:* Photo provided by UNAIDS/A. Gutman.

Another difficulty is that AIDS cannot yet be prevented with a pill or a shot. The only way to prevent transmission is by changing people's behavior (Schneider, 2006). That is a tremendous challenge. And the issue can't wait. The average age of sub-Saharan African residents has already plummeted from 62 to 47, mostly because of premature deaths from AIDS (AVERT, 2008).

Some health communication specialists have concluded that it's naive to assume most people *won't* have sex. The trick, they feel, is to make safer sex sexier. The Pleasure Project, based in Oxford, England, is a cooperative effort to emphasize the erotic appeal of safer sex. The project's website explains:

> While most safer sex and HIV prevention programs are negative and disease-focused, The Pleasure Project is different: We take a positive, liberating, and sexy approach to safer sex. Think of it is as sex education … with the emphasis on "sex." (www. thepleasureproject.org)

Project coordinators present condoms and alternatives to sexual intercourse as exciting and erotically stimulating. The website includes a racy 76-page directory of related organizations and programs, erotic tips for safer sex, and links to organizations that sell condoms and sex toys and donate the proceeds to the safer-sex campaign. *(Fair warning if you care to look it up: The Pleasure Project website is sexually explicit.)*

The safer-sex-is-better-sex effort has been applauded by a range of public health experts. After reviewing relevant research, the authors of a Viewpoint article in *The Lancet* concur:

> Since pursuit of pleasure is one of the main reasons that people have sex, this factor must be addressed when motivating people to use condoms and participate in safer sexual behaviour. (Philpott, Knerr, & Maher, 2006, p. 3)

These are just a few of the many approaches to preventing HIV and AIDS. Some lessons suggested by recent efforts include the following.

- *Listen and learn.* Knowing what the public believes and is willing to do is just as important (sometimes more important) than knowing what experts think people *should* do (Covello, 2003).
- *Vary your approach.* Fear appeals can be highly motivational. But particularly for frightening and long-term crises such as AIDS, people may tune out fear messages because they are overwhelming or overly familiar. Innovative, culturally sensitive appeals may regain people's attention.

## SARS

One of the great success stories in managing a public health crisis arose from worldwide efforts to contain severe acute respiratory syndrome (SARS). The issue first drew attention in February 2003, when a man in Vietnam entered the hospital with a respiratory disorder. His condition deteriorated, and, although he was transferred to a Hong Kong medical center, he died within 4 days. Soon, seven caregivers who'd been involved with the patient became sick as well. The disorder spread so quickly that, in slightly more a month, there were 150 cases of SARS in eight countries (WHO, 2003, March 16).

By May 2003, SARS had become a pandemic. New cases were emerging at the rate of 200 a day. The disease had spread to every continent. A total of 8,000 people in 28 countries were infected (WHO, 2003, June 18). SARS was especially hard to contain because it was easily spread from person to person, it was infectious for more than a week before symptoms appeared, and it was hard to diagnose because the initial symptoms were similar to those of many other illnesses. Worst of all, SARS was deadly. About 10% of people who were infected (many of them hospital personnel) died.

The authors of the World Health Report (2007) recall:

> SARS incited a degree of public anxiety that virtually halted travel to affected areas and drained billions of dollars from economies across entire regions.... It showed that the danger arising from emerging diseases is universal. No country, rich or poor, is adequately protected from either the arrival of a new disease on its territory or the subsequent disruption this can cause. (p. xix)

However, it might have been worse. Remarkably, just 100 days into the crisis (June 18, 2003), spokespersons for WHO announced that the pandemic was under control and that new cases had dwindled to handful a day. The crisis was over by July. How was that possible? Lessons from the experience illustrate how it happened.

- *Develop strong teams.* WHO credits "monumental efforts" by governments, health professionals, and public health agencies. Because officials around the world reported cases promptly, WHO and other agencies were able to monitor and contain new outbreaks as much as possible. WHO dubbed it "solidarity" and "interdependence" on a global scale never seen before (WHO, 2003, June 18, paragraph 8).
- *Don't forget the basics.* One of the world's oldest methods of limiting contagion, quarantines, worked. Officials worked internationally to limit travel that might expose people to SARS. At the same time,

hospitals designated isolated SARS wards to keep those patients away from others.
- *Make the most of communication technology.* Technology allowed researchers and health experts to share data and new developments quickly and accurately. Because of this, they figured out how SARS was transmitted "in record time" (WHO, 2003, June 18, paragraph 11).
- *Keep everyone informed.* Although experts did a good job communicating with each other, members of some affected populations were out of the loop. In China, because of tight government controls on media content, many people were frustrated by the lack of SARS news coverage. Zixue Tai and Tau Sun (2007) report that Chinese people, desperate for news, used the Internet to seek and share information about SARS that they couldn't get otherwise.
- *Stop it at the source.* Once officials knew that SARS was transmitted via droplets spread during coughing and sneezing, they were able to educate health care workers about how to minimize the risk of infection.

In just a few months SARS took a heavy toll. By the time it was contained, 8,098 people had been infected and 774 of those had died (CDC, 2005). However, containing the disease so quickly saved millions of lives. The SARS case is regarded as a model response to a nearly unthinkable public health threat.

## Anthrax

Some public health crises are the result of intentional acts. The CDC (2007a) defines **bioterrorism** as "the deliberate release of viruses, bacteria, or other germs (agents) used to cause illness or death in people, animals, or plants" (paragraph 1). Bioterrorism is not new. Schneider (2006) points out that when the American settlers purposely gave Native Americans blankets from people with smallpox, they were engaging in (tragically effective) germ warfare. Today, dense population centers are especially vulnerable to bioterrorism. Since 2001, the U.S. government has spent $50 billion on preparedness efforts, yet hospital personnel warn that a widespread attack could easily overwhelm the health care system ("Threat," 2008). Bioterrorism, understandably, incites a great deal of fear.

One act of bioterrorism on American soil occurred in 2001, when 22 people were sickened and 5 died after contact with letters containing anthrax spores. Anthrax is a potentially deadly disease that people can get by breathing in, touching, or digesting a rare bacterium. In September and October 2001, someone sent four envelopes containing anthrax spores to media professionals and government officials. In doing so, the terrorist put many people, including postal workers and mailroom employees, at grave risk.

Because the anthrax attacks occurred soon after the terrorist attacks of September 11, public anxiety was particularly high. And because the attack occurred through the mail, it was difficult to know who had been or might be exposed to anthrax. Potentially, anyone in the country might be next. As Haider and Aravindakshan (2005) put it: "The threat turned junk mail into potential parcels of danger" (p. 393). In contrast to a typical illness, which begins in one place and then may spread, this one was immediately a nationwide concern (Gursky et al., 2003). At one point, health officials put 32,000 people on antibiotics, a preemptive move that experts speculate saved many lives.

In the article "Order Out of Chaos," Freimuth (2006) describes how the CDC Office of Communication (of which she was director) functioned in the high-pressure weeks following the anthrax attacks. The CDC is the arm of the U.S. Department of Health and Human Services in charge of public health efforts, education, information, and more. One component of the communication division, the media relations office, usually fields about 55 calls a week. But it received an average of 1,283 calls a week in the 6 weeks following the anthrax attacks (Freimuth). On top of that, the staff coordinated a total of 373 press briefings, press statements, and broadcast interviews in that time. "It was common in a single day to have interview requests

from every network morning show, every network evening news hours, and the Larry King Hour," recalls Freimuth (p. 144). Since there was no way the 10-person media relations staff could meet the demands on their own, Freimuth oversaw a temporary reorganization in which the staff was tripled to 30 people and organized into two teams that each worked four days a week, overlapping one day in the middle.

As with many public health crises, one of the greatest hurtles was managing uncertainty. Scientific evidence about inhalable anthrax was scant, and information that emerged was sometimes incomplete and inaccurate. As new information was released, the media sometimes treated the old information as "mistakes" (Freimuth, p. 142). And, in their eagerness to get information, some reporters turned to untrustworthy sources who were willing to offer speculative and self-serving information. The CDC staff, which prides itself on a "slow, thoughtful scientific" process, was forced to work quickly and with less deliberation than usual (Freimuth, 2006, p. 142). Friction sometimes resulted when scientists were concerned that their research might be oversimplified but others quickly had to summarize scientific findings and make them easy to understand. All the while, the FBI (which was officially in charge of the case) wanted some details kept secret to avoid compromising the investigation.

To keep up with demands and to make sure stakeholder groups were not overlooked, members of the CDC communication staff organized themselves into teams. One team communicated with clinicians, another with concerned citizens, still others with media professionals, policy-makers, and the like. As in most crises, success was defined largely by communication. "Not all of these staff had to be communication specialists, but they needed to be managed by communication staff so that messages could be consistent across the agency and delivered in a timely manner," writes Freimuth (2006, p. 146).

Another challenge was to identify and prepare spokespeople. Freimuth (2006) reflects that the public naturally looks to political leaders for information and updates. But those leaders are often not well informed about scientific details, and they tend to comfort audiences rather than level with them. Scientists, although more knowledgeable, often err in the other direction, coming off as "logical and unemotional" (Freimuth, p. 142). Choosing and preparing spokespeople was difficult but was worth the extra effort. Kristen Swain's (2007) study of news coverage during the anthrax crisis shows that audiences responded most favorably when information was specific and clearly linked to trustworthy sources.

The anthrax case involved people from many agencies and organizations. At the height of the crisis, when a suspicious substance was reported in the western United States, Freimuth was awakened at 3 a.m. to take part in a conference call involving nearly 15 people from a wide range of agencies. "It was impossible to sort out who was with what organization and what position they held," she says, "yet in that phone call, decisions had to be reached" (Freimuth, 2006, p. 143).

Many of the same confounders emerged in the anthrax case as in the mad cow disease saga: uncertainty, tension between agencies, the temptation to comfort, reluctance to frighten the public unduly, and so on. The anthrax case occurred over a shorter, more intense interval, however. And, although the anthrax case revealed serious deficits in the government's preparedness for a bioterrorist attack, the CDC Office of Communication was lauded as doing an admirable job during extremely trying circumstances.

The following lessons about public health and risk/crisis communication emerge from the anthrax case.

- *Crisis is a matter of perception.* In the same year that anthrax killed 5 people, 30,000 others died from influenza (Lovett, 2003). It's a phenomenon that risk and crisis communicators know well: Fear and uncertainty elevate some health concerns to crisis status while far more prevalent killers such as the flu and diabetes often fail to make headlines.
- *Even if you don't specialize in crisis management, learn as much as you can about it and be prepared to take part.* The media relations restructuring was possible because the CDC staff pulled communication experts from a range of other duties and partnered them with content experts. Freimuth (2006) advises: "Health communicators working in any public health context need to add risk communication and crisis management skills to their repertoire" (p. 148).
- *Even in the midst of a crisis, don't be afraid to restructure the system if it helps you respond to stakeholders more effectively.*
- *Show genuine compassion.* Empathize with people's fears, sadness, and frustration. Crisis communication expert Vincent Covello (2003) advises: "Avoid using distant, unfeeling language when discussing harm, deaths, injuries, and illness" (p. 7).
- *Speaking with many voices is sometimes okay.* This lesson runs counter to crisis management advice for companies, individuals, and political campaigns. In those instances, it is important to deliver a clear, consistent message to the public. But a public health campaign is usually far more complex, and evidence suggests that allowing a range of viewpoints is sometimes effective and even preferable. After studying the anthrax case, L. Clarke and colleagues (2006) concluded that the situation was "naturally given to the expression of many voices" and that "a single voice with a single message would have been so discordant with actual circumstances that it could only misrepresent the risks that people might face" (p. 167). Experience shows that, even in a crisis, people expect and can cope with a range of expert viewpoints on complex issues. One caveat is that audiences who are already distrustful of public health messages may assume sources are being dishonest if they provide inconsistent information (Meredith, Eisenman, Rhodes, Ryan, & Long, 2007). For this reason, it is important not to hide inconsistencies, but to acknowledge and explain why they exist (Seeger, 2006).

# Risk/Crisis Communication Centers

Center for Risk Communication: www. centerforriskcommunication.com/home.htm

The Communication Initiative Network: www. comminit.com

Peter Sandman's interactive blog about crisis and risk communication: www.psandman.com/ gst2006.htm

Also check university websites. Many schools have developed centers for risk and crisis communication as well as degree programs in the field.

---

- *Don't go it alone.* Covello (2003) advises organizations to "coordinate, collaborate, and partner with other credible sources" (p. 6). Such teamwork can help offset overwhelming demands on any one organization and can demonstrate to the public that multiple sources agree on key issues.
- *Don't overlook "forgotten publics."* In the anthrax case, postal workers were particularly sensitive to any implication that their safety was less important than the people to whom the dangerous letters were addressed. Similar tensions arose on a much greater scale during the Hurricane Katrina crisis, when government agencies were accused of devaluing New Orleans residents on the basis of race and socioeconomic status (L. B. Fisher, 2007; Littlefield & Quenette, 2007; Waymer & Heath, 2007).

Next we turn to an issue that, as of this writing, is still in the precrisis phase.

## Avian Flu

If you vowed never to eat another hamburger after reading the mad cow disease saga, take a deep breath. Like mad cow disease, avian flu has been passed from animals (in this case, birds) to people. But the effects are far more devastating. Compared to 10% of infected people who died from SARS, some 65% of people who get this version of bird flu (known so far as H5N1) die from it. In serious cases, there is nothing doctors can do. Within days, lung tissue dies, and so does the patient.

The first documented case of H5N1 occurred in Hong Kong in 1997. After that, the government oversaw the killing of every chicken in Hong Kong (about 1.5 million birds) (Appenzeller, 2005). The disease seemed to go away. But it resurfaced in 2003, killing millions of birds and affecting some humans. By 2007 more than 350 human cases had been diagnosed, and 230 people had died from it (WHO, 2007e).

The virus often kills birds in a matter of hours by destroying their lungs, brains, muscles, and intestines (Appenzeller, 2005). So far, people with H5N1 seem to have caught it from animals. Although scientists are not certain how the disease jumps to humans, they caution people to cook poultry fully, to use gloves and masks when handling live or dead birds, and not to use bird-dropping fertilizer.

But the real danger—and one that has public health officials around the world on high alert—is that this virus or a similar one will mutate so that it can spread from human to human. Flu viruses in the past have been remarkably adept at doing that. "It's bound to happen," predicts Jeremy Farrar, an Oxford University physician who specializes in avian flu, "and when it does, the world is going to face a truly horrible pandemic" (quoted by Appenzeller, 2005, paragraph 11).

If H5N1 becomes a pandemic, millions of people could die. It has happened before. During World War I, some 50 million people died from Spanish flu. That is more than three times the number of soldiers who died in the war (Appenzeller, 2005). Like avian flu, Spanish flu probably jumped from animals to people. That type of mutation is very dangerous because humans have few antibodies to protect them from the novel virus.

And if you're thinking that you rarely get the flu or that you get over it quickly when you do, beware. The H5N1 version of the flu is especially dangerous for people who have well-functioning immune

## BOX 12.5 ETHICAL CONSIDERATIONS

# Who Should Be Vaccinated?

The good news is that researchers have created a vaccine for H5N1. It's not perfect, because they don't know exactly how the virus will mutate. And researchers must still make sure there are no harmful side effects. But even if the vaccine is approved, there is not likely to be enough for everyone. So public health experts face a dilemma. After reading about bird flu in this chapter, consider what you would do in their shoes.

1. If you had to choose, which of the following populations would you vaccinate and why? (a) people who are most likely to die from the disease if they get it, (b) service providers such as health care professionals, fire fighters, and police officers, or (c) another population of your choosing.
2. Would you first vaccinate people in communities in which avian flu cases have already been diagnosed? Why or why not? If those citizens

or their governments are unable to afford the vaccine, do you believe people in other countries should help pay for it? Why or why not?
3. Viruses such as the flu often spread quickly among children. Would you vaccinate them early on? Why or why not?
4. Are you in favor of *requiring* people at high risk for avian flu (such as those who regularly handle birds) to get vaccinated? Why or why not?
5. Depending on how the virus mutates, the vaccine might not be especially effective. Do you feel governments should invest in it anyway? Why or why not?
6. Given the opportunity, would you choose to be vaccinated? Why or why not?

To see how the WHO representatives weighed these issues at their 2007 conference in Geneva, see the conference report at: www.who.int/csr/resources/publications/WHO_HSE_EPR_GIP_2008_1d.pdf

---

systems. In serious cases, avian flu so overstimulates the body's immune system that the lungs become grossly inflamed with white blood cells and life-sustaining tissues die (Appenzeller, 2005).

It is difficult to imagine overplanning for a crisis such as avian flu. As Barbara Reynolds (2006) points out, in any health crisis, "the devil is most certainly in the details" (p. 249). WHO (2007d) has released rapid-response guidelines for containing a deadly flu pandemic. Public health personnel in your community are probably already working on the local plan. WHO guidelines include the following: (1) Create a geographic "containment zone" when the first cases surface, to separate people who have the disease as well as those who have been exposed to it from other people, (2) create a "buffer zone" around the containment zone to reduce further the risk of contagion, and (3) communicate effectively with the public to maintain barriers, keep people informed,

ensure that people within the containment zone have adequate care and supplies, and minimize stigmatization of people with the disease.

How will this work exactly? It sounds a bit frightening, but it's not as scary as the alternative. Imagine your community partitioned with roadblocks, warning signs, and guarded screening stations. No one except essential personnel will go in or out of containment zones for at least 20 days. It sounds like something from a movie, but it's no exaggeration. Health officials realize that the only way to save lives is to limit the spread of the virus. Inside the containment zone—which could be your neighborhood or a portion of your hometown—health officials will monitor people's health, care for and quarantine (in a hospital or at home) people who are infected, watch for new outbreaks, and help distribute antiviral medication to those who are still healthy. (See Box 12.5 for more about ethical

## BOX 12.6 RESOURCES

### Pandemic Response Plans

To view WHO's 6-minute video *Global Alert, Global Response,* go to www.who.int/csr/en

WHO's rapid-response protocol for a pandemic flu is available at www.who.int/csr/disease/avian_ influenza/guidelines/RapidContProtOct15.pdf

The official U.S. government pandemic response plan is available at pandemicflu.gov

To find out what individuals should do to prepare for a flu pandemic, see www.pandemicflu.gov/ plan/individual/checklist.html

## BOX 12.7

### Can You Guess?

1. Which state has the highest percentage of uninsured residents?
2. Which states have the lowest percentage of uninsured residents?
3. If you were buying health insurance for your family in the Philippines, how much would you pay per year?
4. If you were buying health insurance for your family in the United States, how much would you pay per year?

*See answers at the end of the chapter.*

dilemmas concerning who should receive the limited number of vaccines available.)

This means that, if a person in your household becomes ill, you may all be voluntarily confined to your home until officials can be sure you are not contagious. And even if everyone in your household is healthy, if an outbreak occurs in your area, it is advisable to remain in your home. Public health experts recommend that everyone maintain a 2-week supply of food, water, and needed medications just in case. They also recommend washing the hands frequently and covering the mouth when sneezing or coughing.

Because we are currently in a precrisis, planning phase concerning the next pandemic flu, it is difficult to know what lessons will emerge. But it is interesting to note that health officials are consciously building on what worked well in the SARS case. A visit to the WHO, CDC, or PandemicFlu.gov website reveals an extensive collection of materials, including health-tracking software, government agency contact lists, brochures and checklists for a wide range of stakeholder groups, and more. (See Box 12.6.)

As with many other components of public health and risk/crisis management, success depends largely on effective communication (Seeger, 2006). It is no longer defensible to think of avian flu as an Asian crisis or a future scenario. Sandman (2006b) advises

crisis communicators to imagine "that the crisis has just begun and to make a list of things they wish the public had already learned or already done" (p. 259). As members of the public, we might ask ourselves: Are we aware and prepared for a deadly flu pandemic? If containment zones were created in our community next week or next month, would we understand what was happening? Are we (and our neighbors) prepared to stay in our homes for 2 weeks or longer? Ideally, the public should answer yes to these questions well in advance of the crisis.

### Wrapping It Up

Public health can feel overwhelming at the best of times. Add a crisis, and the demands are even greater. Sometimes it helps to remember that challenges are happening all the time, but so are victories. In his article "Still a Privilege to Be a Doctor," pediatrician Lawrence Rifkin (2008) pauses to reflect on the small miracles health advocates accomplish every day:

Ashley's in Room 3, with a positive rapid strep. It doesn't get more commonplace than that. Then, with a sense of wonder, I remember: A century ago, rheumatic fever complications from strep were the No. 1 cause of death in school-age children. Now, we hardly see rheumatic fever in this country; a few generations ago, Ashley may have been one of the victims. As I write out yet another prescription for amoxicillin, I think maybe I just saved a life. (Rifkin, p. 28)

On that note, we shift to another zone of opportunity in the quest for public health.

## HEALTH CARE REFORM

Many Americans assume the U.S. healthcare system is the best in the world. And it is, in some respects. It is the world leader in terms of spending. And it is the #1 most responsive health system on the planet, meaning it is quickest to adapt to changing health needs.

But the United States doesn't begin to reach its full potential in terms of keeping people alive and healthy (ranked 72 among 191 nations in health performance), charging a fair amount for health services relative to other life expenses (ranked 54/55 in a tie with Fiji), or providing equitable treatment for everyone (ranked 32 in health distribution). Overall, the United States health system doesn't make the Top 5 In the World list. Not even the Top 20. It comes in 37th.

These are the conclusions of the *World Health Report 2000*, created by WHO. It is the latest—and, for most purposes, the only—worldwide ranking of health systems. In Table 12.1 you can see that the United States is ranked far behind France, Italy, Japan, the United Kingdom, and even some lesser-known nations, such as Andorra in southwest Europe.

And WHO isn't alone in its assessment. When researchers at The Commonwealth Fund—a New York-based foundation dedicated to improving health care—issued their *National Scorecard on U.S. Health Systems Performance,* they gave the United States a D (65%) on overall health, quality of care, access to care, efficiency, and equity (Commonwealth Fund, 2008c). The report's authors concluded: "The U.S. health system is on the wrong track" (paragraph 3).

In this section, we take a closer look at some of the lessons we can learn by considering what works

### Table 12.1 World Health Systems Performance Ranking

| | Ranking Among World Health Systems* | Type of health coverage |
|---|---|---|
| 1 | France | Universal |
| 2 | Italy | Universal |
| 3 | San Marino | Universal |
| 4 | Andorra | Universal |
| 5 | Malta | Universal |
| 6 | Singapore | Universal |
| 7 | Spain | Universal |
| 8 | Oman | Universal |
| 9 | Austria | Universal |
| 10 | Japan | Universal |
| 11 | Norway | Universal |
| 12 | Portugal | Universal |
| 13 | Monaco | Universal |
| 14 | Greece | Universal |
| 15 | Iceland | Universal |
| 16 | Luxembourg | Universal |
| 17 | Netherlands | Universal |
| 18 | United Kingdom | Universal |
| 19 | Ireland | Universal |
| 20 | Switzerland | Universal |
| 21 | Belgium | Universal |
| 22 | Colombia | Universal |
| 23 | Sweden | Universal |
| 24 | Cyprus | Universal |
| 25 | Germany | Universal |
| 26 | Saudi Arabia | Universal |
| 27 | United Arab Emirates | Universal |
| 28 | Israel | Universal |
| 29 | Morocco | |
| 30 | Canada | Universal |
| 31 | Finland | Universal |
| 32 | Australia | Universal |
| 33 | Chile | Universal |
| 34 | Denmark | Universal |
| 36 | Costa Rica | Universal |
| 37 | United States | |
| 38 | Slovenia | Universal |
| 39 | Cuba | Universal |
| 40 | Brunei | Universal |

\* Based on WHO World Health Report, 2000 (the latest worldwide ranking available)

well and what does not. As we go, keep in mind the words of the great management theorist Peter Senge (2006): "When placed in the same system, people, however different, tend to produce similar results" (p. 42). If health care is not performing well, it's usually the fault of the system itself, not the individuals in it. Very often, health professionals are the most vocal of anyone about the needs for improvement. They, like all of us, want the best results possible, but they can't achieve that by themselves.

## Analyzing the Issues

If health equaled wealth, citizens of the United States would live twice as long as the rest of the world. The United States spends more on health care, per capita, than any other nation and eight times the world average (see Figure 12.1). Yet 28 countries, many of which spend less on health care, have longer life expectancies (WHO, 2008b). What's more, despite how much the United States spends, it has fewer physicians per citizen than many industrialized nations (see Figure 12.2). And many countries that spend far less than the United States offer health care to *all* their citizens, whereas about 47 million Americans go largely without. So what's not working?

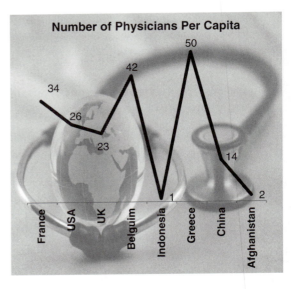

**Figure 12-2** Off the Charts: The numbers above don't even tell the whole story. In many African nations there is less than 1 doctor for every 10,000 people. In Sierra Leone, there is only 1 doctor for every 36,574 people. If the doctor saw 15 patients a day and worked 7 days a week, it would still take more than 6 1/2 years to see them all

Source: WHO World Health Statistics, 2008. © Günay Mutlu / iStockPhoto

The problem, say many experts, is that part of the money is being wasted, and too much of it goes to the people who are already health rich. Let's take a closer look at these issues.

**Waste** Part of the waste results from excessive bureaucracy. "Lowering insurance administrative costs alone could save up to $100 billion a year," according to the *National Scorecard* (Commonwealth Fund, 2008c, paragraph 6). The report's authors gave the United States an F (53%) on overall efficiency.

Waste also results from hospital visits and other care that could be avoided with better preventive efforts and more effective access and communication. Americans receive recommended levels of preventive care only about 55% of the time, despite predictions that 150 million Americans will have

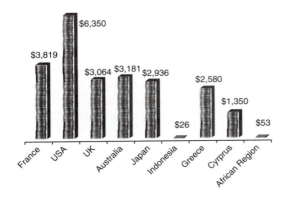

**Figure 12-1** Health Care Spending per Capita, in US. Dollars

Source: WHO World Health Statistics, 2008. © Luca di / Filippo / iStockPhoto

chronic health conditions such as obesity, diabetes, and cardiovascular disease by 2015 (American College of Physicians, 2008, p. 55). Treating chronic conditions is typically more expensive than preventing them. However, judged against prevention programs in 19 other industrialized nations, the United States came in last (Commonwealth Fund, 2008c).

Moreover, money spent on medical care is sometimes wasted. Americans are three to four times more likely than residents of other countries to report that their doctors order duplicate tests and do not have test results when they show up for appointments (Commonwealth Fund, 2008c).

A major culprit is the lack of medical information technology. In contrast to countries such as the Netherlands and New Zealand, in which nearly all physicians (98% and 92%, respectively) use **electronic medical records (EMRs),** only about 28% of U.S. physicians utilize them (Schoen, Osborne, et al., 2007). EMRs (also called *EHRs,* for electronic health records) are similar to the traditional patient records, in that they indicate medical visits, concerns, diagnoses, treatments, prescribed drugs, and so on. But because EMRs can be viewed and shared by a number of caregivers, they allow doctors more easily to identify (and avoid) treatment overlaps and drug interactions and to track patients' overall progress. They are also invaluable in emergencies, when paper records might be unavailable or when waiting for them would waste precious time. As a result, EMRs save time, money, and lives. (On the bright side, the U.S. figure is up significantly from 17% in 2001.)

***Inequities and Oversights*** Although the United States is the wealthiest nation on earth, the gap between haves and have-nots is large, and that gap often determines who gets care. For example, about 26% of families who earned at least $84,000 in 2007 said they would have sought more medical care if they could have afforded it. That is alarming enough. But among families that made half that much, 61% went without needed care (Commonwealth Fund, 2008a). By contrast, citizens of countries such as

Canada, the Netherlands, and the United Kingdom seldom report that money is a concern, because their governments guarantee medical care for everyone (Commonwealth Fund, 2007).

In the United States, access to health care has worsened, not improved. Health insurance premiums have risen 10 times faster than wages since 2001 (Robert Wood Johnson Foundation, 2008). As a result, more than 4 in 10 adults under age 63 are uninsured or underinsured. That's an increase of 14 million people in just four years (Commonwealth Fund, 2008c).

And if you have lived in different states you may have noticed that care varies even within the United States. If you grew up in Massachusetts, for example, there is a 93% chance you got all of the recommended vaccines when you were a toddler. But your odds are lower if you grew up in Nevada, where only 66.7% of youngsters get all their shots (State Scorecard, 2007, Table 3.4). The inequities begin at birth and last until death. In Maine, about 4.3 of 1,000 babies die each year, compared to 10 infant deaths per 1,000 births in Mississippi (State Scorecard, 2007, Table 6.3). And you might want to get involved with health reform now to avoid the dilemma of people who need long-term care. In North Dakota, fewer than 8 in 100 high-risk nursing home residents get pressure sores, but more than twice that, 19 in 100, get pressure sores in District of Columbia nursing homes (State Scorecard, 2007, Table 3.14). To find out how your state and country compare to others, see Box 12.8.

***Less Costs More*** You might think that restricted access saves money on health care. But the opposite is true. In the long run, it usually costs less to provide ongoing care than to wait until people's health deteriorates. In states with the lowest number of insured residents, the cost of health care is up to five times greater than in well-insured states (Cantor, Schoen, Belloff, How, & McCarthy, 2007).

Some countries have built their systems on this conviction. When I was in Japan studying their health system a few years ago, I was surprised to

BOX 12.8 **RESOURCES**

## Health System Assessments

An interactive U.S. map provides data from the *Commonwealth Fund State Scorecard on Health System Performance* at www.commonwealthfund.org/statescorecard.

Also see the U.S. Census Bureau's report "Income, Poverty, and Health Insurance Coverage in the United States: 2006," available at www.census.gov/hhes/www/hlthins/hlthin06.html.

For information on health systems throughout the world, visit WHO's Countries index at www.who.int/countries/en/ or the International Institute for Health Promotion at www.american.edu/academic.depts/cas/health/iihp/iihpcountryprofile.html.

learn that most Japanese citizens see a doctor at least once month. The visits are often brief—just a few minutes long. But regular contact keeps lines of communication open and allows caregivers to monitor changes in people's health very closely. (This is a built-in feature of the Japanese system because doctors dispense prescription medication, usually in 2- or 4-week increments.)

As further evidence of Japan's commitment to prevention, consider this: The United States spends about 11% of its health care budget on preventive care; Japan devotes 30% of its budget to prevention (Colby, 1997). This may be one reason that, although the Japanese spend less than half as much money per capita as the Unites States, they live an average of 5 years longer (WHO, 2008b).

*Out of Pocket, Out of Luck?* Even paying a fraction of personal medical costs can be financially devastating. Worldwide, 100 million people a year sink into poverty because of out-of-pocket medical bills (WHO, 2008b). The problem is worst in countries that require citizens to pay more than 15% of medical costs out-of-pocket. (The U.S. is dangerously close to that at 13% [American College of Physicians, 2008].)

About half of U.S. residents who file for bankruptcy do so because of medical bills (Himmelstein, Warren, Thorne, & Woolhandler, 2005). Middle-class families with children are especially hard hit. Three-quarters of those who go bankrupt because of medical costs are insured when their health crisis begins, but many lose their insurance when they are unable to continue working. The resulting spiral of lost wages and mounting bills is too much. And it doesn't take huge bills to drain the budget. The average out-of-pocket medical debt for those who go bankrupt is $11,854 (Himmelstein et al.).

*Hope* There is hope. A range of successful health care models exists around the world and within the United States. Policy analyst Joel Cantor and colleagues (2007) calculate that, if every U.S. state matched the national best in terms of avoidable mortality rates, care for chronic conditions, coverage for the uninsured, and efficiency, we could:

- Save 90,000 people a year who otherwise die from avoidable medical errors,
- Cut the number of uninsured Americans from 47 million to 23.5 million,
- Prevent 4 million people with diabetes from facing catastrophic outcomes such as kidney failure and limb amputation, and
- Save between $22 billion and $38 billion a year—on Medicare costs alone!

Cantor and coauthors observe that Rhode Island leads the nation in quality of care, thanks partly to its initiative to build quality incentives into the state Medicaid plan. Likewise, Hawaii long had the smallest percentage of uninsured residents of any state (10%), even with its large number of seasonal and part-time jobs, largely because Hawaii took the lead in 1974 to pass the first laws requiring employers to offer health plans. (As you will see, Massachusetts recently set a new record, only 7% uninsured, by implementing universal coverage.) Observations such as these inspire many to call for health care reform.

## The American Model

Before we talk about reform, let's quickly survey the current system. The United States is a **multi-payer** (also known as a *pluralistic*) **system**. That means that, when someone receives medical care, the bill may be paid by a number of sources, including government-sponsored programs, private insurance companies (about 24% of the time), and, in some cases, individuals. Publicly funded programs, such as Medicare, Medicaid, and the State Children's Health Insurance Program, as well as some private and local efforts are known as the **safety net**, a diverse collection of efforts to help provide for vulnerable and underserved populations.

Table 12.2 lists the strengths and weaknesses of the American system. After you review these, it should be easier to evaluate the pros and cons of health care reform models, which we discuss next.

## Universal Coverage Models

Imagine knowing that, from the moment you are born until you die, you can get health care any time you need it. **Universal coverage** means that all citizens and sometimes all residents and visitors are assured of health benefits. Universal coverage is based on a commitment to offer health services to everyone who needs them, regardless of age, ability to pay, or any other factor.

In some countries, universal coverage means that everyone is required to buy health insurance. In others, health care is funded through taxes or through contributions to a single national insurance plan, and people pay little or nothing when they need care. When my friend Andrea was in Italy recently, her son Zack got food poisoning. Local residents escorted them to the emergency room of a Roman hospital. "They immediately gave him a stretcher," Andrea recalls. "He had two rounds of antibiotics, several liters of IV fluids, an ultrasound, and three blood tests, and he spent a night in the ER." There was no charge for the visit.

In many countries, health care is regarded as a human right and as a foundation for the nation's

### Table 12.2 Strengths and Weaknesses of the U.S. Health Care System

| Strengths | Weaknesses |
|---|---|
| High-quality care is available for those who can afford it. | Limited care is available for 47 million uninsured Americans. |
| The medical workforce is well trained. | A critical shortage of nurses and primary care physicians plagues the system. |
| A wide range of services, including elective procedures, is available to those who can afford it. | There is minimal emphasis on prevention and health maintenance. |
| The system is highly responsive to emerging health concerns. | Limited access contributes to health disparities by age, race, income, and literacy level. |
| The nation is willing to make huge expenditures on health care. Between 1980 and 2003, the portion of the U.S. gross domestic product spent on health care nearly doubled—from 8.8% to 15.2% (Henry J. Kaiser, 2007). | Waste limits the usefulness of the large budget. The disproportionate rise in health care spending means the United States has less to spend on education, roads, housing, and other concerns. |
| The system is known for investing in expensive treatment technology. | The system has been sluggish about adopting communication technology such as electronic medical records. |

overall success. As you can see from Table 12.1, nearly all of the top 40 health systems offer universal coverage. In fact, the United States is the only wealthy industrialized nation that does not offer universal coverage.

It's not that Americans haven't considered it. Proposals to implement universal coverage date as far back as 1915 (Dranove, 2008). However, there has not been a great deal of support until recent years. A 2002 survey revealed that 49% of physicians favored national health insurance (Ackermann & Carroll, 2003). Within five years, physician support jumped to 60% (Carroll & Ackermann, 2008). And currently, about 81% of Americans support universal coverage in which all citizens are enrolled in either affordable public insurance or private insurance (Commonwealth Fund, 2008b).

## BOX 12.9 RESOURCES

## Health Care Reform in the States

For regular updates on state initiatives to institute universal coverage, see the Henry J. Kaiser Family Foundation website at www.kff.org.

In the past few years some U.S. cities and states have launched their own universal coverage plans. San Francisco, Massachusetts, and Vermont launched universal coverage in 2007. Maine has pledged to begin universal provisions, and similar proposals have been or will be considered in Connecticut, Illinois, Iowa, Kansas, Minnesota, New Jersey, New Mexico, New York, Oregon, Pennsylvania, Washington, and Wisconsin. Proposals in Colorado and California were considered but not approved by state legislators. (Box 12.9 provides a link to updates about state health reform efforts.) To get an idea what the plans implemented so far look like, let's sample a few.

*Massachusetts and Vermont* Let's imagine you live in Massachusetts or Vermont and you don't have health insurance. You have a few options.

- You can enroll in a public program for people in financial need who are not eligible for employer-based health insurance. MassHealth is such a public program. About 70% of members pay no premium. The most anyone pays is $105 per month for single coverage (Kaiser Commission, 2008, p. 9).
- Or you can apply for subsidies that help pay the cost of your insurance premiums. The amount of your subsidy depends on your income as it compares to the federal poverty line. For example, families whose annual incomes are 200% of the federal poverty line pay about $60 per month in Vermont, whereas families above 300% pay $1,100 per month. (See Box 12.10 for an explanation of the federal poverty line.)

## BOX 12.10

## What Is the Federal Poverty Line?

Every year since 1963, the U.S. Census Bureau has calculated a **federal poverty line** based on the cost of living. The poverty line is expressed in terms of annual family income. Families whose income is less than the specified amount are considered unable to pay for basic necessities. For example, in 2008 the poverty line for a family of four was $21,200 per year. This amount is applied to residents of the 48 continental sates and the District of Columbia. (The poverty line for Alaska and Hawaii are calculated separately.) You will sometimes see thresholds of poverty expressed in percentages, as in "200% of the federal poverty line." This means the family earns two times the poverty-line income (in our example, $42,400 for a family of four).

- Or the state will help you find an affordable private insurance plan.

In Vermont and Massachusetts, companies with 10 or more employees are required to **play or pay**. That is, they must either provide company-sponsored health plans that meet state regulations for minimum coverage or contribute to the state program. In Massachusetts, contributions equate roughly to $295 per employee per year, in Vermont $365 per employee per year. Rates are set to increase over time; but even so, the state contribution is typically less than a small company would pay for health benefits on its own.

The Massachusetts plan also includes an **individual mandate**, meaning that all residents of the state (with a few exceptions for religious reasons and other factors) are required by law to maintain health insurance. State residents must either submit proof of insurance with their annual income tax returns or pay a fine. (The penalty was $912 in 2008.) The fines help pay for participation in the state system.

So far, results are encouraging but mixed. In Massachusetts, nearly 93% of adults younger than 65 are now insured, making it the best-insured state in the country (Long, 2008). Enrollment in Vermont has been lower than expected, however. Sponsors had hoped to enroll 4,245 new subscribers by the end of 2007, but they enrolled only 1,352 (Kaiser Commission, 2008). Six months into the new plan, enrollment was at 2,764 (O'Connor, 2008). We may see lower numbers in Vermont because there is no individual mandate as there is in Massachusetts.

*Overview, Pros, and Cons*  Here's a quick overview of universal coverage proposals American-style (so far).

- People who like their current insurance can keep it.
- Conversely, those who are dissatisfied with their coverage, don't qualify for private coverage, or can't afford private coverage can enroll instead in public programs or get help paying for private coverage.
- The most successful model so far requires individuals to enroll in either public or private insurance or to pay a tax penalty that doubles as buy-in to the public health plan.
- Employers either offer health plans or contribute to the national plan.

If these reforms were implemented on a national scale, the U.S. health system would more closely resemble the Australian, Belgian, Dutch, French, German, and Swiss systems (to name just a few), which rely on a mixture of public and private programs to provide universal coverage.

The American reform model has a number of advantages, articulated by Cathy Schoen and colleagues (2008) as follows:

- *Little disruption.* People who are happy with the current system wouldn't notice much change.
- *Continuity of coverage.* National health insurance would prevent coverage interruptions for people who switch or lose their jobs. This would result in less of what economist David Dranove (2008) calls **job lock,** the tendency to stay with less-than-desirable jobs just to keep one's health coverage.
- *Equitable employer contributions.* The play-or-pay option would allow businesses, both large and small, to contribute a fair amount. (Currently small businesses carry a larger per-employee burden if they offer company health plans.)
- *Dramatic improvement in coverage.* Experts predict that the plan described would result in an 80/20 mix of private and public insurance, with 99% of the U.S. population being insured.
- *Cost effective.* Schoen and colleagues estimate, based on the Health Benefits Simulation Model, that total annual health care spending would increase by only about 1% ($15 billion), although the new plan would offer an additional $51.5 billion per year in health services. Based on their proposal, savings would come from lower administrative costs, more consistent employer contributions, and lower provider reimbursements. (The reimbursement plan would represent a slight drop in overall revenue for providers who currently serve mostly privately insured patients but an increase for those who now serve Medicaid and/or uninsured patients.)

Here are a few disadvantages of this model:

- *Continued disparities.* Even though nearly all Americans would be insured, their coverage and out-of-pocket burdens might differ substantially.
- *Uncertain tax burden.* Although overall health costs are not expected to increase much under the proposed plan and although gains in public health are expected to save money over time, it is possible that the initial tax burden would be greater.
- *Resources taxed.* If, overnight, 47 million uninsured Americans were suddenly able

to visit the doctor, we might see schedule overloads until the system adjusts. Likewise, there might be slightly longer waits for elective and nonemergency procedures. (On a brighter note, better ongoing care would reduce avoidable hospital and ER visits, helping to save money overall.)

Now that we have reviewed the common features of American universal coverage reform proposals, let's look at one more option.

### Single-Payer Model

In some countries, universal coverage is funded through a **single-payer system**. That means that one source—often the government, though it can be another source, such as a national health insurance company—pays all the bills. This can be accomplished through taxes or by collecting subscription fees from individuals and/or employers. A few of the countries with single-payer systems are Canada, the United Kingdom, Japan, and the Philippines.

In the Philippines a national health insurance corporation, PhilHealth, covers all sectors of the population, including people who are employed, unemployed, retired, rich, or poor. Employers help fund the system for workers, and unemployed families can get coverage for about 100 Filipino pesos per month (about $2.26 in American currency). The system is not perfect. Enrollment is voluntary, hospital access in some rural areas is still quite limited, and residents may find themselves billed for "surpluses," which are portions of their medical bills not covered by PhilHealth. But at least 70% of the nation's residents are enrolled, no small feat in a country of 82 million people—many of them poor, rural residents—spread across more than 7,000 islands (Obermann, Jowett, Alcantara, Banzon, & Bodard, 2006). The program is regarded as a model for developing countries, proof that a nation need not wait for economic prosperity to begin offering health care to all citizens.

Some reformers in the United States advocate switching to a single-payer system. This idea is sometimes referred to as "Medicare for all." Although Medicare has some faults (most notably gaps and complexities in its drug coverage policy), it has been quite successful overall. It covers 99% of people above retirement age, a group that, prior the 1960s, was largely out in the cold where health insurance was concerned. Research suggests that the health of many older adults improves once they are on Medicare (N. Anderson, 2008).

Here are some advantages of a single-payer system:

- *Large, diverse risk pool.* People pay into the system for most of their lives while they are healthy and draw from the system when they need medical care. This provides a better risk pool than in systems that serve mostly high-need or short-term subscribers.
- *Better access.* In contrast to private insurance companies, which sometimes deny coverage to people with preexisting conditions, a single-payer system includes everyone.
- *Wellness incentive.* When system administrators know they will care for a person all his or her life, they have a vested interest in maintaining that person's health from an early age.
- *Lower administrative costs.* It costs less to administer one system than many. And providers benefit from having one approval and billing procedure to follow (rather than dozens of them).
- *Less need for expensive advertising.*
- *Less likelihood that health care dollars will fund extravagant salaries for CEOs and other corporate leaders.*
- *Clearer benefits.* If you have ever asked your doctor if a procedure is covered by your insurance plan, you may realize the answer isn't always easy or foolproof. Some providers say they can't answer the question, and no wonder. They often deal with a mind-boggling number of plans and providers, each with its own parameters.
- *Fewer coverage interruptions because of job changes or retirement.*

- *Easier-to-maintain national standards for health coverage.*

There are some disadvantages of a single-payer system, however.

- *May involve a higher tax burden.*
- *May result in longer waits for elective and nonemergency procedures.*[2]
- *Less consumer choice than in free market systems.*
- *Fewer luxuries.* In a free market system, hospitals and medical centers often vie for patients who can pay top dollar by offering lavish amenities and surroundings. If everyone's care is funded at the same level, some of the amenities may disappear.

## Wrapping Up Talk About Universal Coverage

As you can see, universal coverage isn't a single model so much as underlying idea. In some cases, it means never having to pay out-of-pocket for medical care. In others, it means one national health plan serves everyone. So far, where universal coverage does exist in the United States, it mostly involves public assistance coupled with compulsory enrollment in either a public or a private health plan.

Many people argue the merits of universal coverage in terms of money. But some feel that it is an issue of human rights. Physician Joseph Swedish (2008) argues for universal coverage on humanitarian grounds:

> We know firsthand what happens when an uninsured diabetic postpones treatment and ends up in the emergency room, or is hospitalized for a preventable

complication. We treat the cancer patient who convinced himself to ignore early warning signs, fearing the expense associated with the lack of insurance coverage. These are human tragedies as well as avoidable costs. (p. 22)

Others join Swedish in arguing that financial considerations are well and good but that the bottom line is doing what is *right*:

> Questions of reform should be seen as ethical choices, as political options for what sort of society we seek to have, and not primarily as issues of economic or organizational adjustments.... Health care reforms must be comprehensive morally and not just economically. Health policy must engage us in terms of common civic purpose, not only as individual consumers of health services. (Churchill, 1994, p. 3).

Indeed, in many regions of the world, health care is considered an inalienable right.

It's also important to note that universal coverage usually has limits. Even in some "cradle to grave" health systems there are out-of-pocket expenses. In the United Kingdom, these average about 1,200 pounds a year (about $2,200 in American currency) in addition to 3,850 pounds (about $7,000) in annual taxes to support the National Health System (Donnelly, 2008). That's less than most U.S. citizens pay for premiums and deductibles (not to mention taxes), but it goes to show that health care is never free. It must be funded in some way—through taxes, premiums, out-of-pocket fees, employer contributions, or some other windfall. In the end, universal coverage isn't meant to make health care free but, rather, to make sure everyone is under the umbrella.

Anywhere you look, a natural impediment to reform is skepticism about the unfamiliar.

- Even as Americans are wary of becoming "like Canada," Canadians are afraid of becoming "like America." To many Canadians the U.S. system seems "too free market, too expensive and too inefficient" (Gratzer, 2008, p. A21).
- Some U.S. newspaper columnists caution against moving closer to "socialized

---

[2] Although this is a common argument against universal care, research is actually mixed. In a recent study, several universal-coverage nations outranked the United States in terms of wait time to see a doctor. Some 30% of U.S. residents surveyed said they could get same-day appointments with their doctors, whereas at least 50% of the residents of Germany, the Netherlands, and New Zealand had same-day access (Commonwealth, 2007). Americans seldom wait more than a month for elective and nonemergency surgeries, but that is also true in Germany, New Zealand, and Australia, all of which have universal coverage (Commonwealth, 2007).

medicine," whereas their counterparts in the London media worry that the U.K. system is subject to "creeping privatization" (Donnelly, 2008, p. 6).

- Meanwhile, the Japanese react with horror when Americans allow the poor to suffer, and many Japanese urge their leaders not to entrust health care to free market corporations, which they feel will be oriented to profits rather than humanitarianism (Kakizoe, 2008).

It is still too soon to say whether universal coverage is the wave of the future. But it's safe to say that you will be involved in the debate and its outcome no matter what lies ahead.

## SUMMARY

A collection of case studies illustrates the complexities and interrelatedness of public health, risk communication, crisis communication, and health care reform. From the mad cow disease saga we learn that, even when scientists cannot provide definitive answers, it is dangerous and unethical to keep the public in the dark about a potential health threat. Public officials naturally worry about creating panic, but there is little to suggest that people do panic in crises. The majority of evidence suggests just the opposite: People try to help each other. This desire to help others can actually make it difficult to convince citizens and rescue workers to use safety precautions, as we saw following the 9/11 terrorist attacks. Although people seldom panic, public health experts are advised to use fear appeals with sensitivity. Overloading the public with frightening messages can cause undue worry. Conversely, offering false reassurance can mislead the public and damage their trust in public officials. A different challenge is keeping an ongoing health crisis such as AIDS on the public agenda. Prevention efforts are complicated by the sensitive nature of transmission-related behaviors and the wide diversity of cultures affected. The AIDS case reminds us to listen to, respect, and understand the people we are trying to help.

The global nature of commerce and travel makes it imperative that health advocates around the world work together to monitor emerging concerns, track their incidence, and stop the spread of contagious illnesses as quickly as possible. The SARS case represents a successful effort to do just that. Efforts are already under way to respond to an avian fly pandemic if it occurs.

Although these lessons look easy on paper, the stress and demands of an actual crisis make them difficult to follow. The risk management/communication framework reminds us that the best crisis communicators lay solid groundwork before a crisis emerges so that they have information at hand, trusting and open relationships with stakeholders, and well-developed and well-rehearsed plans in place. Also keep in mind that crisis management involves everyone, whether a member of the affected public, a journalist, or a health professional. The anthrax case study reminds us that a wide range of professionals is likely to be enlisted for help, making crisis management skills an important part of anyone's professional portfolio. At the same time, ethical dimensions of risk and crisis communication are everyone's businesses. In this chapter, we debated the question: Who should receive the limited number of vaccines in the case of a deadly pandemic?

Health care reform efforts are designed to create structures and processes that nurture good health among the population. The United States—despite its reputation for offering highly skilled, high-tech care—does not lead the world on most health indicators, mostly because, while people of means get excellent care, millions go without. This disparity occurs even though the United States spends more than 8 times the per capita average of other nations. The United States is unique among peer nations in that it does not guarantee universal care. However, a number of states within the country are considering or have implemented their own universal coverage plans. So far, these build on the multipayer system already in place and offer assistance to citizens in need so that everyone in the state may be adequately insured. Some plans involve individual mandates requiring all citizens to be insured, either through a private company or a public health plan. One alternative, which has been implemented by many countries, is universal coverage funded by a single payer such as the government or a national health insurance company. All in all, it is difficult to imagine systems that are different than the one to which we are accustomed, but people who can knowledgeably debate and guide reform efforts will have powerful influence over the future of health care.

## KEY TERMS

public health
social mobilization
risk communication
crisis communication
risk management/communication framework (RMCF)
bioterrorism
electronic medical records (EMRs)
multipayer system
safety net
universal coverage
federal poverty line
play or pay
individual mandate
job lock
single-payer system

## DISCUSSION QUESTIONS

1. Do you remember when mad cow disease was frequently in the news? If so, did you feel adequately informed about it? Did you feel personally at risk? Why or why not?

2. What lessons can we learn from the BSE case study?

3. Describe some of the career options and resources relevant to public health. Are any of these interesting to you? Why or why not?

4. What is public health? How does it compare to individual medical care?

5. What is social mobilization? Can you think of an effort to mobilize the public that has affected you (e.g., a don't-drink-and-drive campaign that involves active participation, involvement in a community effort to pass a local tax, a health education class, a political campaign, or the like)? If so, describe your experience.

6. What is risk communication? How does it differ from health promotion?

7. This chapter contains about 27 lessons for risk and crisis communication. Name at least 15 of them. Try to think of examples from the book as well as examples that do not appear in the book.

8. What advice do you have for health crisis communicators who are worried about creating panic?

9. What are the three risk communication traditions presented by Peter Sandman? Which is most descriptive of risk communication? Of crisis communication?

10. What factors should health communicators consider when using fear appeals?

11. Describe the risk management/communication framework (RMCF) that Scott Ratzan and Wendy Meltzer present.

12. Discuss the ethical implications raised by the Andrew Speaker and Mary Mallon (Typhoid Mary) cases. Why might such public health risks be even more salient today than in Mallon's time? What do you think we should do to protect individual liberties while preserving the public's health interest?

13. Describe the Pleasure Project's approach to preventing HIV transmission. Do you find this approach appealing or offensive? Why?

14. Give a basic timeline of events in the SARS case. How were the officials able to contain the disease so quickly?

15. Do you remember news coverage about SARS? Do you feel you were adequately informed? Did you feel personally at risk? Why or why not?

16. If an incident of bioterrorism occurs in your state or community, what spokespeople will you trust most? What type of information will you want? Through what channels are you most likely to seek information?

17. Give the opportunity, would you like to be part of a crisis management team such as the CDC communication team? Why or why not? What aspects of the job appeal to you most? What do you think would be most difficult?

18. Trace the development of the H5N1 avian flu case so far. Would you be frightened if a containment zone is declared in your area? Why

or why not? Do you feel adequately informed about and prepared for such a crisis? Why or why not?

19. Discuss the ethical implications of administering to a limited number of people a vaccine against a deadly epidemic. Who do you think should be vaccinated first? Why?

20. Were you surprised that the United States health system ranks 37th in the world? Why or why not? What factors, if improved, might move the United States higher on the list?

21. How does the United States compare to other countries in terms of charges for health services relative to other expenses, equitable care, health care spending, life expectancy, physician–citizen ratio, and use of electronic medical records?

22. In what ways are health care dollars wasted in the United States? Have you ever experienced these or other wasteful practices yourself? If so, explain how.

23. What is an electronic medical record? Why are EMRs valuable?

24. Describe some of the factors that lead to inequities in the U.S. health care system.

25. How does your state compare to others in terms of health indicators and insurance coverage for all citizens?

26. Describe the typical chain of events that leads a family in the United States to go bankrupt because of medical bills.

27. What does it mean to be a multipayer health system? When you get medical care, who pays the bill—you or your family, a private insurance company, a public or school-based health program, or some other entity?

28. Outline at least five strengths and five weaknesses of the U.S. health care system. Which of these are most important to you? Why?

29. What does the term *universal coverage* mean? Are you in favor of universal coverage? Why or why not?

30. Describe your options for health coverage if you lived in Vermont or Massachusetts. In what ways are these two states' plans alike? How are they different? Which plan has enrolled a greater percentage of citizens? Why?

31. What does the term *play or pay* mean relative to the Vermont and Massachusetts programs?

32. What does it mean to have an individual mandate? What is the penalty for violating this mandate in Massachusetts?

33. What are the advantages of a multipayer universal coverage plan with an individual mandate and "play or pay" requirements for employers? What are the disadvantages?

34. What is the significance of a risk pool?

35. What are the advantages and disadvantages of a single-payer program? Do you prefer multipayer or single-payer models? Why?

## ANSWERS TO *CAN YOU GUESS?*

1. Texas has the highest percentage of uninsured residents (24.1%) of any state.

2. Massachusetts wins, with only 7% uninsured as of 2008. But, based on the latest census statistics (released in 2006), a number of states are close behind. The following states tie for second, with 8% to 10% uninsured residents: Minnesota, Hawaii, Iowa, Wisconsin, Maine.

3. Insurance premiums for a family in the Philippines total about 1,200 Filipino pesos per year (equivalent to about $27 in the United States).

4. Insured families in the United States pay about $10,728 in premiums per year (Robert Wood Johnson Foundation, 2008).

# CHAPTER 13

# Planning Health Promotion Campaigns

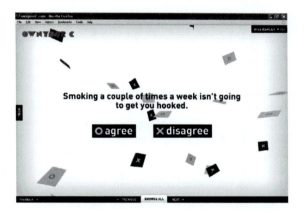

**Own Your C - Smoking Graphic**
Photo courtesy of Cactus Marketing and Communications

*Do you agree or disagree with the question posed above?* Click your answer on the Own Your C website (ownyourC.com) and see how your response compares to those of others. Then try your hand at a variety of other questions on smoking, nutrition, fashion, UFOs, friendship, and more:

*Does fast food make teens fat?*
*Does how you dress define who you are?*
*Do UFOs exist?*
*Do your friends know the real you?*

Indicate your answers to questions such as these, and they become part of a running tally. (When I went online, 56% agreed that "the cigarette is dead" and 47% agreed that "I'm more stressed than most others.") It's an interactive, ongoing peer opinion poll that invites teens to comment on key issues and read others' comments. In the end, it's all about *choices*—represented by the letter *C*. The Own Your C campaign began as a statewide effort in Colorado to dissuade teens from smoking but has since expanded into an interactive "choice-making community." The campaign reflects the powerful impact of audience analysis. It's designed to capture the attention of 12- to 18-year-olds—not so that adults can tell them what to do, but to empower teens to make healthy decisions for themselves. Own Your C has caught young people's attention and won numerous awards. (See Box 13.1 for more about the campaign.)

As you will see in this chapter, different audiences have different preferences. Designing health promotion messages that are both advantageous and audience-oriented is a multistage process.

In the previous chapter, we discussed the overlap between public health and crisis communication. Here we turn our attention to another side of the same coin—efforts to help people protect themselves from more chronic health threats, such as cancer, obesity, diabetes, and accidents. Whereas crisis communicators typically try to assuage people's fears, the goal in health promotion is usually to alert people that they may be more vulnerable than they think. As you will

BOX 13.1

## Campaign Spotlight: Own Your C

*I think if you were born outside a major metropolis, you're not as easily stressed out. Life is good, enjoy it people, relax. In with the good air, out with the bad, lol*

*'Hate to shatter the dream, but it's gonna take longer than our lifetimes to restore the environment to its original state. However, a difference can be made, and it's possible that even the ozone layer can be completely repaired in 40 to 50 years…*

*I only smoked a couple times a week. These were the best times of smoking, and led to me buying pack after pack after pack, faster and faster. Don't think it'll happen to you? Try it. I've been smoking a pack a day for three years now.*

These are just a few of the comments teens have posted on ownyourC.com. Forget your stereotypes of what being a teenager is all about. These young people are sometimes stressed and sometimes playful, but mostly they are…smart! And amazingly witty.

The idea for Own Your C emerged after the Colorado State Tobacco Education & Prevention Partnership (STEPP) commissioned the Denver-based Cactus Marketing Communications firm to create an antitobacco campaign for teens. Before they made another move, members of the Cactus team got to work learning more about the youth they hoped to reach. They witnessed, through teens' eyes, the allure of high-fashion tobacco ads promoting tantalizing products such as flavored cigarettes named Kauai Kolada and Mandarin Mint (Cactus, 2007, p. 3). They got a close-up look at today's teen lifestyle, in which MP3 players, cell phones, and handheld computers are indispensable.

The researchers soon realized that, while they were trying to put a finger on which brands

teens like most, the teens were creating their own "brands"—sophisticated online profiles on MySpace and Facebook. Through these personal profiles, the teens play an active role in creating and promoting identities for themselves (Cactus, p. 3). Virtual environments their grandparents could never have imagined are as familiar as the bus stop or the cafeteria. And if teens aren't sure what to expect beyond college, they are at least clear on the tenor of their future plans. The research team came to appreciate that most young people today feel "surrounded by negative messages and want to see things that reflect their optimism" (Cactus, p. 4). They enjoy envisioning idealized futures for themselves, and they like the sense that they can accomplish anything.

Today's teens are not entirely unrecognizable from generations past, however. As it was when their parents were younger, dire predictions typically bounce off them. Teens tend to believe they are immune to harm or at least long decades away from it (Cactus, 2007). They typically focus on the present and the immediate future. Consequently, they can be impulsive and get caught up following the "in crowd." And although some teens are inclined to do what adults tell them (therefore it *is* important to say, "Don't smoke"), the older they get, the more likely teens are to crave a sense of personal freedom and empowerment. At that point, the very idea that cigarettes are dangerous and against the rules can make them enticing "forbidden fruit" (Cactus, p. 3).

With these insights, Cactus and STEPP created, not just a health communication campaign, but a full-fledged brand capable of breaking through the "advertising clutter" that surrounds teens today. In the fall of 2006, they unveiled Own Your C. The *C* stands for "choices," a key word in the campaign and the concept behind it. The campaign designers explain:

> "Choice" was selected as a message because it is universal to all youth, regardless of gender, geographic location, ethnicity, sexual orientation, income or age. Choice is relevant

to all teens since it connects to them on an emotional level. While youth are impulsive by nature, they demonstrate that they are receptive to messages that provide perspective and empower them. (Cactus, 2007, p. 4)

The "own it" message reflects teens' own wording. "Among young adults, *own it* means to step up and take accountability for your actions" (Cactus, p. 4).

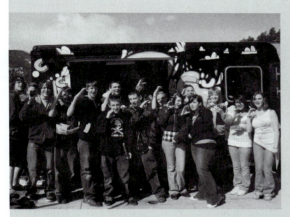

Photo courtesy of Cactus Marketing and Communications

Own Your C is a multimedia, interactive experience that involves an engrossing website (developed in partnership with New York-based Agency Net), irreverent TV spots, and a tricked-out ice cream truck (the C-ride, pictured above) that travels to youth events around the state. Campaign directors say the idea is not for adults to tell youth what to do but, instead, "to share responsibility and power with young people" (Cactus, 2007, p. 2). The emphasis is on teens' ability to make good choices for themselves. Own Your C creators remind website visitors:

Our role is to simply start the conversation around topics you care about. Like tobacco, health, self-image, culture, alcohol, relationships and school.... This site belongs to you. Meaning everyone here has a voice

and the power to own his or her choice. You will be heard. Come C for yourself.

Registered users can post comments on a wide range of issues and read others' responses. They can also sort responses in terms of answer (for example, comments from people who agree that "relationships get in the way of friendships") or authors' sex, age, or geographic location. If you want to know what teens your age, in your zip code, think about smoking, it's there with a click of a button.

The website includes a schedule of C-Ride events around the state and quick facts about tobacco use, including photos of stained teeth and the hard facts about cancer. Teens can click on links to resources on substance abuse, sexual assault, and suicide prevention. They can also sign up for *Fixnixer*, which guides them in personalizing a 21-day program to quit smoking or chewing tobacco. Participants receive information and tips, take part in blogs, and receive personalized e-mails and text messages designed to strengthen their resolve.

Own Your C television spots (available on the website) are spoofs with clear messages about the importance of choice. In one, a teen furtively runs into a grassy field and flings three large *C*s into the sky. One year later, as he is walking down a city sidewalk, *C*s begin pelting down on all sides of him. As the menacing and quickly multiplying *C*s split the sidewalk, break glass, and set off car alarms, the youth dashes into a phone booth, terrified and out of breath. The phone rings, and a maniacal horror-movie voice on the line warns: "Be careful with your choices. They may come back to haunt you."

The Own Your C campaign has been recognized as a leader among health campaigns and as a brand name in league with Adidas, Gillette, and others. It has won a long list of awards and was presented as an exemplar at the 2008 National Conference on Health Communication, Marketing, and Media. Even better, in the first month of launch, the website attracted visitors from 143 countries, and it has experienced high levels of engagement with target

*(continued)*

BOX 13.1 (*continued*)

audience members, who spend an average of 5 minutes or more viewing about 18 pages per visit. Campaign representatives have visited more than 150 schools in 49 counties across Colorado. When program sponsors asked teens to submit original video vignettes about smoking, they received more than 100 entries. An Australian student wrote to campaign leaders to thank them for being "refreshing" and "nonpreachy." Another young person wrote to say, "Thanks for not lecturing." Health officials in at least five other states are interested in bringing Own Your C to their communities.

see, keeping health issues on the public agenda and working with people to change their everyday behaviors can be as challenging as managing a crisis.

**Health-promoting behaviors** are those that "enhance health and well-being, reduce health risks, and prevent disease" (Brennan & Fink, 1997, p. 157). These behaviors include lifestyle choices, medical care, prevention efforts, and activities that foster an overall sense of well-being.

**Health promotion campaigns** are systematic efforts to influence people to engage in health-enhancing behaviors (Backer & Rogers, 1993). These efforts may involve the use of many communication channels, from face-to-face communication to mass media. The term **health promoter** includes anyone involved in the process of creating and distributing health promotion messages. This includes volunteers in the community, employees of nonprofit health agencies, public relations and community relations professionals, production artists, media decision makers, and more. As this list suggests, health promotion offers diverse career opportunities for communication specialists (See Box 13.2).

In this chapter we consider the challenges of promoting health behaviors among diverse members of the population. We'll begin with a brief overview of health campaigns, describing some particularly notable ones. Then we'll follow the first four stages of designing a health promotion campaign:

*Step 1:* Defining the situation and potential benefits

*Step 2:* Analyzing and segmenting the audience

*Step 3:* Establishing campaign goals and objectives

*Step 4:* Selecting channels of communication

Steps 5 through 7, on designing and implementing a campaign, are covered in the next chapter. Keep in mind that it is important to know all the steps before you actually begin. Although evaluating and refining the campaign is the final step, you must consider from the beginning how you will accomplish those goals later on. The steps in these chapters are based on recommendations by J. D. Brown and Einsiedel (1990) and reflect an abbreviated version of the steps recommended by the CDC and the National Cancer Institute.

## BACKGROUND ON HEALTH CAMPAIGNS

"Live long and prosper," the Vulcan salutation on *Star Trek*, seems to say it all. A long and healthy existence—isn't that what life is all about? You might think so. But it turns out that Vulcan logic is not always able to explain human behavior, as Mr. Spock discovered.

Early health campaigns were designed with the confidence that humans want nothing so much as their own health and longevity. From that viewpoint it follows that, if people know a behavior is unhealthy, they will not act that way. Likewise, they should go to great lengths to pursue health-enhancing outcomes. Seen this way, persuasion was not an issue. People only needed reliable information. The motivation to comply with it was presumably already there, as innate as the animal instinct for survival.

## BOX 13.2 CAREER OPPORTUNITIES

# Health Promotion and Education

Hospital-based health educator
School-based health educator
Community health educator
Director of nonprofit organization
Patient advocate or patient navigator
Professor/educator
Health information publication designer
Corporate wellness director
Fitness instructor

## Career Resources and Job Listings

American Association for Health Education: aahperd.org/aahe

Society for Public Health Education: sophe.org
Area Health Education Centers: nationalahec.org/main/ahec.asp
Society for Public Health Education: sophe.org
Health Care Job Store, Inc.: Healtheducationjobs.com
National Commission for Health Education Credentialing (NCHEC): nchec.org
NCHEC: Health Educators Working for Wellness: nchec.org/forms/OOQ_health_educators.pdf
U.S. Bureau of Labor Statistics Occupational Outlook: bls.gov/oco/ocos063.htm
Chronicle of Higher Education: chronicle.com/jobs
Center for Disease Prevention and Control Division of Health Communication: cdc.gov/od/oc/hcomm/aboutdivision.html
National Institutes of Health: nih.gov
World Health Organization: who.int/employment/vacancies/en

## Motivating Factors

It turns out that influencing human behavior is not that simple. People are motivated by a number of factors that make them more or less receptive to health information and more or less motivated to change their behavior. Sometimes people do things they know to be unhealthy because the behavior is inexpensive, convenient, socially rewarding, or fun (Brown & Einsiedel, 1990). For instance, research indicates people may drink alcoholic beverages even though they believe them to be unhealthy because they are reluctant to give up the social ritual of drinking with friends. Conversely, people sometimes change their behavior without knowing much about the change or the reasons for it. They may try a behavior (like taking vitamins) simply because someone in authority tells them to or because the change seems interesting, easy, fashionable, or so on. In these instances, knowledge may *follow* behavior change.

Research has not always been encouraging about health campaigns' actual effects. Campaigns have

been criticized for naively seeking to change people's behavior without changing their circumstances (J. Green, 1996) and for assuming that knowledge reaches and affects all people equally (J. D. Brown & Walsh-Childers, 1994).

In reality, campaigns may raise awareness, but, unless the recommended behaviors are compatible with people's beliefs and are supported within their social networks, campaigns are unlikely to change people's behavior. Health promoters have discovered they cannot simply educate people about health and presume they will adjust their lifestyles accordingly. A range of factors must be taken into account. This means the promoter must know the audience, and he or she must consider, not just why audience members should act in recommended ways, but also why they may find it difficult to do so.

## Exemplary Campaigns

This section describes five exemplary health promotion campaigns. Each provides an inspiring lesson for promoters. Together, these examples illustrate that health promoters must often do more than simply give out information if they are to succeed. Sensitivity to audience needs, problem-solving skills, assessment, and careful planning and follow-through are required as well.

*Go to the Audience*  A health promoter interviewed by a student of mine once said, "You can't talk to people where you wish they were. You have to talk to them where they really are." His words characterize one quality of good campaigners: *They know their audiences well and design campaigns to suit those audiences.*

One example of this is the "Powerful Girls Have Powerful Bones" campaign, sponsored by the National Bone Health Campaign. The website (girlshealth.gov/bones) features a bright pink background, photos of young girls having fun, and an invitation to join "Carla and Friends" in a series of interactive, animated computer games. In one game, the challenge is to choose and move high-calcium snacks from a conveyer belt onto the girls' lunch trays before time runs out. One reward for participating in the games is the choice of a new outfit for the animated character, available in a colorful virtual boutique. The website is carefully designed to appeal to young girls, its target audience.

Another exemplary campaign was designed to reach elderly African American women, who are at high risk for breast cancer but are often unable to afford cancer screening and are hard to reach via traditional media. In the 1990s, campaigner designers noted that the women they most wanted to reach had a favorite place for swapping stories and sharing information—the beauty salon (Forte, 1995). With this in mind, they arranged for salons in Los Angeles to show throughout the day an educational video about breast cancer. The video featured African American women and emphasized that they are at high risk for cancer. Salon clients were also given pamphlets about breast cancer and were offered free mammograms at a local clinic or in a mobile unit scheduled to visit the salon on a regular basis. According to Deirdra Forte,

the beauty of this program was that, "by showing the video where African American women already exchange information and socialize, they are more likely to understand and accept the benefit of mammography" (paragraph 22). The campaign was honored as one of the year's best by the U.S. Department of Health and Human Services. Similar programs have since been launched in numerous locations around the country (Linnan & Ferguson, 2007).

*Take Action*  Another lesson is that health promotion comes in many forms, and *sometimes actions are as important as words.* When the leaders of an extensive heart health campaign in New York City realized that preschoolers in the area received 40% of their daily saturated fat from whole milk served at school, they put down their pens for a while and rolled up their sleeves (Shea, Basch, Wechsler, & Lantigua, 1996; Wechsler & Wernick, 1992). In addition to public education, community involvement, and a multimedia campaign, the health promoters convinced school officials to serve low-fat milk. The program won awards for its open-eyed, innovative approach.

*Measure Your Success*  The value of combining media exposure, community outreach, and scientific research was demonstrated by the Minnesota Heart Health Program (MHHP), which was one the most extensive health campaigns in American history (Luepker et al., 1994). It was conducted for 13 years (1980–1993) and involved nearly half a million people in the upper Midwest (Luepker et al.). The goal of MHHP was to lower heart-disease risk factors (cholesterol, high blood pressure, and smoking) and increase heart-healthy behaviors such as exercise. It included an extensive mass media campaign, educational programs in schools, and the involvement of local organizations.

What made MHHP extraordinary was its dedication to charting the health outcomes of people exposed to campaign messages. It is a good example of how to *establish goals and measure your success.* Researchers monitored people's behavior over a period of years and compared people touched by the campaign to people in other communities. Over time, they found modest but significant decreases in high blood pressure, high cholesterol, and smoking in communities involved in the program (Luepker et al., 1994). There was also a notable increase in physical activity among female schoolchildren involved in the heart-healthy education programs (Kelder, Perry, & Klepp, 1993).

*Encourage Social Support* An award-winning program called the 90-Second Intervention is being used to lower some Americans' risk of high blood pressure (Fishman, 1995). The intervention program is based on the principle that *recruiting social support for healthy behaviors increases the likelihood that people will stick to them*. The 90-Second Intervention was designed considering that many Americans (about 50 million) are at risk for high blood pressure but that compliance with medical advice is notoriously low, mostly because people with high blood pressure feel OK most of the time so that they do not perceive a reason to change their lifestyle or continue medication. (Despite the lack of symptoms, high blood pressure can lead to strokes, heart disease, and kidney disease.)

The campaign planners reasoned that people would be more likely to follow medical advice if their doctors were not the only ones imploring them to eat right, exercise, and stay on medication and if they received daily encouragement. Therefore, they designed a simple intervention program that takes place in the doctor's office. During a checkup, the doctor asks the patient to call a loved one and ask that person to commit to becoming a "health partner." The partner's role is to exercise with the patient, help maintain a healthy diet, and so on. The genius of the plan is that it makes healthy behaviors socially rewarding. The health partner and patient both benefit from the healthy activities they enjoy together, and the doctor is no longer the only one concerned about the problem. The 90-second phone call is presumably well worth the effort.

Next let's consider how we would create our own health campaign.

## PLANNING A HEALTH CAMPAIGN

To illustrate the steps in planning a health campaign, imagine that staff members of a university sports recreation department have asked you to help recruit new participants. Specifically, they would like to increase the number of people who go to the campus gym in their free time. The recreation department will not benefit financially from the added enrollment, but the staff wishes to increase participation because physical activity improves people's health. In accepting this project, you take on the role of health promoter. The rest of the chapter guides you through the initial steps of creating a campaign. The hypothetical sports recreation campaign is admittedly a small-scale effort, but many influential campaigns are aimed at limited audiences, and improving health habits among even a small group is a momentous goal. Furthermore, the steps given apply well to large and small campaigns.

### Step 1: Defining the Situation and Potential Benefits

If you are like many people, your first instinct is to post fliers and to send a story about the recreation program to the campus newspaper. Those may be effective steps; but before you begin, take the advice of professional campaign planners and do some preliminary research to assess potential benefits and the current situation (Nowak & Siska, 1995).

*Benefits* At this stage, you should be interested in learning what benefits (if any) your efforts might achieve. Following are some questions you might research.

- Would exercising at the gym actually improve people's health?
- Would everybody benefit?
- Are there some people who would not benefit?
- Are there alternative ways to get the same benefits?

Answers to these questions can be obtained by reading published literature and talking with experts in the field. Such preliminary research will prepare you to share useful knowledge with others and may help you decide if the project is worthwhile.

*Current Situation* Assuming that you find reasonable evidence to believe that people might benefit from exercising at the gym, the next step is to assess the current situation. Following are some questions to guide your preliminary research. The same questions will be useful later in guiding audience analysis. Remember that experts, program leaders, current participants, and nonparticipants are all valuable sources of information. In addition to these general questions, you may want to add some specific questions relevant to your campaign.

- How many people currently participate in the recommended behavior?
- What types of people participate and for what reasons? (Of interest is demographic information, such as age, sex, and income, as well as cultural, personal, social, or personality variables that might be relevant.)
- What are the strengths and weaknesses of the program (from the perspective of participants and nonparticipants)?
- What types of people do not participate?
- What are their reasons for not participating?
- What factors are most important to participants and nonparticipants (e.g., cost, convenience, social interaction)?
- Do people consider the potential benefits of this behavior important? Why or why not?
- Are there any conditions under which nonparticipants might participate?
- How do the people in your audience usually receive information (i.e., fliers, newspaper, radio, e-mail, etc.)?
- Through what channels do they prefer to get information?
- What information sources do they trust?

Preliminary answers to your questions may surprise you. You may find, for instance, that current sports recreation participants are not primarily concerned about health benefits. They go to the gym because their friends are there and they enjoy the social interaction. Or you might find that some people will not participate no matter how healthy physical activity is because they are afraid of looking foolish on the basketball court or out of shape in aerobics classes. Perhaps recreational programs are scheduled when many people cannot attend them. If these factors are important, simply educating people about the health benefits of exercise may not do much good.

*Diverse Motivations* Keep in mind that health concerns are not people's only motivation. People are most receptive to options that satisfy them on many levels (intellectual, emotional, personal, social, etc.). In assessing the situation, it is important not to assume that everyone is motivated in the same way as you. Consider (and ask about) the diversity among people who might participate in the sports recreation program. Your audience is probably not just traditional college students (a diverse group in itself), but international students, people with disabilities, middle-aged and older adults, experienced students and newcomers, university faculty and staff members, and maybe even community members and children.

In Step 2, you will attempt to learn about your audience and choose a portion of it to target. Being sensitive to diverse beliefs and motivations can help you understand why people behave as they do. This understanding is crucial to your success as a health promoter.

## Step 2: Analyzing and Segmenting the Audience

After assessing the health benefits and the current situation at the sports recreation department, you are ready to analyze the audience. This will involve asking a larger number of people many of the questions you asked in preliminary research.

Audience research may seem an unnecessary step, but experienced campaign planners know better. Audience analysis allows health promoters to collect important data about people's behaviors and preferences. It pays to know, in advance, what sources target audiences members use and trust, how they view their overall health, what their main concerns are, and more (Ledlow, Johnson, & Hakoyama, 2008). Edward Maibach and Roxanne Parrott (1995) applaud promoters for considering the audience's needs before they determine campaign goals. As they put it, audience-centered analysis "means that health messages are designed primarily to respond to the needs and situation of the target audience, rather than to the needs and situation of the message designers or sponsoring organizations" (p. 167).

*Data Collection* There are several ways to learn about potential audience members. Preexisting databases are a good place to start (Salmon & Atkin, 2003). For example, you might request demographics about the student body and usage statistics from the campus recreation department.

You should also seek more specific information about the target audience's beliefs, values, and habits. This section describes the comparative advantages of using interviews, questionnaires, and focus groups to learn about the people you hope to help.

**INTERVIEWS** Interviews are a useful way to collect information. Here are different interview strategies and the advantages and limitations of each (based on Frey, Botan, Friedman, & Kreps, 1991).

- **Highly scheduled interviews.** Interviewers are given specific questions to ask and are not allowed to make comments or ask additional questions. This helps minimize the interviewers' influence on respondents' answers, but it does not allow for follow-up questions or clarifications. Answers are typically brief but easy to tally and compare.
- **Moderately scheduled interviews.** Interviewers are given a set of questions but are allowed to ask for clarification and additional information as they see fit. These interviews are more relaxed and conversational, but less precise, than highly scheduled interviews.

- **Unscheduled interviews.** Interviewers are given a list of topics but are encouraged to phrase questions as they wish and to probe for more information when it seems useful and appropriate. These interviews are useful for collecting information about respondents' feelings, but they do not yield answers that can easily be compared or tallied.

**QUESTIONNAIRES** Questionnaires are another popular way to collect audience information, because they can be administered to large numbers of people in less time than it would take to interview them. A **questionnaire** asks respondents to write down their answers to a list of questions. In general, written responses are more limited than interview responses, but people may be more willing to answer sensitive questions in writing, especially if surveys are conducted anonymously.

**COMMUNICATION SKILL BUILDERS: DESIGNING A QUESTIONNAIRE** Here are some guidelines for designing an effective questionnaire (based on Arnold & McClure, 1989, and Frey et al., 1991).

- *Keep it brief.* People are most likely to complete the questionnaire if it is no longer than one page.
- *Seek immediate response.* If people take time to complete the survey right away, the response rate will be higher.
- *Collect demographic information.* Demographic information includes age, sex, income, college major, occupation, and the like. Ask respondents to select the appropriate responses from a list of all possibilities. (These are called **fixed-alternative questions.**) This will make it easy for respondents to answer and easy for you to count and compare answers.
- *Ask about knowledge and behaviors.* A mixture of open and closed questions will yield the most useful information. **Open questions** allow respondents to express ideas in their own words (e.g., How do you

feel about basketball and aerobics?). **Closed questions** require very brief answers (e.g., Do you prefer basketball or aerobics?).

- *Pilot (pretest) the questionnaire.* Try the questionnaire on a few people before making a full set of copies. Ask them to indicate if any questions are confusing or leading, if the fixed-alternative questions include all possible answers, and if they can think of other questions that should be added.
- *Allow for anonymity.* If you think people may wish to respond anonymously, provide a way for them to fill out questionnaires privately and to submit them without revealing their identity (as in a drop box or through the mail).

FOCUS GROUPS  A third option for collecting information is the use of focus groups. A **focus group** involves a small number of people who respond to questions posed by a moderator (Berko, Wolvin, & Curtis, 1993). The moderator tries to encourage the group members to speak openly on topics relevant to the campaign. Members' comments are usually recorded so that they can be studied later. Focus groups are useful for learning the target audience's feelings about an issue. Myra Crawford and colleagues (2005) used focus groups to gauge how nurses and social workers felt about a proposed quit-smoking campaign for pregnant women (M. A. Crawford, Woodby, Russell, & Windsor, 2005), and Kim Witte (1997) used focus groups to ask teenage mothers about the impact of peer pressure and education on young people's sexual behavior.

Whether you use surveys, questionnaires, or focus groups, it is important to think carefully about whom you include. Choosing people to include is called **sampling** the population. Interviews and surveys allow you to collect information from a large number of people. Make sure your sample reflects the diversity in the population you are considering. By contrast, focus group members are usually chosen because they are members of a target group (like nontraditional students or freshmen). Too much diversity can make it hard to develop a focused discussion. For example, when M. F. Casper and colleagues (2006) conducted

focus groups about coed drinking patterns, they had student participants fill out questionnaires in advance. Then they assigned students to one of three focus groups. The students didn't know it, but the groups reflected their typical drinking levels—nondrinkers, moderate, and more-than-average drinkers (Casper, Child, Gilmour, McIntyre, & Pearson, 2006). The researchers knew that participants were more likely to engage in open discussion if it emerged that other people in the room had similar feelings.

In your case, you might choose to conduct separate focus groups with people who use the workout facilities and those who do not. Too much diversity among participants in any one group makes it difficult to develop key ideas and may discourage some people from participating. Just be careful not to assume that one group speaks for the others or for the population overall.

COMMUNICATION SKILL BUILDERS: CONDUCT-ING FOCUS GROUPS  Experts offer the following tips for conducting effective focus groups (based mostly on Greenbaum, 1991, and Katcher, 1997):

- Determine what type of information you most want to collect. Bruce Katcher (1997) advises: "You must be clear from the outset what you really want to learn from the participants and how you will use the information" (p. 222). For example, are you more interested in the opinions of people who already use the sport recreation center or people who are not yet involved?
- Design a list of open questions to get the information you most want.
- Appoint (or hire) a facilitator to lead the focus group discussion. A good facilitator helps people feel comfortable expressing their opinions, allows everyone to contribute to the discussion, and does not influence members' responses. Many experts recommend using a facilitator not associated with the promotion effort because focus group members may feel more comfortable voicing criticisms and because the facilitator may be more objective.

- Choose 7 to 10 people from your target audience to make up each focus group.
- Arrange to conduct the focus group in a conference room or another comfortable area. (It is customary to provide refreshments for focus group participants.)
- Arrange to audiotape and videotape the session unobtrusively (with participants' permission).
- Review the information collected.
- Consider conducting multiple focus groups with different members of your target audience.

*Segmenting the Audience* The next step is to use the data you have collected to identify a target audience, also called a *focus community*. Following are some questions to consider.

- Who is currently involved (and not involved) in the recommended activity?
- What are people's reasons for participating (or not)?
- Who stands to benefit from the recommended behaviors?
- Who is in most need of these benefits?
- Who might reasonably be expected to adopt these behaviors?
- Is there anyone who should *not* be encouraged to participate?

Remember that some campaigns do more harm than good by recommending behaviors inappropriate for the audience. For example, vigorous exercise is not right for everybody. As you consider who should receive information about the sports recreation program, it may be tempting to target everyone possible. However, research suggests that appealing to an entire population at one time does not usually pay off. Because people tend to evaluate information based on its relevance to them, a broad message may seem too general for anyone to take personally (Slater, 1995). Furthermore, tastes differ, and what appeals to one group does not necessarily appeal to others. Messages that try to satisfy everyone very often become so generic that they do not interest anyone. The odds are that, even on small

campuses, the population is varied enough to make audience segmentation preferable.

**Segmenting the audience** means identifying specific groups who are alike in important ways and whose involvement is important to the purpose of the campaign (Slater, 1995). As you attempt to segment the audience, avoid grouping people based on superficial attributes. Characteristics such as race and income are not reliable indicators of how people think and behave (J. E. Williams & Flora, 1995). People within those categories may have very divergent viewpoints. Identifying groups on the basis of similar goals and experiences is harder to do, but it is more productive.

Keep in mind that indirect approaches sometimes work well. People who plan campus lectures often ask professors to publicize them in class and to consider offering students extra credit for attendance. They recognize that students might be more influenced by their professors' encouragement than by fliers or word-of-mouth. A similar effect seems to hold true for teenagers and drug use. Parents with authoritative communication styles are more likely than others to be effective in discouraging their teenagers from using illegal drugs (Quick & Stephenson, 2007; Stephenson, Quick, Atkinson, & Tschida, 2005). This knowledge underscores the importance of including parents in antidrug campaigns.

Also be open to unexpected combinations. For instance, freshmen and university staff members may be alike in feeling out of place at the campus gym. Where the campaign is concerned, this similarity may be more important than the differences between these groups. Based on these similarities, you might decide that both freshman and staff members would respond more enthusiastically to personal invitations than to bulletin board notices.

It is sometimes difficult to decide where to draw the line in segmenting an audience. The choice may be to target a small audience of high-need individuals or a large audience whose needs are less severe. Sometimes campaign designers overlook great opportunities to help small audiences. For example, tobacco harvesters are a relatively isolated and overlooked community within the overall population. But they have serious health concerns. For one, they often suffer from nausea, dizziness, and heart rate disruptions caused by exposure to green tobacco leaves (Parrott & Polonec, 2008). They can minimize their risk simply by wearing thicker clothing and changing into dry clothes when moisture from the plants soaks them, but little effort has been devoted to educating farmers about this (Parrott & Polonec). This health concern might not be as widespread as some others, but it is a serious issue for the people involved, and results are readily attainable. All in all, there is no definitive rule for choosing between highly focused and more generalized approaches, but health promoters who are sensitive to audience needs and health benefits are most likely to make reasonable judgments.

Based on your audience analysis, you might decide to target your sports recreation campaign toward people new on campus (students, staff, or both), to community members, or to nontraditional students. You might find that current participants do not reflect the racial and ethnic diversity on campus, or that the current membership is mostly men or women, or that people with disabilities are not as involved as they could be. Consequently, you might direct the campaign toward groups that are currently underutilizing the sports recreation program or those people who have the greatest need of the benefits it offers. And do not forget the current participants. Maybe their involvement can be improved. The possibilities are numerous, making it especially important to know the audience well before choosing a segment of it to target.

*Audience as a Person*  Once a target focus community has been identified, then, as Lefebvre et al. (1995) recommend, imagine the audience as a single person, complete "with name, gender, occupation, and lifestyle" (p. 221). With this "person" in mind, Lefebvre and colleagues suggest, pose the following questions for consideration.

- What is important to this person?
- What are the person's feelings, attitudes, and beliefs about the behavior change (including perceived benefits and barriers)?
- What are his or her media habits?

Lefebvre and coauthors say that imagining the audience as a person is useful in focusing the campaign and in creating messages that seem personal and immediate.

Every audience and every audience member is unique, but some overall characteristics may help guide your efforts. Here is some information that may be useful to you as you attempt to understand your focus community.

*Young Audiences*  Age may have some affect on how members perceive health messages. Although it is difficult to make generalizations about adult audiences, the developmental stages of youth often have relatively predictable effects.

Children are an important audience. As Erica Weintraub Austin (1995) points out, it is easier to prevent bad habits than to break them. Sending consistent messages to children early on may prevent them from developing unhealthy behaviors. Evidence supports that children are strongly influenced by adults. On the bright side, young people tend to follow their parents' advice (Henriksen & Jackson, 1998). However, children often seek to emulate adult behaviors—even the unhealthy ones. As you learned in the Own Your C case study (Box 13.1), portraying behaviors such as smoking as "adult-only" may actually make them seem more appealing to youngsters.

Adolescents often believe they are unlike other people and that others do not understand them (this is called **personal fable**). Consequently, they are likely to assume health warnings do not apply to them (K. Greene, Rubin, Hale, & Walters, 1996). Teenagers also tend to be extremely self-conscious and feel that people are scrutinizing their appearance and behavior (this is called **imaginary audience**). This makes them sensitive to peer pressure and social approval, which can work for or against health promotion efforts (K. Greene et al., 1996). A third factor, called **psychological reactance**, characterizes adolescents' desire to assert their independence and sense of personal control (Brehm, 1966). They often resent the sense that other people are telling them what to do, and they may rebel just to avoid feeling controlled.

Despite the challenges, there is some promising research about reaching children and adolescents.

- *Focus on immediate concerns.* Austin (1995) reminds health promoters that teens' immediate social concerns may outweigh their long-term health considerations. In Austin's words, adolescents may "care more that smoking will make their breath smell bad than that they could develop cancer" (p. 115).
- *Emphasize personal choice.* Adolescents tend to react negatively to messages that restrict their freedom of choice (Rains & Turner, 2007). Claude Miller and colleagues (2007) found that adolescents responded favorably when health messages included a "restoration of freedom" passage at the end emphasizing their right to make healthy choices for themselves. The restoration postscript the researchers used included the following: "You've probably heard a lot of messages telling you to exercise for good health.... You know what is best for yourself.... Everybody is different. We all make our own decisions and act as we choose to act. Obviously, you make your own decisions too. The choice is yours. You're free to decide for yourself" (C. H. Miller, Lane, Deatrick, Young, & Potts, 2007, p. 240).
- *Remember, there are many stages of youth.* A few years can make a big difference in how youth audiences respond. Hye-Jin Paek's (2008) data indicate that younger children respond well to school-based programs, whereas older teens benefit more from high-sensation appeals and truth-based information that portrays tobacco companies as deceptive members of "the establishment" (p. 98).

**Sensation-Seekers** The **activation model for information exposure** proposes that persuasive messages will be most effective when they stimulate an optimal amount of arousal in the reader/viewer, and what is "optimal" for one person may be boring or too intense for another (Donohew, Palmgreen, & Duncan, 1980). Here is a case in point. In the 1990s, *Rolling Stone* magazine ran an advertisement that proclaimed, "Why Women Find a Little Prick Attractive." Beside the headline was a photograph of a beautiful woman in black lingerie. Smaller wording explained that "the prick" in question was a small mark on a man's finger where he had drawn blood to verify he was not HIV-positive (Ivinski, 1997). The advertisement was for an at-home HIV test. It concluded: "And if the woman in your life is having any doubts—don't worry. That little prick is sure to satisfy her."

As you might imagine, "The Little Prick" ad drew considerable comment. At least one critic considered it irresponsible to portray a serious subject such as HIV in such a whimsical (some would say tasteless) manner. As Pamela Ivinski (1997) expressed it:

> Using sex to sell a test that determines whether someone has contracted a virus that's often transmitted during sex, and then subtly implying in the copy that the user shouldn't worry because he'll probably test negative, and he can use that fact to attract women for more sex, is a little bit creepy, not to mention misleading and even cynical. (paragraph 8)

The advertisement's creators acknowledged that the ad was not for everyone, but they argued that it was shocking and sexy enough to make young men pay attention to an important topic.

The activation model can apply to audiences of any age or description. So far researchers and campaign designers have used it most extensively for adolescent and young adult audiences, who are more likely than others to be high **sensation-seekers**, meaning they enjoy new and intense experiences (Everett & Palmgreen, 1995; Zuckerman, 1994). The danger with high sensation-seekers is that risky behaviors appeal to them. Not only are they less likely than others to take precautions, they are more apt to be in dangerous situations in the first

BOX 13.3 **ETHICAL CONSIDERATIONS**

# The Politics of Prevention— Who Should Pay?

Health promotion may seem like a win–win situation. If people can be encouraged to prevent disease and injuries, they will enjoy better health and the nation's health costs will be minimized. How far should we carry this line of reasoning? Should people who work hard to be healthy get discount prices on health care and insurance? Should they be given advantages when competing for jobs? If people knowingly engage in unhealthy behaviors, should society help pay for their medical bills?

About 75 cents of every dollar spent on health care in the United States goes to treating chronic illnesses, many of which could have been avoided with healthier diets, more exercise, and abstention from tobacco use ("Interview," 2007). And that figure doesn't even include the cost of treating preventable *injuries*. The added expense eats up tax money and leads to hikes in health insurance rates. As Daniel Wikler (1987) puts it, "The person who takes risks with his [or her] own health gambles with resources which belong to others" (p. 14). Some theorists argue that people who continue risky behavior (like smoking, overeating, or driving without seatbelts) when they know it is bad for them should pay from their own pockets when their behavior leads to medical expenses.

In a related issue, some feel that companies that profit from selling unhealthy products should pay part of the health bill. State and federal governments have sought damages from tobacco companies, charging that it is unfair for tobacco companies to make huge profits while others foot the enormous bill of treating tobacco-related illnesses. At least 50 chemicals in tobacco smoke are known to cause cancer (WHO, 2007b). Around the world, more than 5 million people a year die from tobacco-related illnesses, including 200,000 who are killed by the effects of secondhand smoke (WHO, 2007b, 2007c). Experts estimate that smoking costs Americans $167 billion a year in medical expenses and lost productivity (CDC, 2007b). Some companies now refuse to hire smokers or people who

are extremely overweight because they are at greater health risk, thus likely to cost the company more money than others in terms of health benefits and sick leave. Similarly, some insurance companies offer a discount to people who do not smoke and those who remain accident-free or who complete informational programs such as defensive-driving courses.

On the other side of the issue, some worry that government and employers are becoming too involved in people's lifestyle decisions. Some charge that groups like Mothers Against Drunk Driving (MADD) are taking a good thing too far by seeking to punish people for drinking even small amounts of alcohol (DiLorenzo & Bennett, 1998). Similarly, policy analyst Will Crawford (1997) warns that the government may soon be telling people what to eat in the name of controlling obesity. Some people say that increasing the "sin taxes" on alcohol and tobacco will hurt consumers, not companies, and they are afraid the taxes will be extended to cover snack foods and other not-so-healthy items. A third argument is that health concerns such as obesity are not always matters of individual control. Obesity has many causes, including social norms and heredity. People may gain weight because of medications or other health conditions. However, media coverage tends to sway the public toward considering obesity as either an individualistic or a societal issue (Kim & Willis, 2007). All in all, opponents of tighter health requirements say you cannot assume people are fully in control of their health, and you cannot control the risks people take without controlling their freedom to choose.

## What Do You Think?

1. Should people who knowingly take health risks pay more for health insurance? Should they be denied insurance? Should they be denied health services?
2. Should people be required by law to engage in healthy practices (like being immunized or exercising regularly)?
3. Should it be against the law to sell or advertise products known to have a high health risk? Does it matter if such products are addictive?

4. Do you agree with the rationale behind many states' seatbelt and motorcycle helmet laws—that people who neglect safety precautions not only endanger their own lives but increase the trauma and expense for everybody?

5. How do you weigh the argument that some people are not well informed about health issues (perhaps because they cannot read or cannot afford a computer) and that it is unfair to expect them to follow health guidelines about which they know little or nothing?

6. In your opinion, which of the following behaviors (if any) should be grounds for denying or limiting

health benefits? On what criteria do you make your judgments?

Smoking
Engaging in unprotected sex
Exceeding the speed limit
Snow skiing
Neglecting to exercise regularly
Overeating
Playing football
Rescuing accident victims

7. If a person has a family history of a disease, should he or she be required by society to take extra health precautions?

---

place. For instance, compared to their peers, high sensation-seekers are more likely to think smoking is appealing (Paek, 2008). They are typically more impulsive about having sex yet less willing than others to use condoms (Noar, Zimmerman, Palmgreen, Lustria, & Horosewski, 2006). And they tend to associate with other high sensation-seekers, which can make their behaviors seem normal rather than dangerous or extreme (Yanovitzky, 2006).

Here are a few promising lines of research about appealing to high sensation-seekers.

- *Make messages varied and intense.* Messages that have quick and vivid visual edits and loud and fast music typically have the most impact on high sensation-seekers, teens, and tweens (9- to 12-year-olds) (Lang, Schwartz, Lee, & Angelini, 2007; Niederdeppe, Davis, Farrelly, & Yarsevich, 2007).

- *Make the most of low-distraction environments.* Donald Helme and colleagues (2007) successfully influenced middle school students' attitudes about smoking when they used laptop computers in the classroom to expose students to three episodes of *Friends* in which the researchers had interspersed antismoking PSAs (Helme, Donohew, Baier, & Zittleman, 2007). Interestingly,

both intense and mild-content PSAs made an impact on high sensation-seekers in the sample, perhaps because the PSAs were embedded in entertainment programming and the classroom offered relatively few distractions.

- *Run PSAs during popular programs.* High sensation-seekers who watch a lot of television don't necessarily remember a lot about the PSAs they see. But they do typically remember the PSAs that appear during their favorite programs (typically sports, comedy, and cartoons for 16- to 25-year-olds) (D'Silva & Palmgreen, 2007).

Part of the dilemma, of course, is that the intense messages that sensation-seekers enjoy may be too much for most audiences, making it difficult to target high-risk individuals without offending others. (For ethical considerations about health promotion, see Box 13.3).

**Underinformed Audiences** In their article "Lessons From the Field," three noted health promotion specialists urge campaign designers not to overlook marginalized members of society. They write:

Conducting communication research within diverse ethnic/racial/underserved communities will be

**BOX 13.4 THEORETICAL FOUNDATIONS**

# The Knowledge Gap Hypothesis

The **knowledge gap hypothesis** proposes that people with plentiful information resources (such as newspapers, televisions, computers, and well-informed friends and advisors) are likely to know more and to continue learning more than people with fewer information resources (Tichenor, Donohue, & Olien, 1970). Income and education are highly linked to resource availability and media habits. Consequently, people of high socioeconomic status tend to be knowledge rich, and people of low status tend to be knowledge poor. The gap remains even when less educated persons are highly motivated to learn the information (Viswanath, Kahn, Finnegan, Hertog, & Potter, 1993). New information often increases the knowledge gap rather than diminishing it. In other words, the people who already know a lot learn more, and the others fall farther behind.

Unfortunately, people who are information poor are often most in need of health information. Here are just a few examples.

- Three years after a state medical assistance program for the uninsured was implemented in their community, 50% of low-income families were still unaware of it (Rucinski, 2004).
- Mexican American women in rural areas more frequently die from breast cancer than other women, but they often know little about breast self-exams and the severity of the disease (Hubbell, 2006).
- Although members of minority cultures in the United States are at highest risk for contracting AIDS, African Americans and Hispanic Americans are typically less informed than others about AIDS (Ebrahim, Anderson, Weidle, & Purcell, 2003).

These knowledge gaps typically reflect socioeconomic status. The knowledge gap narrows or disappears for members of racial and cultural minorities who are affluent and well educated (Ebrahim et al.).

There are several reasons underprivileged persons are hard to reach with health messages. One barrier is ethnic. Underprivileged audiences tend disproportionately to be people from minority cultures. They may be skeptical about mainstream messages, either because they seem irrelevant (aimed at whites rather than blacks, for example) or because they mistrust the sources (Matthews, Sellergren, Manfredi, & Williams, 2002). Researchers note that African American men, although at higher-than-normal risk for prostate cancer, are relatively uninformed about the symptoms and risk factors. Men in one study said they largely distrust doctors, are unable to get much preventive care, and are culturally averse to being tested for or diagnosed with a disease, such as prostate cancer, that they consider emasculating (Allen, Kennedy, Wilson-Glover, & Gilligan, 2007).

Second, underprivileged people are more likely than others to rely on television than on more detailed sources, such as newspapers and online medical information. A so-called digital divide separates the information rich who have high-speed broadband Internet access (predominantly young, well-educated city dwellers) and the information-poor, who are often rural residents with no online access or who rely on dial-up connections (Rains, 2008b). As you might expect, people with quick, ready access to online sources are more likely to use them to access health information (Rains). Thus, underprivileged persons' media habits often put them at a disadvantage.

Third, although they may watch television, members of ethnic co-cultures are more likely to trust interpersonal sources (like friends and health professionals) than the mainstream media (Cheong, 2007). This is okay if they have ready access to health experts, but many don't. Female African American and Latina adolescents in one study were familiar with breast and lung cancer because they knew of people with those diseases. However, most of the girls had never heard of cervical cancer, even though it was getting abundant media attention in connection with a new human papillomavirus (HPV) vaccine (Mosavel & El-Shaarawi, 2007). Their lack of knowledge is especially unfortunate because the vaccine is designed primarily for girls their age (Mosavel & El-Shaarawi).

Fourth, people may filter out new information because it doesn't mesh with what they know or believe. "Individuals selectively orient their attention to those stimuli in their environments that match their existing predispositions, values, and behaviors," explains Dutta-Bergman (2005, p. 112), "Campaign materials that propose to alter the belief structure of the receiver of the message are not likely to be adhered to. Instead, those individuals who are already interested in the issue end up learning more from the message."

Finally, underprivileged audiences may have different priorities than others. People worried about violence and hunger may feel long-term health issues are the least of their worries (Holtgrave, Tinsley, & Kay, 1995).

---

especially important in the future. Attention to these audiences is a necessity, not a nicety. . . . Working with an audience for the first time inevitably brings frustrations as one discovers that principles applied successfully in the past with other populations do not necessarily fit in other contexts. Our experience has been that the potential payoff is worth the initial frustration. (Edgar, Freimuth, & Hammond, 2003, p. 627)

Unfortunately, people most in need of health resources and information are often the least likely to benefit from health messages in the media. (See Box 13.4 for more on the knowledge gap hypothesis.)

Typically, the use of mass media—particularly news viewing—is associated with being more informed and resource rich. But the benefits are not equal, even among media users. Christopher Beaudoin and Esther Thorson (2006) found that, in terms of social capital, watching television news benefits European Americans significantly more than African Americans. They define **social capital** as the benefits possible when members of a community build positive social connections and a mutual sense of trust. Beaudoin and Thorson observe that African American communities often enjoy negative or less-than-optimal benefits from media use because they are so often portrayed negatively in the news and entertainment media. For them, media images may strengthen prejudice and powerlessness rather than provide information they feel they can trust and use.

The challenge for health promoters is to earn trust, respond to community needs, and inform and enable people, at the same time being careful to avoid stigmatizing communities at risk (R. Smith, 2007). Here are a few suggestions.

- *Focus on social capital.* Recognize that health is not merely a matter of individual control. Prejudice, trust, community resources, social networks, and confidence have profound affects as well. (We will cover this idea more thoroughly in Chapter 14.)

- *Tailor materials to audiences' literacy levels.* For example, Satya Krishnan (1996) recommends that clinics educate people with low reading skills by showing instructional health videos in medical waiting rooms.

- *Help build online skills and confidence.* For some people, access to health information is limited because they lack a computer or online capability. Even for those with access, however, a sense of self-efficacy is often missing (Rains, 2008a). Evidence suggests that underinformed audiences benefit profoundly if they are coached to use the Web knowledgeably and confidently. The National Cancer Institute has helped fund a number of projects to "narrow the digital divide" by designing websites tailored to the needs of underserved populations and offering community workshops to teach people how to use them (Kreps, 2005).

As you complete Step 2 in creating a health campaign, it may seem that, though you have already done a lot of work, you still do not know what the campaign will involve. Your efforts will not go to waste. Research shows that campaigns launched without a clear understanding of the audience, current situation, and potential benefits are often frustrating to create and ineffective at reaching their goals. With a focus community in mind, you are ready for Step 3.

## Step 3: Establishing Campaign Goals and Objectives

By this point you should have a fairly clear impression of the sports recreation department, its potential benefits, and the people you most want to reach with your campaign. Collecting and analyzing data has prepared you to establish specific objectives for your campaign. **Objectives** state in clear, measurable terms exactly what you hope to achieve with the campaign. You might consider the following questions.

- What exactly do you want people to start/stop/continue doing?
- If you are hoping to encourage a particular behavior, when (and for how long) should it occur to be of benefit?
- How will you know if your campaign has been successful?

Relevant to the sports recreation campaign, you may decide that signing up 40 freshmen in 3 months would constitute success. Or perhaps you have decided to focus on students with disabilities or newcomers. Your objective may be to get at least 20 current participants to bring an individual from one of those groups to an event.

Make sure your objectives are oriented to the overall purpose of the campaign. For instance, if people participate in aerobics only once, will there be health benefits? If not, it may be important to aim for continued participation—perhaps attendance once a week for at least 2 months.

Think ahead about exactly how you will measure campaign affects. This may involve follow-up surveys or sign-up sheets to keep track of participation. Setting measurable goals allows you (and others) to determine if the campaign has been a success.

---

**BOX 13.5 RESOURCES**

## Disease Maps on the Web

Visit the CDC Map Gallery at cdc.gov/gis/gallery.htm

View U.S. Department of the Interior disease maps at diseasemaps.usgs.gov/index.html

---

Health promoters are increasingly being held accountable for their efforts. **Accountability** means demonstrating how the results of a project compare to the money and time invested in it. For example, a hospital I know of reorganized its marketing and public relations department because patient surveys showed that people chose the hospital based on their doctor's advice, not on advertising. The hospital did not discontinue advertisements completely. (The same study revealed that billboards, while they didn't bring in new patients, significantly raised workplace morale!) But the public relations staff redirected part of their effort into marketing services directly to physicians.

In the larger population, a useful means of tracking health risks and changes is the use of **disease maps**, which look like regular maps but are color-coded to show the incidence of disease in geographical areas. These maps present a great deal of information in a way that is clear and visually appealing (Parrott, Hopfer, Ghetian, & Lengerich, 2007). (See Box 13.5 for links to online disease maps.) For example, you might look up a cancer map of the United States and feel alarmed that your state is shaded in a color that, according to the map key, signifies high cancer incidence. With some maps, you can click on regions and get more detailed information, such as cancer rates in your hometown or neighborhood, links to charts and graphs, even relevant photographs. If they are accurate and up to date, disease maps have an advantage over complex reports. Imagine scanning tables of disease statistics about every area of your community and state! It might take you

BOX 13.6

## Can You Guess?

One challenge of health promotion is monitoring what diseases are most prevalent and most deadly. Rank the following from highest (1) to lowest (10) in terms of annual deaths around the world.

| | |
|---|---|
| _____ | lung cancer |
| _____ | Alzheimer and other dementias |
| _____ | stomach cancer |
| _____ | colon and rectal cancers |
| _____ | AIDS |
| _____ | diabetes |
| _____ | heart disease |
| _____ | stroke |
| _____ | chronic obstructive pulmonary artery disease (COPD) |
| _____ | breast cancer |

*See answers at the end of the chapter.*

hours and many volumes of paperwork to show what a simple map can convey in a few minutes. And even if you carefully reviewed the data in table format, it would be easy to overlook health patterns that show up vividly on a disease map—like cancer rates that are particularly high around an industrial plant or river. This information is useful in accomplishing what some researchers call *environmental justice* or environmental *equity*, meaning that attention is given to demographically situated populations that lag behind others or require more resources than they currently have to ensure citizens' health (Waller, Carlin, Xia, & Gelfand, 1997).

## Step 4: Selecting Channels of Communication

A **channel** is a means of communicating information, either directly (in person) or indirectly (through media like TV or radio or computers).

To select the best channels for your campaign, consider what channels your target audience uses most and trusts most.

Sometimes channel selection is limited by time or money. Your sports recreation enrollment effort will probably not involve full-color magazine ads or sophisticated television commercials. Nevertheless, as a health promoter, you should be familiar with all types of channels. Moreover, do not assume too quickly that a channel is out of your reach. For example, you may not produce television commercials, but you might book appearances on local television talk shows.

*Channel Characteristics* You should also consider the advantages and limitations of different channels. Experts suggest that channels for a health campaign be evaluated in terms of reach, specificity, and impact (Schooler, Chaffee, Flora, & Roser, 1998). **Reach** refers to the number of people who will be exposed to a message via a particular channel. **Specificity** refers to how accurately the message can be targeted to a specific group of people. **Impact** is how influential a message is likely to be.

Television has a larger and more diverse audience than any other medium (Warner, 1987). As such, it has immense reach. However, because the audience is so large and diverse, it is hard to tailor messages to particular viewers. Thus, television has low specificity (although that is changing somewhat with the creation of special-interest cable and satellite programs). Radio stations and large-circulation newspapers also have broad reach.

Although it may be tempting to aim for the broadest reach possible, it is advisable to focus on your target audience. Exposure that is broader than necessary can waste resources and contribute to information overload, making it difficult for people to identify which messages are most important and relevant to them (Lang, 2006). One solution is to use channels, such as magazines and direct mail, that have high specificity. Magazines are often marketed to people with specific interests, such as health, family, entertainment, automobiles, hobbies, travel, and so on (Biagi, 1999). Direct mail is sent directly to people at their homes or businesses. Direct mail is inexpensive compared to mass media and offers more assurance that campaign messages are actually reaching target audience members, even people who do not use traditional media much (Dignan, Michielutte, Jones-Lighty, & Bahnson, 1994).

Impact is usually related to arousal and involvement. **Arousal** refers to how emotionally stimulating and exciting a message is (Schooler et al., 1998). When we view words and images about risky products, such as condoms, liquor bottles, and cigarettes, we typically experience greater emotional and physical arousal than with more innocuous products, such as pop cans and juice bottles (Lang, Chung, Lee, & Zhao, 2005). We tend to identify the risky products more quickly and remember them longer (Lang et al.). This can make it difficult for healthy campaign messages (especially if they are sedate) to compete with advertisements for unhealthy products.

Interactive computer programs are a good example of high-arousal messages that can be used to promote healthy behaviors. Interactive, on-screen messages are often very engrossing, with colorful graphics, moving images, and sound (Street & Rimal, 1997). Roberto and colleagues (2007) report great success using an interactive computer program to involve high school students in safer-sex and pregnancy-prevention efforts. Compared to other students, those who took part in the online program were more knowledgeable about STDs, more aware of their personal risk, more reluctant to have sex, and more confident about their ability to use safer-sex practices if they did have sex.

**Involvement** is the amount of mental effort required to understand a message (Parrott, 1995). Interpersonal communication is high involvement. It requires a great deal of thought and action. Thus, health professionals, family members, and friends tend to have high impact. Newspapers are also high-involvement channels, because people must read and use their imaginations. Television is low involvement, because viewers passively observe the sounds and sights displayed for them.

The **elaboration likelihood model** proposes that when we are highly involved with a message we

pay close attention to details and evaluate the message thoroughly. As a consequence, we remember high-involvement messages longer than others and are more likely to act on them (Briñol & Petty, 2006; Petty & Cacioppo, 1981). In short, people usually pay closer attention when using high-involvement channels, like reading and talking, and this affects how much they are influenced by the information. Surveys show that people who use high-involvement channels are usually better informed about health than people who rely on low-involvement channels, like television (for literature review, see Parrott, 1995).

### Communication Technology: Using Computers to Narrowcast Messages

We often speak of *broadcasting* messages to large audiences. Messages in the mass media draw people's attention to health topics. However, there are advantages to *narrowcasting* as well.

**Narrowcasting**, or tailored communication, is designed to meet the specific needs of individual consumers. Matthew Kreuter and colleagues (1999) use the example of a doctor's visit to treat high cholesterol. As usual, the physician offers advice on diet and exercise, but this time the doctor also provides a printout tailor-made for the patient:

> It seems like the cold weather has been keeping you from walking every day like you had hoped to in your physical activity plan. Did you know that many of the local malls open early in the winter for walkers? Crestwood Mall is the one closest to your house, and it opens for walkers at 6:30 every morning. Mall walking might also help with your recent lack of motivation. You've been struggling with exercise because your walking partner moved away, and this might be a way for you to meet some new people, and not feel like you're exercising alone. (Kreuter, Farrell, Olevitch, & Brennan, 1999, p. 2)

The information might also include healthy recipes suited to your family's preferences and tips for finding healthy food in the local supermarket.

Before receiving tailored health messages from a physician, people typically fill out questionnaires about their health, habits, preferences, and environments. The questions go beyond simple demographics such as age and sex (Rimal & Adkins, 2003). For example, if the goal is to help older adults avoid harmful falls, the questions may ask about the presence of stairs, handrails, and rugs and the need to do lawn work and home repairs (Kreuter et al., 1999). This information is entered into computer databanks (either online or in the doctor's office) that produce individualized profiles and suggestions. For example, the tailored response might suggest ways to reorganize one's home to minimize the chance of falling and community resources to help with riskier activities, such as house painting and snow shoveling (Kreuter et al., 1999). It is also possible to key in information about an individual's education and literacy level so that the resulting printout is usable and comprehensible, perhaps showing mostly pictures and diagrams if the client is not proficient at reading (Bernhardt & Cameron, 2003).

The idea is that people are more likely to act on customized information than to sift through data that may or may not apply to them or that may exceed their comprehension level. Kreuter and colleagues (1999) compare tailored health messages to a realtor who provides a list of homes that meet a client's wishes rather a realtor who says, "Here's a street map of our entire city. By going up and down all the streets, you're sure to find something that meets your needs" (p. 4).

Health promoters in charge of large campaigns may not have license to be quite so specific. But they can still tailor messages to some extent. For example, Valerie Pilling and Laura Brannon (2007) tried a tailored approach in creating a responsible-drinking website for college students. Some students in the study viewed a version of the website tailored to suit their personalities (either responsible, communicative, logical, or adventuresome), while others viewed more general messages about the danger of binge drinking. Students who viewed the tailored messages were significantly more likely than the others to consider the website interesting, to predict that it would be effective, and to say that

the materials affected their attitudes about drinking. In their review of the literature, Barbara Rimer and Matthew Kreuter (2006) applaud such efforts and encourage health promoters to continue refining tailored messages to suit recipients' cultural and motivational preferences. In tailored-information websites, a spokesperson of the same race as the reader might present the information, artwork and graphics might vary, and information might be more or less complex based on the recipient's preference.

Unfortunately, many health websites have not realized the full potential for narrowcasting. A review of 21 safer-sex websites revealed that most of them were moderately targeted at best (Noar, Clark, Cole, & Lustria, 2006). Noar and coauthors suggest that health-oriented web developers might invite users to complete a brief questionnaire when they register and then use that information to highlight key health information throughout the rest of the site.

*Multichannel Campaigns* As you have seen, broadcasting and narrowcasting have advantages. Many times, the best chance of making a difference is to reach people through several channels (Flay & Burton, 1990). Multichannel efforts are important because people have different communication patterns and preferences. What appeals to some people may not appeal to others. For example, Richard Street Jr. and Timothy Manning (1997) found that women who were highly interested in breast cancer preferred to get information about it through an interactive, multimedia computer program. However, women who were less interested preferred to watch a videotape about breast cancer, presumably because it required less effort. In this study, women learned about the same amount from both formats.

Other researchers suggest that culture may affect channel preferences. Traditional Hispanics typically consider health an intimate topic, not to be discussed outside one's close social network (Alcalay & Bell, 1996). African Americans often get health messages and health-related assistance at church. The 635 African American churches included in one study sponsored a total of 1,804 outreach programs, offering such services as food, shelter, substance abuse counseling, and AIDS education (S. B. Thomas, Quinn, Billingsley, & Caldwell, 1994). The researchers suggest that health promoters work with churches when trying to reach and assist African Americans.

Mass-mediated and interpersonal channels are also complementary, in that the media messages typically influence what people think about and talk about (see E. M. Rogers & Dearing, 1988), but people do not simply buy into everything the media says. They are also likely to be influenced by discussions with neighbors and family members. The phrase **diffusion of innovations** refers to the process through which new information is filtered and passed along throughout a community (E. M. Rogers, 1983). Researchers suggest that some community members act as opinion leaders who have credibility by virtue of their expertise or social standing. Often, opinion leaders pass along new ideas or information from the media to other people. In this way, media messages may influence people indirectly whether they use the media or not. The process by which people relay media messages to others is called **two-step flow** (Brosius & Weimann, 1996; Lazarsfeld, Burleson, & Gaudet, 1948). For example, physicians can be powerful change agents. In the 1990s, citizens of Milwaukee were warned via pamphlets and news stories that lead pipes might be poisoning the water in their homes. Although inundated with information, the people at highest risk (low-income residents living in older homes) did not perceive their risk to be any higher than that of others, and they were relatively unwilling to take precautions (Griffin & Dunwoody, 2000). However, these residents *did* respond when their doctors told them they were personally at risk.

## SUMMARY

Successful health promotion recognizes that people do not necessarily change their behaviors because they are presented with new health information.

Campaigners must take into account the concerns, habits, and preferences of the people they wish to influence. Campaigns with the best chance of succeeding talk to people where they are, whether it is the beauty salon, the athletic field, or the doctor's office. They make it practical for people to adopt healthy behaviors, even if it means changing public policy or offering free treatment. Good health campaigns are thorough and backed by long-term commitment. The best campaigns involve members of the focus population as active participants and recruit social support for healthy behaviors. Furthermore, they speak with many voices, including the concerned tones of loved ones, the calm assurance of experts, and the printed and recorded messages of mass media.

Because people are inclined to pay more attention to messages that seem relevant to them, campaigns directed at "everyone" may not pique the interest of anyone. Health campaign success stories show that it is important to know the audience well, take positive action, establish clear goals, measure success, and make behaviors socially rewarding.

Whereas illness and disease prevention seem to benefit everyone, ethical dilemmas are involved, such as: Should people be rewarded or penalized based on their health-related behavior? How should we balance people's right to choose for themselves with society's interest in keeping costs down? Where do we draw the line between healthy and unhealthy behaviors?

The first step in creating a health campaign is to research potential benefits of the campaign. Find out who stands to gain, who is already behaving according to campaign recommendations, and what alternatives exist.

The second step is to choose a target audience. Interviews, questionnaires, and focus groups are useful ways to learn about potential audience members—what they like, what they know, how they typically behave, what they consider important, and more. You may wish to target people in great need or those who are most likely to respond to the campaign. At the same time, keep in mind audience characteristics such as self-consciousness, sensation hunger, confidence, need for independence, and psychological reactance. It is typically difficult to reach audiences who are culturally different from the mainstream. However, considering the knowledge gap hypothesis, these audiences are often the most in need of health information and assistance.

With a target audience in mind, the third step in creating a health campaign is to establish clear and measurable objectives so you can accurately assess the campaign's effects. Fourth, health promoters select channels through which to communicate campaign messages. Channels typically differ in terms of reach, specificity, and impact. Sometimes narrowcasting is more effective than broadcasting, in that it helps message recipients focus on information that is tailored to their interests, abilities, and resources. Often, the best campaigns make use of several channels. All in all, the media play an important role in promoting health issues, but media impact is limited without interpersonal reinforcement.

## KEY TERMS

health-promoting behaviors
health promotion campaigns
health promoter
highly scheduled interviews
moderately scheduled interviews
unscheduled interviews
questionnaire
fixed-alternative questions
open questions
closed questions
focus group
sampling
segmenting an audience
personal fable
imaginary audience
psychological reactance
activation model for information exposure
sensation-seekers
social capital
knowledge gap hypothesis
objectives
accountability
disease maps
channel
reach
specificity
impact
arousal
involvement
elaboration likelihood model
narrowcasting
diffusion of innovations
two-step flow

## DISCUSSION QUESTIONS

1. What is your opinion of the Own Your C campaign? Do you think it is well designed to appeal to teenagers? Why or why not?
2. Name some of the factors that influence people's behavior.
3. What are some careers in the field of health promotion and education?
4. Name and describe the first four steps in creating a health promotion campaign.
5. What are four qualities of good campaigns, as illustrated by the exemplary campaigns in this chapter?
6. What questions might you address as you research the current situation and potential benefits of a health campaign?
7. Why is it important to select a target audience?
8. What are three types of interviews? How do they compare?
9. Provide some guidelines for designing an effective questionnaire.
10. What is the difference between an open question and a closed question?
11. Give some guidelines for conducting effective focus groups.
12. Why is sampling important?
13. What are some questions to consider when segmenting an audience?

14. What are some factors to keep in mind if your target audience includes children? If it includes adolescents?

15. What type of health promotion messages are likely to appeal to high sensation-seekers?

16. Do you believe people should pay more for health insurance if they engage in risky or unhealthy behaviors? Why or why not?

17. Using the knowledge gap hypothesis, explain why people of low socioeconomic status are often underinformed about health issues.

18. What factors make it particularly difficult to influence underprivileged persons with conventional promotion efforts?

19. What are some questions to consider when determining campaign goals?

20. Explain how channels differ in terms of reach, specificity, and impact.

21. Describe the process of creating narrowcast messages. What are the advantages of narrowcasting?

22. Why are multichannel efforts recommended?

## ANSWER TO *CAN YOU GUESS?*

1—heart disease, 2—stroke, 3—lung cancer, 4—lower respiratory infections, 5—COPD, 6—colon and rectal cancer, 7—Alzheimer's disease, 8—diabetes, 9—breast cancer, 10—stomach cancer (WHO, 2007a).

*NOTE: AIDS doesn't make the top-10 list yet, but it is expected to be the third leading cause of death, worldwide, by the year 2031.*

# CHAPTER
# 14

# Designing and Implementing
# Health Campaigns

One of the most famous and most widely emulated campaigns on college campuses is the RU SURE campaign, developed in the 1990s at Rutgers University to curb the incidence of dangerous alcohol consumption. The campaign is based on evidence that college students usually overestimate the amount their peers drink. By providing students with more accurate statistics, campaign sponsors try to clarify that the norm is less extreme than students think. Thus, students need not drink excessively to fit in with their peers (Lederman & Stewart, 2005; Lederman, Stewart, Barr, Powell, Laitman, & Goodhart, 2001).

The RU SURE campaign is famous for its high level of student involvement and its novel ways of integrating campaign messages in everyday campus life. Through the years, campaign designers have distributed free T-shirts featuring a Top Ten Misperceptions list about life at Rutgers that features three misperceptions about drinking as well as humorous myths such as "You don't need shower shoes for the dorms." They have also engaged students in RU SURE Bingo games, developed curricula supplements for campus courses, and developed partnerships with community leaders and others.

Evidence on the Rutgers campus indicates that student estimates of peer drinking have dropped considerably since the RU SURE campaign began (Stewart, Lederman, Golubow, Cattafesta, Godhart,

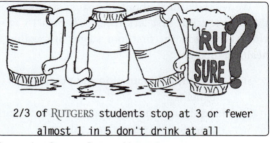

2/3 of RUTGERS students stop at 3 or fewer
almost 1 in 5 don't drink at all

Source: Lea Stewart, Rutgers University

Powell & Laitman, 2002). "Communication majors are involved in all aspects of this campaign, from designing ways to deliver campaign messages to gathering evaluation data," says Lea Stewart, professor and director of the Rutgers Center for Communication and Health Issues. "Since no one works on the campaign without first learning about the scope and consequences of dangerous drinking among college students we reach two audiences: our target audience of first-year students and a secondary audience of upper-level students."

Like many health promotion efforts, the RU Sure campaign is based partly on social marketing. **Social marketing** means that campaign designers apply the principles of commercial advertising to prosocial campaigns, such as health promotion efforts (Lefebvre & Flora, 1988). The rationale is that many of the techniques used to sell goods and services

361

work equally well when promoting healthy lifestyles. From a social marketing perspective, health-related behaviors have a price tag of sorts. They "cost" something in terms of money, time, energy, or some other investment. Although the cost does not translate into profits for the health promoter, the promoter is a type of salesperson who tries to keep the costs as low as possible and convince people that the "price" of the recommended behavior is worth paying.

Because the concern in social marketing is primarily with what the "consumer" needs, health promoters make a great effort to understand the audience, assess its needs, and target specific people. Social marketing also involves using multiple channels and conducting follow-up research to measure the success of campaign efforts.

We will talk more about campaign strategies in this chapter. But first let's recap. Chapter 13 provided a guide to the first four stages of creating a health campaign:

*Step 1:* Defining the situation and potential benefits
*Step 2:* Analyzing and segmenting the audience
*Step 3:* Establishing campaign goals and objectives
*Step 4:* Selecting channels of communication

The process continues in this chapter with a description of key theories and techniques to create health promotion campaigns. The hypothetical sports recreation campaign helps illustrate how a health promotion effort comes together. Keep in mind that the same steps apply to campaigns of various sizes on any number of health topics.

This chapter begins by introducing five influential models of behavior change: the health belief model, social cognitive theory, the embedded behaviors model, the theory of reasoned action, and the transtheoretical model. We will then explore the critical-cultural approach and describe the three final stages in campaign development:

*Step 5:* Designing campaign messages
*Step 6:* Piloting and implementing the campaign
*Step 7:* Evaluating and maintaining the campaign

Along the way, we will touch on a number of message design perspectives, including the role of affect, social norms theory, the theory of normative social behavior, and the extended parallel process model.

## THEORIES OF BEHAVIOR CHANGE

The theories described here emphasize that people make lifestyle decisions based on a complex array of factors, including personal perceptions, skills, social pressure, convenience, and more. Each of these theories has earned considerable respect among health communication scholars and health promoters. Space is not available to discuss each model in great detail, but this introduction should help orient you to the rich scholarship behind health campaign efforts and provide opportunities for further investigation. Applying these theories to health campaigns can have a positive effect—at least sometimes. Keep in mind that theories are only guiding principles, not magic formulas. No one theory works all of the time or with every audience.

### Health Belief Model

The **health belief model** proposes that people base their behavior choices on five primary considerations (Rosenstock, 1960; Stretcher & Rosenstock, 1997). Namely, people are most motivated to change their behaviors if they believe that:

- they will be adversely affected if they do not change,
- the adverse effects will be considerable,
- behavior change will be effective in preventing the undesired outcome,
- the effort and cost of preventive behavior is worthwhile, and
- they are moved to action by a novel or eye-opening occurrence, such as a brush with danger, a compelling warning message, or an alluring incentive.

In short, motivation is based on an individual's perception of personal susceptibility, serious consequences, worthwhile benefits, justifiable costs, and cues to actions.

The health belief model is used widely for assessing audiences and organizing campaigns (Kohler, Grimly, & Reynolds, 1999). For example, Kami Silk and colleagues (2006) used components of the model to guide focus groups with female adolescents and adults prior to developing breast cancer prevention materials. They found that participants of all ages understood the severity of breast cancer, but they defined the consequences somewhat differently. The adolescents tended to emphasize the appearance-altering effects of the disease, such as hair loss during chemotherapy. The mothers were more likely to know someone with breast cancer, to know a lot about the disease, and to feel personally susceptible.

The health belief model also reminds us to keep renewing our familiarity with target audiences. Jon Krosnick and coauthors report that, although the adverse affects of smoking are well known to many, about 34% of the public is still unaware that smoking causes or worsens oral cancer, and 35% is not aware that smoking increases one's risk for stroke (Krosnick, Chang, Sherman, Chassin, & Presson, 2006). Campaign designers who overlook these knowledge gaps may miss important opportunities.

Considering all of these factors, it seems naive to assume people will change simply because someone tells them to do so. A campaign message may be a cue to action, but unless someone has reason to believe the recommended behavior is useful and worthwhile and that it will prevent an outcome that is otherwise likely to occur, the recommendation will probably not be motivation enough.

If you are trying to increase participation in your university's sports recreation program, you might consider how strongly members of your target audience believe the benefits you propose would actually help them. Let's say audience analysis reveals a number of statements such as "I know exercise is good for people. But I'm young and healthy. I don't have to worry about that yet." According to the health belief model, people who feel this way will not be motivated to seek the benefits proposed because they do not believe they need them. Your job as a health promoter might be to show them

more compelling evidence or to appeal to them on the basis of other goals, such as looking good, meeting people, and winning awards. Conversely, if people do not know about the benefits of exercise, the model advocates educating them. Knowledge does not ensure behavior change, but it is an important foundation for it. Research shows that people sometimes change their behavior without being well informed. However, these people are less likely to maintain the new behavior than others, especially if the change requires effort or discomfort (Valente, Paredes, & Poppe, 1998).

### Social Cognitive Theory

Returning to the sports recreation campaign, imagine that everything seems to be in your favor. People are aware of the recreation program. They know about the benefits. They even feel they would benefit personally. Yet they do not plan to participate. This may seem very puzzling. What's a health promoter to do?

A promoter familiar with social cognitive theory would consider the environment. **Social cognitive theory** holds that people make decisions by considering the interplay of internal and environmental factors (Bandura, 1986, 1994). **Internal factors** include knowledge, skills, emotions, habits, and so on. **Environmental factors** include social approval, physical environment, institutional rules, and the like. According to the theory, people are most comfortable when internal and environmental factors are in sync. This may explain why changing people's minds does not necessarily change their behavior (Maibach & Cotton, 1995). Environments are persuasive as well. In your campaign, for example, people may not participate in recreational activities because they perceive that others will laugh at them, the hours are not convenient, or they do not know anyone at the gym.

Social concerns sometimes outweigh personal concerns, even if the behavior in question is particularly risky. When Donna Rouner and Rebecca Lindsey (2006) interviewed female college students, the researchers were impressed by how poised the women seemed. The students rated their knowledge of STDs highly, but they were mostly uncomfortable talking about condoms. The gap between knowing and doing is consistent with previous evidence that people sometimes wish to use condoms during sex, even plan to use them, but abandon their intentions because they are too embarrassed to bring up the subject. Especially for new partners who do not know each other well, it may seem more socially acceptable for sex "just to happen" than to talk about it in advance (M. R. Dennis, 2006). Significantly, people who *do* insist on condom use are typically good communicators—skillful at asserting themselves, understanding other people's feelings, self-disclosing, and managing conflict (Edgar, 1992; Monohan, Miller, & Rothspan, 1997). The implications are that communication skills and well-developed relationships can sometimes help people overcome environmental challenges.

Let's apply social cognitive theory to your sports recreation campaign. Social cognitive theory suggests that health promoters must do more than make people aware of health risks. They must make healthy behaviors practical and socially acceptable. If you find that people in your target audience want to participate in recreational activities but are reluctant to do so, your job may be to help them develop new skills, improve the social atmosphere at the gym, suggest different hours, or make other changes that build their confidence and reduce the risks of participating.

### Embedded Behaviors Model

The embedded behaviors model (Booth-Butterfield, 2003) is similar to social cognitive theory, in that it recognizes internal and external influences on health-related behavior. However, the embedded behaviors model also includes consideration of the behavior itself: its frequency, complexity, familiarity or novelty, and links to other behaviors. In short, the **embedded behaviors model** suggests that behaviors are enduring to the extent that they are an integral part of an individual's lifestyle or self-image and are supported by internal and external factors.

Some behaviors, such as switching to a salt substitute, are relatively easy to make happen because

---

**BOX 14.1**

## Can You Guess?

1. People who smoke tend to die at a younger age than others. How many years of their lives do smokers usually lose?
2. How much does the tobacco industry spend every day to advertise its products?
3. The World Health Organization has named tobacco one of the most severe health threats of modern times. In what percentage of the world is tobacco advertising banned?

*Answers appear at the end of the chapter.*

---

the change does not alter one's lifestyle and because equally desirable alternatives are available. However, other behaviors (such as tobacco use) may be extremely difficult to give up. In a study of teen smoking, Melanie Booth-Butterfield (2003) reports that "smoking is much more complex than simply buying cigarettes and smoking them" (p. 179). Some teen smokers say they feel a sense of belonging around others who smoke (although they typically insist peer pressure has not influenced them). They report that cigarettes become like friends who are "always there" (p. 178) and that smoking is a way to manage their moods by relieving boredom and either soothing or energizing them.

### Theory of Reasoned Action

The **theory of reasoned action (TRA)** is based on the assumption that people are rational decision makers. They do not just *happen* to behave one way or another. Instead, they make decisions and deliberate choices based on two primary considerations: (1) how strongly they believe a behavior will lead to positive outcomes and (2) the perceived social implications of performing that behavior (Ajzen & Fishbein, 1980).

TRA is similar to social cognitive theory, in that both consider personal and social influences. However, TRA is more global in focus. Its predictive power lies in assessing the attitudes and behaviors of large numbers of people (Ajzen & Fishbein, 1980). Because TRA is designed to make generalizations, its founders do not consider it necessary (or even helpful) to focus on specifics such as personality, rules, and emotions. The effects of these variables tend to even out over large populations. By the same token, TRA does not assume that small changes will make much difference overall. As Ajzen and Fishbein put it, "Changing one or more beliefs may not be sufficient to bring about change in the overall attitude" (p. 81).

It may seem that the macro focus of TRA is not very helpful in planning your sports recreation campaign. Indeed, your target audience may be too small to make broad generalizations very useful. But TRA is of interest theoretically because it suggests that people make behavior changes based on their *overall* beliefs and perceptions. Small changes may not have much effect if they are outweighed by larger concerns. For example, imagine a new study suggests it is healthy for men to wear panty hose every day. Do you suppose you could get the men on your campus to do so? Probably not. Their belief in the health benefits of panty hose is probably outweighed by their desire to be socially acceptable. Luckily for you, physical exercise *is* widely accepted. What you propose is already in line with most people's overall intentions.

## Transtheoretical Model

In analyzing the audience for your sports recreation campaign, imagine that you find some people *want* to exercise but that many of them are not doing so. You may even find that people *plan* to go to the gym but do not make it there. This is an important finding because it helps you understand your audience's state of mind. According to the **transtheoretical model**, people may not proceed directly from thinking about a problem to changing their behavior (Holtgrave, Tinsley, & Kay, 1995; Prochaska & DiClemente, 1983; Prochaska, DiClemente, & Norcross, 1992). Instead, they tend to change in stages. According to the model, change typically involves the following five stages:

*Precontemplation:* Not aware of a problem
*Contemplation:* Thinking about a problem
*Preparation:* Deciding to take action
*Action:* Making a change
*Maintenance:* Sticking to the change for 6
    months or more

The implication is that people react differently to health promotion efforts depending on their current stage. Attention-getting information is called for when people are unaware of a problem. But skills training and encouragement may be more useful for those who are already prepared to make a change. Furthermore, people who have already adopted the recommended behavior should be encouraged to continue it.

Hyunyi Cho and Charles Salmon (2006) found support for this concept when they exposed students to a variety of messages about skin cancer. Participants in precontemplation stages who viewed highly threatening messages were highly motivated to protect themselves, but they also reported higher-than-average feelings of hopelessness and fatalism. The authors concluded that fear appeals can call attention to previously unattended issues, but they may be counterproductive unless accompanied by clear and useful guidance.

From the perspective of the transtheoretical model, people choose options by weighing the relative pros and cons among a complex array of considerations. For example, Alan DeSantis (2002) described the camaraderie in a cigar shop in which the regulars met to smoke and drink, seemingly impervious to the antismoking messages of loved ones and media campaigns and even to the smoking-related death of one their own members.

> Within days, and sometimes hours, after wives and children have implored their husbands and fathers to quit smoking, the local press has reported on the "latest findings from the *New England Journal of Medicine*," or *20/20* has broadcasted its latest investigative report on the hazards of cigar smoking, the regulars at the cigar shop light back up, with only the smell of cigar smoke on their minds. (DeSantis, p. 169)

## BOX 14.2 THEORETICAL FOUNDATIONS

# Synopsis of Campaign-Related Theories

**cultural-critical perspective:** Health is not simply a matter of personal agency, but is inextricably linked to larger issues of culture, power, control, identity, and social consciousness.

**embedded behaviors model:** The likelihood for behavior change is related to the behavior itself—how frequent, complex, familiar, or novel it is and how interwoven it is with other valued behaviors.

**health belief model:** People are more or less motivated to change their behavior based on their perception of personal susceptibility, serious consequences, worthwhile benefits, justifiable costs, and cues to actions.

**extended parallel process model:** People evaluate threatening messages, first, to determine if they are personally at risk and, second, to judge whether they can prevent a harmful outcome. If they perceive a risk but do not feel they can avoid a bad outcome, they are likely to avoid the issue.

**normative social behavior theory:** People are influenced by social norms to a greater or lesser degree depending on how much they value the social approval to be gained by conforming, what outcomes they expect from the behavior, and how much they identify with the group.

**social cognitive theory:** People make decisions by considering the interplay of internal factors, such as skills and knowledge, and environmental factors, such as environment and social approval.

**theory of reasoned action:** People make rational and deliberate choices based on how strongly they believe a behavior will lead to positive outcomes and the perceived social implications of performing that behavior.

**transtheoretical model:** People tend to change in stages, ranging from precontemplation to contemplation, preparation, action, and maintenance.

---

DeSantis described how cigar shop regulars justified their habit through collective arguments that cigar smoking was poorly understood by the medical establishment, was actually no more dangerous than mowing the lawn or driving on the freeway, and was beneficial, in that it relieved their stress. Members regularly talked about cigar smokers (such as George Burns and Milton Berle) who lived long lives and of health advocates who died young. Everyone in the shop knew the story of a heart surgeon who stopped by one day and reportedly asked, through a "relaxing" exhale, "Now how can that be bad for you?" (p. 185).

The cigar shop study illustrates the tenacity of behaviors embedded in social and environmental contexts. It also emphasizes that change is not automatic or linear. The stages described are only a general guide. People may remain in one stage indefinitely, lose interest, or skip steps.

Considering change as a stage-based process reveals some key challenges and opportunities for health campaign managers. One challenge is that people do not simply overhaul their behavior as soon as they hear new information (Maibach & Cotton, 1995). Change agents must be sensitive to barriers and motivations as well. Second, the transtheoretical model reveals why prevention efforts are particularly challenging. Campaign planners are wise to seek incremental change rather than radical transformations (Prochaska, Johnson, & Lee, 1998). Edward Maibach and David Cotton (1995) report that inundating audience members with messages inappropriate to their stage of change may actually discourage them from proceeding. Rather than accelerate the change process, people may avoid the issue entirely.

The transtheoretical model presents opportunities for important contributions as well. Without motivational health campaigns, members of at-risk populations are likely to "remain stuck in the early stages" (Prochaska et al., 1998, p. 64). The model also suggests that changes, once made, must be supported. Effective campaigns are not simply one-shot affairs, but ongoing programs that support change and commitment.

## Wrapping It Up

In closing our discussion of behavior change theories, it's important to point out that health promoters need not limit themselves to any one model. The beauty of these theories is that they often overlap and call attention to different shades of meaning within the same process. Theories are like camera lenses, in that they help us achieve focus and clarity. This can be immensely helpful. But if we're not careful, a focus can be a limitation. In the next section we explore a different perspective.

## CRITICAL-CULTURAL PERSPECTIVE

Return for a moment to the idea of a camera. When you look through the viewfinder you can zoom in on elements of the environment. But while you are focusing on one thing—even a very big thing like a sunset—there are other things you don't see. That's natural. The problem occurs when it begins to feel that what we see in the viewfinder is all there is. No matter what our perspective, there is usually more there than meets the eye. In this spirit, critical theorists remind us that—for all the many contributions of the cognitive theories we have just discussed—they share a common focus: They treat health as primarily the product of choices we make as individuals (Dutta-Bergman, 2005). Granted, cognitive theories acknowledge that our choices are influenced by a range of factors. But the nexus is still individual thought and decision making. What if we assume that this is only part of the story and look at health issues through a wider-angle lens?

Communication theorist Mohan J. Dutta has emerged as a leading advocate of the **critical-cultural approach**, which proposes that health is not merely the result of individual choices, but is intertwined with issues of culture, power, control, identity, and social consciousness. From this perspective, health-related behaviors are profoundly influenced by dynamics that are larger and more pervasive than any individual (Dutta-Bergman, 2005).

There is plentiful evidence to support the idea that health is, to a great extent, a socially enacted phenomenon. As you may remember from Chapter 6, health disparities typically observe social boundaries. The overall health of some groups is worse or better than the health of others, for a range of reasons that includes resources, prejudice and discrimination, trust, cultural mores, information, stress, living and working conditions, and more. Assuming that people who are information- and resource-poor have the same choices as other people requires that we overlook a host of factors that are very real to the people who experience them.

Moreover, it is not simply a question of having or not having. Cultural values and identities influence what is "good," "healthy," and "acceptable." The way a health expert views a particular behavior (such as smoking, drug use, driving fast, wearing a helmet, monogamy, or so on) may be very different than the way members of diverse cultures view it. Slater (2006) observes that health-related behaviors are often tied to issues of personal identity:

> Risk-taking teens may believe that alcohol or marijuana experimentation is part of what defines them as adventurous, fun party people. Farmers may believe that accepting risk of injury [as in deciding not to have roll-bars mounted on their tractors] in the interest of keeping costs low is part of what makes them farmers. (p. 155)

Conversely, scientific evidence suggests that these behaviors are dangerous. And health-related behaviors may also be attributed moral qualities such that they are considered bad, irresponsible, or evil. (This is especially true of issues such as drug use and sex.)

Considering these diverse viewpoints, a number of questions present themselves: Whose view is right? Who should decide how people ought behave? And how is one's quality of life improved or diminished by the behaviors in question? These are difficult questions. The answers, say critical theorists, are not simple or universal. Rather than privileging one perspective over another, they advocate open and respectful dialogue about the issues involving theorists, practitioners, and, most notably, members of the social group themselves (Dutta-Bergman, 2005).

Critical-cultural theorists observe that health promotion efforts that do not recognize the social contexts in which people live often fail to do much good. In fact, they often do harm—by reifying power differences, dominating the cultural landscape, and reinforcing the idea that people whose health is "poor" are not trying very hard or are like children who should be instructed by others. (See Box 14.3 for more on these ethical dilemmas.)

This is not to say that health promoters mindfully oppress the people they are trying to serve. It's more that their good intentions are often based on tacitly held assumptions about whose ideas are most valuable and who should be telling whom how to behave. You may say, "But they are only trying to teach people how to have better health." That's undoubtedly true. But let's unpack the baggage within that assertion. The idea of teaching implies that one person has knowledge or insight that he or she helps others comprehend. That is relatively unproblematic if we assume the information is straightforward and value-free. One thing we know about health: It is never impersonal or value-free. So who defines what "better health" means? And who decides the best ways to accomplish that? When health promoters assume they have the answers to these questions, the result is often a paternalistic "I know what is best for you" mindset. Actually, critical theorists argue, what is "best" is largely a matter of interpretation and value. Deborah Lupton (1998) asserts that health promotion experts are often so confident about the importance of their scientific knowledge and worldview that the values and

goals of the target community are "discounted as irrelevant and ignorant, as barriers to public health goals" (p. 4).

In the end, privileging one perspective, even if it seems to be "for people's own good," is an exercise in power and often serves to marginalize and alienate people who see the world differently. Dutta and Rebecca de Souza (2008) trace the history of health promotion efforts, showing that the tradition has largely been for those "in the center" to assist those "in the margins." They write:

> This position was based on the assumption of the expertise of those at the center, who could examine an underdeveloped community, evaluate its needs based on scientific instruments, and propose solutions that would supposedly propel the community toward development; the category of the "underdeveloped" was fixed in its position as the object of interventions, its people portrayed as the "primitive" receivers of campaign messages who were incapable of development without the helping hand of the interventionists. (p. 327)

Such efforts have often been experienced as insulting and naive, and, despite (and perhaps partly because of) widespread health promotion campaigns, the gap between the health rich and the health poor around the world continues to widen at a staggering pace (Dutta & de Souza, 2008).

One approach recommended by the critical-cultural perspective involves embracing the notion of "many realities," none more correct or dominant than another (Dutta-Bergman, 2005, p. 117). This means shedding the notion that health promoters should set the agenda. Instead, it requires that they immerse themselves in the communities they serve, acting as facilitators who support community members' efforts to decide for themselves what they consider important and how they can best attain their goals (Dutta-Bergman, 2005). Health experts can share what they know of science and theory, but it is important not to presume (or behave as if) that information is more right or important than participants' own perspectives. In other words, knowledge is one of many resources to be shared,

## BOX 14.3 ETHICAL CONSIDERATIONS

# Three Issues for Health Promoters to Keep in Mind

Health promoters are faced with a number of ethical considerations. Among them is deciding how to warn audiences without needlessly frightening them. They must also be careful not to blame people for ill health, while at the same time encouraging people to prevent any illnesses and injuries they can. All the while, they must walk a fine line between making people concerned about illness and making them worried sick.

## Timing

When early evidence of a health risk surfaces, is it better to warn the public right away or to wait for more conclusive evidence? This question poses a dilemma for health promoters. On the one hand, researchers suggest people are wary of premature announcements that are later shown to be inaccurate. Health news writer Alan Rees (1994) contends that "the average individual is caught in a withering crossfire of conflicting health messages and is inclined to disregard them all" (paragraph 7). For example, people were long urged to increase their exposure to sunlight to ensure sufficient amounts of vitamin D. Now people are encouraged to avoid sunlight to lower their risk of skin cancer (Parrott, 1995). Conflicting messages such as these may confuse people and cause them to ignore health advisories.

On the other hand, it may take months or years to compile conclusive evidence. All the while, people may be exposed to health risks they might have avoided. People are likely to be angry if health officials are aware of potential risks yet do not warn the public.

## Scapegoating

It is difficult to know where the responsibility for personal health lies. For example, if children are not vaccinated, is it (1) the parents' fault for not bringing them to a doctor, (2) the government's fault for not providing neighborhood health services, (3) the city's fault for not providing better public transportation to the health unit, or (4) health officials' fault for not educating parents about the need for immunization? Although all of these factors probably contribute to the problem, part of a health promoter's job is to identify what conditions most need improvement. In doing so, however, it is easy to **scapegoat** (blame one person or group for the whole problem).

Scapegoating presents an ethical dilemma. It makes sense to focus attention on the condition or people with the greatest chance of making a difference. The typical health promotion message cannot describe all the factors that contribute to a problem. However, focusing on one aspect or group of people may seem to place blame (Burdine, McLeroy, & Gottlieb, 1987). For example, a campaign that admonishes parents to bring their children in for vaccinations may alienate parents who do not have transportation to the public health unit and cannot afford private care. These parents may feel frustrated and criticized, and they may resent promoters' efforts. Second, people not held to blame may feel the problem is no longer their responsibility. Ruth Faden (1987) asserts that government promotes the idea that people are personally responsible for their health partly because this lets government off the hook. There is little imperative to make sweeping social changes or health care reform if it seems that health is solely the product of voluntary lifestyle changes.

Evidence fuels both sides of the debate, suggesting that personal choices and empowerment are important to health but that, at the same time, personal efforts are often constrained by environmental factors beyond individuals' control (such as money to afford medical care or sanitary living conditions). Health promoters may find themselves trying to identify key objectives without ignoring that every objective is intertwined with others.

## Stigmatizing

Prevention is the process of avoiding undesirable outcomes. People wear helmets to avoid head injuries, they

*(continued)*

BOX 14.3 (continued)

are immunized to avoid diseases, and so on. Typically, the worse the potential outcome, the more people try to prevent it. Therefore health promoters try to motivate people by showing them how bad undesirable outcomes can be.

The dilemma is that, in portraying some *conditions* as undesirable, promoters may stigmatize some *people* as undesirable. Guttman (1997) warns that campaigners' good intentions sometimes backfire when they make people so frightened of diseases that they avoid the people who have them. For instance, an image of a child with a disability may be frightening enough to make children observe safety rules, but how are they likely to feel about children with disabilities? The same dilemma applies to AIDS publicity. People may become so frightened that they overprotect themselves by avoiding people who have AIDS.

## What Do You Think?

1. Should health promoters release information about potential health risks immediately or wait for more conclusive evidence?
   a. How long is it reasonable to wait?
   b. What constitutes conclusive evidence?
2. Can you think of a way to promote public health without seeming to place the blame on certain people or groups?
3. Do you think it is possible to warn people about health hazards without stigmatizing people who have already been affected? Why or why not?

not a tool used in the process of controlling others (Dutta, 2008). The goal is an interactive, ongoing process in which "problems are configured and reconfigured; solutions are generated and worked on based on the needs of the community as defined by community members" (Dutta-Bergman, 2005, p. 116). One objective is to build social consciousness about health and engender a sense of **collective efficacy**, a communal sense that positive change can be accomplished. Dutta-Bergman (2005) also emphasizes the necessity of **community capacity,** the resources needed for good health, such as healthful food and water, safe shelter, and medical care. These basics are lacking in many parts of the country and the world.

Considering your campus campaign, you might choose to work with people who are frequently "in the margins" of fitness efforts. For example, you might focus on students and employees with physical disabilities. To accomplish this, you will want to immerse yourself, as best you can, in the concerns and viewpoints of the people in your focus community. (Even if you have a disability yourself, it's risky to make assumptions from your own perspective.) Perhaps there is an organization or support group at which people with disabilities openly discuss their goals and concerns. You might attend meetings, or, if such a format does not already exist, you might organize a series of meetings yourself. The process of encouraging people with disabilities to talk about fitness goals may be powerful in itself. There is likely to be great diversity among the people who participate, but you might learn that they share some common goals and face some common barriers they would like to overcome. Perhaps they are already involved in fitness efforts you don't know about. You may find that, like many other people, they dread feeling conspicuous at the gym. Or perhaps they require specialized equipment or spacing between pieces of equipment that isn't currently available. It may be that health professionals focus mostly on their other concerns and don't encourage them to pursue fitness goals much, so they don't feel confident about exercising. Already, you can probably imagine how issues of collective efficacy and community capacity might emerge and how you

## BOX 14.4 CAREER OPPORTUNITIES

# Health Campaign Design and Management

Campaign director
Publication designer
Communication director
Media relations specialist
Public relations specialist
Director of nonprofit organization
Professor/educator

## Career Resources and Job Listings

Social Marketing Institute: social-marketing.org
Healthpromotionjobs.com

HPCareer.Net
    wellnessconnection.com
Chronicle of Philanthropy: philanthropy.
    com/jobs
Wellness Council of America:
    welcoa.org
American Journal of Health Promotion:
    healthpromotionjournal.com
Centers for Disease Prevention and Control,
    Division of Health Communication: cdc.gov/od/
    oc/hcomm/aboutdivision.html
National Institutes of Health: nih.gov
World Health Organization: who.int/employment/
    vacancies/en

---

might help. Also keep in mind that—while it might seem patently audacious to tell people with disabilities how to behave if you don't understand their worldview—it can be equally as presumptuous to tell people from cultures and communities different than our own how to think and act. Critical-cultural theory requires us to be respectful of "diverse realities" at every level.

Systems theory (see Chapter 9) is consistent with the critical-cultural approach in recognizing that nothing happens in isolation. What seem to be individual choices are often patterns of behavior shaped and reinforced by the systems in which they occur (Bohm, 1996; Senge, 2006). Ignoring the larger patterns can result in unproductive attempts at localized change. For example, health campaign designers frequently appeal to people to avoid or quit smoking, but they rarely tackle the larger issues of public policy and tobacco industry standards (Dutta, 2008; K. C. Smith & Wakefield, 2006). Health promoters can help equalize disparities by advocating for community resources, public policies, and issues of social justice to help communities overcome their marginalized status.

The medical director of a free, walk-in clinic I know is able to recite a long list of systems-level dilemmas. For one, the clinic recently received a grant to publicize its services to people who can't afford medical care. But the grant doesn't cover operating expenses, and the staff is already overwhelmed. "It's kind of crazy to think publicity will solve the problem," he says. "Before we can serve more people, we need more staff." Another dilemma is that patients often cannot make scheduled appointments. "Maybe their boss won't let them off, or they don't have reliable transportation, or they work assorted day jobs and they can't afford to pass up an opportunity," explains the medical director, adding, "If we make appointments, the staff ends up sitting around when we could have been caring for other people." So the clinic maintains a come-anytime policy. But he says that is problematic as well: "You might get in right away, or you might have to wait for hours to see a doctor. People on hourly wages can't afford to do that. We're in a fix. We're here to serve, but limitations pop up every day." The issues the clinic faces (e.g., its own limited budget and the restricted resources and circumstances of the people it serves) are large ones. They bring us back to the central tenets of the critical-cultural approach. For one, health is partly a matter of personal agency. Theories of individual behavior change are important. But there are also larger forces at work that are frequently inequitable and pervasive. Experts unaware of the systems, structures, and assumptions that relegate some people to "the margins" and others to "the center" risk being ineffective in accomplishing true change. And even worse, they may contribute to the very disparities they are trying to overcome.

## DESIGNING AND IMPLEMENTING A CAMPAIGN

This section discusses the three final stages in developing a health campaign: designing campaign messages, piloting and implementing the campaign, and evaluating and maintaining the effort.

### Step 5: Designing Campaign Messages

As we discussed in Chapter 13, the first step in designing an effective campaign is to listen and ask questions. Holtgrave and colleagues (1995) recommend that campaign designers work closely with members of the focus community to determine what aspect of the problem is most important to them and then make that concern a focal point. Critical-cultural theory also behooves us to look at cultural values and the macro-level, systemic factors that affect the people we want to help.

It may turn out that your campaign does not involve the traditional step of creating messages that will be widely distributed to audience members. Instead, you might advocate for new hours at the fitness center, specialized fitness classes, more space or resources, skills training, or some other effort. Most campaigns, however, involve some degree of message creation and dissemination. Even if your principal effort is changing the structure, you will want to get the word out somehow. And members of the focus community will probably be interested in involving people who are not already onboard.

In this section we focus on the central principles of message design.

*Choosing a Voice*    Campaign messages have a voice. The voice may seem masculine, feminine, young, old, friendly, casual, stern, or so on. Whatever its character, this voice embodies the mood and personality of the campaign. Here are some questions to consider in finding that voice.

- What is the campaign's personality and mood?
- Is this an authority figure or a friend?
- Is this a logical person or an emotional person?
- Is this the sort of person to whom the audience is likely to respond?

Even when words appear in print, the tone of the message gives the reader a sense of who is "talking" and what type of relationship the writer wishes to establish with the reader. Lefebvre and colleagues (1995) described how carefully Nike considered the presentation of its "Just do it" advertising slogan. They say the creators decided not to use an exclamation mark after the statement and not to have an announcer say it aloud. "The concern was that the wrong voice, the wrong delivery, and the wrong inflection could have doomed the ads for many viewers" (Lefebvre et al., p. 224).

Of course, the source is even more apparent when the audience can see or hear a spokesperson deliver the message. Messages typically have more impact when the target audience trusts the spokesperson and thinks he or she is capable and attractive. Celebrities can sometimes fill the bill. Michael J. Fox has been successful at calling attention to Parkinson's disease, raising money for research, and testifying before Congress (Beck, 2005). Basketball star Magic Johnson changed the public perception of HIV and AIDS when he announced in 1991 that he was HIV-positive. In the wake of his announcement, the National AIDS Hotline received 10 times as many calls as usual. New coverage and public knowledge about HIV transmission increased, especially among young people, and the number of people seeking HIV testing increased dramatically (Casey et al.,

2003). After studying public reaction to Johnson's announcement, William Brown and Michael Basil (1995) concluded that people reacted so strongly because they felt they knew Magic Johnson.

There are drawbacks to using well-known spokespersons, however. Public role models sometimes behave in ways that contradict or cloud health campaign messages. For example, when Mark McGwire broke the major league home run record in 1998, even people who did not follow baseball knew about it. Then it was revealed that McGwire had used androstenedione, a dietary supplement meant to speed muscle development. About 24% of the people who heard about his use of androstenedione wanted to learn more about it, and about 22% said they would like to try it (W. J. Brown, Basil, & Bocarnea, 2003). This was certainly not a practice health experts wanted to promote! In another case, a pharmaceutical company in Australia paid a well-known soccer star the equivalent of $123,000 to stop smoking. He didn't. Fortunately for the promoters, the publicity surrounding the failed attempt nonetheless increased sales of nicotine- replacement therapies (Chapman & Leask, 2001).

There is also considerable evidence that audiences are most likely to believe people who are similar to them, an effect called **source homophily** (E. M. Rogers, 1973). Not only do people pay more attention when the spokesperson is similar to them, they feel more personally vulnerable to the health risk (Rimal & Morrison, 2006). For example, African Americans typically prefer and are more likely to trust PSAs that feature African Americans rather than people of other races (Wang & Arpan, 2008). In a national survey, 50% of African Americans interviewed said they trust black-oriented media, but only 34% trusted mainstream media sources (Brodie, Kjellson, Hoff, & Parker, 2008). This may be partly because 78% of the African American respondents felt that they are often left out of health-related news stories, and 76% felt they are overrepresented in stories about crime (Brodie et al.).

*Designing the Message* In designing an effective health campaign message, it is important to consider community expectations and the role of logic, emotion, and novelty. Box 14.5 describes the different ways that messages about the same health behavior can be framed. Here we talk more about the art of matching messages to audience needs and emotions.

*Community Expectations* A message is effective only if people consider it relevant and meaningful. When she studied campaigns about prostate cancer screening, Juanne Nancarrow Clarke (1999) found that nearly all the campaign messages embodied themes of male sexuality, machismo, and brotherhood. Although these messages may appeal to some men, others are probably turned off by an image they do not feel applies to them. The same can be true of other audiences. A good deal of research has focused on college students' alcohol consumption. There is consistent evidence that students who drink typically consider that alcohol frees their inhibitions and makes them less shy and more socially engaging (Sopory, 2005). This is a tough perception to overcome. And it is one reason that students and health advocates often disagree about how much drinking is too much. Although researchers tend to define five or more drinks as "binge drinking," students typically perceive that five drinks are within the normal range for their peers (Lederman, Stewart, Goodhart, & Laitman, 2008). They define a binge in more extreme terms. Consequently, researchers who survey students about "binge drinking" may be measuring something different than they think. And students may feel that warnings about "binge drinking" do not apply to them because their behavior is within "normal" bounds (Lederman et al.). (For more on social norms as the basis for safe-drinking campaigns, see Box 14.6.)

*Logical and Emotional Appeals* A **logical appeal** attempts to educate people and demonstrate a clear link between a behavior and a result. For example, it is logical to eat less if it will result in greater health and a longer life. An **emotional appeal** (also called *affect appeal*) suggests that people should *feel* a certain way regarding their health or their

**BOX 14.5**

# Framing Health Choices: What Do We Lose? What Do We Gain?

You're walking through the mall with a friend when you come upon a booth proclaiming "Free Health Screening." The health professionals staffing the booth say they can give you a relatively accurate cholesterol score. They just need a drop or two of blood from your finger. And they can tell your body fat percentage by gently pinching and measuring the skin on your upper arm. One of you says, "Sure! What do I have to lose?" and steps up to participate. The other says, "No thanks," and backs away quickly. Why do you respond so differently?

Message-frame theorists are interested in the way people interpret health-related behaviors and in health promoters' efforts to affect those interpretations (Slater, 2006). A famous example involves smoking. For years, health promoters tried to get people to quit because it was bad for their health. But the real turning point occurred when researchers proved the dangers of secondhand smoke. The issue was reframed from endangering self to endangering others. Whereas the personal risk seemed acceptable—even cool and rebellious to some—many people found it unacceptable to put others at risk. It was the same behavior, but framed differently. As Michael Slater (2006) puts it, relative to health, message framing "refers to the social priorities and the values with which a topic is implicitly associated" (p. 155). He proposes that it is unrealistic to expect people to adopt behaviors that are inconsistent with their personal or social identity.

As with most things health-related, effects are not simple or predictable. Men are still at particularly high risk for smoking. One reason may be that advertisers have done a good job framing smoking in culturally masculine terms. In a study of smoking references in men's magazines, Dutta and Josh Boyd (2007) found that smoking was consistently framed as a sensual pleasure, as independent and mysterious, and as occurring in places of power, in exotic lands,

or in appealing outdoor locations. The researchers suggest that antismoking campaigns might turn around the masculine appeal of these themes by framing antismoking messages in similar ways.

One way messages are framed is with respect to potential gains, losses, and risks (Rothman & Salovey, 1997). A **gain-frame appeal** illustrates the advantages of performing the recommended behavior. For example, people might be persuaded that eating a low-carbohydrate diet will keep their weight down and help prevent diabetes and heart disease. They gain something by following the diet. Conversely, a **loss-frame appeal** emphasizes the negative repercussions of not taking action, as in "People who eat a lot of processed carbohydrates are at risk for disease that can shorten their lives."

There is some evidence that gain-frame appeals are more effective than loss-frame appeals at getting people to engage in preventive behaviors (O'Keefe & Jensen, 2007; Rothman, Bartels, Wlaschin, & Salovey, 2006). For example, you might use sunscreen, brush your teeth twice a day, take vitamins, and so on. These are gain-related behaviors without much risk.

But it gets a little more complicated when the goal shifts from disease prevention to disease detection. For example, you may willingly stock your beach bag with sunscreen, but imagine that you notice a suspicious mole on your shoulder. If you're like most people, you will feel a range of complicated emotions. Seeking a diagnosis is emotionally risky. You might learn that you have cancer and need treatment. It's emotionally self-protective to avoid what might be an anxiety-producing outcome. In fact, such avoidance can, and often does, last months or years.

But perhaps something else happens. You hear about someone who died of skin cancer, or you see an alarming PSA. These are loss-frame messages, in that they highlight bad things that might happen if you don't take action. It's possible that you will become so frightened about what might be happening with your body that your anxiety will outweigh your desire to ignore the issue. Perhaps you'll make the doctor's appointment after all.

The rule of thumb is to promote disease prevention with gain-frame messages and disease-detection behaviors (such as doctor visits and health screenings) with loss-frame messages. But actual evidence on the value of loss-frame messages is inconclusive (O'Keefe & Jensen, 2007). This is probably because of the complex interplay of factors and emotions that surround health decisions. In our hypothetical example of the health booth, one of you is willing to be tested but the other isn't. Research is filled with such inconsistencies. In the suspicious mole scenario, maybe you wouldn't delay seeing a doctor if you noticed a suspicious mole. Perhaps you don't like uncertainty, you want to be sure it doesn't get any worse, you're pretty sure it's no big deal, or you have a checkup scheduled anyway so you'll mention the mole to avoid a second visit. By contrast, another person might see the same frightening PSA yet still put the issue off, perhaps reasoning that "If it hasn't killed me yet, it must not be too bad" or "I'll die when it's my time to die and there's not much I can do about it anyway." People are complicated, to say the least. Although we seem to share the basic desire to maximize gains and minimize losses, there are numerous reasons we might weigh these factors differently.

Some theorists argue that loss- and gain-framing is valid even though the evidence is mixed. They propose that aggregate-level trends are not apparent because the effects are felt on an individual level (Latimer, Salovey, & Rothman, 2007). In other words, what motivates you might not motivate the person next to you, so the overall numbers look like a wash even if some people benefited. The challenge, these theorists say, is for researchers and health promoters to focus on individuals and small groups who share common concerns rather than trying to reach large numbers of people with the same message.

## What Do You Think?

1. What factors might influence your decision to take part in a free health screening at the mall? Are you more likely to participate or to say "No, thanks"? Why? What might you gain if you are tested? On the other hand, what unpleasant outcomes might result if you participate?

2. What if the stakes were higher? If you suspected you had been exposed to HIV, what factors would influence whether you got tested or not? Would frightening information about HIV make you more inclined or less inclined to get tested? Why?

3. List some prevention behaviors you engage in every day. Why do you do these things? Is it mostly because of positive effects or mostly to avoid bad outcomes?

behaviors. For example, they should be frightened if they are exposed to AIDS, proud if they have quit smoking, or guilty if they are endangering others. Ellen Peters and colleagues (2006) propose that affect appeals serve four purposes: (1) to provide information, as when we think, "The people in that commercial look really happy; it must be a good product," (2) to grab or hold our attention, (3) to motivate us to think carefully or take action, and (4) to link behaviors with community values, as when a message encourages us to recycle because it is good for the earth or to stop smoking because it puts our children in danger (Peters, Lipkus, & Diefenbach, 2006). Although emotions occur along a complex continuum, Peters and colleagues observe that there are two basic "flavors"—positive and negative. For the most part, campaigns encourage people to strive for positive outcomes and avoid

## BOX 14.6 THEORETICAL FOUNDATIONS

# What Does Science Say About Peer Pressure?

*"I think that alcohol is a huge part of adult life. It's like a rite of passage when you finally turn 21."*
*"Every college student I know drinks."*
*"College students love to party. It's tradition."*

Thinking of your own undergraduate experience, you might find yourself nodding in agreement as you read these comments made by college students in Casper and colleagues' (2006) study (p. 295). Or you might shake your head in doubt. Experiences vary. And conventional wisdom suggests that your experience has a lot to do with the company you keep. It feels normal for partiers to party and nondrinkers not to drink. But in some instances, some people don't follow the crowd. What *does* science say about fitting in with the crowd?

On the one hand, there is ample evidence that people are more likely to engage in risky behaviors if their friends do. Having peers who smoke and approve of smoking is the single greatest predictor of a teen's decision to smoke cigarettes (Grandpre & Alvaro, 2006; Krosnick et al., 2006; C. H. Miller, Burgoon). The same goes for kicking the habit. The overall decline in smoking hasn't occurred so much here and there as in distinct social clusters. In studying the issue, Nicholas Christakis and James Fowler (2008) found that smoking had persisted in some circles but that in others "whole groups of people were quitting in concert" (p. 2249).

One foundation for the RU SURE campaign that begins this chapter is **social norms theory**, which suggests that people base their behavior partly on what they consider appropriate and socially acceptable (Haines & Spear, 1996). The idea is that such campaigns may be especially influential in settings such as college campuses, where students are part of novel situations in which they are not immediately aware of cultural expectations. As you know, that campaign has had demonstrable success curbing student alcohol abuse.

But some social norm campaigns have been less successful. In a study of students at 37 colleges, Wechsler and colleagues (2003) found that drinking was the same on campuses with social norm campaigns as on those without them. In another study, 72.6% of college students surveyed disbelieved the assertion that "most students drink 0 to 4 drinks when they party" (Polonec, Major, & Atwood, 2006, p. 23). And Shelly Campo and Kenzie Cameron (2006) found that, after viewing social-norming messages, light drinkers were even more determined to keep their drinking within healthy bounds, but heavier drinkers often went the other way. Their drinking intentions were *more* intense after viewing the normative messages. Another challenge to the power of social norms is that, in some cases, people find nonconformity appealing. People of varying ages who rank high on individualism or rebellious tendencies are likely to go *against* the norm (Lapinski, Rimal, DeVries, & Lee, 2007; M. J. Lee & Bichard, 2006).

Rajiv Rimal and Kevin Real (2005) have sought to make sense of the complexity with their **theory of normative social behavior (TNSB)**. The theory proposes that we *are* influenced by perceived social norms but that a variety of factors either strengthen or weaken how much those perceptions affect us. These include (1) how much we value the social approval to be gained from conforming, (2) the outcomes we expect from engaging in the behavior, and (3) the degree to which we identify with the group. In other words, if we like and value the group, we may want to "fit in" by acting in accordance with its norms, especially if the behavior offers rewards we like. However, our desire to fit in may be outweighed by other factors—as when the behavior seems inconsequential, we don't value or identify with the group very much, we enjoy being different, or we like the behavior so much we are willing to buck convention to do it. There is evidence that college students drink if/when they perceive that the rewards (such as loss of social inhibitions) outweigh the potential for negative repercussions, such as getting in trouble or getting hurt. And this is particularly true if they also perceive that drinking is accepted and approved of by their friends (Rimal & Real, 2005).

So back to the initial question: Does believing that "most people drink" or "drink a lot" mean we are likely to do the same? So far, the best answer is that it depends. For one, it depends on how we define "most people." The "norm" that researchers often use (as in "two of three college students stop at three or fewer drinks") is an aggregate statistic. It might change your mind about typical college student behavior. Or you might think, "They clearly haven't met *my* friends!" or "I'm a grad student. That doesn't apply." Evidence suggests that, if the overall statistic seems different than what you perceive strongly within your own social network, you are likely to disbelieve or disregard it (Polonec et al., 2006; Yanovitzky, Stewart, & Lederman, 2006). A second consideration concerns the perceived value of the behavior (Rimal, 2008). Whereas a **descriptive norm** describes what "what most people do," an **injunctive norm** characterizes the perception that people *should* do it based on particular values (Boer & Westhoff, 2006; Rimal, 2008). For example, even if you believe that most of your friends occasionally drink and drive, you may refuse to do so yourself because you consider it wrong or irresponsible. Finally, TNSB suggests that norms affect us to the degree that it is socially and personally rewarding to live up to them. If any of a complex array of factors change (rewards, penalties, group membership, or so on), the power of the norm may change considerably.

Here are a few implications for health campaigns.

- *Correct misperceptions about descriptive norms.* Although descriptive norms do not tell the whole story, nearly everyone agrees that people who overestimate the prevalence of risky behaviors are more likely than others to feel that the behaviors are acceptable and even socially preferred.

- *Emphasize descriptive <u>and</u> injunction norms.* For example, a sun-safety program was particularly effective when the health promoters presented both an injunctive norm (photos that showed undesirable skin damage) and a descriptive norm (information that most people now use sunscreen) (Mahler, Kulik, Butler, Gerrard, & Gibbons, 2008).

- *Don't rely solely on norming messages.* Norms sometimes take a backseat to other factors, such as personal enjoyment. College students in Cameron and Campo's (2006) study were most likely to smoke, exercise, and drink if they enjoyed those behaviors, even when there was no strong peer support for them. It may help to emphasize the negative repercussions of unhealthy behaviors as well as social norms.

- *Target social networks.* A common suggestion among social norm researchers is that campaigns address alcohol abuse as a social network issue. This often involves developing partnerships with sororities and fraternities, sports teams, student governments, and other groups.

The debate continues to be a lively and productive one. The success of Rutgers' RU SURE campaign may be based partly on its social norm foundation and partly on the integrated and multifaceted nature of the campaign itself. TNSB offers a rich, contextual understanding of the facets that figure into social norming, a concept that continues to evolve and to influence theorists as well as practitioners.

negative ones. Research discussed in this section describes the usefulness and the limitations of various emotional appeals.

**POSITIVE AFFECT APPEALS** Campaigns may promote positive emotional rewards in the form of popularity, a sense of accomplishment, honor, fun, or happiness. For example, a nutrition information program helped people feel confident and optimistic about their ability to reduce fat intake (Chew, Palmer, & Kim, 1998). These people were subsequently more concerned about nutrition than others and were more likely to monitor their diets. The researchers concluded that providing nutrition information was not very helpful unless people felt empowered to make a difference.

Campaigns may also inspire positive affect because the messages themselves are pleasant or entertaining. Evidence suggests that relatively uninterested individuals are likely to judge information on a superficial level, perhaps based on the music, humor, or graphics or the attractiveness of the spokesperson (Petty & Cacioppo, 1986). If the announcement is not interesting and appealing, they may ignore it altogether. By contrast, people who are already concerned about an issue may want more detailed information. All in all, research shows that pleasant messages grab people's attention but that people may not take these messages as seriously as fearful ones (Monohan, 1995).

NEGATIVE AFFECT APPEALS Some campaigns attempt to motivate people by making them feel anxious, fearful, or guilty. There is evidence that fearful appeals are effective at convincing people to be tested for AIDS and to take other health precautions (E. C. Green & Witte, 2006; Hullett, 2006). But fearsome appeals can also inspire avoidant behaviors (Lang, 2006). In one study, women responding to a cancer screening campaign said they would not like to hear messages that escalated their fears about cancer or mammography (Marshall, Smith, & McKeon, 1995). They were already frightened by these topics, and they wanted clear information. Likewise, in a study involving Hispanic women, participants who believed that cancer was God's will did not want information about the disease (Oetzel, DeVargas, Ginossar, & Sanchez, 2007). However, people who are not anxious about health risks are often not very interested in prevention information (Millar & Millar, 1998). Intense messages might *get* their attention.

Communication theorist Kim Witte proposes that, if people are not at all anxious about a health topic, then they probably are not motivated to learn about it or to take action. However, if they are overly anxious, they may avoid the subject. Witte's **extended parallel process model** (EPPM) proposes that people evaluate a threatening message, first, to determine if they are personally at risk and, second, to judge whether they can prevent a harmful outcome. If they perceive a risk but do not feel they can avoid a bad outcome, they are likely to soothe their anxiety by avoiding the issue (Witte, 1997, 2008). For example, David Buller and colleagues (2000) found that parents of elementary school students responded favorably to a highly intense message about sun protection *if* the message presented an acceptable solution. The messages began by describing the problem in intense language: "A bad sunburn is embarrassing. So is the peeling skin that follows a sunburn. Worse than peeling skin and redness are the deadly problems which can follow these annoyances..." (p. 273). Readers were then presented with a solution (using sunscreen year-round). The authors speculate that this message was effective because it was arousing enough to be memorable and because it provided a clear, culturally appropriate solution. On the other hand, a highly intense message without a promising solution might dissuade audience members from changing their attitudes or behaviors (H. Cho & Salmon, 2007).

Simon-Arndt and associates (2006) used EPPM principles to test an online program for Marines. Marines in the study answered online questions about their alcohol consumption. Then they received online feedback about their risk levels and potential ways to prevent unhealthy outcomes (note the EPPM components). About 85% of the Marines who took part preferred this program to other alcohol-use campaigns, perhaps because it seemed highly targeted to their own behaviors (Simon-Arndt, Hurtado, & Patriarca-Troyk, 2006).

**Guilt,** a feeling of remorse about having done something wrong, is a particularly strong emotion. Consequently, it is a useful tool for advertisers and health campaigners. Bruce Huhmann and Timothy Brotherton (1997) assert that people typically feel sorry or ashamed when they have behaved badly, especially when others are hurt by their actions. Advertisers who bring these feelings to the surface and offer a way to make retributions may find that people are willing to cooperate to soothe their consciences. Huhmann and Brotherton found that 1 in 20 magazine advertisements included a guilt appeal, ranging from "I wish I had started saving for my children's college education when they were young" (p. 36) to "Last night, 2 million children in the U.S. went to bed hungry" (p. 37). Guilt often seems to work. For example, warnings about the deadly effects of secondhand smoke are particularly effective at getting people to quit or to change their smoking habits (Goldman & Glantz, 1998).

Overall, negative affect is a popular component of persuasive messages, but it must be used carefully. Health promoters have overshot the mark in some cases. Women in the United States now consistently overestimate their risk of breast cancer (K. O. Jones, Denham, & Springston, 2007). And it isn't easy to reassure them. Amanda Dillard and colleagues found that it was just as difficult to reduce women's sense of breast cancer danger as it was to *stimulate* their concern about other health risks (Dillard, McCaul, Kelso, & Klein, 2006).

**NOVEL AND SHOCKING MESSAGES Novel messages** tend to catch people's attention and stick in their memory (Parrott, 1995). Some messages are novel (new or different) without being **shocking** (intense or improper) **messages**. For instance, posting health warnings in public restrooms is an effort to use an unexpected format to reinforce the risks of smoking and drinking during pregnancy. It is a novel approach, but not particularly shocking. At other times, novel messages may be shocking because they deal with topics not usually discussed in public or because they are purposefully controversial to attract attention. One difficulty about using novel images to attract attention is that the novelty wears off (Walters, Walters, Kern-Foxworth, & Priest, 1997). Keeping novelty alive may mean becoming ever more risqué. It is sometimes difficult to balance decorum with the need for public awareness.

One difficulty surrounding AIDS awareness is that health promoters must deal with delicate issues like premarital sex and anal intercourse. Even when promoters do not mean to be shocking, they often

---

**BOX 14.7 RESOURCES**

## More About Designing Health Campaigns

For guidance on creating your own health campaign, visit the following websites.

The Community Tool Box: ctb.ku.edu

The American Public Health Association: apha.org

www.Healthbehavior.com

social-marketing.com/HELinks.html

Global Dialogue for Effective Stop Smoking Campaigns: stopsmokingcampaigns.org/index. php?page=campaign_tool_kit

*Making Health Communication Programs Work: A Planner's Guide* is available at cancer.gov/pinkbook

*Communication Planning with CDCynergy* is available at cdc.gov/healthmarketing

---

are. Particularly when AIDS first became a health concern, condoms and gay sex were not socially acceptable topics for mass media campaigns. In the 1990s, controversy arose concerning a poster campaign in New York City. The posters (which were hung in subway terminals) read "Young, Hot, Safe!" and showed images of homosexual couples kissing while holding condoms, gloves, and spermicide ("Controversy Heats Up," 1994). Some people felt the posters were indecent, while others argued that they communicated an important message to a high-risk group. (The poster campaign was discontinued soon thereafter.)

**LESSONS ABOUT EMOTIONAL APPEALS** Here are a few guidelines, suggested by research, about using emotional appeals.

- *Match the emotion to the goal.* Emotional appeals are most persuasive when they are appropriate to the desired response. For example, fear appeals can alert people to danger, disgust appeals can make unhealthy behaviors unappealing, hope appeals can convince people it is worth taking action, and so on (Dillard & Nabi, 2006).

- *Build empathy.* "It won't happen to me" is a common response to health messages, even when they are highly arousing. For example, we may feel concerned about intravenous drug users because they are at risk for AIDS but perceive our own risk to be negligible because we are not part of that group. We usually feel a sense of personal relevance only if we understand the message cognitively, the speaker effectively conveys his or her feelings of vulnerability, and we perceive that those feelings are relevant to our own situation (Campbell & Babrow, 2004).
- *Don't overdo it.* Too much affect can be counterproductive and cause people to avoid the issue or to worry unnecessarily (Peters et al., 2006, p. S155).

## Step 6: Piloting and Implementing the Campaign

It is important to pilot (pretest) a campaign before launching it full-scale. **Piloting** usually involves selecting members from the target audience to review the campaign materials and comment on them. Salmon and Atkin (2003) say early feedback is crucial:

> The feedback from the audience can reveal whether the tone is too righteous (admonishing unhealthy people about their incorrect behavior), the recommendations too extremist (rigidly advocating unpalatable ideas of healthy behavior), the execution too politically correct (staying within tightly prescribed boundaries of propriety to avoid offending overly sensitive authorities and interest groups), and the execution too self-indulgent (letting creativity and style overwhelm substance and substantive content). (p. 453)

Some questions to consider include these (adapted from Donohew, 1990):

- Are written messages easy to read and understand?
- Are recorded messages easy to understand?
- Do messages seem relevant and important?
- Are the messages appealing? Why or why not?
- Is the spokesperson effective?
- Does the information seem controversial or offensive?

It may be useful to survey people before and after they are exposed to the campaign materials to see if there is any change in their knowledge, attitudes, and intentions. When possible, it is also advisable to survey people a week or a month after they are initially exposed to campaign materials to see how much they remember and whether message effects are still present. Remember to allow time to refine campaign messages based on the results of pretesting. Planning ahead will improve the campaign's likelihood of success.

Once campaign messages have been created, piloted, and refined, it is time to distribute them through chosen channels. In some cases (as with one-on-one communication and community presentations), health promoters have direct contact with community members. With the majority of channels, however, health promoters must rely on others to share their messages. For instance, editors and news directors choose what PSAs to publicize and when, and what topics to cover in the news. On a social level, community opinion leaders focus on some issues more than others, affecting what the people around them think and believe. People in the media and the community who decide what information will be publicized and how are known as **gatekeepers**.

Good campaign designers employ a variety of communication channels to help ensure that messages make it to focus community members through one gate or another. The wise health promoter realizes the importance of gatekeepers, includes them in campaign planning, and considers their points of view. John McGrath (1995) observes that media gatekeepers are bound by multiple pressures (e.g., operating budgets, community demands, and time constraints). The promoter who gets to know gatekeepers personally and makes it easy for them to pass along information has a better chance of getting through to a community.

## Step 7: Evaluating and Maintaining the Campaign

A campaign is not over when it has been released to the public. Effective health promotion requires that campaign managers evaluate the success of the project, help community members maintain any positive changes they may have made, and refine and develop future campaign messages.

*Evaluation*  The effects of a campaign may be evaluated in several ways. A **pretest–posttest design** means that campaigners survey people before the campaign is released and then survey them again afterwards (Wimmer & Dominick, 1997). The survey may indicate if people's attitudes, knowledge, or actions have changed since the campaign. Keep in mind that if changes have occurred, they may or may not be the result of campaign exposure.

To evaluate the impact of the **truth°** campaign (Box 14.9), researchers conducted telephone surveys with 6,897 youth ages 12 to 17 before the campaign began (Farrelly et al., 2002). The survey participants were chosen to represent teens in different ethnic and racial groups, urban and nonurban areas, and areas with and without other antitobacco campaigns. The youth were asked to indicate their level of agreement or disagreement with statements about the tobacco industry, the social acceptability of smoking, and their intention to smoke within the next year. In follow-up interviews after the campaign's release, researchers asked 10,692 youth if they remembered seeing any antitobacco campaigns and, if so, what they remembered about them. They also asked about perceptions of the tobacco industry, the social acceptability of smoking, and the youths' intention to smoke in the next year. To factor out as many intervening variables as possible, researchers statistically controlled for such factors as the number of parents in the household, amount of television viewing, the presence of smokers in the household, and parental messages about smoking. With the data collected, researchers were able (1) to gauge the extent to which community members saw and remembered the campaign and (2) to compare youth attitudes before and after the campaign.

---

**BOX 14.8 RESOURCES**

## More About Assessing the Impact of Health Campaigns

The following sources offer excellent advice about measuring the effect of your campaign.

Hornik, R. C. (Ed.). (2002). *Public health communication: Evidence for behavior change.* Mahwah, NJ: Lawrence Erlbaum.

Murray-Johnson, L., & Witte, K. (2003). Looking toward the future: Health message design strategies. In T. L. Thompson, A. M. Dorsey, K. I. Miller, & R. Parrott (Eds.), *Handbook of health communication* (pp. 473–495). Mahwah, NJ: Lawrence Erlbaum.

---

Another way to evaluate a campaign's success is to study actual behavior changes, such as the number of people who sign up for basketball or the number of hospital admissions or calls to a hotline. These evaluation techniques are useful, but it is always difficult to know precisely what effects a campaign has had. For one thing, the campaign is not the only factor influencing people's attitudes and behavior. They may be affected by personal experiences, news stories, or other occurrences. Imagine trying to evaluate the impact of an AIDS awareness program that happened to coincide with Magic Johnson's public announcement that he had HIV! Second, campaigns often have indirect effects. For instance, the campaign may have reached influential members of the community, who in turn spread the word to others. Thus, people who were not exposed to campaign messages personally may be affected by them. Third, sometimes the success of a health campaign is reflected in what does *not* occur over the long run. For example, the coordinators of a drug-free program in elementary schools may not know if they have been successful until the children involved are adolescents or adults, by which time they will have been influenced by many other factors as well. When undesired behaviors do not occur, it is difficult to

**BOX 14.9**

## Campaign Spotlight: The truth® About Smoking

*"In 1971, when one tobacco executive was reminded that smoking can lead to underweight babies, he said, 'Some women prefer smaller babies.'"*

*"According to the New York Times, in 1998, one tobacco executive said: 'Nobody knows what you'd turn to if you didn't smoke. Maybe you'd beat your wife.'"*

*"Tobacco kills 20 times more people than murder."*

These are just a few of the facts presented by **truth**®, the nation's largest youth smoking-prevention campaign. Messages like those shown appear in advertising campaigns and on the campaign website (www.thetruth.com), which is loaded with interactive games, downloads, and videos, including one of a singing cowboy who breathes through a hole in his throat and speaks through an electronic device since his larynx was removed because of cancer. The American Legacy Foundation®, a national public health foundation devoted to keeping young people from smoking and to helping all smokers quit, launched **truth**® in 2000. The American Legacy Foundation was founded as a result of the 1998 Master Settlement Agreement between the tobacco industry and 46 states and 5 U.S. territories. Payments to the American Legacy Foundation are made on behalf of the settling states.

Teens' awareness of antitobacco messages nearly doubled in the first 10 months of the **truth**® campaign (Farrelly, Healton, Davis, Messeri, & Haviland, 2002). Youth exposed to campaign messages were significantly less likely than others to consider smoking "cool" and more likely to believe that tobacco companies lie to sell their products (Farrelly et al.). The effects have endured. Prior to **truth**®, about 45% of youth in the target audience perceived that their peers smoked. Three years into the campaign, the percentage had dropped to 38% (K. C. Davis, Nonnemaker, & Farrelly, 2007).

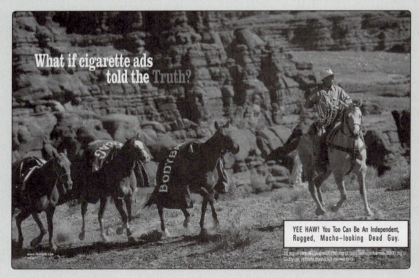

Photo courtesy of Patricia McLaughlin, American Legacy Foundation

Analysts say **truth®** has been successful largely because campaign designers took time to understand the target audience, youth ages 12 to 17. Matthew Farrelly and colleagues (2002) write:

> The "truth" brand builds a positive, tobacco-free identity through hard-hitting advertisements that feature youths confronting the tobacco industry. This rebellious rejection of tobacco and tobacco advertising channels youths' need to assert their independence and individuality, while countering tobacco marketing efforts. (p. 901)

By contrast, the *"Think. Don't Smoke."* campaign by the Philip Morris tobacco company, launched in 1998, has not hurt cigarettes' image. Exposure has not influenced youth's perception of peer smoking rates (K. C. Davis, Nonnemaker, & Farrelly, 2007).

Indeed, there is evidence that young people exposed to *"Think. Don't Smoke."* messages are *more* likely than others to intend to smoke in the next year (Farrelly et al., 2002). Farrelly and coauthors conclude that the purpose of the *"Think. Don't Smoke."* campaign was "to buy respectability and not to prevent youth smoking" (p. 906). Phillip Morris began another campaign (*Talk. They'll Listen.*") in 1999, focused on parental responsibility for talking to children about smoking. Researchers found that that campaign was also associated with increased intent to smoke and lower levels of antitobacco attitudes among those exposed to the campaign messages (Wakefield et al., 2006). While *"Think. Don't Smoke."* eventually went off the air (in 2002), public health advocates continue to urge the tobacco industry to remove all its PSAs from television, due to their ineffectiveness (Farrelly et al., 2002; "Trick or Treat," 2006; Wakefield et al., 2006).

know how many people might have adopted those behaviors if not for the campaign.

Sometimes health campaigns have unintended or undesirable consequences. Audiences may be so turned off by the message that they actively avoid the subject or lose trust in the sender. Here is an extreme example. When I was in college, the 1936 film *Reefer Madness* made a comeback, not as the frightening documentary it was originally designed to be but as a comedy. College students flocked to the local midnight movie to see the jerky-action black-and-white film in which young people smoke what the narrator (a high school principal) calls "demon weed" and immediately become shaky, wild-eyed, and demented. The students subsequently listen to "evil jazz" music and become serial killers—threats so unbelievable that the movie dialogue was often drowned out by the audience's laughter. We can only imagine the extent to which the outdated movie damaged the credibility of antidrug messages at the time.

For better or worse, sometimes the best that campaigners can do is evaluate the **reach** (number of people exposed to campaign messages) and

**specificity** (the type of people exposed to the campaign) of a campaign. For this purpose, promoters can survey community members and keep track of when and where campaign messages are publicized.

*Maintenance* Maintaining behaviors that have been positively influenced by a campaign involves continued encouragement and skills training. Keep in mind that people are most likely to continue new behaviors if they fully understand the benefits of doing so (Valente et al., 1998). Because some people try new behaviors without first fully understanding them, do not assume that people who begin a behavior are fully educated about it. Encouragement, incentives, and continued skills training can help people overcome setbacks they are likely to encounter (Maibach & Cotton, 1995).

## SUMMARY

Social marketers conduct extensive audience analyses and strive to create messages with the same appeal as commercial messages. The results of social marketing are measured, not in sales figures or profit margins, but in public awareness and improved health. These outcomes are often realized in subtle ways over long periods of time, but social marketers work hard to gauge the success of their efforts and apply what they learn to future campaigns.

Theories of behavior change explain the conditions under which people are likely to make lifestyle changes. The overall message is that behavior is influenced by a complex array of factors, both internal and external. Failing to consider these can lead to health campaigns that may look good but have very little social value. What's more, campaign designers who fail to consider and accommodate audience members' beliefs and opportunities can alienate the people they hope to influence and can actually make things worse by promoting behaviors that people find offensive, puzzling, or even impossible to carry out. One alternative is for health advocates to serve as facilitators and enablers who help communities set their own agendas and build collective efficacy and social capacity.

In designing campaign messages, health promoters should consider ethical implications concerning timing, scapegoating, and stigmatizing as well as audience needs, campaign goals, and benefits of the recommended behaviors.

Campaign messages have different voices ranging from stern to casual and friendly. Often, the spokesperson influences the way the message is perceived. Research suggests that people typically respond most favorably to spokespersons who are similar to them, likable, and attractive. A celebrity may be an effective spokesperson or a public liability.

The same behavior may be framed in a number of ways to emphasize potential gains, losses, or social implications. Campaign messages also appeal to our logic and emotions. Some campaigns motivate people through positive affect, such as the promise of pleasure and happiness or the desire to fit in with social norms. Negative affect appeals may induce people to change by stirring up feelings of anxiety, fear, and guilt. According to the extended parallel process model, anxiety is a powerful motivator except when the threat is so overwhelming

that people would rather avoid the issue. Novel and shocking messages typically create interest, but they may be controversial and offensive to some people.

Experts recommend that health promoters pilot new campaigns before implementing them. Testing campaign messages on sample community members can reveal unanticipated reactions and ambiguities in time to improve the messages before they are publicly released. Finally, health promoters should evaluate campaigns once they are released, apply what they have learned to future efforts, and compare the results with their stated goals.

## KEY TERMS

social marketing
health belief model
social cognitive theory
internal factors
environmental factors
embedded behaviors model
theory of reasoned action (TRA)
transtheoretical model
critical-cultural approach
scapegoat
collective efficacy
community capacity
source homophily
game-frame appeal
loss-frame appeal
social norms theory
theory of normative social behavior (TNSB)
descriptive norm
injunctive norm
logical appeal
emotional appeal
extended parallel process model (EPPM)
guilt
novel messages
shocking messages
piloting
gatekeepers
pretest–posttest design
reach
specificity

# DISCUSSION QUESTIONS

1. What is involved with social marketing? Can you think of health messages that are as appealing as regular commercials? Which are your favorites and why? Do they influence the choices you make? Why or why not? What might motivate you to visit a website?

2. According to the health belief model, what five criteria affect people's decision to make behavior changes? Can you think of a time when a certain event or message spurred you to action? If so, why do you think it had that affect?

3. Explain what role internal and environmental factors play in social cognitive theory. What internal and environmental factors influence your health-related behavior?

4. You might be a member of the target audience for the sports recreation campaign. Take a moment to reflect on your own characteristics as an audience member. Do you exercise frequently? Why or why not? How do your considerations match up with the theories in this chapter?

5. According to the embedded behaviors model, what factors influence how likely people are to change particular behaviors? What behaviors are embedded in your lifestyle? What would it take to change those behaviors?

6. According to the theory of reasoned action, what factors influence people's behavior?

7. What are the stages of change in the transtheoretical model? What can result if campaigners expose community members to messages inconsistent with their stage of change?

8. Have you ever seen a PSA you didn't like? If so, what made it unappealing?

9. Summarize the critical-cultural perspective.

10. What factors influence your own health-related behaviors (e.g., how often you visit a doctor, whether you exercise everyday, eat right, and so on)? In what ways are these behaviors affected by larger issues such as resources, culture, and social support?

11. What do you think of the idea that health promotion experts, although they mean well, often reinforce a group's marginal status by adopting a paternalistic "This is what you should do" mindset?

12. Have you ever felt misunderstood or belittled by people who were trying to help you? If so, describe the experience.

13. Can you think of behaviors you engage in even though you know they are unhealthy? What are the rewards of these behaviors? What would it take (if anything) to get you to quit? What advice do you have for health campaign designers trying to target this behavior?

14. Does a career in health campaign design appeal to you? What aspects would you most enjoy? Not enjoy?

15. What are the implications of blaming (scapegoating) people for engaging in risky health behaviors?

16. What are some questions to consider when choosing a "voice" and "personality" for your campaign?

17. What factors should you keep in mind when choosing a spokesperson?

18. What is meant by source homophily?

19. Do you look at campaign messages differently depending on who the spokesperson is? Does it matter if the person is similar to you? Why or why not?

20. What does it mean to frame a health message?

21. Think of a health-related behavior (e.g., drinking water, avoiding sweets, getting enough sleep). Brainstorm ways you can frame the behavior in terms of potential losses, gains, and risks. What do you think would be most effective?

22. Have you noticed social norm campaigns similar to RU Sure on your campus? If so, what do you think of them?

23. In your experience, how much alcohol do most college students imbibe? How often? Why? What if you learned that your estimates were inaccurate? Would it influence the way you behave? If people just entering college received the same information, do you think it would influence them? Why or why not?

24. Describe the components of the theory of normative social behavior.

25. In what circumstances are positive affect messages usually effective? Negative affect appeals? Think of as many examples as you can. Which type of appeal do you typically prefer, and why?

26. Explain the extended parallel process model as it relates to negative affect appeals. How might this theory apply to our hypothetical sports recreation campaign?

27. What types of audiences are likely to respond favorably to shocking or intense messages?

28. What are some tips for using affect appeals effectively?

29. What are some questions to consider when piloting campaign materials?

30. What role do gatekeepers play in health promotion efforts?

31. Why is it often difficult to assess accurately the impact of a health campaign?

32. What do you think of the **truth**® campaign? Has it influenced the way you regard the tobacco industry? What is appealing (or unappealing) about the campaign to you?

## ANSWERS TO *CAN YOU GUESS?*

1. Smoking cuts an average of 15 years off a person's life (WHO, 2008a).

2. Tobacco companies spend $36 million a day on advertising—in the United States alone. Their *daily* budget is more than the *annual* budget of the **truth**® campaign, which is the largest antitobacco campaign in history ("New Research," 2008).

3. Only 5% of the world's population is shielded from tobacco advertising ("WHO Wants Total Ban," 2008).

Abbe, M., Sudano, J. J., Jr., Demko, C. A., Victoroff, K. Z., Williams, K., Lalumandier, J. A., & Wotman, S. (2007). Revisiting comfort: Strategies observed in the direct observation study. *General Dentistry, 55*(5), 420–425.

About 11 million children below the age of five die every year. (2002, September 7). *The Economist,* NA.

Abramson, J. S., & Mizrahi, T. (1996). When social workers and physicians collaborate: Positive and negative interdisciplinary experiences. *Social Work, 41,* 270–281.

Accreditation Council to Graduate Medical Education. (2006, April). Introduction to competency-based education. Facilitator's guide. Chicago: Author. Retrieved November 5, 2008, from http://www.acgme.org/outcome/e-learn/21M1_FacManual.pdf

Achterberg, J. (1991). *Woman as healer.* Boston: Shambhala.

Ackerknecht, E. H. (1968). *A short history of medicine.* New York: Ronald Press.

Ackermann, R. T., & Carroll, A. E. (2003). Support for national health insurance among U.S. physicians: A national survey. *Annals of Internal Medicine, 139,* 795–801.

Adams, M. O., & Osho, G. S. (nd). A comprehensive evaluation of mad-cow disease: Evidence from public administration perspective. El Cajon, CA: National Social Science Association. Retrieved August 27, 2008, from http://www.nssa.us/journals/2007-28-2/2007-28-2-01.htm

Adams, N., & Field, L. (2001). Pain management 1: Psychological and social aspects of pain. *British Journal of Nursing, 10*(14), 903–911.

Adams, R. J., & Parrott, R. (1994, February). Pediatric nurses' communication of role expectations to parents of hospitalized children. *Journal of Applied Communication Research, 22,* 36–47.

Adelman, M. B., & Frey, L. R. (1997). *The fragile community: Living together with AIDS.* Mahwah, NJ: Lawrence Erlbaum.

Adelman, S. A. (2008, January 4). Be careful what you promise. *Medical Economics, 85*(1), 14.

Advance data from vital and health statistics. Staffing, capacity, and ambulance diversion in emergency departments: United States, 2003–2004. (2006, September 27). Atlanta: Centers for Disease Control and Prevention. Retrieved October 10, 2008, from http://www.cdc.gov/nchs/data/ad/ad376.pdf

Ahmad, N. N. (2004, April 15). Arab-American culture and health care. Online publication. Retrieved December 19, 2008, from http://www.cwru.edu/med/epidbio/mphp439/Arab-Americans.htm

Ahmed, A. T., Mohammed, S. A., & Williams, D. R. (2007). Racial discrimination & health: Pathways & evidence. *The Indian Journal of Medical Research, 126*(4), 318–327.

Ajzen, I., & Fishbein, M. (1980). *Understanding attitudes and predicting behavior.* Englewood Cliffs, NJ: Prentice Hall.

Albrecht, T. L. (1982). Coping with occupational stress: Relational and individual strategies of nurses in acute health care settings. In M. Burgoon (Ed.), *Communication yearbook 6* (pp. 832–849). Beverly Hills, CA: Sage.

Albrecht, T. L., & Adelman, M. B. (1987). Communicating social support: A theoretical perspective. In T. L. Albrecht & M. B. Adelman (Eds.), *Communicating social support* (pp. 18–39). Newbury Park, CA: Sage.

Alcalay, R., & Bell, R. A. (1996). Ethnicity and health knowledge gaps: Impact of the California

*Wellness Guide* on poor African American, Hispanic, and non-Hispanic white women. *Health Communication, 8,* 303–330.

Alcohol Concern. (2007, July). *Not in front of the children—child protection and advertising.* London: Author. Retrieved October 6, 2008, from http://www.alcoholpolicy.net/files/Not_in_front_of_the_children.pdf

Al-Janabi, H., Coast, J., & Flynn, T. N. (2008). What do people value when they provide unpaid care for an older person? A meta-ethnography with interview follow-up. *Social Science & Medicine, 67,* 111–121.

Allen, J. D., Kennedy, M., Wilson-Glover, A, & Gilligan, T. D. (2007, June). African-American men's perceptions about prostate cancer: Implications for designing educational interventions. *Social Science & Medicine, 64*(11), 2189–2200.

Allman, J. (1998). Bearing the burden of baring the soul: Physician self-disclosures and boundary management regarding medical mistakes. *Health Communication, 10,* 175–197.

Alston, S. (2007). Nothing to laugh at: Humour as a means of coping with pain and stress. *Australian Journal of Communication, 34*(1), 77–89.

American Association of Colleges of Nursing. (2008, September). Nursing shortage. Washington, DC: Author. Retrieved October 23, 2008, from http://www.aacn.nche.edu/Media/FactSheets/NursingShortage.htm

American Association of Medical Colleges (AAMC). (2007, October 16). 2007 U.S. medical school entering class is largest ever. Washington, DC: Author. Retrieved October 20, 2008, from http://www.aamc.org/newsroom/pressrel/2007/071016.htm

American College of Healthcare Executives. (2002). A race/ethnic comparison of career attainments in health care management. Retrieved August 12, 2003, from www.ache.org

American College of Physicians. (2008, January). Achieving a high-performance health care system with universal access: What the United Sates can learn from other countries. *Annals of Internal Medicine, 148*(1), 55–75.

American Foundation for Suicide Prevention (AFSA). (2008). Struggling in silence: Physician depression and suicide. Fact sheet. New York: Author. Retrieved November 8, 2008, from http://www.afsp.org/index.cfm?fuseaction=home.viewPage&page_ID=9859BF59-CF1C-2465-128DAE02D3C9B309

American Hospital Association (AHA). (1994). *Hospital closures, 1980 through 1993, a statistical profile.* Chicago: Health Care Information Resources Group.

American Hospital Association (AHA). (2008, March). Hospital facts to know. Washington, DC: Author. Retrieved October 10, 2008, from http://www.aha.org/aha/content/2008/pdf/08-issue-facts-to-know-.pdf

American Medical Association (AMA). (2003). Low literacy has a high impact on patients' ability to follow doctors' orders. American Medical Association. Retrieved July 30, 2003, from www.ama-assn.org/ama/pub/print/article/4197-7395.html

American Medical Association Minority Affairs Consortium. (2008). Board of Trustees report 15, "Diversity in medical education." Chicago: Author. Retrieved October 21, 2008, from http://www.ama-assn.org/ama/pub/category/12938.html

Americans value the health benefits of prescription drugs, but say drug makers put profits first, new survey shows. (2005, February 25). Menlo Park, CA: The Henry J. Kaiser Family Foundation. Retrieved October 2, 2008, from, http://www.kff.org/kaiserpolls/pomr022505nr.cfm

Amundsen, D. W., & Ferngren, G. B. (1983). *The clinical encounter.* Dordrecht: D. Reidel.

An, S. (2007, September). Attitude toward direct-to-consumer advertising and drug inquiry intention: The moderate role of perceived knowledge. *Journal of Human Communication, 12*(6), 567–580.

Anderlink, M. R. (2001). *The ethics of managed care: A pragmatic approach.* Bloomington, IN: Indiana University Press.

Andersen, R. E., Crespo, C. J., Bartlett, S. J., Cheskin, L. J., & Pratt, M. (1998). Relationship of physical activity and television watching with body weight and level of fatness among children. Results from the Third National Health and Nutrition Examination Survey. *Journal of the American Medical Association, 279,* 938–942.

Anderson, J. O., & Geist Martin, P. (2003). Narratives and healing: Exploring one family's stories of cancer survivorship. *Health Communication, 15*(2), 133–143.

Anderson, N. (2008, September 17). Product placement still huge as advertisers fight DVRs. *Ars Technica,* np. Retrieved October 2, 2008, from http://arstechnica.com/news.ars/post/20080917-product-placement-still-huge-as-advertisers-fight-dvrs.html

Añez, L. M., Silva, M. A., Paris, M., Jr., & Bedregal, L. E. (2008). Engaging Latinos through the integration of cultural values and motivational interviewing principles. *Professional Psychology: Research and Practice, 39*(2), 153–159.

Angell, M. (2004, July 15). The truth about drug companies. *The New York Review of Books, 51*(12), np. Retrieved September 30, 2008, from http://www.nybooks.com/articles/17244

Apker, J. (2001). Role development in the managed care era: A case in hospital-based nursing. *Journal of Applied Communication Research, 29*(2), 117–136.

Appenzeller, T. (2005, October). Tracing the next killer flu. *National Geographic, 208*(4), 2–31. Retrieved August 30, 2008, through Academic OneFile via Gale.

Arab American Institute Foundation. (2000). Arab American population highlights. Washington, DC: Author. Retrieved December 20, 2008, from http://aai.3cdn.net/9298c231f3a79e30c6_g7m6bx9hs.pdf

Arab Americans. Famous Arab Americans. (2006, February 18). Washington, DC: Arab American Institute. Retrieved December 19, 2008, from http://www.aaiusa.org/arab-americans/23/famous-arab-americans

Armstrong, K., McMurphy, S., Dean, L. T., Micco, E., Putt, M., Halbert, C. H., Schwartz, J. S., Sankar, P., Pyeritz, R. E., Bernhardt, B., & Shea, J. A. (2008). Differences in the patterns of health care system distrust between blacks and whites. *Journal of General Internal Medicine, 23*(6), 827–833.

Arnold, W. E., & McClure, L. (1989). *Communication training and development.* Prospect Heights, IL: Waveland Press.

Arnst, C. (1998, May 18). Of mice, men, and cancer cures. *Business Week, 3578,* 44.

Arrington, M. I. (2003). "I don't want to be an artificial man": Narrative reconstruction of sexuality among prostate cancer survivors. *Sexuality & Culture, 7*(2), 30–58.

Ashley, B. M., & O'Rourke, K. D. (1997). *Health care ethics: A theological analysis* (4th ed.). Washington, DC: Georgetown University Press.

Ashraf, H. (2000, November). BSE inquiry uncovers "a peculiarly British disaster." *The Lancet, 356,* 1579–1580.

Astin, J. A. (1998). Why patients use alternative medicine: Results of a national study. *Journal of the American Medical Association, 279,* 2548–2553.

Atherly, A., Kane, R. L., & Smith, M. A. (2004). Older adults' satisfaction with integrated capitated health and long-term care. *The Gerontologist, 44*(3), 348–357.

Aulagnier, M., Verger, P., Ravaud, J. F., Souville, M., Lussault, P. Y., Garnier, J. P., & Paraponaris, A. (2005). General practitioners' attitudes towards patients with disabilities: The need for training and support. *Disability and Rehabilitation, 27*(22), 1343–1352.

Austin, E. W. (1993). Exploring the effects of active parental mediation of television content. *Journal of Broadcasting & Electronic Media, 37,* 147–158.

Austin, E. W. (1995). Reaching young audiences: Developmental considerations in designing health messages. In E. Maibach & R. L. Parrott

(Eds.), *Designing health messages* (pp. 114–144). Thousand Oaks, CA: Sage.

Austin, E. W., & Hust, S. J. T. (2005). Targeting adolescents? The content and frequency of alcoholic and nonalcoholic beverage ads in magazine and video formats November 1999–April 2000. *Journal of Health Communication, 10*(8), 769–785.

Austin, E. W., & Johnson, K. K. (1997). Immediate and delayed effects of media literacy training on third graders' decision making for alcohol. *Health Communication, 9,* 323–350.

Austin, E. W., & Meili, H. K. (1994). Effects of interpretations of televised alcohol portrayals on children's alcohol beliefs. *Journal of Broadcasting & Electronic Media, 38,* 417–435.

Austin, E. W., & Nach-Ferguson, B. (1995). Sources and influences of young school-aged children's general and brand-specific knowledge about alcohol. *Health Communication, 7,* 1–20.

Austin, E. W., Roberts, D. F., & Nass, C. I. (1990). Influences of family communication on children's television-interpretation process. *Communication Research, 17,* 545–564.

AVERT: Averting HIV and AIDS. (2008, July 30). HIV and AIDS in Africa. West Sussex, UK: Author. Retrieved September 1, 2008, from http://www.avert.org/aafrica.htm

Ayres, J., & Hopf, T. (1995). An assessment of the role of communication apprehension in communication with the terminally ill. *Communication Research Reports, 12,* 227–234.

Azevedo, D. (1996). Taking back health care: Doctors must work together. *Medical Economics, 73,* 156–162.

Babin, L. A., & Carder, S. T. (1996, May). Viewers' recognition of brands placed within a film. *International Journal of Advertising, 15,* 140–151.

Babrow, A. S. (1992). Communication and problematic integration: Understanding diverging probability and value, ambiguity, ambivalence, and impossibility. *Communication Theory, 2,* 95–130.

Babrow, A. S. (2001). Uncertainty, value, communication, and problematic integration. *Journal of Communication, 51*(3), 553–573.

Bachenheimer, E. A., & DeKoven, M. (2003). The view from the middle. *Healthcare Executive, 18*(2), 73–74.

Backer, T. E., & Rogers, E. M. (1993). Introduction. In T. E. Backer & E. M. Rogers (Eds.), *Organizational aspects of health communication campaigns: What works?* (pp. 1–9). Newbury Park, CA: Sage.

Bae, H.-S., & Kang, S. (2008). The influence of viewing an entertainment-education program on cornea donation intention: A test of the theory of planned behavior. *Health Communication, 23*(1), 87–95.

Baglia, J. (2005). *The Viagra ad venture.* New York: Peter Lang.

Baldwin, D. M. (2003). Disparities in health and health care: Focusing on efforts to eliminate unequal burdens. *Online Journal of Issues in Nursing, 8*(1), 2.

Balint, J., & Shelton, W. (1996). Regaining the initiative: Forging a new model of the patient–physician relationship. *Journal of the American Medical Association, 275,* 887–892.

Ballantine, J. H., Roberts, K. A., & Ritzer, G. (2008). *Our social world + the McDonaldization of society.* Thousand Oaks, CA: Pine Forge Press.

Baltes, M. M., & Wahl, H.-W. (1996). Patterns of communication in old age: The dependence-support and independence-ignore script. *Health Communication, 8,* 217–231.

Bandura, A. (1986). *Social foundations of thought and action: A social cognitive approach.* Englewood Cliffs, NJ: Prentice Hall.

Bandura, A. (1994). Social cognitive theory of mass communication. In J. Bryant & D. Zillman (Eds.), *Media effects: Advances in theory and research* (pp. 61–90). Hillsdale, NJ: Lawrence Erlbaum.

Banerjee, S. C., & Greene, K. (2006). Analysis versus production: Adolescent cognitive and attitudinal responses to antismoking interventions. *Journal of Communication, 56,* 773–794.

Banja, J. D. (2005). *Medical errors and medical narcissism.* Boston: Jones and Bartlett.

Banja, J. D., & Amori, G. (2005). The empathic disclosure of medical error. In *Medical errors and medical narcissism* (pp. 173–192). Boston: Jones and Bartlett.

Bao, Y., Fox, S. A., & Escarce, J. J. (2007). Socioeconomic and racial/ethnic differences in the discussion of cancer screening: "between-" versus "within-" physician differences. *Health Services Research, 42*(3), 950–970.

Bardbard, L. (1993, November). Cosmetics and reality. *FDA Consumer, 27,* 32–33.

Barkley, T. (2008, March 26). How Social Security, Medicare? *Wall Street Journal,* p. A8

Barnard, A. (2003, January 22). Doctors brace for changes on patient privacy. *Boston Globe,* National/Foreign, p. A1.

Barnes, M. K., & Duck, S. (1994). Everyday communicative contexts for social support. In B. R. Burleson, T. L. Albrecht, & I. G. Sarason (Eds.), *Communication of social support: Messages, interactions, relationships, and community* (pp. 175–194). Thousand Oaks, CA: Sage.

Barrett, B. (2003). Alternative, complementary, and conventional medicine: Is integration upon us? *Journal of Alternative and Complementary Medicine, 9*(3), 417–427.

Basil, M. D. (1997). The danger of cigarette "special placements" in film and television. *Health Communication, 9,* 191–198.

Bass, A. (1990, November 25). Health care marketing seeks gain from pain. *Boston Globe,* National/Foreign section, p. 1.

Basu, A., & Dutta, M. J. (2007). Centralizing context and culture in the co-construction of health: Localizing and vocalizing health meanings in rural India. *Health Communication, 21*(2), 187–196.

Basu, A., & Dutta, M. J. (2008). The relationship between health information seeking and community participation: The roles of health information orientation and efficacy. *Health Communication, 23*(1), 70–79.

Bates, D. W., & Komaroff, A. L. (1996). A cyberday in the life. *Journal of the American Medical Association, 275,* 753–755.

Baur, C. (2000). Limiting factors on the transformative powers of e-mail in patient–physician relationships: A critical analysis. *Health Communication 12*(3), 239–259.

Beach, W. A. (2002). Between dad and son: Initiating, delivering, and assimilating bad cancer news. *Health Communication, 14*(3), 271–298.

Beach, W. A., & Japp, P. (1983). Storyifying as time-traveling: The knowledgeable use of temporarily structured discourse. In R. N. Bostrom (Ed.), *Communication yearbook 7* (pp. 867–889). New Brunswick, NJ: Transaction Book.

Bean-Mayberry, B. A., Chang, C. C., McNeil, M. A., Whittle, J., Hayes, P. M., & Scholle, S. H. (2003). Patient satisfaction in women's clinic versus traditional primary care cares in the Veterans Administration. *Journal of General Internal Medicine, 18*(3), 175–181.

Beaudoin, C. E., & Thorson, E. (2006). The social capital of Blacks and Whites: Differing effects of the mass media in the United States. *Human Communication Research, 32,* 157–177.

Beck, C. S. (2005). Personal stories and public activism: The implications of Michael J. Fox's public health narrative for policy and perspectives. In E. B. Ray (Ed.), *Health communication in practice: A case study approach* (pp. 335–345). Mahwah, NJ: Lawrence Erlbaum.

Beck, C. S., & Ragan, S. L. (1992). Negotiating interpersonal and medical talk: Frame shifts in the gynecologic exam. *Journal of Language and Social Psychology, 11,* 47–61.

Beck, C. S., Ragan, S. L., & du Pré, A. (1997). *Partnership for health: Building relationships between women and health caregivers.* Mahwah, NJ: Lawrence Erlbaum.

Becker, G., & Newsom, E. (2003). Socioeconomic status and dissatisfaction with health care among chronically ill African Americans. *American Journal of Public Health, 93*(5), 742–748.

Beckman, H. B., & Frankel, R. M. (1984). The effect of physician behavior on the collection of data. *Annals of Internal Medicine, 101,* 692–696.

Beebe, S. A. (1995). Nurses' perception of beeper calls: Implications for resident stress and patient care. *Archives of Pediatrics & Adolescent Medicine, 149,* 187–191.

Begany, T. (1995). Do you get the respect you deserve? *RN, 58,* 32–33.

Bell, D. J., Bringman, J., Bush, A., & Phillips, O. P. (2006). Job satisfaction among obstetrician-gynecologists: A comparison between private practice physicians and academic physicians. *American Journal of Obstetrics and Gynecology, 195*(5), 1474–1478.

Benzil, D. L., Abosch, A., Germano, I., Gilmer, H., Maraire, J. N., Muraszko, K., Pannullo, S., Rosseau, G., Schwartz, L., Todor, R., Ullman, J., & Zusman, E. (2008, September). The future of neurosurgery: A white paper on the recruitment and retention of women in neurosurgery. *Journal of Neurosurgery, 109*(3), 378–386.

Berger, P., & Luckmann, T. (1966). *The social construction of reality.* New York: Doubleday.

Bergstrom, M. J., & Holmes, M. E. (2000). Lay theories of successful aging after the death of a spouse: A network text analysis of bereavement advice. *Health Communication, 12*(4), 377–406.

Bergstrom, M. J., & Nussbaum, J. F. (1996). Cohort differences in interpersonal conflict: Implications for the older patient–younger care provider interaction. *Health Communication, 8,* 233–248.

Berko, R. M., Wolvin, A. D., & Curtis, R. (1993). *The business of communicating* (5th ed.). Madison, WI: Brown & Benchmark.

Bernhardt, J. M., & Cameron, K. A. (2003). Accessing, understanding, and applying health communication messages. The challenge of health literacy. In T. L. Thompson, A. M. Dorsey, K. I. Miller, & R. Parrott (Eds.), *Handbook of health communication* (pp. 583–605). Mahwah, NJ: Lawrence Erlbaum.

Bernheim, S. M., Ross, J. S., Krumholz, H. M., & Bradley, E. H. (2008). Influence of patients' socioeconomic status on clinical management decisions: A qualitative study. *Annals of Family Medicine, 6*(1), 53–59.

Bernstam, E. V., Walji, M. F., Sagaram, S., Sagaram, D., Johnson, C. W., & Meric-Bernstam, F. (2008, March). Commonly cited website quality criteria are not effective at identifying inaccurate online information about breast cancer. *Cancer, 112*(6), 1206–1213.

Berry, L. L., & Seltman, K. D. (2008). *Management lessons from Mayo Clinic: Inside one of the world's most admired service organizations.* New York: McGraw-Hill.

Berry, T. R., Wharf-Higgins, J., & Naylor, P. J. (2007). SARS wars: An examination of the quantity and construction of health information in the news media. *Health Communication, 21*(1), 35–44.

Best places to work in Illinois, 2007. A workplace analysis and competition. (2007). *The Business Ledger* (Chicago), p. 1. Retrieved October 20, 2008, from http://www.resourcebrokerage.com/PDFs/BPTW_07.pdf

Bethea, L. S., Travis, S. S., & Pecchioni, L. (2000). Family caregivers' use of humor in conveying information about caring for dependent older adults. *Health Communication, 12*(4), 361–376.

Betts, K. (2002, March 31). The tyranny of skinny, fashion's insider secret. *New York Times,* p. 1, section 9.

Beware of online cancer fraud. (2008, September 18). Washington, DC: U.S. Food and Drug Administration. Retrieved October 6, 2008, from http://www.fda.gov/consumer/updates/cancerfraud061708.html

Bhopal, P. (1998, June 27). Spectre of racism in health and health care: Lessons from history and the United States. *British Medical Journal, 7149,* 1970–1973.

Biagi, S. (1999). *Media/impact: An introduction to mass media.* Belmont, CA: Wadsworth.

Bibace, R., & Walsh, M. E. (1981). Children's conceptualizations of illness. In R. Bibace & M. E. Walsh (Eds.), *Children's conceptualizations of health, illness, and bodily functions* (pp. 31–48). San Francisco: Jossey-Bass.

Bille, D. A. (1981). The approach to health care in three American minorities. In D. A. Bille (Ed.), *Practical approaches to patient teaching* (pp. 85–94). Boston: Little, Brown & Company.

Blanch, D. C., Hall, J. A., Roter, D. L., & Frankel, R. M. (2008, September). Medical student gender and issues of confidence. *Patient Education and Counseling, 72*(3), 374–381.

Blank, R., & Slipp, S. (1998, July). Managers' diversity workbook. *HR Focus, 75,* S7–S8.

Block, S. D. (2001). Psychological considerations, growth, and transcendence at the end of life. *Journal of the American Medical Association, 285*(22), 2898–2905.

Bochner, S. (1983). Doctors, patients and their cultures. In D. Pendleton & J. Hasler (Eds.), *Doctor-patient communication* (pp. 127–138). London: Academic Press.

Bock, B. C., Becker, B. M., Niaura, R. S., Partridge, R., Fava, J. L., & Trask, P. (2008). Smoking cessation among patients in an emergency chest pain observation unit: Outcomes of the Chest Pain Smoking Study (CPSS). *Nicotine & Tobacco Research, 10*(10), 1523–1531.

Boden, W. E., & Diamond, G. A. (2008, May 22). DTCA for PTCA—crossing the line in consumer health education? *The New England Journal of Medicine, 358*(21), 2197.

Boer, H., & Westhoff, Y. (2006, February). The role of positive and negative signaling communication by strong and weak ties in the shaping of safe sex subjective norms of adolescents in South Africa. *Communication Theory, 16*(1), 75–90.

Bohm, D. (1980). *Wholeness and the implicate order.* London: Routledge & Kegan Paul.

Bohm, D. (1996). *On dialogue.* L. Nichol (Ed.). London: Routledge & Kegan Paul.

Bonner, T. N. (1992). *To the ends of the earth. Women's search for education in medicine.* Cambridge, MA: Harvard University Press.

Bonsteel, A. (1997, March–April). Behind the white coat. *The Humanist, 57,* 15–19.

Boodman, S. (1997, February 25). Silent doctors more likely to be sued; malpractice study suggests that physicians' manner affects patients' readiness to go to court. *Washington Post,* p. WH9.

Booth-Butterfield, M. (2003). Embedded health behaviors from adolescence to adulthood: The impact of tobacco. *Health Communication, 15*(2), 171–184.

Booth-Butterfield, M., Anderson, R., & Booth-Butterfield, S. (2000). Adolescents' use of tobacco, health locus of control, and self-monitoring. *Health Communication, 12*(2), 137–148.

Borreani, C., Brunelli, C., Miccinesi, G., Morino, P., Piazza, M., Piva, L., & Tamburini, M. (2008). Eliciting individual preferences about death: Development of the end-of-life preferences interview. *Journal of Pain and Symptom Management, 36(4),* 335–350.

Botta, R. A., & Dumlao, R. (2002). How do conflict and communication patterns between fathers and daughters contribute to or offset eating disorders? *Health Communication, 14*(2), 199–219.

Bottorf, J. L., Gogag, M., & Engelberg-Lotzkar, M. (1995). Comforting exploring the work of cancer nurses. *Journal of Advanced Nursing, 22,* 1077–1084.

Bowen, D. J., Singal, R., Eng, E., Crystal, S., & Burke, W. (2003). Jewish identity and intentions to obtain breast cancer screening. *Cultural Diversity and Ethnic Minority Psychology, 9*(1), 78–87.

Boyd, R. S. (1997, June 21). Medical aids, media reports 'a flood of confusing advice': Marketing hype, thirst for the news among causes of bewilderment. *Houston Chronicle,* p. 7.

Boylstein, C., Rittman, M., & Hinojosa, R. (2007). Metaphor shifts in stroke recovery. *Health Communication, 21*(3), 279–287.

Bradac, J. J. (2001). Theory comparison, uncertainty reduction, problematic integration, uncertainty management, and other curious constructs. *Journal of Communication, 51*(3), 456–476.

Brady, M. J., & Cella, D. F. (1995, May 30). Helping patients live with their cancer. *Patient Care,* pp. 41–49.

Braithwaite, D. O. (1996). "Persons first": Expanding communicative choices by persons with disabilities. In E. B. Ray (Ed.), *Communication and disenfranchisement: Social health issues and implications* (pp. 449–464). Mahwah, NJ: Lawrence Erlbaum.

Braithwaite, D. O., & Harter, L. M. (2000). Communication and the management of dialectic tensions in the personal relationships of people with disabilities. In D. O. Braithwaite & T. L. Thompson (Eds.), *Handbook of communication and people with disabilities: Research and applications* (pp. 17–36). Mahwah, NJ: Lawrence Erlbaum.

Braithwaite, D. O., & Japp, P. (2005). "They make us miserable in the name of helping us": Communication of persons with visible and invisible disabilities. In E. B. Ray (Ed.), *Health communication in practice: A case study approach* (pp. 171–179). Mahwah, NJ: Lawrence Erlbaum.

Braithwaite, D. O., & Thompson, T. L. (Eds.). (2000). *Handbook of communication and people with disabilities: Research and applications.* Mahwah, NJ: Lawrence Erlbaum.

Braithwaite, D. O., Waldron, V. R., & Finn, J. (1999). Communication of social support in computer-mediated groups for people with disabilities. *Health Communication, 11*, 123–151.

Branch, W. T., Jr., Arky, R. A., Woo, B., Stoeckle, J. D., Levy, D. B., & Taylor, W. C. (1991). Teaching medicine as a human experience: A patient–doctor relationship course for faculty and first-year medical students. *Annals of Internal Medicine, 114*, 482–489.

Branch W. T., Jr., Levinson, W., & Platt, F. W. (1996). Diagnostic interviewing: Make the most of your time. *Patient Care, 30*(12), 68–76.

Branch, W. T., Jr., & Malik, T. K. (1993). Using "windows of opportunities" in brief interviews to understand patients' concerns. *Journal of the American Medical Association, 269*, 1667–1668.

Brann, M. (2007). Health care providers' confidentiality practices and perceptions: Expanding a typology of confidentiality breaches in health care communication. *Qualitative Research Reports in Communication, 8*(1), 45–52.

Brann, M., & Mattson, M. (2004). Toward a typology of confidentiality breaches in health care communication: An ethic of care analysis of provider practices and patient perceptions. *Health Communication, 16*(2), 229–251.

Brashers, D. E., & Babrow, A. S. (1996). Theorizing health communication. *Communication Studies, 47*, 237–251.

Brashers, D. E., Haas, S. M., & Neidig, J. L. (1999). The patient self-advocacy scale: Measuring patient involvement in health care decision-making interactions. *Health Communication, 11*(2), 97–121.

Brehm, J. W. (1966). *A theory of psychological reactance.* New York: Academic Press.

Brennan, P. F., & Fink, S. V. (1997). Health promotion, social support, and computer networks. In R. L. Street Jr., W. R. Gold, & T. Manning (Eds.), *Health promotion and interactive technology: Theoretical implications and future directions* (pp. 157–169). Mahwah, NJ: Lawrence Erlbaum.

Bresnahan, M., Lee, S. Y., Smith, S. W., Shearman, S., Nebashi, R., Park, C. Y., & Yoo, J. (2007a). A theory of planned behavior study of college students' intention to register as organ donors in Japan, Korea, and the United States. *Health Communication, 21*(3), 201–211.

Bresnahan, M., Lee, S. Y., Smith, S. W., Shearman, S., & Yoo, J. H. (2007b). Reservations of the spirit: The development of a culturally sensitive spiritual beliefs scale about organ donation. *Health Communication, 21*(1), 45–54.

Breton, A., Miller, C. M., & Fisher, K. (2008). Enhancing the sexual function of women living with chronic pain: A cognitive-behavioural treatment group. *Pain Research & Management: The Journal of the Canadian Pain Society, 13*(3), 219–224.

Brett, R. (2003, February 21). Life's great, say area survivors. *The Plain Dealer*, p. B1.

Brice, J. H., Travers, D., Cowden, C. S., Young, M. D., Sanhueza, A., & Dunston, Y. (2008). Health literacy among Spanish-speaking patients in the emergency department. *Journal of the National Medical Association, 100*(11), 1326–32.

Briñol, P., & Petty, R. E. (2006). Fundamental processes leading to attitude change: Implications for career prevention communications. *Journal of Communication. 56*, S81–S104.

Britton, P. C., Williams, G. C., & Conner, K. R. (2008). *Journal of Clinical Psychology, 64*(1), 52–66.

Brodie, M., Kjellson, N., Hoff, T., & Parker, M. (2008). Perceptions of Latinos, African

Americans, and Whites on media as a health information source. In L. C. Lederman (Ed.), *Beyond these walls: Readings in health communication* (pp. 378–394). New York: Oxford University Press.

Brody, H. (1987). *Stories of sickness.* New Haven, CT: Yale University Press.

Broom, A. (2008). Virtually healthy: The impact of Internet use on disease experience and the doctor–patient relationship. In L. C. Lederman (Ed.), *Beyond these walls: Readings in health communication* (pp. 92–109). New York: Oxford University Press.

Brosius, H., & Weimann, G. (1996). Who sets the agenda? Agenda-setting as a two-step flow. *Communication Research, 23*, 561–580.

Brotman, S., Ryan, B., & Cormier, R. (2003). The health and social service needs of gay and lesbian elders and their families in Canada. *Gerontologist, 43*(2), 192–202.

Brown, H., Cassileth, B. R., Lewis, J. P., & Renner, J. H. (1994). Alternative medicine—or quackery? *Patient Care, 28*, 80–90.

Brown, J., & Addington-Hall, J. (2007). How people with motor neuron disease talk about living with illness: A narrative study. *Journal of Advanced Nursing, 62*(2), 200–208.

Brown, J. B., Weston, W. W., & Stewart, M. (1995). The first component: Exploring both the disease and the illness experience. In M. Stewart, J. B. Brown, W. W. Weston, I. R. McWhinney, C. L. McWilliams, & T. R. Freeman (Eds.), *Patient-centered medicine: Transforming the clinical method* (pp. 31–43). Thousand Oaks, CA: Sage.

Brown, J. D., & Einsiedel, E. R. (1990). Public health campaigns: Mass media strategies. In E. B. Ray & L. Donohew (Eds.), *Communication and health: Systems and applications* (pp. 153–170). Hillsdale, NJ: Lawrence Erlbaum.

Brown, J. D., & Walsh-Childers, K. (1994). Effects of media on personal and public health. In J. Bryant & D. Zillmann (Eds.), *Media effects: Advances on theory and research* (pp. 389–415). Hillsdale, NJ: Lawrence Erlbaum.

Brown, S. J. (1995, May 15). Rethink how medical schools pick "best" students. *American Medical News, 19*, 29.

Brown, T. N., Ueno, K., Smith, C. L., Austin, N. S., & Bickman, L. (2007). Communication patterns in medical encounters for the treatment of child psychosocial problems: Does pediatrician–parent concordance matter? *Health Communication, 21*(3), 247–256.

Brown, W. J., & Basil, M. D. (1995). Media celebrities and public health: Responses to "Magic" Johnson's HIV disclosure and its impact on AIDS risks and high-risk behaviors. *Health Communication, 7*, 345–370.

Brown, W. J., Basil, M. D., & Bocarnea, M. C. (2003). The influence of famous athletes on health beliefs and practices: Mark McGwire, child abuse prevention, and androstenedione. *Journal of Health Communication, 8*(1), 41–57.

Bruck, L. (1996, September). Today's issues in tax exemption. *Nursing Homes, 45*, 43–46.

Buchholz, B. (1992, January–February). Psyching yourself: How to prepare for medical procedures. *Arthritis Today, 6*(1), 20–24.

Buckman, R., Lipkin, M., Jr., Sourkes, B. M., Toole, S. W., & Talarico, L. D. (1997). Strategies and skills for breaking bad news. *Patient Care, 31*, 61–78.

Bucknall, T., & Thomas, S. (1996). Critical care nurse satisfaction with level of involvement in clinical decisions. *Journal of Advanced Nursing, 23*, 571–577.

Buller, D. B., Burgoon, M., Hall, J. R., Levine, N., Taylor, A. M., Beach, B., Buller, M. K., & Melcher, C. (2000). Long-term effects of language intensity in preventive messages on planned family solar protection. *Health Communication, 12*(3), 261–275.

Burda, D. (2008, April 28). The perfection injection; not paying for "never events" is a slippery slope. *Modern Healthcare, 38*(17), 20.

Burdine, J. N., McLeroy, K. B., & Gottlieb, N. H. (1987). Ethical dilemmas in health promotion: An introduction. *Health Education Quarterly, 14*, 7–9.

Burgoon, M. H., & Burgoon, J. K. (1990). Compliance-gaining and health care. In J. P. Dillard

(Ed.), *Seeking compliance: The production of interpersonal influence messages* (pp. 161–188). Scottsdale, AZ: Gorsuch Scarisbrick.

Burleson, B. R. (1990). Comforting as social support: Relational consequences of supportive behaviors. In S. Duck & R. C. Silver (Eds.), *Personal relationships and social support* (pp. 66–82). London: Sage.

Burleson, B. R. (1994). Comforting messages: Significance, approaches, and effects. In B. R. Burleson, T. L. Albrecht, & I. G. Sarason (Eds.), *Communication of social support: Messages, interactions, relationships, and community* (pp. 175–194). Thousand Oaks, CA: Sage.

Bute, J. J., Donovan-Kicken, E., & Martins, N. (2007). Effects of communication-debilitating illnesses and injuries on close relationships: A relational maintenance perspective. *Health communication, 21*(3), 235–246.

By the numbers. (2007, April 20). *WR News, Edition 4, 88*(23), 2.

Byck, R. (1986). *The encyclopedia of psychoactive drugs: Treating mental illness.* New York: Chelsea House.

Bylund, C. L. (2005). Mothers' involvement in decision making during the birthing process: A quantitative analysis of women's online birth stories. *Health Communication, 18*(1), 23–39.

Cactus Marketing Communications. (2007). Redefining empowerment: A case study of effectively marketing to teens without turning them off. Unpublished white paper. Denver: Author.

Cadogan, M. P., Franzi, C., Osterweil, D., & Hill, T. (1999). Barriers to effective communication in skilled nursing facilities: Differences in perception between nurses and physicians. *Journal of the American Geriatrics Society, 47,* 71–75.

Caldroney, R. D. (2008, March 21). Why we've never been sued: This doctor and his partners have stayed out of the courtroom for nearly 30 years. Learn how to follow their lead. *Medical Economics, 85*(6), 30–32.

Calfee, J. E. (2002, Fall). Direct-to-consumer advertising of prescription drugs: Evaluating regulatory policy in the United States and New Zealand. *Journal of Public Policy & Marketing, 21*(2), 174.

Cameron, K. A., & Campo, S. (2006). Stepping back from social norms campaigns: Comparing normative influences to other predictors of health behaviors. *Health Communication, 20*(3), 277–288.

Campbell, R. G., & Babrow, A. S. (2004). The role of empathy in responses to persuasive risk communication: Overcoming resistance to HIV prevention messages. *Health Communication, 16*(2), 159–182.

Campbell-Heider, N., & Hart, C. A. (1993). Updating the nurse's bedside manner. *Image: Journal of Nursing Scholarship, 25,* 133–139.

Campo, S., & Cameron, K. A. (2006). Differential effects of exposure to social norm campaigns: A cause for concern. *Health Communication, 19*(3), 209–219.

Campo, S., & Mastin, T. (2007). Placing the burden on the individual: Overweight and obesity in African American and mainstream women's magazines. *Health Communication, 22*(3), 229–240.

Candib, L. M. (1994). Reconsidering power in the clinical relationship. In E. S. More & M. A. Milligan (Eds.), *The empathic practitioner: Empathy, gender, and medicine* (pp. 135–155). New Brunswick, NJ: Rutgers University Press.

Cantor, J. C., Schoen, C., Belloff, D., How, S. K. H., & McCarthy, D. (2007, June). Aiming higher: Results from a State Scorecard on Health System Performance. New York: The Commonwealth Fund Commission on a High Performance Health System. Retrieved August 12, 2008, from www.commonwealthfund.org/publications/publications_show.htm?doc_id=494551

Caplan, S. E., Haslett, B. J., & Burleson, B. R. (2005). Telling it like it is: The adaptive function of narratives in coping with loss in later life. *Health Communication, 17*(3), 233–251.

Capossela, C., Warnock, S., & Miller, S. (1995). *Share the care: How to organize a group to care for someone who is seriously ill.* New York: Fireside.

Capriotti, T. (1999, February 1). Exploring the "herbal jungle." *MedSurg Nursing, 8,* 53.

Carlzon, J. (1987). *Moments of truth: New strategies for today's customer-driven economy*. New York: Harper & Row.

Carpiac-Claver, M. L., & Levy-Storms, L. (2007). In a manner of speaking: Communication between nurse aides and older adults in long-term care settings. *Health Communication*, 22(1), 59–67.

Carroll, A. E., & Ackerman, R. T. (2008). Support for national health insurance among U.S. physicians: 5 years later. *Annals of Internal Medicine*, 148, 566–567.

Cartner-Morley, J. (2007, September 15). Catwalk inquiry wants medicals for models: Investigation paints disturbing picture: Passport checks reinforce London ban on under-16s. *The Guardian* (London), Final Edition, p. 7.

Casey, M. K., Allen, M., Emmers-Sommer, T., Sahlstein, E., Degooyer, D., Winters, A. M., Wagner, A. E., & Dun, T. (2003). When a celebrity contracts a disease: The example of Earvin "Magic" Johnson's announcement that he was HIV positive. *Journal of Health Communication*, 8(1), 249–256.

Casper, M. F., Child, J. T., Gilmour, D., McIntyre, K. A., & Pearson, J. C. (2006). Healthy research perspectives: Incorporating college student experiences with alcohol. *Health Communication*, 20(3), 289–298.

Cassedy, J. H. (1991). *Medicine in America: A Short history*. Baltimore: Johns Hopkins University Press.

Cassell, E. J. (1991). *The nature of suffering*. New York: Oxford University Press.

Catlin, A., Armigo, C., Volat, D., Vale, E., Hadley, M. A., Gong, W., Bassir, R., & Anderson, K. (2008). Conscientious objection: A potential neonatal nursing response to care orders that cause suffering at the end of life? Study of a concept. *Neonatal Network*, 27(2), 101–8.

Cawyer, C. S., & Smith-du Pré, A. (1995). Communicating social support: Identifying supportive episodes in an HIV/AIDS support group. *Communication Quarterly*, 43, 243–258.

Cegala, D. J. (2006). Emerging trends and future directions in patient communication skills training. *Health Communication*, 20(2), 123–129.

Cegala, D. J., & Broz, S. L. (2003). Provider and patient communication skills training. In T. L. Thompson, A. M. Dorsey, K. I. Miller, & R. Parrot (Eds.), *Handbook of health communication* (pp. 95–119). Mahwah, NJ: Lawrence Erlbaum.

Cegala, D. J., Post, D. M., & McClure, L. (2001). The effects of patient communication skills training on the discourse of older patients during a primary care interview. *Journal of the American Geriatrics Society*, 49(11), 1505–1511.

Cegala, D. J., Street, R. L., Jr., & Clinch, C. R. (2007). The impact of patient participation on physicians' information provision during a primary care medical interview. *Health Communication*, 21(2), 177–185.

Centers for Disease Control and Prevention (CDC). (2005, May 3). Frequently asked questions about SARS. Atlanta: Author. Retrieved September 1, 2008, from http://www.cdc.gov/ncidod/sars/faq.htm

Centers for Disease Control and Prevention (CDC). (2007a, February 12). What is bioterrorism? Atlanta: Author. Retrieved September 1, 2008, from http://emergency.cdc.gov/bioterrorism/overview.asp

Centers for Disease Control and Prevention (CDC). (2007b, July). Economic facts about U.S. tobacco use and tobacco production. Atlanta: author. Retrieved September 12, 2008, from http://www.cdc.gov/tobacco/data_statistics/fact_sheets/economics/economic_facts.htm

Centers for Disease Control and Prevention (CDC). (2008, July 1). Overview of crisis & emergency risk communication. Atlanta: Author. Retrieved September 1, 2008, from http://emergency.cdc.gov/cerc

Chamberlain, M. A. (1994). New technologies in health communication: Progress or panacea? *American Behavioral Scientist*, 38, 271–285.

Chapman, S., & Leask, J. A. (2001, December). Paid celebrity endorsement in health promotion: A case study from Australia. *Health Promotion International, 16*(4), 333–338.

Charchuk, M., & Simpson, C. (2005). Hope, disclosure, and control in the neonatal intensive care unit. *Health Communication, 17*(2), 191–203.

Charlton, C. R., Dearing, K. S., Berry, J. A., & Johnson, M. J. (2008). Nurse practitioners' communication styles and their impact on patient outcomes: An integrated literature review. *Journal of the American Academy of Nurse Practitioners. 20*(7), 382–388.

Charmaz, K. (1987). Struggling for a self: Identity levels of the chronically ill. In J. Roth & P. Conrad (Eds.), *Research in the sociology of health care* (pp. 283–321). Greenwich, CT: JAI Press.

Charski, M. (1998, June 29). Now on the Net: Live birth. Next: The operating room. *U. S. News & World Report, 124,* 36.

Chatterjee, P. (2003). Spreading the word about HIV/AIDS in India. *The Lancet, 361*(9368), 1526–1527.

Chen, M.-J., Grube, J. W., Bersamin, M., Waiters, E., & Keefe, D. B. (2005). Alcohol advertising: What makes it attractive to youth? *Journal of Health Communication, 10*(6), 553–565.

Cheong, P. H. (2007). Health communication resources for uninsured and insured Hispanics. *Health Communication, 21*(2), 153–163.

Chesler, M. A., & Barbarin, O. A. (1984). Difficulties of providing help in a crisis: Relationships between parents of children with cancer and their friends. *Journal of Social Issues, 40,* 113–134.

Chew, F., Palmer, S., & Kim, S. (1998). Testing the influence of the health belief model and a television program on nutritional behavior. *Health Communication, 8,* 227–246.

Chieh, L. H., & Tan, J. (2007, August 24). Medical schools see an influx of women; more women are studying medicine here since the quota was lifted in 2002. *Straits Times* (Singapore), np.

Childhood obesity. (2008, August 20). Atlanta: Centers for Disease Control and Prevention. Retrieved October 3, 2008, from http://www.cdc.gov/HealthyYouth/obesity/

Children in developing world bear the burden of cancer. (2003, March 18). *Cancer Weekly, 125.*

Cho, H., & Salmon, C. T. (2006). Fear appeals for individuals in different stages of change: Intended and unintended effects and implications on public health campaigns. *Health Communication, 20*(1), 91–99.

Cho, H., & Salmon, C. T. (2007). Unintended effects of health communication campaigns. *Journal of Communication, 57,* 293–317.

Cho, S. (2006). Network news coverage of breast cancer. *Journalism and Mass Communication, 83*(1), 116–130.

Christakis, N. A., & Fowler, J. H. (2008, May 22). The collective dynamics of smoking in a large social network. *New England Journal of Medicine, 358*(21), 2249.

Christen, R. N., Alder, J., & Bitzer, J. (2008). Gender differences in physicians' communicative skills and their influence on patient satisfaction in gynecological outpatient consultations. *Social Science & Medicine, 66*(7), 1464–1483.

Christmas, C., Park, E., Schmaltz, H., Gozu, A., & Durso, S. C. (2008). A model intensive course in geriatric teaching for non-geriatric educators. *Journal of General Internal Medicine, 23*(7), 1048–1052.

Chung, S. (2008, April 18). When a balance makes patients avoid you. Letter to the editor. *Medical Economics, 85*(8), 17.

Churchill, L. R. (1994). *Self-interest and universal health care: Why well-insured Americans should support coverage for everyone.* Cambridge, MA: Harvard University Press.

Ciechanowski, P., & Katon, W. J. (2006). The interpersonal experience of health care through the eyes of patients with diabetes. *Social Science & Medicine, 63,* 3067–3079.

Cipher, D. J., Hooker, R. S., & Sekscenski, E. (2006). Are older patients satisfied with physician assistants and nurse practitioners? *Official Journal of the American Academy of Physician Assistants, 19*(1), 39–40, 42–44.

Clarke, J. N. (1999). Prostate cancer's hegemonic masculinity in select print mass media depictions

(1974–1995). *Health Communication*, *11*(1), 59–74.

Clarke, J. N., & Binns, J. (2006). The portrayal of heart disease in mass print magazines, 1991–2001. *Health Communication*, *19*(1), 39–48.

Clarke, L. (2002, Fall). Panic: Myth or reality? *Contexts*, *1*(3), 21–26.

Clarke, L. Chess, C., Holmes, R., & O'Neill, K. M. (2006, September). Speaking with one voice: Risk communication lessons from the U.S. anthrax attacks. *Journal of Contingencies and Crisis Management*, *14*(3), 160–169.

Clarke, L. H., & Griffin, M. (2008). Visible and invisible ageing: Beauty work as a response to ageism. *Aging & Society*, *28*(5), 653–674.

Clements, B. (1996). Talk is cheaper than three extra office visits. *American Medical News*, *39*, 17–20.

Cline, R. J. W., & Boyd, M. F. (1993). Communication as threat and therapy: Stigma, social support, and coping with HIV infection. In E. B. Ray (Ed.), *Case studies in health communication* (pp. 131–148). Hillsdale, NJ: Lawrence Erlbaum.

Cline, R. J. W., & Young, H. N. (2004). Marketing drugs, marketing health care relationships: A content analysis of visual cues in direct-to-consumer prescription drug advertising. *Health Communication*, *16*(2), 131–157.

Cohen, J. (1997). The media's love affair with AIDS research: Hope vs. hype. *Science*, *275*, 289–299.

Cohen, J., Collins, R., Darkes, J., & Gwartney, D. (2007). A league of their own: Demographics, motivations and patterns of use of 1,955 male adult non-medical anabolic steroid users in the United States. *Journal of the International Society of Sports Nutrition*, *4*(12), 1–14.

Cohen, S., & Wills, T. A. (1985). Stress, social support, and buffering hypothesis. *Psychological Bulletin*, *98*, 310–357.

Cohn, F., Harrold, J., & Lynn, J. (1997). Medical education must deal with end-of-life care. *Chronicle of Higher Education*, *43*, A56.

Colby, M. A. (1997). *Negotiating the gray maze: The business of medicine in Japan*. Warren, CT: Floating World Editions.

Collins, J. (2001). *Good to great: Why some companies make the leap ... and others don't*. New York: HarperCollins.

Collins, R. L., Elliott, M. N., Berry, S. H., Kamouse, D. E., Kunkel, D., Hunter, S. B., & Miu, A. (2004). Watching sex on television predicts adolescent initiation of sexual behavior. *Pediatrics*, *114*, e280–e289.

The Commonwealth Fund. (2007). International health policy survey in seven countries. New York: Author. Retrieved August 19, 2008, from www.commonwealthfund.org/surveys/surveys_show.htm?doc_id=568326

The Commonwealth Fund. (2008a). Cost-related access problems, by race/ethnicity, income, and insurance status, 2007. New York: Author. Retrieved September 23, 2008, from http://www.commonwealthfund.org/chartcartcharts/chart-cartcharts_show.htm?doc_id=694054www.commonwealthfund.org/surveys/surveys_show.htm?doc_id=568326

The Commonwealth Fund. (2008b, January 15). National survey on public's health care reform views: Americans favor keeping employer role in paying for health insurance; believe covering all should be shared responsibility of employers, individuals, and government. New York: Author. Retrieved August 21, 2008, from http://www.commonwealthfund.org/newsroom/newsroom_show.htm?doc_id=646974

The Commonwealth Fund. (2008c, July). Why not the best? Results from the National Scorecard on U.S. Health System Performance, 2008. New York: Author. Retrieved August 12, 2008 at www.commonwealthfund.org/publications/publications_show.htm?doc_id=69268

Conan, N. (2002, April 12). Medical privacy. National Public Radio's *Talk of the Nation*. Retrieved August 31, 2003, from LexisNexis.

Conlee, C. J., Amabisca, W., & Vagim, N. N. (1995). *Gender differences for patient satisfaction: The clash between medical socialization and patient expectations*. Paper presented at the annual meeting of the Speech Communication Association, San Antonio.

Conrad, C. (1994). *Strategic organizational communication: Toward the twenty-first century.* New York: Holt, Rinehart & Winston.

Conrad, P. (1988). Learning to doctor: Reflections on recent accounts of the medical school years. *Journal of Health and Social Behavior, 29,* 323–332.

Controversy heats up over subway's safer sex ads. (1994, February 7). *AIDS Weekly, 9,* 9–10.

Cooper, R. A., & Stoflet, S. J. (1996). Trends in the education and practice of alternative medicine clinicians. *Health Affairs, 15,* 226–237.

Corbin, J., & Strauss, A. L. (1988). Experiencing body failure and a disrupted self image. In J. Corbin & A. L. Strauss (Eds.), *Unending work and care: Managing chronic illness at home* (pp. 49–67). San Francisco: Jossey-Bass.

Costello, D. (2008, May 17). Billing issue has patients feeling ill: Policyholders are being pressured by hospitals and doctors when insurers don't full pay for services. *Los Angeles Times,* Business Desk, Part C, p. 1.

Cottingham, H. (1992). Cartesian dualism: Theology, metaphysics, and science. In J. Cottingham (Ed.), *The Cambridge companion to Descartes* (pp. 236–257). Cambridge, MA: Cambridge University Press.

Council on Foreign Relations. (2005, January 7). Tsunami disaster: Relief effort. New York: Author. Retrieved September 1, 2008, from http://www.cfr.org/publication/7792/tsunami_disaster.html

Council on Physician and Nurse Supply. (2007). Survey: Hospital CEOs see doctor shortage as a serious problem. More than 95% call for more physician and nurse training. Philadelphia: Author. Retrieved October 23, 2008, from http://www.physiciannursesupply.com/Articles/council-survey-2007-release.pdf

Coupland, N., Coupland, J., & Giles, H. (1991). *Language, society & the elderly.* Oxford, UK: Blackwell.

Coupland, N., Coupland, J., Giles, H., & Coupland, D. (2003, March). *Language, society, and the elderly: Discourse, identity, and aging* (Language in Society, No. 18). Malden, MA: Blackwell.

Covello, V. T. (2003). Best practices in public health risk and crisis communication. *Journal of Health Communication, 8,* 5–8.

Cowan, C. A., & Hartman, M. B. (2005, July). Financing health care: Businesses, households, and governments, 1987–2003. *Health Care Financing Review, 1*(2), np. Centers for Medicare & Medicaid Services, Washington, D.C. Retrieved July 23, 2008, from www.cms.hhs.gov/healthcarefinancingreview

Coward, D. D. (Fall 1990). The lived experience of self-transcendence in women with advanced breast cancer. *Nursing Science Quarterly, 3*(3), 162–169.

Cowart, D., & Burt, R. (1998). Confronting death: Who chooses, who controls? *The Hastings Center Report, 28,* 14–24.

Cox, T. H., Jr. (1991). The multicultural organization. *Academy of Management Executive, 5,* 34–47.

Cox, T. H., Jr. (2001). *Creating the multicultural organization: A strategy for capturing the power of diversity.* San Francisco: Jossey-Bass.

Crandall, S. J., Volk, R. J., & Loemker, V. (1993). Medical students' attitudes toward providing care for the underserved: Are we training socially responsible physicians? *Journal of the American Medical Association, 269,* 2519–2523.

Crawford, M. A., Woodby, L. L., Russell, T. V., & Windsor, R. A. (2005). Using formative evaluation to improve a smoking cessation intervention for pregnant women. *Health Communication, 17*(3), 265–281.

Crawford, W. (1997, October). Taxing for health? *Consumers' Research Magazine, 80,* 34.

Creutzfeldt-Jakob Disease (CJD) Statistics. (2008, August 4). National Creutzfeldt-Jakob Disease Surveillance Unit: Edinburgh, Scotland. Retrieved August 26, 2008, from http://www.cjd.ed.ac.uk/figures.htm

Croft, J. B., Giles, W. H., Pollard, R. A., Kennan, N. L., Casper, M. L., & Anda, R. F. (1999). Heart failure survival rate among older adults in the United States. *Archives of Internal Medicine, 159,* 505.

Cross, M. L., Wright, S. W., Wrenn, K. D., Ishihara, K. K., Socha, C. M., & Higgins, J. P. (1996). Interaction between the trauma team and families: Lack of timely communication. *American Journal of Emergency Medicine, 14,* 548–550.

Cullen, L. A., & Barlow, J. H. (2004). A training and support programme for caregivers of children with disabilities: An exploratory study. *Patient Education and Counseling, 55*(2), 203–209.

Curtin, R. B., Walters, B. A., Schatell, D., Pennell, P., Wise, M., & Klicko, K. (2008). Self-efficacy and self-management behaviors in patients with chronic kidney disease. *Advances in Chronic Kidney Disease, 15*(2), 191–205.

Cutrona, C. E., & Suhr, J. A. (1994). Social support communication in the context of marriage: An analysis of couples' supportive interactions. In B. R. Burleson, T. L. Albrecht, & I. G. Sarason (Eds.), *Communication of social support: Messages, interactions, relationships, and community* (pp. 113–135). Thousand Oaks, CA: Sage.

Daly, A., Jennings, J., Beckett, J. O., & Leashore, B. R. (1995). Effective coping strategies of African Americans. *Social Work, 40,* 240–248.

Daniels, D. Y. (1996, October). An open ICU. *RN, 59,* 30–33.

Davenport, T. H., Prusak, L., & Wilson, H. J. (2003). Who's bringing you hot ideas and how are you responding? *Harvard Business Review, 81*(2), 58–64, 124.

Davis, J. (2007). The effect of qualifying language on perceptions of drug appeal, drug experience, and estimates of side-effect incidence in DTC advertising. *Journal of Health Communication, 12*(7), 617–622.

Davis, K. C., Nonnemaker, J. M., & Farrelly, M. C. (2007). Association between national smoking prevention campaigns and perceived smoking prevalence among youth in the United States. *Journal of Adolescent Health, 41,* 430–436.

Davis, K., Schoen, C., Schoenbaum, S. C., Audet, A. J., Doty, M. M., Holmgren, A. L., & Kriss, J. L. (2006, April). Mirror, mirror on the wall: An update on the quality of American health care through the patient's lens. The Commonwealth Fund. Retrieved November 17, 2008, from http://www.commonwealthfund.org/publications/publications_show.htm?doc_id=364436

Davis, R. M. (2008). Achieving racial harmony for the benefit of patients and communities: Contrition, reconciliation, and collaboration. *Journal of the American Medical Association, 3003*(3), 323–325.

Davison, W. P. (1983). The third-person effect in communication. *Public Opinion Quarterly, 47,* 1–13.

Deary, I. J., Whiteman, M. C., & Fowkes, F. G. R. (1998). Medical research and the popular media. *The Lancet, 351,* 1726–1727.

deBusk, C., & Rangle, A., Jr. (nd). Creating a lean Six Sigma hospital discharge process. An iSixSigma case study. iSix Sigma Healthcare. Retrieved October 16, 2008, from http://healthcare.isixsigma.com/library/content/c040915a.asp

Delate, T., Simmons, V., & Motheral, B. (2004). Patterns of use of sildenafil among commercially insured adults in the United States: 1998–2002. *International Journal of Impotence Research, 16*(4), 305–312.

Deloitte Center for Health Solutions. (2008). Embracing disruption: How consumers are transforming the U.S. health care system. Retrieved July 23, 2008, from www.deloitte.com/dtt/article/0,1002,cid=203518,00.html

DeLorne, D. E., Huh, J., & Reid, L. N. (2006). Age differences in how consumers behave following exposure to DTC advertising. *Health Communication, 20*(3), 255–265.

Dennis, B. P., & Small, E. B. (2003). Incorporating cultural diversity in nursing care: An action plan. *Association of Black Nursing Faculty Journal, 14*(1), 17–25.

Dennis, M. R. (2006). Compliance and intimacy: Young adults' attempts to motivate health-promoting behaviors for romantic partners. *Health Communication, 19*(3), 259–267.

Dennison, B. A., Erb, T. A., & Jenkins, P. L. (2002, June). Television viewing and television in bedroom associated with overweight risk among low-income preschool children. *Pediatrics, 109*(6), 1028–1035.

Dens, N., Eagle, L. C., & De Pelsmacker, P. (2008). Attitudes and self-reported behaviors of patients, doctors, and pharmacists in New Zealand and Belgium toward direct-to-consumer advertising of medication. *Health Communication, 23,* 45–61.

de Ridder, D. T. D., Theunissen, N. C. M., & van Dulmen, S. M. (2007). Does training general practitioners to elicit patients' illness representations and action plans influence their communication as a whole? *Patient Education and Counseling, 66*(3), 327–336.

Dervin, B. (1999, May). Sense-making's theory of dialogue: A brief introduction. Paper presented at a nondivisional workshop held at the meeting of the International Communication Association, San Francisco.

Dervin, B., & Frenette, M. (2001). Sense-making methodology: Communicating communicatively with campaign audiences. In R. Rice, & C. Atkin (Eds.), *Public Communication Campaigns* (3rd ed., pp. 69–87). Thousand Oaks, CA: Sage Publications.

DeSantis, A. D. (2002). Smoke screen: An ethnographic study of a cigar shop's collective rationalization. *Health Communication, 14*(2), 167–198.

Desloge, R. (1997, October 20). Optometry school sets sights on elderly vision loss. *St. Louis Business Journal,* online. Retrieved September 3, 2000, from www.amcity.com//stlouis/stories/102097/focus7.html

de Souza, R. (2007). The construction of HIV/AIDS in Indian newspapers: A frame analysis. *Health Communication, 21*(3), 257–266.

Desrochers, D. M., & Holt, D. J. (2007). Children's exposure to television advertising: Implications for childhood obesity. *Journal of Public Policy & Marketing, 26*(2), 182–201.

Diem, S. J., Lantos, J. D., & Tulsky, J. A. (1996). Cardiopulmonary resuscitation on television: Miracles and misinformation. *New England Journal of Medicine, 334,* 1578–1582.

DiFranza, J. R., Richard, J. W., Paulman, P. M., Wolf-Gillespie, N., Fletcher, C., Jaffe, R. D., & Murray, D. (1991). RJR Nabisco's cartoon camel promotes Camel cigarettes to children. *Journal of the American Medical Association, 266,* 3149–3153.

Dignan, M. B., Michielutte, R., Jones-Lighty, D. D., & Bahnson, J. (1994). Factors influencing the return rate in a direct mail campaign to inform university women about prevention of cervical cancer. *Public Health Reports, 109,* 507–511.

Dillard, A. J., McCaul, K. D., Kelso, P. D., & Klein, W. M. P. (2006). Resisting good news: Reactions to breast cancer risk communication. *Health Communication, 19*(2), 115–123.

Dillard, J. P., Carson, C. L., Bernard, C. J., Laxova, A., & Farrell, P. M. (2004). An analysis of communication following newborn screening for cystic fibrosis. *Health Communication, 16*(2), 195–206.

Dillard, J. P., & Nabi, R. L. (2006). The persuasive influence of emotion in cancer prevention and detection messages. *Journal of Communication, 56,* S123–S139.

Dillard, J. P., Shen, L., Laxova, A., & Farrell, P. (2008). Potential threats to the effective communication of genetic risk information: The case of cystic fibrosis. *Health Communication, 23*(3), 234–244.

DiLorenzo, T. J., & Bennett, J. T. (1998, May). The U.S. is becoming a nanny state. *USA Today Magazine, 126,* 12–15.

Do, T.-P., & Giest, P. (2000). Embodiment and disembodiment: Identity transformation and persons with physical disabilities. In D. O. Braithwaite & T. L. Thompson (Eds.), *Handbook of communication and people with disabilities: Research and applications* (pp. 49–65). Mahwah, NJ: Lawrence Erlbaum.

Doctor–patient communication by race/ethnicity, family income, insurance, and residence, 2004. (2008). Results of the National Scorecard on U.S. Health System Performance, 2008. New York: The Commonwealth Fund. Retrieved December 3, 2008, from http://www.commonwealthfund.org/chartcartcharts/chartcartcharts_show.htm?doc_id=694048

Domar, A. D., & Dreher, H. (2000). *Self-nurture: Learning to care for yourself as effectively as you care for everyone else.* New York: Penguin Books.

Donelle, L., & Hoffman-Goetz, L. (2008). An exploratory study of Canadian Aboriginal online health care forums. *Health Communication, 23*(3), 270–281.

Donnelly, J. (2003, January 26). Lives lost; none of them had to die. *Boston Globe,* p. 1.

Donnelly, L. (2008, February 17). Families pay 1,2000 pounds a year to supplement NHS medical care. *Sunday Telegraph* (London), News, p. 6. Retrieved August 20, 2008, through LexisNexis Academic.

Donohew, L. (1990). Public health campaigns: Individual message strategies. In E. B. Ray & L. Donohew (Eds.), *Communication and health: Systems and applications* (pp. 136–170). Hillsdale, NJ: Lawrence Erlbaum.

Donohew, L., Palmgreen, P., & Duncan, J. (1980). An activation model of information exposure. *Communication Monographs, 47,* 295–303.

Donovan, G. (2008, May 19). Well-versed in diversity; adapting a workforce to the melting pot it serves. *Modern Healthcare, 38*(20), 27.

Dorsey, J. L., & Berwick, D. M. (2008, February 27). Dirty words in healthcare. *Boston Globe,* Op-Ed, p. A9.

Douglas, C. (1994). The barber trembles. *British Medical Journal, 68,* 184.

Douglas, J. E. (2008, May). NightHawk Teleradiology Services: A template for pathology? *Bnet,* np. Retrieved November 2, 2008, from http://find-articles.com/p/articles/mi_qa3725/is_200805/ai_n25500303

Douki, S., Zineb, S. B., Nacef, F., & Halbreich, U. (2007). Women's mental health in the Muslim world: Cultural, religious, and social issues. *Journal of Affective Disorders, 102*(1–3), 177–189.

Dowling, C. G. (1997, February). Through the ages, artists and doctors have confronted the mysteries of anatomy. *Life, 20,* 48–56.

Drucker, P. F. (1993). *Post-capitalistic society.* New York: HarperCollins.

Drum, D. (1997, November 17). Product placement matures into placement of nonprofit causes. *Variety, 369,* S27–S28.

D'Silva, M. U., & Palmgreen, P. (2007). Individual differences and context: Mediating recall of anti-drug public service announcements. *Health Communication, 21*(1), 65–71.

Dora, C. (Ed.). (2006). *Health, hazards, and public debate: Lessons for risk communication from the BSE/CJD saga.* Copenhagen: World Health Organization Europe.

Dranove, D. (2008). *Code red: An economist explains how to revive the healthcare system without destroying it.* Princeton: NJ: Princeton University Press.

Dudo, A. D., Dahlstrom, M. F., & Broussard, D. (2007). Reporting a potential pandemic: A risk-related assessment of avian influenza coverage in U.S. newspapers. *Science Communication, 28*(4), 429–454.

Duewald, M. (2003, June 22). Body and image; one size definitely does not fit all. *New York Times,* np. Retrieved October 6, 2008, from http://query.nytimes.com/gst/fullpage.html?sec=health&res=9F0DE7DD1638F931A15755C0A9659C8B63

Duffy, J. (1979). *The healers: A history of American medicine.* Urbana, IL: University of Illinois Press.

Duggan, A. (2006). Understanding interpersonal communication processes across health contexts: Advances in the last decade and challenges for the next decade. *Journal of Health Communication, 11,* 93–108.

Duggleby, W. (2003). Helping Hispanic/Latino home health patients manage their pain. *Home Healthcare Nurse, 21*(3), 174–179.

du Pré, A. (1998). *Humor and the healing arts: Multimethod analysis of humor use in health care.* Mahwah, NJ: Lawrence Erlbaum.

du Pré, A. (2002). Accomplishing the impossible: Talking about body and soul and mind during a medical visit. *Health Communication, 14*(1), 1–22.

du Pré, A. (2005). Making empowerment work: Medical center soars in satisfaction ratings. In E. B. Ray (Ed.), *Health communication in practice: A case study approach* (pp. 311–322). Mahwah, NJ: Lawrence Erlbaum.

du Pré, A., & Beck, C. S. (1997). "How can I put this?" Exaggerated self-disparagement as alignment strategy during problematic disclosures by patients to doctors. *Qualitative Health Research, 7*, 487–503.

du Pré, A., & Ray, E. B. (2008). Comforting episodes: Transcendent experiences of cancer survivors. In L. Sparks, H. D. O'Hair, & G. L. Kreps (Eds.), *Cancer, communication and aging* (pp. 99–114). Cresskill, NJ: Hampton Press.

Dutta, M. J. (2006). Theoretical approaches to entertainment education campaigns: A subaltern critique. *Health Communication, 20*(3), 221–231.

Dutta, M. J. (2007). Health information processing from television: The role of health orientation. *Health Communication, 21*(1), 1–9.

Dutta, M. J. (2008). *Communicating health: A culture-centered approach.* Cambridge, MA: Polity Press.

Dutta, M. J., & Boyd, J. (2007). Turning "smoking man" images around: Portrayals of smoking in men's magazines as a blueprint for smoking cessation campaigns. *Health Communication, 22*(3), 253–263.

Dutta, M. J., & de Souza, R. (2008). The past, present, and future of health development campaigns: Reflexivity and the critical-cultural approach. *Health Communication, 23*(4), 326–339.

Dutta, M. J., & Feng, J. (2007). Health orientation and disease state as predictors of online health support group use. *Health Communication, 22*(2), 181–189.

Dutta-Bergman, M. J. (2005). Theory and practice in health communication campaigns: A critical interrogation. *Health Communication, 18*(2), 103–122.

Dyche, L., & Swiderski, D. (2005). The effect of physician solicitation approaches on ability to identify patient concerns. *Journal of General Internal Medicine, 20*(3), 267–270.

Dyer, J. (1996). *In a tangled wood: An Alzheimer's journey.* Dallas: Southern Methodist University Press.

Dym, H. (2008). Risk management techniques for the general dentist and specialist. *Dental Clinics of North America, 52*(3), 563–77.

Eastin, M. S., & Griffiths, R. P. (2006). Beyond the shooter game: Examining presence and hostile outcomes among male game players. *Communication Research, 33*, 448–466.

Eastman, J. K., Eastman, K. L., & Tolson, M. A. (1997). The ethics of managed care: An initial look at physicians' perspectives. *Marketing Health Services, 17*, 26–40.

Eating disorder statistics: 9 million Americans, hundreds dying each year. (2007). Washington, DC: Eating Disorders Coalition. Retrieved October 6, 2008, from http://www.eatingdisorderscoalition.org/reports/FactSheet9Million.pdf

Eaton, L., & Dyer, O. (2003, March 15). African women at high risk of death in pregnancy. *British Medical Journal, 326*, 567.

Ebrahim, S. H., Anderson, J., Weidle, P., & Purcell, D. W. (2003). Race-related knowledge gap about treatment for HIV/AIDS, United States, 2001. Paper presented at the National HIV Prevention Conference, Atlanta.

Economic Research Initiative on the Uninsured. (2005, December). Rising health care costs frustrate efforts to reduce uninsured rate, No. 10. Retrieved July 18, 2008, from eriu.sph.umich.edu/pdf/highlight-chernew.pdf

Edelstein, L. (1967). *Ancient medicine.* Baltimore: Johns Hopkins University Press.

Edgar, T. (1992). A compliance-based approach to the study of condom use. In T. Edgar, M. A. Fitzpatrick, & V. S. Freimuth (Eds.), *AIDS: A communication perspective* (pp. 47–67). Hillsdale, NJ: Lawrence Erlbaum.

Edgar, T., Freimuth, V., & Hammond, S. L. (2003). Lessons learned from the field on prevention and health campaigns. In T. L. Thompson, A. M. Dorsey, K. I. Miller, & R. Parrott (Eds.), *Handbook of health communication* (pp. 625–636). Mahwah, NJ: Lawrence Erlbaum.

Edgar, T. M., Satterfield, D. W., & Whaley, B. B. (2005). Explanations of illness: A bridge to understanding. In E. B. Ray (Ed.), *Health communication in practice: A case study approach* (pp. 95–109). Mahwah, NJ: Lawrence Erlbaum.

Educational programs in U.S. medical schools, 2001–2002. (2002, September 4). *Journal of the American Medical Association, 288*(9), 1067–1072.

Edwards, H., & Noller, P. (1998). Factors influencing caregiver–care receiver communication and the impact on the well-being of older care receivers. *Health Communication, 10*, 317–342.

Egan, T. (1988, May 1). Rebuffed by Oregon, patients take their life-or-death cases public. *New York Times*, online. Retrieved December 7, 2008, from http://query.nytimes.com/gst/fullpage.html?res=940DE4DC1638F932A35756C0A96E948260&sec=health&spon=&pagewanted=all

Egbert, N., Koch, L., Coeling, H., & Ayers, D. (2006). The role of social support in the family and community integration of right-hemisphere stroke survivors. *Health Communication, 20*(1), 45–55.

Egbert, N., Sparks, L., Kreps, G. L., & du Pré, A. (2008). Finding meaning in the journey: Methods of spiritual coping for aging patients with cancer. In L. Sparks, H. D. O'Hair, & G. L. Kreps (Eds.), *Cancer, communication and aging* (pp. 277–291). Cresskill, NJ: Hampton Press.

Egerton, J. (2007, September 21). 11 ways to keep your patients satisfied: Your front-desk staff can make the patient experience positive or turn them off. Here's how to make sure that all goes well. *Medical Economics, 84*(18), 50–52.

Eggly, S. (2002). Physician–patient co-construction of illness narratives in the medical interview. *Health Communication, 14*(3), 339–360.

Eisenberg, E. M., Baglia, J., & Pynes, J. E. (2006). Transforming emergency medicine through narrative: Qualitative action research at a community hospital. *Health Communication, 19*(3), 197–208.

Eisenberg, E., & Goodall, H., Jr. (2004). *Organizational communication: Balancing creativity and constraint.* New York: Bedford/St. Martin's.

El Nasser, H. (2007, September 27). Fewer seniors live in nursing homes. *USA Today*, online. Retrieved December 14, 2008, from http://www.usatoday.com/news/nation/census/2007-09-27-nursing-homes_N.htm

Ellingson, L. L. (2007). The performance of dialysis care: Routinization and adaptation on the floor. *Health Communication, 22*(2), 103–114.

Elliott, C. (2007). Assessing "fun foods": Nutritional content and analysis of supermarket foods targeted at children. *Obesity Reviews, 9*(4), 368–377.

Elliott, S. (2003, April 4). Changes requested in ads for youth. *New York Times*, p. 5C.

Ellis, B. H., & Miller, K. I. (1993). The role of assertiveness, personal control, and participation in the prediction of nurse burnout. *Journal of Applied Communication, 17*, 327–342.

Ely, J. W., Levinson, W., Elder, N. C., Mainous, A. G., III, & Vinson, D. C. (1995). Perceived causes of family physicians' errors. *Journal of Family Practice, 40*, 337–344.

The e-mail advantage. (2007, September 7). *Medical Economics, 84*(17), 28.

Emanuel, E. J., & Emanuel, L. L. (1995). Four models of the physician–patient relationship. In J. D. Arras & B. Steinbock (Eds.), *Ethical issues in modern medicine* (4th ed., pp. 67–76). Mountain View, CA: Mayfield.

Emanuel, E. J., & Emanuel, L. L. (1998, May 16). The promise of a good death. *The Lancet, 351*, S21–S29.

Eng, T. R., Maxfield, A., Patrick, K., Deering, M. J., Ratzan, S. C., & Gustafson, D. H. (1998). Access to health information and support. *Journal of the American Medical Association, 279*, 1371.

English, J., Wilson, K., & Keller-Olaman, S. (2008). Health, healing and recovery: Therapeutic landscapes and the everyday lives of breast cancer survivors. *Social Science & Medicine, 67*, 68–78.

English, V., Critchley-Romano, G., Sheather, J., & Sommerville, A. (2002). Medicine as entertainment. *Journal of Medical Ethics, 28*(5), 327–328.

Entertainomercials. (1996, November 4). *Forbes, 158*, 322–323.

Erdelyi, M, H., & Zizak, D. M. (2004). Beyond gizmo subliminality. In L. J. Shrum (Ed.), *The psychology of entertainment media: Blurring the lines between entertainment and persuasion* (pp. 13–44). Mahwah, NJ: Lawrence Erlbaum.

Erdman, L. (1993). Laughter therapy for patients with cancer. *Journal of psychosocial oncology, 11*, 55–67.

Erickson, S. (2008, May 16). The day I received my final verdict: A lawsuit left the author with worries about his reputation, until a surprising visit took place. *Medical Economics, 85*(10), 32–33.

Evans, R. L., & Connis, R. T. (1995). Comparison of brief group therapies for depressed cancer patients receiving radiation treatment. *Public Health Reports, 110*, 306–312.

Everett, M. W., & Palmgreen, P. (1995). Influences of sensation seeking, message sensation value, and program context on effectiveness of anticocaine public service announcement. *Health Communication, 7*, 225–248.

Exposure to stress: Occupational hazards in hospitals. (2008, July). Atlanta: Centers for Disease Control and Prevention (CDC). Retrieved November 8, 2008, from http://www.cdc.gov/niosh/docs/2008-136/default.html

Faden, R. R. (1987). Ethical issues in government sponsored public health campaigns. *Health Education Quarterly, 14*, 27–37.

Fagin, L., Carson, J., Lear, J., De Villiers, N., Bartlett, H., O'Malley, P., West, M., Mcelfatrick, S., & Brown, D. (1996). Stress, coping and burnout in mental health nurses: Findings from three research studies. *International Journal of Social Psychiatry, 42*, 102–111.

Fahey, K. F., Rao, S. M., Douglas, M. K., Thomas, M. L., Elliott, J. E., & Miaskowski, C. (2008). Nurse coaching to explore and modify patient attitudinal barriers interfering with effective cancer pain management. *Oncology Nursing Forum, 35*(2), 234–240.

Fanning, M. M. (1997). A circular organization chart promotes a hospital-wide focus on teams. *Hospital & Health Services Administration, 42*, 243–264.

Farber, N. J., Novack, D. H., & O'Brien, M. K. (1997). Love, boundaries, and the patient–physician relationship. *Archives of Internal Medicine, 157*, 229–294.

Farley, M. J., & Stoner, M. H. (1989). The nurse executive and interdisciplinary team building. *Nursing Administration Quarterly, 13*, 24–30.

Farrar, K. M., Krcmar, M., & Nowak, K. L. (2006). Contextual features of violent video games, mental models, and aggression. *Journal of Communication, 56*, 387–405.

Farrelly, M., Healton, C. G., Davis, K. C., Messeri, P., & Haviland, M. L. (2002, June). Getting to the truth: Evaluating national tobacco countermarketing campaigns. *American Journal of Public Health, 92*(6), 901–907.

Fearn-Banks, K. (1996). *Crisis communication: A casebook approach*. Mahwah, NJ: Lawrence Erlbaum.

Feldman, S. (2008). 2007 DrScore.com annual report card on patient satisfaction in the U.S. DrScore.com. Retrieved November 17, 2008, from http://www.drscore.com/press/report/012508.pdf

Ferguson, J. A., Weinberger, M., Westmoreland, G. R., Mamlin, L. A., Segar, D. S., Green, J. Y., Martin, D. K., & Tierney, W. M. (1998). Racial disparity in cardiac decision making: Results from patient focus groups. *Archives of Internal Medicine, 158*, 1450–1453.

Ferguson, T. (1997, November–December). Health care in cyberspace: Patients lead a revolution. *The Futurist, 31*(6), 29–34.

Ferguson, W. J. (2008). Un poquito. *Health Affairs, 27*(6), 1695–1700. Retrieved December 21, 2008, from http://content.healthaffairs.org/cgi/content/full/27/6/1695

Festinger, L. (1957). *A theory of cognitive dissonance*. Stanford, CA: Stanford University Press.

Finally, an antidote to TV drug ads. (2007, November 1). Yonkers, NY: Consumer Reports. Retrieved September 30, 2008, from http://blogs.consumerreports.org/health/2007/11/finally-an-anti.html?resultPageIndex=1&resultIndex=

2&searchTerm=patient%20requests%20for%20 advertised%20drugs

Fischer, P. M., Schwartz, M. P., Richard, J. W., & Goldstein, A. O. (1991). Brand logo recognition by children aged 3 to 6 years: Mickey Mouse and Old Joe the Camel. *Journal of the American Medical Association, 266,* 3154–3158.

Fisher, B. (2008, April 18). Hospitalists: Look a bit deeper. Letter to the editor. *Medical Economics, 85*(8), 17.

Fisher, J. A. (1994). *The plague makers.* New York: Simon & Schuster.

Fisher, J. D., Goff, B. A., Nadler, A., & Chinsky, J. M. (1988). Social psychological influences on help seeking and support from peers. In B. H. Gottlieb (Ed.), *Marshaling social support: Formats, processes, and effects* (pp. 267–304). Newbury Park, CA: Sage.

Fisher, L. B. (2007, March). President Bush's major post-Katrina speeches: Enhancing image repair. Discourse theory applied to the public sector. *Public Relations Review, 33*(1), 40–48.

Fisher, S. (1984). Institutional authority and the structure of discourse. *Discourse Processes, 7,* 201–224.

Fishman, T. (1995). The 90-second intervention: A patient compliance medical technique to improve and control hypertension. *Public Health Reports, 110,* 173–178.

Flay, B. R., & Burton, D. (1990). Effective mass communication strategies for health campaigns. In C. Atkin & L. Wallack (Eds.), *Mass communication and public health* (pp. 129–146). Newbury Park, CA: Sage.

Flores, G., Abreu, M., Olivar, M. A., & Kastner, B. (1998, November). Access barriers to health care for Latino children. *Archives of Pediatric & Adolescent Medicine, 152*(11), 1119–1125.

Florida hospital surgeons mistakenly amputate wrong leg of patient. (1995, March 20). *Jet* online. Retrieved August 22, 2008, from http://findarticles.com/p/articles/mi_m1355/is_n19_v87/ai_16717100

Floyd, K., Hesse, C., & Haynes, M. T. (2007, January). Human affection exchange: SV. Metabolic and cardiovascular correlates of trait expressed affection. *Communication Quarterly, 55*(1), 79–94.

Fonarow, G. C., Abraham, W. T., Albert, N. M., Stough, W. G., Gheorghiade, M., Greenberg, B. H., O'Connor, C. M., Pieper, K., Sun, J. L., Yancy, C. W., & Young, J. B. (2008). Factors identified as precipitating hospital admissions for heart failure and clinical outcomes: Findings from OPTIMIZE-HF. *Archives of Internal Medicine, 168*(8), 847–854.

Ford, L. A., Babrow, A. S., & Stohl, C. (1996). Social support messages and the management of uncertainty in the experience of breast cancer: An application of problematic integration theory. *Communication Monographs, 63,* 189–208.

Ford, L. A., & Christmon, B. C. (2005). "Every cancer is different": Illness narratives and the management of identity in breast cancer. In E. B. Ray (Ed.), *Health communication in practice: A case study approach* (pp. 157–170). Mahwah, NJ: Lawrence Erlbaum.

Ford, L. A., & Yep, G. A. (2003). Working along the margins: Developing community-based strategies for communicating about health with marginalized groups. In T. L. Thompson, A. M. Dorsey, K. I. Miller, & R. Parrott (Eds.), *Handbook of health communication* (pp. 241–261). Mahwah, NJ: Lawrence Erlbaum.

Former UCLA employee indicted for HIPAA violations over celebs. (2008, May 5). *Modern Healthcare, 38*(18), 4.

Forrest, C. B., Shadmi, E., Nutting, P. A., & Starfield, B. (2007). Specialty referral completion among primary care patients: Results from the ASPN referral study. *Annals of Family Medicine, 5*(4), 361–367.

Forte, D. A. (1995). Community-based breast cancer intervention programs for older African American women in beauty salons. *Public Health Reports, 110,* 179–183.

Forte, P. S. (1997, May–June). The high cost of conflict. *Nursing Economics, 15,* 119–123.

Foster, E. (2007). *Communicating at the end of life: Finding magic in the mundane.* Mahwah, NJ: Lawrence Erlbaum.

Foubister, V. (1997). Advisory panel encourages minority doctor involvement. *American Medical News, 40*, 24.

Fowler, B. A. (2006). Claiming health: Mammography screening decision making of African American women. *Oncology Nursing Forum, 33*(5), 969–975.

Fowler, C., & Nussbaum, J. (2008). Communicating with the aging patient. In K. B. Wright & S. D. Moore (Eds.), *Applied health communication* (pp. 159–178). Cresskill, NJ: Hampton Press.

Frampton, S., Gilpin, L., & Charmel, P. (Eds.) (2003). *Putting patients first: Designing and practicing patient-centered care.* San Francisco: Jossey-Bass.

Frank, E., Carrera, J. S., Stratton, T., Bickel, J., & Nora, L. M. (2006). Experiences of belittlement and harassment and their correlates among medical students in the United States: Longitudinal survey. *British Medical Journal, 333*, 682–684.

Frank, E., Modi, S., Elon L., & Coughlin, S. S. (2008). U.S. medical students' attitudes about patients' access to care. *Preventive Medicine, 47*(1), 140–145.

Frankel, R. M., & Beckman, H. B. (1989). Conversation and compliance with treatment recommendations: An application of micro-interactional analysis in medicine. In L. Grossberg, B. J. O'Keefe, & E. Wartella (Eds.), *Rethinking communication: Vol. 2. Paradigm exemplars* (pp. 60–74). Newbury Park, CA: Sage.

Frankl, V. E. (1959). *Man's search for meeting.* Boston: Beacon Press.

Frasier, P. Y., Savard-Fenton, M., & Kotthopp, M. E. (1983). The education of primary care residents in team health care delivery. In T. L. Thompson & R. L. Byyny (Eds.), *Primary and team health care education* (pp. 126–133). New York: Praeger.

Frates, J., Bohrer, G. G., & Thomas, D. (2006). Promoting organ donation to Hispanics: The role of the media and medicine. *Journal of Health Communication, 11*(7), 683–698.

Freeborn, D. K., & Hooker, R. S. (1995) Satisfaction of physician assistants and other nonphysician providers in a managed care setting. *Public Health Reports, 110*, 714–720.

Freimuth, V. S. (2006). Order out of chaos: The self-organization of communication following the anthrax attacks. *Health Communication, 20*(2), 141–148.

Frey, L. R., Botan, C. H., Friedman, P. G., & Kreps, G. (1991). *Investigating communication: An introduction to research methods.* Englewood Cliffs, NJ: Prentice Hall.

Fried, L. P., Francomano, C. A., MacDonald, S. M., Wagener, E. M., Stokes, E. J., Carbone, K. M., Bias, W. B., Newman, M. M., & Stobo, J. D. (1996). Career development for women in academic medicine: Multiple interventions in a department of medicine. *Journal of the American Medical Association, 276*, 898–906.

Friedman, D. M. (2003). *A mind of its own: A cultural history of the penis.* New York: Penguin.

Friedman, H. S., & DiMatteo, M. R. (1979). Health care as an interpersonal process. *Journal of Social Issues, 35*, 1–11.

Friedrich, D. D. (2001). *Successful aging: Integrating contemporary ideas, research findings, and intervention strategies.* Springfield, IL: Charles C Thomas Publisher.

Frith, K., Shaw, P., & Cheng, H. (2005). The construction of beauty: A cross-cultural analysis of women's magazine advertising. *Journal of Communication, 55*(1), 56–70.

Fry, R. B., & Prentice-Dunn, S. (2005). Effects of coping information and value affirmation on responses to a perceived health threat. *Health Communication, 17*(2), 133–147.

Fuchs-Lacelle, S., Hadjistavropoulos, T., & Lix, L. (2008). Pain assessment as intervention: A study of older adults with severe dementia. *Clinical Journal of Pain, 24*(8), 697–707.

Gabbard-Alley, A. S. (1995). Health communication and gender: A review and critique. *Health Communication, 7*, 35–54.

Gabbard-Alley, A. S. (2000). Explaining illness: An examination of message strategies and gender. In B. B. Whaley (Ed.), *Explaining illness* (pp. 147–170). Mahwah, NJ: Lawrence Erlbaum.

Galinsky, M. J., Schopler, J. H., & Abell, M. D. (1997). Connecting group members through telephone and computer groups. *Health and Social Work, 22,* 181–189.

Gallagher, S., Phillips, A. C., Ferraro, A. J., Drayson, M. T., & Carroll, D. (2008). Social communication is positively associated with the immunoglobulin M response to vaccination with pneumococcal polysaccharides. *Biological Psychology, 78*(2), 211–215.

Gallo, L. C., Smith, T. W., & Cox, C. M. (2006). Socioeconomic status, psychosocial processes, and perceived health: An interpersonal perspective. *Annals of Behavioral Medicine, 31*(2), 109–119.

Gamlin, R. (1999). Sexuality: A challenge for nursing practice. *Nursing Times, 95*(7), 48–50.

Gany, F., Kapelusznik, L., Prakash, K., Gonzalez, J., Orta, L. Y., Tseng, C.-H., & Changrani, J. (2007). The impact of medical interpretation method on time and errors. *Journal of Internal Medicine, 22,* Supplement 2, 319–323.

Gany, F., & Ngo-Metzger, Q. (2008, January 17). Language barriers in health care: Special supplement. *Journal of General Internal Medicine,* online. Retrieved December 4, 2008, from http://www.commonwealthfund.org/publications/publications_show.htm?doc_id=649185

Gardenswartz, L., & Rowe, A. (1998, July). Why diversity matters. *HR, 75,* S1–S3.

Garfinkel, H. (1967). *Studies in ethnomethodology.* Cambridge, MA: Polity Press/Basil Blackwell.

Garrison, F. H. (1929). *An introduction to the history of medicine* (4th ed.). Philadelphia: W. B. Saunders.

Gaster, B., Unterborn, J. N., Scott, R. B., & Schneeweiss, R. (2007, October). What should students learn about complementary and alternative medicine? *Journal of the Association of American Medical Colleges, 82*(10), 934–938.

Gearon, C. J. (2002). Planetree (25 years older). *Hospitals & Health Networks, 76*(10), 40–43.

Geist, P., & Dreyer, J. (1993). The demise of dialogue: A critique of medical encounter dialogue. *Western Journal of Communication, 57,* 233–246.

Geist, P., & Gates, L. (1996). The poetics and politics of recovering identities in health communication. *Communication Studies, 47,* 218–228.

Geller, G., Bernhardt, B. A., Carrese, J., Rushton, C. H., & Kolodner, K. (2008). What do clinicians derive from partnering with their patients? Reliable and valid measure of "personal meaning in patient care." *Patient Education and Counseling, 72,* 293–300.

Gelsema, T. I., van der Doef, M., Maes, S., Janssen, M., Akerboom, S., & Verhoeven, C. (2006). A longitudinal study of job stress in the nursing profession: Causes and consequences. *Journal of Nursing Management, 14*(4), 289–299.

Gerbner, G. (1996, Fall). TV violence and what to do about it. *Nieman Reports, 50,* 10–12.

Gerbner, G., Gross, L., Morgan, M., & Signorelli, N. (1994). *Living with television: The dynamics of the cultivation process.* In J. Bryant & D. Zillmann (Eds.), *Perspectives on media effects* (pp. 17–40). Hillsdale, NJ: Lawrence Erlbaum.

Getting doctors out in the neighborhoods. (2002, June 17). Davis, CA: UC (University of California) Newsroom. Retrieved November 4, 2008, from http://www.universityofcalifornia.edu/news/article/4472

Getting old is a pain. (2003, August). *National Geographic* (unnumbered Geographica supplement).

Gibson, T. A. (2007, May). WARNING—the existing media system may be toxic to your health: Health communication and the politics of media reform. *Journal of Applied Communication Research, 35*(2), 125–132.

Gidwani, P. P., Sobol, A., DeJong, W., Perrin, J. M., & Gortmaker, S. L. (2002, September). Television viewing and initiation of smoking among youth. *Pediatrics, 110*(3), 505–508.

Giles, H., Ballard, D., & McCann, R. M. (2002). Perceptions of intergenerational communication across cultures: An Italian case. *Perceptual and Motor Skills, 95,* 583–591.

Giles, L. C., Glonek, G. F., Luszcz, M. A., & Andrews, G. R. (2005, July). Effect of social networks on 10-year survival in very old Australians: The Australian longitudinal study of aging. *Journal* of *Epidemiology & Community Health, 59*(7), 574–579.

Gill, E. A., & Babrow, A. S. (2007). To hope or to know: Coping with uncertainty and ambivalence in women's magazine breast cancer articles. *Journal of Applied Communication Research, 35*(2), 133–155.

Gillespie, S. R. (2001). The politics of breathing: Asthmatic Medicaid patients under managed care. *Journal of Applied Communication Research, 29*(2), 97–116.

Gillisen, A. (2007). Patient's adherence in asthma. *Journal of Physiology and Pharmacology, 58,* Supplement 5, 205–222.

Ginossar, T. (2008). Online participation: A content analysis of differences in utilization of two online cancer communities by men and women, patients and family members. *Health Communication, 23*(1), 1–12.

Gitomer, J. (1998). *Customer satisfaction is worthless: Customer loyalty is priceless.* Austin, TX: Bard Press.

Giuffrida, A., & Torgerson, D. J. (1997). Should we pay the patient? Review of financial incentives to enhance patient compliance. *British Medical Journal, 315,* 703–707.

Glass, R. M. (1996). The patient–physician relationship: JAMA focuses on the center of medicine. *Journal of the American Medical Association, 275,* 147–148.

Glenn, D. R. J., McClure, N., Cosby, L., Path, F. R. C., Stevenson, M., & Lewis, S. E. M. (in press). Sildenafil citrate (Viagra) impairs fertilization and early embryo development in mice. *Fertility and Sterility.*

Glenn, D. R. J., McVicar, C. M., McClure, N., & Lewis, S. E. M. (2007). Sildenafil citrate improves sperm motility but causes a premature acrosome reaction in vitro. *Fertility and Sterility, 87*(5), 1064–1070.

Glik, D. C. (2007, April). Risk communication for public health emergencies. *Annual Review of Public Health, 28,* 33–54.

Global Health Reporting.com. (2008). TB overview. Menlo Park, CA: The Henry J. Kaiser Family Foundation. Retrieved August 27, 2008, from http://www.globalhealthreporting.org/tb.asp?gclid=CO7InYaprpUCFQQiIgod6gf2aw

Global population profile: 2002. (2004). Washington DC: U.S. Census Bureau. Retrieved December 21, 2008, from http://www.census.gov/ipc/www/world.html

Goffman, E. (1963). *Stigma: Notes on the management of spoiled identity.* Englewood Cliffs, NJ: Prentice Hall.

Goffman, E. (1967). *Interaction rituals.* New York: Pantheon Books.

Goffman, E. (1974). *Frame analysis: An essay on the organization of experience.* New York: Harper Colophon.

Goldhaber, G. M. (1993). *Organizational communication* (6th ed.). Dubuque, IA: Wm. C. Brown.

Goldman, L. K., & Glantz, S. A. (1998). Evaluation of antismoking advertising campaigns. *Journal of the American Medical Association, 279,* 772–778.

Goldsmith, D. J. (1994). The role of facework in supportive communication. In B. R. Burleson, T. L. Albrecht, & I. G. Sarason (Eds.), *Communication of social support: Messages, interactions, relationships, and community* (pp. 29–49). Thousand Oaks, CA: Sage.

Goldstein, J. (2008, May 13). Insurers pay caregivers to track patients. *Philadelphia Inquirer,* Health Daily, p. A01.

Goode, E. E. (1993, February 15). The cultures of illness. *U.S. News & World Report, 114,* 74–76.

Gorawara-Bhat, R., Gallagher, T. H., & Levinson, W. (2003). Patient–provider discussions about conflicts of interest in managed care: Physicians' perceptions. *American Journal of Managed Care, 9*(8), 564–571.

Gordon, E. J., Leon, J. B., & Sehgal, A. R. (2003). Why are hemodialysis treatments shortened and skipped? Development of a taxonomy and relationship to patient subgroups. *Nephrology Nursing Journal, 30*(2), 209–217.

Gordon, R. G., Jr. (Ed.), 2005. *Ethnologue: Languages of the world* (15th ed.). Dallas, TX: SIL

International. Retrieved December 21, 2008, from http://www.ethnologue.com

Gorter, R. C., Bleeker, J. C., & Freeman, R. (2006). Dental nurses on perceived gender differences in their dentist's communication and interaction style. *British Dental Journal. 201*(3), 159–164.

Gotcher, J. M. (1995). Well-adjusted and maladjusted cancer patients: An examination of communication variables. *Health Communication, 7*, 21–33.

Gouin, J. P., Hantsoo, L., & Kiecolt-Glaser, J. K. (2008). Immune dysregulation and chronic stress among older adults: A review. *Neuroimmunomodulation, 15*(4–6), 251–259.

Govindarajan, A., & Schull, M. (2003). Effect of socioeconomic status on out-of-hospital transport delays of patients with chest pain. *Annals of Emergency Medicine, 41*(4), 481–490.

Grady, M., & Edgar, T. (2003). Racial disparities in healthcare: Highlights from focus group findings. In. B. D. Smedley, A. Y. Stith, & A. R. Nelson (Eds.), *Unequal treatment: Confronting racial and ethnic disparities in health care* (pp. 392–405). Board on Health Sciences Policy. Institute of Medicine. Retrieved December 3, 2008, from http://books.nap.edu/openbook.php?isbn=030908265X

Grant, C. J., III, Cissna, K. N., & Rosenfeld, L. B. (2000). Patients' perceptions of physicians' communication and outcomes of the accrual to trial process. *Health Communication, 12*(1), 23–39.

Gratzer, D. (2008, April 30). Don't believe the health hype: Enemies of Canadian health reform endlessly fret over the "Americanization" of our medical system. But the facts from south of the border suggest we have nothing to fear. *National Post* (Canada), National Edition, Issues & Ideas, p. A21.

Green, E. C., & Witte, K. (2006). Can fear arousal in public health campaigns contribute to the decline of HIV prevalence? *Journal of Health Communication, 11*(3), 245–259.

Green, F. (2003, June 20). Booze ads target Black teens, report finds. *San-Diego Union-Tribune,* p. C1.

Green, J. (1996, September 15). Flirting with suicide. *New York Times Magazine,* p. 39.

Green, J. O., & Burleson, B. R. (Eds.). (2003). *Handbook of communication and social interaction skills.* Mahwah, NJ: Lawrence Erlbaum.

Green, K. C. (1988, January). Who wants to be a nurse? *American Demographics, 10,* 46–49.

Green R. (1994, Summer). Healthcare public relations shift gears. *Public Relation Quarterly, 39,* 33–36.

Green, R. (1999). *The Nicholas Effect: A boy's gift to the world.* Cambridge, MA: O'Reilly.

Green, R. (2003). A child's legacy of love. The Nicholas Green Foundation. Retrieved December 15, 2008, from http://www.nicholasgreen.org/articles.html

Greenbaum, T. L. (1991, September). Outside moderators maximize focus group results. *Public Relations Journal, 47,* 31–33.

Greenberg, L. (2004, May). Addressing the Accreditation Council for Graduate Medical Education competencies: An opportunity to impact medical education and patient care. *Pediatrics, 113*(5), 1398–1400.

Greene, J. (2008, February 25). Turning the tables: Insurers win low marks in doc-satisfaction survey. *Modern Healthcare, 38*(8), 58.

Greene, K., Rubin, D. L., Hale, J. L., & Walters, L. H. (1996). The utility of understanding adolescent egocentrism in designing health promotion messages. *Health Communication, 8,* 131–152.

Greene, M. C. (2006). Narratives and cancer communication. *Journal of Communication, 56,* S163–S183.

Greene, M. C., Strange, J. J., & Brock, T. C. (Eds.). (2002). *Narrative impact: Social and cognitive foundations.* Mahwah, NJ: Lawrence Erlbaum.

Greene, M. G., Adelman, R. D., & Majerovitz, S. D. (1996). Physician and older patient support in the medical encounter. *Health Communication, 8,* 263–279.

Grensing-Pophal, L. (1997, Spring). Dealing with diversity in the workplace: Learn how to keep differences from being divisive. *Nursing, 27,* 28.

Griffin, R. J., & Dunwoody, S. (2000). The relation of communication to risk judgment and preventive behavior related to lead in tap water. *Health Communication, 12*, 81–107.

Groopman, J. (2007). *How doctors think.* Boston: Houghton Mifflin.

Gross, R., McNeill, R., Davis, P., Lay-Yee, R., Jatrana, S., & Crampton, P. (2008). The association of gender concordance and primary care physicians' perceptions of their patients. *Women & Health, 48*(2), 123–144.

Grube, J. W., & Wallack, L. (1994). Television beer advertising and drinking knowledge, beliefs, and intentions among school children. *American Journal for Public Health, 84*, 254–259.

Guidelines for preventing workplace violence for health care and social service workers. (1997, March–May). *Prairie Rose, 66*, 11a–18a.

Gunther, A. C., Bolt, D., Borzekowski, D. L. G., Liebhart, J. L., & Dillard, J. P. (2006). Presumed influence on peer norms: How mass media indirectly affect adolescent smoking. *Journal of Communication, 56*, 52–68.

Gursky, E., Inglesby, T. V., & O'Toole, T. (2003). Anthrax 2001: Observations on the medical and public health response. *Biosecurity and Bioterrorism, 1*(2), online version, np. Retrieved August 29, 2008, from http://www.upmc-biosecurity.org/website/resources/publications/2003_orig-articles/2003-06-15-anthrax2001observations.html

Guttman, N. (1997). Ethical dilemmas in health campaigns. *Health Communication, 9*, 155–190.

Haas, S. (2002). Social support as relationship maintenance in gay male couples coping with HIV or AIDS. *Journal of Social and Personal Relationships, 18*(1), 87–111.

Haider, M., & Aravindakshan, N. P. (2005). Content analysis of anthrax in the media. In M. Haider (Ed.), *Global public health communication: Challenges, perspectives, and strategies* (pp. 391–406). Boston: Jones and Bartlett.

Haines, M. P., & Spear, S. F. (1996). Changing the perceptions of the norm: A strategy to decrease binge drinking among college students. *Journal of American College Health, 45*, 134–140.

Halbesleben, J. R. (2006). Patient reciprocity and physician burnout: What do patients bring to the patient–physician relationship? *Health Services Management Research, 19*(4), 215–22.

Halbesleben, J. R., & Rathert, C. (2008). Linking physician burnout and patient outcomes: Exploring the dyadic relationship between physicians and patients. *Health Care Management Review, 33*(1), 29–39.

Halkowski, T. (2006). Realizing the illness: Patients' narratives of symptom discovery. In J. Heritage & D. W. Maynard (Eds.), *Communication in medical care: Interactions between primary care physicians and patients* (pp. 86–114). Cambridge: Cambridge University Press.

Hall, Y. (2006, March 7). Coming soon: Your personal DNA map? *National Geographic News*, online. Retrieved December 3, 2008, from http://news.nationalgeographic.com/news/2006/03/0307_060307_dna.html

Hamdan, A. (2007). A case study of a Muslim client: Incorporating religious beliefs and practices. *Multicultural Counseling and Development, 35*, 92–100.

Hamilton, C., & Parker, C. (1997). *Communicating for results: A guide for business & the professions* (5th ed.). Belmont, CA: Wadsworth.

Hammad, A., Kysia, R., Rabah, R., Hassoun, R., & Connelly, M. (1999). Guide to Arab culture: Health care delivery to the Arab American community. Dearborn, MI: Arab Community Center for Economic and Social Services. Retrieved December 19, 2008, from http://www.accesscommunity.org/site/DocServer/health_and_research_cente_21.pdf?docID=381

Hanlon, J. M. (1996, April). Teaching effective communication skills. *Nursing Management, 27*, 48B–50B.

Hardey, M. (2008). E-health: The Internet and the transformation of patients into consumers and producers of health knowledge. In L. C. Lederman (Ed.), *Beyond these walls: Readings in health communication* (pp. 154–164). New York: Oxford University Press.

Harding, J. (1994). The role of organizational ethics committees. *Physician Executive, 20*, 19–24.

Haridakis, P. M. (2006). Men, women, and televised violence: Predicting viewer aggression in male and female television viewers. *Communication Quarterly, 54*(2), 227–255.

Harper, J. (1997, September 15). Information overload may be making some Americans sick. *Insight on the News, 13*, 40–41.

Harres, A. (2008). "But basically you're feeling well, are you?" Tag questions in medical consultations. In L. C. Lederman (Ed.), *Beyond these walls: Readings in health communication* (pp. 49–57). New York: Oxford University Press.

Harrington, N. G., Norling, G. R., Witte, F. M., Taylor, J., & Andrews, J. E. (2007). The effects of communication skills training on pediatricians' and parents' communication during "sick child" visits. *Health Communication, 21*(2), 105–114.

Harris, S. R., & Templeton, E. (2001). Who's listening? Experiences of women with breast cancer in communicating with physicians. *The Breast Journal, 7*(6), 444–449.

Harris, T. M., Parrott, R., & Dorgan, K. A. (2004). Talking about human genetics within religious frameworks. *Health Communication, 16*(1), 105–116.

Harrison, K. (2005). Is "fat free" good for me? A panel study of television viewing and children's nutritional knowledge and reasoning. *Health Communication, 17*(2), 117–132.

Hart, C., & Chesson, R. (1998). Children as consumers. *British Medical Journal, 316*, 1600–1603.

Hart, C. N., Kelleher, K. J., Drotar, D., & Scholle, S. H. (2007). Parent–provider communication and parental satisfaction with care of children with psychosocial problems. *Parent Education and Counseling, 68*, 179–185.

Hart, J. L., & Walker, K. L. (2008). Communicating health beliefs and practices. In K. B. Wright & S. D. Moore (Eds.), *Applied health communication* (pp. 125–142). Cresskill, NJ: Hampton Press.

Hartzband, P., & Groopman, J. (2008). Off the record—avoiding the pitfalls of going electronic. *New England Journal of Medicine, 358*(16), 1656.

Harwood, J., & Sparks, L. (2003). Social identity and health: An intergroup communication approach to cancer. *Health Communication, 15*(2), 145–159.

Haskard, K. B., Williams, S. L., DiMatteo, R., Rosenthal, R., White, M. K., & Goldstein, M. G. (2008). Physician and patient communication training in primary care: Effects on participation and satisfaction. *Health Psychology, 27*(5), 513–522.

Haug, M. R. (1996). The effects of physician/elder patient characteristics on health communication. *Health Communication, 8*, 249–262.

Hawkins, R. P., Pingree, S., Gustafo, D. H., Boberg, E. W., Bricker, E., McTavish, F., Wise, M., & Owens, B. (1997). Aiding those facing health crises: The experience of the CHESS project. In R. L. Street, Jr., W. R. Gold, & T. Manning (Eds.), *Health promotion and technology: Theoretical application and future directions* (pp. 79–102). Mahwah, NJ: Lawrence Erlbaum.

Hawkley, L. C., Masi, C. M., Berry, J. D., & Cacioppo, J. T. (2006). Loneliness is a unique predictor of age-related differences in systolic blood pressure. *Psychology and Aging, 21*(1), 152–164.

Health economics: Soaring healthcare premiums seen as threat to managed care. (2003, July 14). *Health & Medicine Week*, p. 56.

Health literacy overview. (2003). American Medical Association. Retrieved July 30, 2003, from www.ama-assn.org/ama/pub/printcat/8577.html

Health Privacy Project. (2003). Myths and facts about the HIPAA privacy rule. U.S. Department of Health and Human Services. Retrieved online August 31, 2003, from www.healthprivacy.org

Health promotion glossary. (1998). World Health Organization. Retrieved July 30, 2003, from www.who.int/hpr/ncp/support.documents.shtml

Hearing and older people. (1998). National Institute on Aging, online. Retrieved July 10, 1999, from www.aoa.dhhs.gov/aoa/pages/agepages/hearing.html

Heath, C. (2006). Body work: The collaborative production of the clinical object. In J. Heritage & D. W. Maynard (Eds.), *Communication in medical care: Interactions between primary care physicians and patients* (pp. 184–213). Cambridge: Cambridge University Press.

Hegedus, K., Zana, Á., & Szabó, B. (2008). Effect of end-of-life education on medical students' and health care workers' death attitude. *Palliative Medicine, 22,* 264–269.

Heideman, M., & Hawley, S. R. (2007, Summer). Preparedness for allied health professionals: Risk communication training in a rural state. *Journal of Allied Health, 36*(2), 72–76.

Helman, C. G. (1985). Communication in primary care: The role of patient and practitioner explanatory models. *Social Science and Medicine, 20,* 923–931.

Helme, D. W., Donohew, R. L., Baier, M., & Zittleman, L. (2007). A classroom-administered simulation of a television campaign on adolescent smoking: Testing an activation model of information exposure. *Journal of Health Communication, 12,* 399–415.

Henahan, S. (1996). Mad cow disease: The BSE epidemic in Great Britain. An interview with Dr. Frederick A. Murphy. Washington, DC: Access Excellence at the National Health Museum. Retrieved August 26, 2008, from http://www.accessexcellence.org/WN/NM/madcow96.php

Hendrich, A., Chow, M., Skierczynski, B. A., & Lu, Z. (2008). A 36-hospital time and motion study: How do medical-surgical nurses spend their time? *The Permanente Journal, 12*(3), 25–34.

Henriksen, L., & Jackson, C. (1998). Anti-smoking socialization: Relationship to parent and child smoking status. *Health Communication, 10,* 87–102.

Henry J. Kaiser Family Foundation and Health Research and Educational Trust. (2007). Employer health benefits: 2007 summary of findings. Retrieved July 21, 2008, from http://www.kff.org/insurance/7672

Henson, N. (2007). Mosquito-style communication. *Dental Assistant, 76*(3), 32–35.

Heritage, J., & Robinson, J. D. (2006). The structure of patients' presenting concerns: Physicians' opening questions. *Health Communication, 19*(2), 89–102.

Hermansen-Kobulnicky, C. J. (2008). Measurement of self-advocacy in cancer patient and survivors. *Support Care Center, 16,* 613–618.

Herselman, S. (1996). Some problems in health communication in a multicultural clinical setting. A South African experience. *Health Communication, 8,* 153–170.

Hetsroni, A. (2007a). Four decades of violent content on prime-time network programming: A longitudinal meta-analytic review. *Journal of Communication, 57,* 759–784.

Hetsroni, A. (2007b). Three decades of sexual content on prime-time network programming: A longitudinal meta-analytic review. *Journal of Communication, 57,* 318–348.

HHS [Health and Human Services] study finds strong link between patient outcomes and nursing staffing in hospitals. (2001, April 20). Washington, DC: U.S. Department of Health and Human Services. Retrieved September 4, 2003, from newsroom.hrsa.gov

Hillier, D. (2006). *Communicating health risks to the public: A global perspective.* Burlington, VT: Gower.

Himmelstein, D. U., Warren, E., Thorne, D., & Woolhandler, S. (2005, February 2). Market watch: Illness and injury as contributors to bankruptcy. *Health Affairs* Web Exclusive, w5–w73. Retrieved August 20, 2008, from http://content.healthaffairs.org/cgi/reprint/hlthaff.w5.63v1

Hines, S. C. (2001). Coping with uncertainties in advance care planning. *Journal of Communication, 51*(3), 498–513.

Hirschmann, K. (2008). Blood, vomit, and communication: The days and nights of an intern on call. In L. C. Lederman (Ed.), *Beyond these walls: Readings in health communication* (pp. 58–73). New York: Oxford University Press.

History of public health. (2002). *Encyclopedia of public health*. Farmington Hills, MI: Gale Cengage. Retrieved August 26, 2008, from http://www.enotes.com/public-health-encyclopedia/history-public-health

Ho, D. (2002, January 18). Eli Lilly settles charges of violating the privacy of Prozac patients. Associated Press, Business News. Retrieved August 31, 2003, from LexisNexis.

Ho, E. Y. (2006). Behold the power of *Qi*: The importance of *Qi* in the discourse of acupuncture. *Research on Language and Social Interaction, 39*(4), 411–440.

Ho, E. Y., & Bylund, C. L. (2008). Models of health and models of interaction in the practitioner–client relationship in acupuncture. *Health Communication, 23*, 506–515.

Hodgman, A. (1998, May 25). Burb's eye-view. *Brandweek, 39*, 38.

Hoffman-Goetz, L., Gerlach, K. K., Marino, C., & Mills, S. L. (1997). Cancer coverage and tobacco advertising in African-Americans' popular magazines. *Journal of Community Health, 22*, 261–270.

Holland, J. C., & Zittoun, R. (1990). Psychosocial issues in oncology: A historical perspective. In J. C. Holland & R. Zittoun (Eds.), *Psychosocial aspects of oncology* (pp. 1–10). New York: Springer-Verlag.

Holmes, O. W. (1891). *Medical essays: 1842–1882*. Boston: Houghton Mifflin.

Holt, C. L., Lee, C., & Wright, K. (2008). A spiritually based approach to breast cancer awareness: Cognitive response analysis of communication effectiveness. *Health Communication, 23*, 13–22.

Holtgrave, D. R., Tinsley, B. J., & Kay, L. S. (1995). Encouraging risk reduction: A decision-making approach to message design. In E. Maibach & R. L. Parrott (Eds.), *Designing health messages: Approaches from communication theory and public health practice* (pp. 24–40). Thousands Oaks, CA: Sage.

Hopkins, H. (2007, May 18). Analysis: Older people fastest growing online segment in the UK. *Digital Media Wire*, online. Retrieved December 7, 2008, from http://www.dmwmedia.com/news/2007/05/18/analysis-older-people-fastest-growing-online-segment-in-the-uk

Hornik, R. C. (Ed.). (2002). *Public health communication: Evidence for behavior change*. Mahwah, NJ: Lawrence Erlbaum.

Horowitz, L. I., Kosiborod, M., Zhenqui, L., & Krumholz, H. M. (2007). Changes in outcomes for internal medicine inpatients after work-hour regulations. *Internal Medicine, 147*(2), 97–104.

Hsiao, A.-F., Ryan, G. W., Hays, R. D., Coulter, I. D., Andersen, R. M., & Wenger, N. S. (2006). Variations in provider conceptions of integrative medicine. *Social Science & Medicine, 62*, 2973–2987.

Hsieh, E. (2006). Understanding medical interpreters: Reconceptualizing bilingual health communication. *Health Communication, 20*(2), 177–186.

Hubbell, A. P. (2006). Mexican American women in a rural area and barriers to their ability to enact protective behaviors against breast cancer. *Health Communication, 20*(1), 35–44.

Hudson, K. L., Holohan, M. K., & Collins, F. S. (2008). Keeping pace with the times—the Genetic Information Nondiscrimination Act of 2008. *New England Journal of Medicine, 358*(25), 2661–2663.

Huesmann, L. R., Moise-Titus, J., Podolski, C., & Eron, L. D. (2003). Longitudinal relations between children's exposure to TV violence and their aggressive and violent behavior in young adulthood: 1977–1992. *Developmental Psychology, 39*(2), 201–221.

Hufford, D. J. (1997). Gender, culture and experience: A painful case. *Southern Folklore, 54*, 114–123.

Huhmann, B. A., & Brotherton, T. P. (1997, Summer). A content analysis of guilt appeals in popular magazine advertisements. *Journal of Advertising, 26*, 35–45.

Hullett, C. R. (2006). Using functional theory to promote HIV testing: The impact of value-expressive messages, uncertainty, and fear. *Health Communication, 20*(1), 57–67.

Hullett, C. R., McMillan, J. J., & Rogan, R. G. (2000). Caregivers' predispositions and perceived organizational expectations for provision of social support to nursing home residents. *Health Communication, 12*(3), 277–299.

Human genome project information. (2008). Website sponsored by the U.S. Department of Energy Office of Science, Office of Biological and Environmental Research, & Human Genome Program. Retrieved December 4, 2008, from http://www.ornl.gov/sci/techresources/Human_Genome/home.shtml

Hummert, M. L., & Nussbaum, J. F. (Eds.), (2001). *Aging, communication, and health.* Mahwah, NJ: Lawrence Erlbaum.

Hummert, M. L., & Shaner, J. L. (1994). Patronizing speech to the elderly as a function of stereotyping. *Communication Studies, 45,* 145–158.

Hust, S. J. T., Brown, J. D., & L'Engle, K. L. (2008). Boys will be boys and girls better be prepared: An analysis of the rare sexual health messages in young adolescents' media. *Mass Communication and Society, 11*(1), 3–23.

Huvane, K. (2008, October). Quick check-in. Kiosks are emerging as a potentially "easy win" that can increase patient satisfaction and improve staff efficiency. *Healthcare Informatics, 25*(10), 22–29.

Hyde, M. J. (1993). Medicine, rhetoric, and euthanasia: A case study in the workings of a postmodern discourse. *Quarterly Journal of Speech, 79,* 201–224.

Hymes, D. H. (1962). The ethnography of speaking. In T. Gladwin & W. C. Sturtevant (Eds.), *Anthropology and human behavior* (pp. 13–53). Washington, DC: Anthropological Society of Washington.

In her own words. (2004). Commentary about *The most dangerous woman in America* [video documentary], Nancy Porter (Writer/Director). NOVA in association with WGBH/Boston. Retrieved August 27, 2008, from http://www.pbs.org/wgbh/nova/typhoid

Interview: Former U.S. Surgeon General Richard Carmona, MD. (2007, November 30). *WebMD.* Retrieved September 12, 2008, from http://blogs.webmd.com/election-2008-expert-view/2007/11/interview-former-us-surgeon-general.html

Investigating continued gender disparities in physician salaries. (2008, August 20). Chicago: American Medical Association. Retrieved October 21, 2008, from http://www.ama-assn.org/ama1/pub/upload/mm/377/cmerpt19.pdf

Irvine, D. H. (1991, March). The advertising of doctors' services. *Journal of Medical Ethics, 17,* 35–40.

Iverson, K. (1997). *Plain talk: Lessons from a business maverick.* Somerset, NJ: John Wiley & Sons.

Ivinski, P. A. (1997, September–October). Test case: Sex and humor in pharmaceutical advertising. *Print, 51,* 44–46.

Jacobson, P. D., Wasserman, J., & Anderson, J. R. (1997, Spring). Historical overview of tobacco legislation. *Journal of Social Issues, 53,* 75–95.

Jadad, A. R., & Rizo, C. A. (2003). I am a good patient believe it or not. *British Medical Journal, 326*(7402), 1293–1294.

James, A. S., Hall, S., Greiner, K. A., Buckles, D., Born, W. K., & Ahluwalia, J. S. (2008). The impact of socioeconomic status on perceived barriers to colorectal cancer testing. *American Journal of Health Promotion, 23*(2), 97–100.

Janis, I. (1972). *Victims of groupthink* (2nd ed.). Boston: Houghton Mifflin.

Jantarakolica, K., Komolsevin, R., & Speece, M. (2002). Children's perception of TV reality in Bangkok, Thailand. *Asian Journal of Communication, 12*(1), 77–99.

Jarrett, N., & Payne, S. (1995). A selective review of the literature on nurse–patient communication: Has the patient's contribution been neglected? *Journal of Advanced Nursing, 22,* 72–78.

Jauhar, S. (2008a, June 17). Eyes bloodshot, doctors vent their frustration. *New York Times,* Late Edition, Section F, Science Desk Essay, p. 5.

Jauhar, S. (2008b). *Intern: A doctor's initiation.* New York: Farrar, Straus and Giroux.

J. D. Power and Associates. (2008, May 23). Satisfaction with health plans varies dramatically from region to region, largely due to poor communication from insurance providers. Retrieved July 21, 2008, from www.jdpower.com/corporate/news/releases/pressrelease.aspx?ID=2008045

Jecker, N. S., Carrese, J. A., & Pearlman, R. A. (1995). Caring for patients in cross-cultural settings. *Hastings Center Report, 25,* 6–15.

Jenkins, H. S. (2008, February 15). Patients love my broken Spanish: This determined ER physician taught himself a second language so he could communicate with all his patients. *Medical Economics, 85*(4), 42–43.

Jennings, M. C., & O'Leary, S. J. (1995). The role of managed care in integrated delivery networks. In S. B. Goldsmith (Ed.), *Managed care* (pp. 11–20). Gaithersburg, MD: Aspen.

Jeong, S.-H. (2007). Effects of news about genetics and obesity on controllability attribution and helping behavior. *Health Communication, 22*(3), 221–228.

Jha, A. K., Orav, E. J., Zheng, J., & Epstein, A. M. (2008, October 30). Patients' perception of hospital care in the United States. *New England Journal of Medicine, 359*(18), *1921.*

Jibaja-Weiss, M. L., & Volk, R. J. (2007). Utilizing computerized entertainment education in the development of decision aids for lower literate and naive computer users. *Journal of Health Communication, 12*(7), 681–697.

Jobes, M., & Steinbinder, A. (1996). Transitions in nursing leadership roles. *Nursing Administration Quarterly, 20,* 80–84.

Johnson, D. (2006, November.) Risk communication in the fog of disaster. Lessons from ground zero. *Industrial Safety & Hygiene News, 40*(11), 58, 60, 62.

Johnson, D. A. (2008). Managing Mr. Monk: Control and the politics of madness. *Critical Studies in Media Communication, 26*(1), 28–47.

Johnson, L. J. (2007, August 3). Patient e-mail perils. *Medical Economics, 84*(15), 30.

Johnson, R. W. (2008, June). The strains and drains of long-term care. *American Medical Association Journal of Ethics, 10*(6), 297–400.

Johnson, R. W., & Wiener, J. M. (2006, March 1). A profile of frail older Americans and their caregivers. Washington, DC: Urban Institute. Retrieved December 14, 2008, from http://www.urban.org/publications/311284.html

Jones, D., Gill, P., Harrison, R., Meakin, R., & Wallace, P. (2003). An exploratory study of language interpretation services provided by videoconferencing. *Journal of Telemedicine and Telecare, 9*(1), 51–56.

Jones, K. O., Denham, B. E., & Springston, J. K. (2007). Differing effects of mass and interpersonal communication on breast cancer risk estimates: An exploratory study of college students and their mothers. *Health Communication, 21*(2), 165–175.

Jordan, S. R. (2001). *The immune spirit: A story of love, loss, and healing.* Deerfield Beach, FL: Health Communications.

Joy, S. V. (2008). Clinical pearls and strategies to optimize patient outcomes. *The Diabetes Educator, 34,* 54S–59S.

Joyce, M. L. (1994). The graying of America: Implications and opportunities for health marketers. *American Behavioral Scientist, 38,* 341–351.

Kahol, K., Leyba, M. J., Deka, M., Deka, V., Mayes, S., Smith, M., Ferrara, J. J., & Panchanathan, S. (2008). Effect of fatigue on psychomotor and cognitive skills. *American Journal of Surgery, 195*(2), 195–204.

Kai, J. (1996). Parents' difficulties and information needs in coping with acute illness in preschool children: A qualitative study. *British Medical Journal, 313,* 987–990.

The Kaiser Commission on Medicaid and the Uninsured. (2008). States moving toward comprehensive health care reform. Menlo Park, CA: Author. Retrieved August 11, 2008, from www.commonwealthfund.org/chartcartcharts/chartcartcharts_show.htm?doc_id=694054&cat_id=2095www.kff.org/uninsured/upload/State%20Health%20Reform.pdf

Kaiser Family Foundation and Pew Research Center's Project for Excellence in Journalism. (2008, December). *Health news coverage in the*

*U.S. media. January 2007–June 2008.* Retrieved December 29, 2008, from http://www.journalism.org/files/HealthNewsReportFinal.pdf

Kaji, A. H., Koenig, K. L., & Lewis, R. J. (2007). Current hospital disaster preparedness. *Journal of the American Medical Association, 298*(18), 2188–2190.

Kakai, H. (2002). A double standard in bioethical reasoning for disclosure of advanced cancer diagnosis in Japan. *Health Communication, 14*(3), 361–376.

Kakizoe, T. (2008, May 18). Insight into the world: Pro-market theory hurts health care. *The Daily Yomiuri* (Tokyo), p. 4. Retrieved through Lexis-Nexis Academic.

Kalichman, S. C., Benotsch, E. G., Weinhardt, L., Austin, J., Luke, W., & Chauncey, C. (2003). Health-related Internet use, coping, social support, and health indicators in people living with HIV/AIDS. *Health Psychology, 22*(1), 111–116.

Kamwendo, G., & Kamowa, O. (1999). HIV/AIDS and a return to traditional cultural practices in Malawi. In K. R. Hope Sr. (Ed.), *AIDS and development in Africa: A social science perspective* (pp. 165–184). New York: Haworth Press.

Kanaka, D. S., & Bhattacharya, J. (2007). Changes in hospital mortality associated with residency work-hour regulations. *Internal Medicine, 147*(2), 73–81.

Kane, C. (2003, February 20). Advertising: BBDP worldwide enters the lucrative category of marketing prescription drugs to consumers. *New York Times*, Section C, p. 4.

Kaplan, M. (2003). Reporting on the business of health care. *Nieman Reports, 57*(1), 24–25.

Kaplan, R. M. (1997). Health outcomes and communication research. *Health Communication, 9*, 75–82.

Katcher, B. (1997). Getting answers from a focus group: Focus groups must be well conceived and conducted if they are to yield useful data. *Folio: The Magazine for Magazine Management, 25*, 222.

Katz, J. (1984). *The silent world of doctor and patient.* New York: Free Press.

Katz, J. (1995). Informed consent: Ethical and legal issues. In J. D. Arras & B. Steinbock (Eds.), *Ethical issues in modern medicine* (4th ed., pp. 87–97). Mountain View, CA: Mayfield.

Kean, L. G., & Prividera, L. C. (2007). Communicating about race and health: A content analysis of print advertisements in African American and general readership magazines. *Health Communication, 21*(3), 289–297.

Kearney, M. (1978). Spiritualistic healing in Mexico. In P. Morley & R. Wallis (Eds.), *Culture and curing* (pp. 19–39). Pittsburgh: University of Pittsburgh Press.

Keeley, M. P. (2004). Final conversations: Survivors' memorable messages concerning religious faith and spirituality. *Health Communication, 16*(1), 87–104.

Kelder, S. H., Perry, C. L., & Klepp, K. (1993). Community-wide youth exercise promotion: Long-term outcomes of the Minnesota Heart Health Program and the Class of 1989 study. *Journal of School Health, 63*, 218–223.

Keller, S. N., Labelle, H., Karimi, N., & Gupta, S. (2002). STD/HIV prevention for teenagers: A look at the Internet universe. *Journal of Health Communication, 7*(4), 341–353.

Kelly, F. (1996, April). Taking time to talk. *Nursing Times, 92*, 28.

Kelly, K. J., & Edwards, R. W. (1998, Spring). Image advertisements for alcohol products: Is their appeal associated with adolescents' intention to consume alcohol? *Adolescence, 33*, 47–59.

Kelly, K. S., Soderlund, K., Albert, C., & McGarrahan, A. G. (1999). Social support and chronic fatigue syndrome. *Health Communication, 11*(1), 21–34.

Kennedy, J., Chi-Chuan, W., & Wu, C.-H. (2007, May 17). Patient disclosure about herb and supplement use and adults in the US. *eCam*, pp. 1–6.

Kenny, R. W. (2001). Toward a better death: Applying Burkean principles of symbolic action to interpret family adaptation to Karen Ann Quinlan's coma. *Health Communication, 13*(4), 363–385.

Kenny, R. W. (2002). The death of loving: Maternal identity as moral constraint in a narrative testimonial advocating physician-assisted suicide. *Health Communication, 14*(2), 243–270.

Kilbourne, J. (2000). *Killing us softly 3: Advertising's image of women.* North Hampton, MA: Media Education Foundation.

Kim, S.-H., & Willis, L. A. (2007, June). Talking about obesity: News framing of who is responsible for causing and fixing the problem. *Journal of Health Communication, 12*(4), 359–376.

King, S. (2002, July 19). Media: *Minority Report*—an expert's view. If product placement works, as it does in *Minority Report*, it can benefit a brand. *Campaign*, np. Retrieved October 2, 2008, from http://www.brandrepublic.com/Campaign/News/151376/

Kirchheimer, B. (2008, April 7). Sustainable diversity; this year's Top 25 Minority Executives in Healthcare highlights leadership diversity, but some question the true level of inclusion. *Modern Healthcare, 38*(14), 6–7, 22, 24, 26, 28, 30–31.

Klass, P. (1987). *A not entirely benign procedure: Four years as a medical student.* New York: Penguin.

Klass, P. (2008, May 29). The moral of the story. *New England Journal of Medicine, 358*(22), 2313.

Kleinman, A., Eisenberg, L., & Good, B. (1978). Culture, illness, and care: Clinical lessons from anthropological and cross-cultural research. *Annals of Internal Medicine, 88,* 251–258.

Kleinmann, L. (1989, February). Code blue. *Health, 21,* 68–73.

Kneebone, R., Nestel, D., Chrzanowska J., Barnet, A. E., Younger, J., Burgess, A., & Darzi, A. (2006). The perioperative specialist practitioner: Developing and evaluating a new surgical role. *Quality & Safety in Health Care, 15*(5), 354–358.

Knobloch-Westerwick, S., & Alter, S. (2006). Mood adjustment to social situations through mass media use: How men ruminate and women dissipate angry moods. *Human Communication Research, 32*(1), 58–73.

Knoerl, A. M. (2007). Cultural considerations and the Hispanic cardiac client. *Home Healthcare Nurse, 25*(2), 83–86.

Koermer, C. D., & Kilbane, M. (2008). Physician sociality communication and its effect on patient satisfaction. *Communication Quarterly, 56,* 69–86.

Koh, G. C., Khoo, H. E., Wong, M. L., & Koh, D. (2008). The effects of problem-based learning during medical school on physician competency: A systematic review. *Canadian Medical Association Journal, 178*(1), 34–41.

Kohler, C. L., Grimley, D., & Reynolds, K. (1999). Theoretical approaches guiding the development and implementation of health promotion programs. In J. M. Raczynski & R. J. DiClemente (Eds.), *Handbook of health promotion and disease prevention* (pp. 23–49). New York: Kluwer Academic/Plenum.

Komaroff, A. L., & Fagioli, J. (1996). *Medical assessment of fatigue and chronic fatigue syndrome: An integrative approach to evaluation and treatment* (pp. 154–181). New York: Guilford Press.

Kopfman, J. E., & Ray, E. B. (2005). Talking to children about illness. In E. B. Ray (Ed.), *Health communication in practice: A case study approach* (pp. 111–119). Mahwah, NJ: Lawrence Erlbaum.

Koplan, J. P. (2002). The small world of global health. *The Mount Sinai Journal of Medicine, 69*(5), 291–298.

Korkki, Phyllis. (2008, February 10). Going global with concerns on health costs. *New York Times*, Late Edition, Section BU, Monday and Business/Financial Desk, p. 2.

Korsch, D. M., & Negrete, V. F. (1972). Doctor-patient communication. *Scientific American, 227,* 66–74.

Kotler, P., & Clarke, R. N. (1987). *Marketing for health care organizations.* Englewood Cliffs, NJ: Prentice Hall.

Kotz, K., & Story, M. (1994). Food advertisements during children's Saturday morning television programming: Are they consistent with dietary recommendations? *Journal of the American Dietetic Association, 94,* 1296–1300.

Kowalski, K. M. (1997, October). On guard against health rip-off. *Current Health, 24,* 6–11.

Kramer, H., & Kramer, K. (1993, March–April). *Psychology Today, 26,* 26–27.

Kreps, G. L. (1990). Applied health communication research. In D. O'Hair & G. L. Kreps (Eds.), *Applied communication theory and research* (pp. 313–330). Hillsdale, NJ: Lawrence Erlbaum.

Kreps, G. L. (2003). The impact of communication on cancer risk, incidence, morbidity, mortality, and quality of life. *Health Communication, 15*(2), 161–169.

Kreps, G. L. (2005). Narrowing the digital divide to overcome disparities in care. In E. B. Ray (Ed.), *Health communication in practice: A case study approach* (pp. 357–364). Mahwah, NJ: Lawrence Erlbaum.

Kreps, G. L., Query, J. L., Jr., & Bonaguro, E. W. (2008). In L. C. Lederman (Ed.), *Beyond these walls: Readings in health communication* (pp. 3–14). New York: Oxford University Press.

Kreps, G. L., & Thornton, B. C. (1992). *Health communication: Theory & practice* (2nd ed.). Prospect Heights, IL: Waveland Press.

Kreuter, M., Farrell, D., Olevitch, L., & Brennan, L. (1999). *Tailoring health messages: Customizing communication with computer technology.* Mahwah, NJ: Lawrence Erlbaum.

Krishna, S., Francisco, B. D., Balas, E. A., Konig, P., Graff, G. R., & Madsen, R. W. (2003). Internet-enabled interactive multimedia asthma education program: A randomized trial. *Pediatrics, 111*(3), 503–510.

Krishnan, S. P. (1996). Health education at family planning clinics: Strategies for improving information about contraception and sexually transmitted diseases for low-income women. *Health Communication, 8,* 353–366.

Kroll, T., Beatty, P. W., & Bingham, S. (2003). Primary care satisfaction among adults with physical disabilities: The role of patient–provider communication. *Managed Care Quarterly, 11*(1), 11–19.

Krosnick, J. A., Chang, L., Sherman, S. J., Chassin, L., & Presson, C. (2006). The effects of beliefs about the health consequences of cigarette smoking on smoking onset. *Journal of Communication, 56,* S18–S37.

Krug, P. (1998). Where does physician-assisted suicide stand today? *Association of Operating Room Nurses Journal, 68,* 869.

Kubler-Ross, E. (1969). *On death and dying.* New York: Macmillan.

Kulich, K. R., Berggren, U., & Hallberg, I, R.-M. (2003). A qualitative analysis of patient-centered dentistry in consultations with dental phobic patients. *Journal of Health Communication, 8*(2), 171–187.

Kundrat, A. L., & Nussbaum, J. F. (2003). The impact of invisible illness on identity and contextual age. *Health Communication, 15*(3), 331–347.

Kunkel, D., Eyal, K., Donnerstein, E., Farrar, K. M., Biely, E., & Rideout, V. (2007). Sexual socialization messages on entertainment television: Comparing content trends 1997–2002. *Media Psychology, 9*(3), 595–622.

Kunkel, D., Eyal, K., Finnerty, K., Biely, E., & Donnerstein, E. (2005). Sex on TV4. Menlo Park, CA: Henry J. Kaiser Family Foundation. Retrieved October 1, 2008, from http://www.kff.org/entmedia/upload/Sex-on-TV-4-Full-Report.pdf

Kush, R. D., Helton, E., Rockhold, F. W., & Hardison, C. D. (2008). Electronic health records, medical research, and the Tower of Babel. *New England Journal of Medicine, 358*(16), 1738.

La Puma, J. (1998). *Managed care ethics: Essays on the impact of managed care on traditional medical ethics.* New York: Hatherleigh Press.

Laframboise, D. (1998). When home is the hospital. *Chatelaine, 71,* 26–31.

Laine, C., & Davidoff, F. (1996). Patient-centered medicine: A professional evolution. *Journal of the American Medical Association, 275,* 152–155.

Lamberg, L. (1996). Knitting up the raveling sleeve of care: Role of sleep and effects of its lack examined. *Journal of the American Medical Association, 276,* 1205–1207.

Lambert, B. L., Street, R. L., Cegala, D. J., Smith, D. H., Kurtz, S., & Schofield, T. (1997). Provider-patient communication, patient-centered care, and the mangle of practice. *Health Communication, 9,* 27–43.

Landon, B. E., Reschovsky, J. D., Pham, H. H., & Blumenthal, D. (2006). Leaving medicine: The consequences of physician dissatisfaction. *Medical Care, 44*(3), 234–242.

Landrigan, C. P., Barger, L. K., Cade, B. E., Ayas, N. T., & Czeisler, C. A. (2006). Interns' compliance with Accreditation Council for Graduate Medical Education work-hour limits. *Journal of the American Medical Association, 296*(9), 1063–1070.

Lang, A. (2006). Using the limited-capacity model of motivated mediated message processing to design effective cancer communication messages. *Journal of Communication, 56,* S57–S80.

Lang, A., Chung, Y., Lee, S., & Zhao, X. (2005). It's the product: Do risky products compel attention and elicit arousal in media users? *Health Communication, 17*(3), 283–300.

Lang, A., Schwartz, N., Lee, S., & Angelini, J. R. (2007, September). Processing radio PSAs: Production pacing, arousing content, and age. *Journal of Health Communication, 12*(6), 581–599.

Lansdale, D. (2002). Touching lives: Opening doors for elders in retirement communities through e-mail and the Internet. In R. W. Morrell (Ed.), *Older adults, health information, and the World Wide Web* (pp. 133–151). Mahwah, NJ: Lawrence Erlbaum.

Lanza, M. L., Zeiss, R. A., & Rierdan, J. (2006). Non-physical violence: A risk factor for physical violence in health care settings. *American Association of Occupational Health Journal, 54*(9), 397–402.

Lapinski, M. K., Rimal, R. N., DeVries, R., & Lee, E. L. (2007). The role of group orientation and descriptive norms on water conservation attitudes and behaviors. *Health Communication, 22*(2), 133–142.

Larkey, L. K. (1996). Toward a theory of communicative interactions in culturally diverse workgroups. *Academy of Management Review, 21,* 463–491.

Lassiter, S. M. (1998). *Cultures of color in America: A guide to family, religion, and health.* Westport, CT: Greenwood.

Latimer, A. E., Salovey, P., & Rothman, A. J. (2007). The effectiveness of gain-framed messages for encouraging disease prevention behavior: Is all hope lost? *Journal of Health Communication, 12,* 645–649.

Lauer, C. S. (2008a, April 28). Rx for local economies; healthcare picks up where manufacturing left off. *Modern Healthcare, 38*(17), 25.

Lauer, C. S. (2008b, March 10). The unwritten curriculum. Writer: Medical students learn from elders' cynicism. *Modern Healthcare, 38*(10), 50.

Laurant, M. G., Hermens, R. P., Braspenning, J. C., Akkermans, R. P., Sibbald, B., & Grol, R. P. (2008). An overview of patients' preference for, and satisfaction with, care provided by general practitioners and nurse practitioners. *Journal of Clinical Nursing, 17*(20), 2690–2698.

Law, D. (1994, January 15). Making diversity work. *Restaurants & Institutions, 104,* 84–86.

Laws, M., & Scott, M. K. (2008, September/October). The emergence of retail-based clinics in the United States: Early observations. *Health Affairs, 27*(5), 1293–1298.

Lazarsfeld, P., Burleson, B., & Gaudet, H. (1948). *The people's choice.* New York: Columbia University Press.

Lederman, L. C., & Stewart, L. P. (2005). *Changing the culture of college drinking: A socially situated health communication campaign.* Cresskill, NJ: Hampton Press.

Lederman, L. C., Stewart, L. P., Barr, S. L., Powell, R. L., Laitman, L., & Goodhart, F. W. (2001). Using communication theory to reduce dangerous drinking on a college campus. In R. E. Rice & C. K. Atkin (Eds.), *Public communication campaigns* (3rd ed., pp. 295–299). Thousand Oaks, CA: Sage.

Lederman, L. C., Stewart, L. P., Goodhart, F. W., & Laitman, L. (2008). A case against "binge" as the term of choice. In L. C. Lederman (Ed.), *Beyond these walls: Readings in health communication* (pp. 292–303). New York: Oxford University Press.

Ledlow, G. R., Johnson, J. A., & Hakoyama, M. (2008). Social marketing and organizational efficacy. In K. B. Wright & S. D. Moore (Eds.), *Applied health communication* (pp. 85–103). Cresskill, NJ: Hampton Press.

Lee, F. (2004). *If Disney ran your hospital: 9½ things you would do differently*. Bozeman, MT: Second River Healthcare Press.

Lee, M. J., & Bichard, S. L. (2006). Effective message design targeting college students for the prevention of binge-drinking: Basing design on rebellious risk-taking tendency. *Health Communication, 20*(3), 299–308.

Leeman-Castillo, B. A., Corbett, K. K., Aagaard, E. M., Maselli, J. H., Gonzales, R., & MacKenzie, T. D. (2007). Acceptability of a bilingual interactive computerized educational module in a poor, medically underserved patient population. *Journal of Health Communication, 12*(1), 77–94.

Lefebvre, R. C., Doner, L., Johnston, D., Loughrey, K., Balch, G. I., & Sutton, S. M. (1995). Use of database marketing and consumer-based health communication in message design: An example for the Office of Cancer Communications' "5 a Day for Better Health" program. In E. Maibach & R. L. Parrott (Eds.), *Designing health messages: Approaches from communication theory and public health practice* (pp. 217–246). Thousand Oaks, CA: Sage.

Lefebvre, R. C., & Flora, J. A. (1988). Social marketing and public health intervention. *Health Education Quarterly, 15*, 299–315.

Legacy Today urged Philip Morris to pull its "Think. Don't Smoke" ads based on research showing the ads make kids more likely to smoke. (2002, June 29). American Legacy Foundation. Retrieved July 4, 2003, from http://pressroom.americanlegacy.org

Lehman, D. R., Ellard, J. H., & Wortman, C. B. (1986). Social support for the bereaved: Recipients' and providers' perspectives on what is helpful. *Journal of Consulting and Clinical Psychology, 54*, 438–446.

Leiss, W., & Powell, D. (with Whitfield, A.). (2004). Mad cows or crazy communications? In L. William & P. Douglas (Authors), *Mad cows and mothers' milk: The perils of poor risk communication* (pp. 3–25, 2nd ed.). Montreal: McGill–Queen's University Press.

Leonard, B. (2006, February). Gallup: Workplace bias still prevalent. *HRMagazine, 51*(2), 34.

Let us put you in the movies. (1996, September 16). *Brandweek, 37*, S3–S9.

Levin, A. (1998). Evidence-based medicine gaining supporters. *Annals of Internal Medicine, 128*, 334–336.

Levinsky, N. (1995). The doctor's master. In J. D. Arras & B. Steinbock (Eds.), *Ethical issues in modern medicine* (4th ed., pp. 116–119). Mountain View, CA: Mayfield.

Levinson, W., Roter, D., L., Mullooly, J. P., Dull, V. T., & Frankel, R. M. (1997). Physician–patient communication: The relationship with malpractice claims among primary care physicians and surgeons. *Journal of the American Medical Association, 277*, 553–559.

Levy, D. R. (1985). White doctors and Black patients: Influence of race on the doctor–patient relationship. *Pediatrics, 75*, 639–643.

Lewis, M., & Haviland-Jones, J. M. (Eds.) (2000). *Handbook of emotions*. New York: Guilford Press.

Li, H. Z., Krysko, M., Desroches, N. G., & Deagle, G. (2004). Reconceptualizing interruptions in physician–patient interviews: Cooperative and intrusive. *Communication & Medicine, 1*(2), 145–157.

Liao, S. S., Schensul, J., & Wolffers, I. (2003). Sex-related health risks and complications for interventions with hospitality women in Hainan, China. *AIDS Education and Prevention, 15*(2), 109–121.

Lief, H. L., & Fox, R. C. (1963). Training for "detached concern" in medical students. In J. I. Lief, V. F. Lief, & N. R. Lief (Eds.), *The psychological basis of medical practice*. New York: Harper & Row.

Lindberg, D. A. B. (2002). Older Americans, health information, and the Internet. In R. W. Morrell (Ed.), *Older adults, health information, and the*

*World Wide Web* (pp. 13–19). Mahwah, NJ: Lawrence Erlbaum.

Lindenauer, P. K., Rothberg, M. B., Pekow, P. S., Kenwood, C., Benjamin, E. M., & Auerbach, A. D. (2007, December 20). Outcomes of care by hospitalists, general internists, and family physicians. *New England Journal of Medicine, 357*(25), 2589.

Lingard, I., Garwood, K., Schryer, C., & Spafford, M. (2003). "Talking the talk": School and workplace genre tension in clerkship care presentations. *Medical Education, 37*(7), 612–620.

Linnan, L. A., & Ferguson, Y. O. (2007). Beauty salons. *Health Education & Behavior, 34*(3), 517–530.

Lippy, C. H., & Williams, P. W. (1988). *Encyclopedia of the American religious experience.* New York: Charles Scribner's Sons.

Liselotte, N. D., Thomas, M. R., Massie, S., Power, D. V., Eacker, A., Harper, W., Durning, S., Moutier, C., Szydlo, D. W., Novotny, P. J., Sloan, J. A., & Shanafelt, T. D. (2008). Burnout and suicide ideation among U.S. medical students. *Annals of Internal Medicine, 149,* 334–341.

Littlefield, R. S., & Quenette, A. M. (2007, February). Crisis leadership and Hurricane Katrina: The portrayal of authority by the media in natural disasters. *Journal of Applied Communication Research, 35*(1), 26–47.

Living with cancer. (1997, September). *Harvard Health Letter, 22,* 4–5.

Lockley, S. W., Barger, L. K., Ayas, N. T., Rothschild, J. M., Czeisler, C. A., & Landrigan, C. P. (2007). Effects of health care provider work hours and sleep deprivation on safety and performance. *Joint Commission Journal on Quality and Patient Safety/Joint Commission Resources, 33*(11), 7–18.

Loe, M. (2004). *The rise of Viagra: How the little blue pill changed sex in America.* New York: New York University Press.

Löffler, W., Kilian, R., Toumi, M., & Angermeyer, M. C. (2003). Schizophrenic patients' subjective reasons for compliance and noncompliance with neuroleptic treatment. *Pharmacopsychiatry, 36*(3), 105–112.

Lombardo, F. A. (1997). If you don't befriend your patients, your competitors will. *Medical Economics, 74,* 121–124.

Long, S. K. (2008, June 3). On the road to universal coverage: Impacts of reform in Massachusetts at one year. *Health Affairs,* Web Exclusive, w270–w284. Retrieved August 21, 2008, from http://www.commonwealthfund.org/publications/publications_show.htm?doc_id=688057

Longino, C. F. (1997, December). Beyond the body: An emerging medical paradigm. *American Demographics, 19,* 14–18.

Lovett, R. A. (2003, May–June). Fact versus fear: We worry too much about man-made catastrophe. *Psychology Today, 36*(3), 14.

Lowes, R. (2008a, May 2). The concierge model: Want to spend more time with your patients? Consider a retainer practice. *Medical Economics, 85*(9), 69–73.

Lowes, R. (2008b, May 2). Open access, extended hours: Seeing patients when they want to be seen helps you respond to their needs and stay competitive. *Medical Economics, 85*(9), 62–72.

Lowes, R. (2008c, May 16). Say goodbye to insurers: It's possible to walk away from third-party payers and still create a satisfying practice. *Medical Economics, 85,* 26–31.

Lowrey, W., & Anderson, W. B. (2006). The impact of Internet use on the public perception of physicians: A perspective from the sociology of professions literature. *Health Communication, 19*(2), 125–131.

Ludtke, M., & Trost, C. (1998). Covering children's health. *American Journalism Review, 20,* 81–88.

Luepker, R. V., Murray, D. M., Jacobs, D. R., Jr., Mittelmark, M. B., Bracht, N., Carlaw, R., Crow, R., Elmer, P., Finnegan, J., Folsom, A. R., Grimm, R., Hannan, P. J., Jeffrey, R., Lando, H., McGovern, P., Mullis, R., Perry, C. L., Pechacek, T., Pirie, P. Sprafka, J. M., Weisbrod, R., & Blackburn, H. (1994). Community education for cardiovascular disease prevention: Risk factor changes in the Minnesota Heart Health Program. *American Journal of Public Health, 84,* 1381–1393.

Lumsdon, K. (1996, February 5). A kinder, gentler ER. *Hospitals & Health Networks, 70*, 43–45.

Lund, C. C. (1995). The doctor, the patient, and the truth. In J. D. Arras & B. Steinbock (Eds.), *Ethical issues in modern medicine* (pp. 55–57). Mountain View, CA: Mayfield.

Lundin, S. C., Christensen, J., Paul, H., & Strand, P. (2002). *Fish! Tales: Real-life stories to help you transform your workplace and your life.* New York: Hyperion Books.

Lundine, K., Buckley, R., Hutchinson, C., & Lockyer, J. (2008). Communication skills training in orthopedics. *Journal of Bone and Joint Surgery, 90*(6), 1393–1400.

Lupton, D. (1998). A postmodern public health? *Australian and New Zealand Journal of Public Health, 22*(1), 3–5.

Lyall, S. (2000, October 27). British wrongly lulled people on "mad cow," report finds. *New York Times*, online version, np. Retrieved August 26, 2008, from http://query.nytimes.com/gst/fullpage.html?res=9C06E7DB1E31F934A15753C1A9669C8B63&n=Top%2FNews%2FScience%2FTopics%2FAnimals

Lyon, A. (2007, November). "Putting patients first": Systematically distorted communication and Merck's marketing of Vioxx. *Journal of Applied Communication Research, 35*(4), 376–398.

MacDonald, M. (1981). *Mystical bedlam: Madness, anxiety, and healing in seventeenth-century England.* Cambridge: Cambridge University Press.

Macias, W., & McMillan, S. (2008). The return of the house call: The role of Internet-based interactivity in bringing health information home to older adults. *Health Communication, 23*(1), 34–44.

Macias, W., Pashupati, K., & Lewis, L. S. (2007). A wonderful life or diarrhea and dry mouth? Policy issues of direct-to-consumer drug advertising on television. *Health Communication, 22*(3), 241–252.

Mad cows and the minister. (1990, May 24). *Nature, 345*, 277–278. Retrieved August 26, 2008, through ProQuest.

Maeda, T., Hobbs, R. M., Marghoub, T., Guernah, I., Zelent, A., Cordon-Cardo, C., Teruya-Feldstein, J., & Pandolfi, P. P. (2005). Role of the proto-oncogene Pokémon in cellular transformation and ARF repression. *Nature, 433*(7023), 278–285.

Magee, M., & D'Antonio, M. (2003). *The best medicine: Stories of doctors and patients who care for each other* (2nd ed.). New York: Spencer Books.

Magrane, D., Lang, J., Alexander, H., Leadley, J., & Bongiovanni, C. (2007, November). Washington, DC: American Association of Medical Colleges. Retrieved October 21, 2008, from http://www.aamc.org/members/wim/statistics/stats07/start.htm

Mahler, H. I. M., Kulik, J. A., Butler, H. A., Gerrard, M., & Gibbons, F. X. (2008). Social norms information enhances the efficacy of an appearance-based sun protection intervention. *Social Science & Medicine, 67*, 321–329.

Maibach, E. W., & Cotton, D. (1995). Moving people to behavior change: A stage social cognitive approach to message design. In E. Maibach & R. L. Parrott (Eds.), *Designing health messages: Approaches from communication theory and public health practice* (pp. 41–64). Thousands Oaks, CA: Sage.

Maibach, E. W., & Parrott, R. L. (Eds.). (1995). *Designing health messages.* Thousand Oaks, CA: Sage.

Major religions of the world ranked by number of adherents. (2007, August). Adherents.com. Retrieved December 20, 2008, from http://www.adherents.com/Religions_By_Adherents.html

Malinski, V. M. (Ed.). (1986). *Explorations on Martha Rogers' science of unitary human beings.* Norwalk, CT: Appleton-Century-Crofts.

Malis, R. S., & Roloff, M. E. (2007). The effect of legitimacy and intimacy on peer interventions into alcohol abuse. *Western Journal of Communication, 71*(1), 49–68.

Managed care change. (2006, August 7). *Modern Healthcare*, p. 20.

Marantz, P. R. (1990). Blaming the victim: The negative consequences of preventive medicine. *American Journal of Public Health, 80*, 1186–1187.

Margolick, D. (1990, August 6). In child deaths, a test for Christian Science. *New York Times*, online. Retrieved December 25, 2008, from http://query.nytimes.com/gst/fullpage.html?se c=health&res=9C0CE0D61030F935A3575BC0 A966958260

Marin, M. J., Sherblom, J. C., & Shipps, T. B. (1994). Contextual influences on nurses' conflict management strategies. *Western Journal of Communication, 58,* 201–228.

Marion, G. S., Hildebrandt, C. A., Davis, S. W., Marin, A. J., & Crandall, S. J. (2008). Working effectively with interpreters: A model curriculum for physician assistant students. *Medical Teacher, 30*(6), 612–617.

Marks, L. I. (1998). Deconstructing locus of control: Implications for practitioners. *Journal of Counseling and Development, 76,* 251–260.

Marshall, A. A., Smith, S. W., & McKeon, J. K. (1995). Persuading low-income women to engage in mammography screening: Source, message, and channel preferences. *Health Communication, 7,* 283–300.

Martin, L. R., Williams, S. L., Haskard, K. B., & Dimatteo, M. R. (2005). The challenge of patient adherence. *Therapeutics and Clinical Risk Management, 1*(3), 189–199.

Marwick, C. (1997). Proponents gather to discuss evidence-based medicine. *Journal of the American Medical Association, 278,* 531–532.

Maslach, C. (1982). *Burnout: The cost of caring.* Englewood Cliffs, NJ: Prentice Hall.

Mast, M. S. (2007). On the importance of nonverbal communication in the physician–patient interaction. *Patient Education and Counseling, 67*(3), 315–318.

Mastin, T., Andsager, J. L., Choi, J., & Lee, K. (2007). Health disparities and direct-to-consumer prescription drug advertising: A content analysis of targeted magazine genres, 1992–2002. *Health Communication, 22*(1), 49–58.

Mastro, D. E., & Atkin, C. (2002). Exposure to alcohol billboards and beliefs and attitudes toward drinking among Mexican American high school students. *Howard Journal of Communications, 12*(2), 129–151.

Matthews, A. K. (1998). Lesbians and cancer support: Clinical issues for cancer patients. *Health Care for Women International, 1993,* 193–203.

Matthews, A. K., Sellergren, S. A., Manfredi, C., & Williams, M. (2002). Factors influencing medical information seeking among African-American cancer patients. *Journal of Health Communication, 7*(3), 205–219.

Mattson, M., & Roberts, F. (2001). Overcoming truth telling as an obstacle to initiating safer sex: Clients and health practitioners planning deception during HIV test counseling. *Health Communication, 13*(4), 343–362.

Matusitz, J., & Breen, G.-M. (2007). Telemedicine: Its effects on health communication. *Health Communication, 21*(1), 73–83.

Mayer, T. A., & Cates, R. J. (2004). *Leadership for great customer service: Satisfied patients, satisfied employees.* Chicago: Health Administration Press.

Maynard, C. (1998, September). How to make peace with your body. *Current Health, 2,* 66–71.

Maynard, D. W., & Frankel, R. M. (2006). On diagnostic rationality: Bad news, good news, and the symptoms residue. In J. Heritage & D. W. Maynard (Eds.), *Communication in medical care: Interactions between primary care physicians and patients* (pp. 248–278). Cambridge: Cambridge University Press.

McCague, J. J. (2001, May 21). On today's older patients. *Medical Economics, 78*(10), 104.

McComas, K. A. (2006). Defining moments in risk communication research: 1996–2005. *Journal of Health Communication, 11*(1), 75–91.

McConatha, D. (2002). Aging online: Toward a theory of e-equality. In R. W. Morrell (Ed.), *Older adults, health information, and the World Wide Web* (pp. 21–41). Mahwah, NJ: Lawrence Erlbaum.

McCormick, T. R., & Conley, B. J. (1995). Patients' perspectives on dying and the care of dying patients. *Western Journal of Medicine, 163,* 236–243.

McCue, J. D. (1995). The naturalness of dying. *Journal of the American Medical Association, 273,* 1039–1044.

McCullough, D. (2008). *My mother, your mother: Embracing "slow medicine"—the compassionate approach to caring for your aging loved ones.* New York: HarperCollins.

McDermott, J. (1995). The first step (universal coverage is foundation for health care reform). *Journal of the American Medical Association, 273,* 251–254.

McGowan, B. (2001). Self-reported stress and its effects on nurses. *Nursing Standard, 15*(42), 33–38.

McGrath, J. (1995). The gatekeeping process: The right combinations to unlock the gates. In E. Maibach & R. L. Parrott (Eds.), *Designing health messages: Approaches from communication theory and public health practice* (pp. 199–216). Thousands Oaks, CA: Sage.

McNeese-Smith, D. (1996). Increasing employee productivity. *Hospital & Health Services Administration, 41,* 160–175.

McWhinney, I. (1989). The need for a transformed clinical method. In M. Stewart & D. Roter (Eds.), *Communicating with medical patients: Vol. 9. Interpersonal communication* (pp. 25–40). Newbury Park, CA: Sage.

Medical records; the growing threat to patient privacy. (2001, November 28). *San Diego Union-Tribune,* p. B8.

Medication errors injure 1.5 million people and cost billions of dollars annually. (2006, July 20). Washington, DC: The National Academies. Retrieved October 16, 2008, from http://www8. nationalacademies.org/onpinews/newsitem. aspx?RecordID=11623

Mehrotra, A., Wang, M. C., Lave, J. R., Adams, J. L., & McGlyn, E. A. (2008, September/October). Retail clinics, primary care physicians, and emergency departments: A comparison of patients' visits. *Health Affairs, 27*(5), 1272–1282.

Mello, F. (2007, August 6). Overworked?—Limiting residents' hours has helped relieve their exhaustion. But patients aren't much better off, and training may be suffering. *Boston Globe,* Health Science, p. C1.

Meredith, L. S., Eisenman, D. P., Rhodes, H., Ryan, G., & Long, A. (2007, April–May). Trust influences response to public health messages during a bioterrorist event. *Journal of Health Communication, 12*(3), 217–232.

*Merriam-Webster WWWebster Dictionary.* (1999). Merriam-Webster Inc. Retrieved January 2, 2000, from www.m-w.com/cgi-bin/dictionary

Messmer, M. (1998, September). Mentoring: Building your company's intellectual capital. *HR Focus, 75,* 511–512.

The MetLife market survey of nursing home & assisted living costs. (2007, October). Westport, CT: MetLife Mature Market Institute. Retrieved December 14, 2008, from http://www.metlife.com/ FileAssets/MMI/MMIStudies2007NHAL.pdf

Metts, S., & Manns, H. (1996). Coping with HIV and AIDS: The social and personal challenges. In E. B. Ray (Ed.), *Communication and disenfranchisement: Social issues and implications* (pp. 347–364). Mahwah, NJ: Lawrence Erlbaum.

Micalizzi, D. A. (2008, March 3). The aftermath of a "never event"; a child's unexplained death and a system seemingly designed to thwart justice. *Modern Healthcare, 38*(9), 24.

Milika, R. M., & Trorey, G. M. (2008). Patients' expectations of the maintenance of their dignity. *Journal of Clinical Nursing, 17,* 2709–2717.

Millar, M. G., & Millar, K. (1998). Processing messages about disease detection and health promotion behaviors: The effects of anxiety. *Health Communication, 10,* 211–226.

Miller, C. H., Burgoon, M., Grandpre, J. R., & Alvaro, E. M. (2006). Identifying principal risk factors for the initiation of adolescent smoking behaviors: The significance of psychological reactance. *Health Communication, 19*(3), 241–252.

Miller, C. H., Lane, L. T., Deatrick, L. M., Young, A. M., & Potts, K. A. (2007). Psychological reactance and promotional health messages: The effects of controlling language, lexical concreteness, and the restoration of freedom. *Human Communication Research, 33,* 219–240.

Miller, J. F. (2000). *Coping with chronic illness: Overcoming powerlessness.* Philadelphia: F. A. Davis.

Miller, K. I. (1999). *Organizational communication: Approaches and processes* (2nd ed.). Belmont, CA: Wadsworth.

Miller, K. I., Birkholt, M., Scott, C., & Stage, C. (1995). Empathy and burnout in human service work: An extension of the communication model. *Communication Research, 22*, 123–147.

Miller, K. I., Stiff, J. B., & Ellis, B. H. (1988). Communication and empathy as precursors to burnout among human service workers. *Communication Monographs, 55*, 250–265.

Miller, V., & Jablin, F. (1991). Information seeking during organizational entry: Influences, tactics, and a model of the process. *Academy of Management Review, 16*, 92–120.

Miller, W. R., & Rollnick, S. (2002). *Motivational interviewing: Preparing people for change.* New York: Guilford Press.

Miller-Day, M., & Marks, J. (2006). Perceptions of parental communication orientation, perfectionism, and disordered eating behaviors of sons and daughters. *Health Communication, 19*(2), 153–163.

Milliken, F. J., & Martins, L. L. (1996). Searching for common threads: Understanding the multiple effects of diversity in organizational groups. *Academy of Management Review, 21*, 402–433.

Mills, C. B. (2005). Catching up with Down syndrome: Parents' experiences in dealing with the medical and therapeutic communities. In E. B. Ray (Ed.), *Health communication in practice: A case study approach* (pp. 195–210). Mahwah, NJ: Lawrence Erlbaum.

Minorities in medical education. Facts and figures 2005. (2005). Washington, DC: American Association of Medical Colleges. Retrieved October 22, 2008, from https://services.aamc.org/Publications/showfile.cfm?file=version53.pdf&prd_id=133&prv_id=154&pdf_id=53

Mishler, E. G. (1981). The social construction of illness. In E. B. Mishler, L. R. Amarasingham, S. D. Osherson, S. T. Hauser, & R. Leim (Eds.), *Social contexts of health, illness, and patient care* (pp. 141–168). Cambridge: Cambridge University Press.

Mishler, E. G. (1984). *The discourse of medicine: Dialectics of medical interviews.* Norwood, NJ: Ablex.

Mitka, M. (1996, August 26). Coalition presses to preserve affirmative action in medicine. *American Medical News, 39*, 1–4.

Mitka, M. (2000). Some men who take Viagra die—why? *Journal of the American Medical Association, 283*(5), 593–594.

Molina, M. A., Cheung, M. C., Perez, E. A., Byrne, M. M., Franceschi, D., Moffat, F. L., Livingstone, A. S., Goodwin, W. J., Gutierrez, J. C., & Koniaris, L. G. (2008). African American and poor patients have a dramatically worse prognosis for head and neck cancer: An examination of 20,915 patients. *Cancer, 113*(10), 2797–2806.

Monohan, J. L. (1995). Thinking positively: Using positive affect when designing health messages. In E. Maibach & R. L. Parrott (Eds.), *Designing health messages: Approaches from communication theory and public health practice* (pp. 81–98). Thousand Oaks, CA: Sage.

Monohan, J. L., Miller, L. C., & Rothspan, C. (1997). Power and intimacy: On the dynamics of risky sex. *Health Communication, 9*, 303–322.

Moonhee, Y., & Roskos-Ewoldsen, D. R. (2007). The effectiveness of brand placements in the movies: Levels of placements, explicit and implicit memory, and brand-choice behavior. *Journal of Communication, 57*, 469–489.

Moore, J. R., & Gilbert, D. A. (1995). Elderly residents: Perceptions of nurses' comforting touch. *Journal of Gerontological Nursing, 21*(6), 6–13.

Moore, L. G., Van Arsdale, P. W., Glittenberg, J. E., & Aldrich, R. A. (1987). *The biocultural basis of health: Expanding views of medical anthropology.* Prospect Heights, IL: Waveland Press.

Moore, L. W., & Miller, M. (2003). Older men's experiences of living with severe visual impairment. *Journal of Advanced Nursing, 43*(1), 10–18.

Morgan, S. E., Harrison, T. R., Afifi, W. A., Long, S. D., & Stephenson, M. T. (2008). In their own words: The reasons why people will (not) sign an organ donor card. *Health Communication, 23*(1), 23–33.

Morgan, S. E., Harrison, T. R., Chewning, L., Davis, L., & DiCorcia, M. (2007). Entertainment (mis)education: The framing of organ donation in entertainment television. *Health Communication*, *22*(2), 143–151.

Morreim, E. H. (1989). Fiscal scarcity and the inevitability of bedside budget-balancing. *Archives of Internal Medicine*, *149*, 1012–1015.

Morrell, R. W. (Ed.). (2002). *Older adults, health information, and the World Wide Web*. Mahwah, NJ: Lawrence Erlbaum.

Morse, D. S., Edwardsen, E. A., & Gordon, H. S. (2008). Missed opportunities for interval empathy in lung cancer communication. *Archives of Internal Medicine*, *168*(17), 1853–1858.

Mosavel, M., & El-Shaarawi, N. (2007, December). "I have never heard of that one": Young girls' knowledge and perception of cervical cancer. *Journal of Health Communication*, *12*(8), 707–719.

Moss, L. (2008, September 15). Cable's product placements drop 20% in first half: Nielsen. *Multichannel News*, np. Retrieved October 2, 2008, from http://www.multichannel.com/article/CA6596200.html

Motl, S. E., Timpe, E. M., & Eichner, S. F. (2005). Evaluation of accuracy of health studies reported in mass media. *Journal of the American Pharmacists' Association*, *45*(6), 720–725.

Mulac, A., & Giles, H. (1996). "You're only as old as you sound": Perceived vocal age and social meanings. *Health Communication*, *8*, 199–215.

Muller, J. H., Jain, S., Loeser, H., & Irby, D. M. (2008). Lessons learned about integrating a medical school curriculum: Perceptions of students, faculty and curriculum leaders. *Medical Education*, *42*(8), 778–785.

Murquia, A., Peterson, R. A., & Zea, M. C. (2003). Use and implications of ethnomedical health care approaches among Central American immigrants. *Health & Social Work*, *28*(1), 43–51.

Murray, D. (2007, November 2). Hospitals vow a better response. *Medical Economics*, *85*(21), 18.

Murray-Johnson, L., & Witte, K. (2003). Looking toward the future: Health message design strategies. In T. L. Thompson, A. M. Dorsey, K. I. Miller, & R. Parrott (Eds.), *Handbook of health communication* (pp. 473–495). Mahwah, NJ: Lawrence Erlbaum.

Muskin, P. R. (1998). The request to die: Role for a psychodynamic perspective on physician-assisted suicide. *Journal of the American Medical Association*, *279*, 323–328.

Myers, P. N., & Biocca, F. A. (1992, Summer). The elastic body images: The effect of television advertisement and programming on body image distortion of young women. *Journal of Communication*, *42*, 108–133.

Nabi, R. L., & Sullivan, J. L. (2001). Does television viewing relate to engagement in protective action against crime?: A cultivation analysis from a theory of reasoned action perspective. *Communication Research*, *28*(6), 802–825.

Nachreiner, N. M., Gerberich, S. G., Ryan, A. D., & McGovern, P. M. (2007). Minnesota Nurses' Study: Perceptions of violence and the work environment. *Industrial Health*, *45*, 672–678.

Naeem, A. G. (2003). The role of culture and religion in the management of diabetes: A study of Kashmiri men in Leeds. *Journal of the Royal Society of Health*, *123*(2), 110–116.

Nathanson, A. I., & Yang, M.-S. (2003, January). The effects of mediation content and form on children's responses to violent television. *Human Communication research*, *29*(1), 111–134.

National Center for Health Statistics. (2007a). Chartbook on trends in the health of Americans. Hyattsville, MD: Author. Retrieved December 6, 2008, from http://www.cdc.gov/nchs/data/hus/hus07.pdf#027

National Center for Health Statistics. (2007b). Health, United States, 2007. U.S. Department of Health and Human Services Centers for Disease Control and Prevention. Hyattsville, MD. Retrieved July 18, 2008, from www.cdc.gov/nchs/fastats/lifexpec.htm

National Coalition on Health Care. (2008). Health insurance costs. Washington, DC: Author. Retrieved December 29, 2008, from http://www.nchc.org/facts/cost.shtml

National Commission on Adult Literacy. (2008, June). Reach higher, America. Overcoming the crisis in the U.S. workforce. New York: Author. Retrieved December 6, 2008, from http://

www.nationalcommissiononadultliteracy.org/ReachHigherAmerica/ReachHigher.pdf

National Institute on Drug Abuse (NIDA). (2007, December). InfoFacts: High school and youth trends Bethesda, MD: Author. Retrieved October 6, 2008, from http://www.drugabuse.gov/infofacts/hsyouthtrends.html

National Research Council. (1989). *Improving risk communication*. Washington, DC: National Academy Press. Retrieved August 28, 2008, from http://www.nap.edu/openbook.php?isbn=0309039436

Needleman, J., Buerhaus, P. I., Stewart, M., Zelevinsky, K., & Marrke, S. (2006, February). Market watch. Nursing staffing in hospitals: Is there a business case for quality? *Health Affairs*, 25(1), 204–211.

Neighbors, L. A., & Sobal, J. (2007). Prevalence and magnitude of body weight and shape dissatisfaction among university students. *Eating Disorders*, 8, 429–439.

Nelkin, D., & Gilman, S. L. (1991). Placing blame for devastating disease. In A. Mack (Ed.), *In time of plague: The history and social consequences of lethal epidemic disease* (pp. 39–56). New York: New York University Press.

Nemeth, S. A. (2000). Society, sexuality, and disabled/able bodied romantic relationships. In D. O. Braithwaite & T. L. Thompson (Eds.), *Handbook of communication and people with disabilities: Research and applications* (pp. 37–48). Mahwah, NJ: Lawrence Erlbaum.

Nestle, M. (1997, March–April). Alcohol guidelines for chronic disease prevention: From prohibition to moderation. *Nutrition Today*, 32, 86–92.

Neuendorf, K. A. (1990). Health images in the mass media. In E. B. Ray & L. Donohew (Eds.), *Communication and health: Systems and applications* (pp. 111–135). Hillsdale, NJ: Lawrence Erlbaum.

Newbart, D., & Grossman, K. N. (2003, June 24). Court rules in the affirmative. *Chicago Sun-Times*, p. 6.

New CDC study finds no increase in obesity among adults; but levels still high. (2007, November 28).

Hyattsville, MD: National Center for Health Statistics. Retrieved October 7, 2008, from http://www.cdc.gov/nchs/pressroom/07newsreleases/obesity.htm

Newman, M. A. (1986). *Health as expanding consciousness*. St. Louis, MO: C. V. Mosby.

Newman, M. A. (1995). *A developing discipline: Selected works of Margaret Newman*. New York: National League for Nursing Press.

Newman, M. A. (2000). *Health as expanding consciousness* (2nd ed.). Boston: Jones & Bartlett.

New research shows the national truth: youth smoking prevention campaign offset negative effects of decreased state tobacco control funding. (2008, April 3). Washington, DC: American Legacy Foundation. Retrieved September 16, 2008, from http://www.americanlegacy.org/2343.aspx

Newton, B. W., Barber, L., Clardy, J., Cleveland, E., & O'Sullivan, P. (2008). Is there hardening of the heart during medical school? *Academic Medicine*, 83(3), 244–249.

Nichols, J. D. (2003, February). Lawyer's advice on physician conduct with malpractice cases. *Clinical Orthopedics and Related Research*, 407, 14–18.

Niederdeppe, J., Davis, K. C., Farrelly, M. C., & Yarsevich, J. (2007). Stylistic features, need for sensation, and confirmed recall of national smoking prevention advertisements. *Journal of Communication*, 57, 272–292.

Niederdeppe, J., Hornick, R. C., Kelly, B. J., Frosch, D. L., Romantan, A., Stevens, R. S., Barg, F. K., Weiner, J. L., & Schwartz, J. S. (2007). Examining the dimensions of cancer-related information seeking and scanning behavior. *Health Communication*, 22(2), 153–167.

Nielsen reports TV, Internet and mobile usage among Americans. (2008, July 8). New York: Nielson Company. Retrieved October 7, 2008, from http://www.nielsen.com/media/2008/pr_080708.html

Noar, S. M., Clark, A., Cole, C., & Lustria, M. L. A. (2006). Review of interactive safer sex web sites: Practice and potential. *Health Communication*, 20(3), 233–241.

Noar, S. M., Zimmerman, R. S., Palmgreen, P., Lustria, M., & Horosewski, M. L. (2006). Integrating personality and psychosocial theoretical approaches to understanding safer sexual behavior: Implications for message design. *Health Communication, 19*(2), 165–174.

Noland, C., & Walter, J. C. (2006). "It's not our ass": Medical resident sense-making regarding lawsuits. *Health Communication, 20*(1), 81–89.

Norling, G. R. (2005). Developing a theoretical model of rapport building: Implications for medical education and the physician–patient relationship. In M. Haider (Ed.), *Global public health communication* (pp. 407–414). Boston: Jones and Bartlett.

Northouse, P. G., & Northouse, L. L. (1985). *Health communication: A handbook for health professionals.* Englewood Cliffs, NJ: Prentice Hall.

Novack, D. H., Suchman, A. L., Clark, W., Epstein, R. M., Najberg, G. E., & Kaplan, C. (1997). Calibrating the physician: Personal awareness and effective patient care. *Journal of the American Medical Association, 278*, 502–510.

Nowak, G. L., & Siska, M. J. (1995). Using research to inform campaign development and message design. In E. Maibach & R. L. Parrot (Eds.), *Designing health messages: Approaches from communication theory and public health practice* (pp. 169–185). Thousand Oaks, CA: Sage.

Nursing homes say Medicare change will cost them $5 billion. (2008, May 5). *Modern Healthcare, 38*(18), 4.

Nursing lobby to address nursing shortage. (2003, February 10). *PR Newswire.* Retrieved August 8, 2003, through LexisNexis.

Nussbaum, J. F. (2007). Life span communication and quality of life. Presidential address. *Journal of Communication, 57*, 1–7.

Nussbaum, J. F., Baringer, D., Fisher, C. L., & Kundrat, A. L. (2008). Connecting health, communication, and aging. In L. Sparks, H. D. O'Hair, & G. L. Kreps (Eds.), *Cancer, communication and aging* (pp. 67–76). Cresskill, NJ: Hampton Press.

Nussbaum, J. F., & Coupland, J. (Eds.). (2004). *Handbook of communication and aging research* (2nd ed.). Mahwah, NJ: Erlbaum.

Nussbaum, J. F., Pecchioni, L., Grant, J. A., & Folwell, A. (2000). Explaining illness to older adults: The complexities of the provider–patient interaction as we age. In B. B. Whaley (Ed.), *Explaining illness* (pp. 171–194). Mahwah, NJ: Lawrence Erlbaum.

Nussbaum, J. F., Pecchioni, L. L., Robinson, J. D., & Thompson, T. L. (2000). *Communication and aging* (2nd ed.). Mahwah, NJ: Lawrence Erlbaum.

Nussbaum, J. F., Ragan, S., & Whaley, B. (2003). Children, older adults, and women: Impact on provider–patient interaction. In T. L. Thompson, A. M. Dorsey, K. I. Miller, & R. Parrott (Eds.), *Handbook of health communication* (pp. 183–204). Mahwah, NJ: Lawrence Erlbaum.

Nussbaum, J. F., Thompson, T., & Robinson, J. D. (1989). *Communication and aging.* Cambridge, MA: Harper & Row.

Obermann, K., Jowett, M. R., Alcantara, M. O. O., Banzon, E. P., & Bodard, C. (2006). Social health insurance in a developing country: The case of the Philippines. *Social Science & Medicine, 62*, 3177–3185.

Occupational Safety & Health Administration, U.S. Department of Labor. (2004). Guidelines for preventing workplace violence for health care and social service workers. Retrieved October 23, 2008, from http://www.osha.gov/Publications/OSHA3148/osha3148.html

O'Connell, B., Bailey, S., & Pearce, J. (2003). Straddling the pathway from pediatrician to mainstream health care: Transition issues experienced in disability care. *Australian Journal of Rural Health, 11*(2), 57–63.

O'Connor, K. (2008, April 13). Catamount health faces six-month checkup. *Rutland Herald* (Rutland, VT). Retrieved August 11, 2008, from www.rutlandherald.com/apps/pbcs.dll/article?AID=/20080413/NEWS04/804130424/-1/LEGISLATURE05

Oetzel, J., DeVargas, F., Ginossar, T., & Sanchez, C. (2007). Hispanic women's preferences for breast health information: Subjective cultural influences on source, message, and channel. *Health Communication, 21*(3), 223–233.

O'Keefe, D. J., & Jensen, J. D. (2007, October). The relative persuasiveness of gain-framed loss-framed messages for encouraging disease prevention behaviors: A meta-analytic review. *Journal of Health Communication, 12*(7), 623–644.

O'Leary, S. C. B., Federico, S., & Hampers, L. C. (2003). The truth about language barriers: One residency program's experience. *Pediatrics, 111*(5), 1100.

Oliver, M. B., & Kalyanaraman, S. (2002). Appropriate for all viewing audiences? An examination of violent and sexual portrayals in movie previews featured on video rentals. *Journal of Broadcasting & Electronic Media, 46*(2), 283–299.

Olson, A. L., Gaffney, C. A., Lee, P. W., & Starr, P. (2008). Changing adolescent health behaviors: The healthy teens counseling approach. *American Journal of Preventive Medicine. 35*(5), S359–S3564.

Olson, L. G., & Ambrogetti, A. (1998). Working harder—working dangerously? Fatigue and performance in hospitals. *Medical Journal of Australia, 168*, 614–616.

O'Malley, A. S., & Reschovsky, J. D. (2006, May). No exodus: Physicians and managed care networks. Center for Studying Health System Change. Retrieved July 23, 2008, from www.hschange.com/CONTENT/838

100 most powerful people in healthcare. (2002, August 26). *Modern Healthcare, 32*, 7.

100 most powerful people in healthcare. (2008, August 25). *Modern Healthcare, 38*, 56.

Online usage: 2008 survey of health care consumers. (2008). Deloitte. Retrieved October 30, 2008, from http://www.deloitte.com/dtt/article/0,1002,cid%253D192702,00.html

Orbe, M. P., & King, G., III. (2000). Negotiating the tension between policy and reality: Exploring nurses' communication about organizational wrongdoing. *Health Communication, 12*(1), 41–61.

Oregon begins paying for assisted suicide. (1998, December 9). *Academic universe* (vol. 2). LexisNexis Mealey Publications.

Organ donation: Don't let these 10 myths confuse you. (2008). Rochester, MN: Mayo Clinic. Retrieved December 15, 2008, from http://www.mayoclinic.com/health/organ-donation/FL00077

OrganDonor.Gov. (2008). Access to U.S. government information on organ & tissue donation and transplantation. Washington, DC: U.S. Department of Health and Human Services. Retrieved December 15, 2008, from http://www.organdonor.gov

Ornish, D., Scherwitz, L., W., Billings, J. H., Gould, K. L., Merritt, T. A., Sparler, S., Armstrong, W. T., Ports, T. A., Kirkeeide, R. L., Hogeboom, C., & Brand, R. J. (1998). Intensive lifestyle changes for reversal of coronary heart disease. *Journal of the American Medical Association, 280*, 2001.

Orr, R. D. (1996). Transcultural medical care. *American Family Physician, 53*, 2004–2007.

Ota, H., Giles, H., & Somera, L. P. (2007). Beliefs about intra- and intergenerational communication in Japan, the Philippines, and the United States: Implications for older adults' subjective well-being. *Communication Studies, 58*(2), 173–188.

Ovalle, P. P. (2008, October 30). Viva Viagra! Or, how race dances around erectile dysfunction. *Flow TV*, online. Retrieved December 22, 2008, from http://flowtv.org/?p=2128

Paek, H.-J. (2008). Mechanisms through which adolescents attend and respond to antismoking media campaigns. *Journal of Communication, 58*, 84–105.

Pahal, J. S. (2006). The dynamics of resident-patient communication: Data from Canada. *Communication & Medicine, 3*(2), 161–170.

Panchak, P. (2003, November 1). Lean health care? It works! *Industry Week*. Retrieved October 16, 2008, from http://www.industryweek.com/ReadArticle.aspx?ArticleID=1331

Pardun, C. J. (2005). Changing attitudes, changing the world. Media's portrayal of people with intellectual disabilities. Special Olympics Report. Retrieved October 6, 2008, from http://www.specialolympics.org/NR/rdonlyres/eptchdrhwvdflwsrgeuegszs3xcau26ggwblw7635ux2ecg6iyahhrm6gtfxenwq7astcfh7dw2jklyfop6ksnzinkh/CACW_Media_A4.pdf

Parker, B. J. (1998, Spring). Exploring life themes and myths in alcohol advertisements through a meaning-based model of advertising experiences. *Journal of Advertising, 27,* 97–112.

Parker-Pope, T. (2002, November 11). Viagra is misunderstood despite name recognition. *Wall Street Journal,* online. Retrieved December 23, 2008, from http://www.usrf.org/breakingnews/bn_111202_viagra/bn_111202_viagra.html

Parkes, C. M. (1998). The dying adult. *British Medical Journal, 316,* 1313–1315.

Parrott, R. L. (1995). Motivation to attend to health messages: Presentation of content and linguistic considerations. In E. Maibach & R. L. Parrott (Eds.), *Designing health messages: Approaches from communication theory and public health practice* (pp. 7–23). Thousand Oaks, CA: Sage.

Parrott, R., Hopfer, S., Ghetian, C., & Lengerich, E. (2007). Mapping as a visual health communication tool: Promises and dilemmas. *Health Communication, 22*(1), 13–24.

Parrott, R., & Polonec, L. (2008). Preventing green tobacco sickness in farming youth: A behavioral adaptation to health communication in health campaigns. In K. B. Wright & S. D. Moore (Eds.), *Applied health communication* (pp. 341–359). Cresskill, NJ: Hampton Press.

Parrott, R., Silk, K., Krieger, J. R., Harris, T., & Condit, C. (2004). Behavioral health outcomes associated with religious faith and media exposure about human genetics. *Health Communication, 16*(1), 29–45.

Pascale, R. T. (1999). Leading from a different place: Applying complexity theory to tap potential. In J. A. Conger, G. M. Spreitzer, & E. E. Lawler, III (Eds.), *The leader's change handbook: An essential guide to setting direction and taking action* (pp. 195–220). San Francisco: Jossey-Bass.

Patel, D. S. (2005). Social mobilization as a tool for outreach programs in the HIV/AIDS crisis. In M. Haider (Ed.), *Global public health communication: Challenges, perspectives, and strategies* (pp. 91–102). Boston: Jones and Bartlett.

Paterniti, D. A., Pan, R. J., Smith, L. F., Horan, N. M., & West, D. C. (2006). From physician-centered to community-centered perspectives on health care: Assessing the efficacy of community-based training. *Academic Medicine, 81*(4), 347–353.

Patient and family perceptions of nursing home care. (2006). The Commonwealth Fund. Retrieved November 17, 2008, from http://www.commonwealthfund.org/snapshotscharts/snapshotscharts_show.htm?doc_id=413504

Patient perceptions of physician interpersonal quality of care. (2006, December). The Commonwealth Fund. Retrieved November 17, 2008, from http://www.commonwealthfund.org/snapshotscharts/snapshotscharts_show.htm?doc_id=381936

Patient satisfaction planner: Unsatisfactory stay sparks Planetree care model. (2007, September 1). *Hospital Peer Review,* np.

Pearson, J. C., & Nelson, P. E. (1991). *Understanding and sharing* (5th ed.). Dubuque, IA: Wm. C. Brown.

Pendleton, D., Schofield, T., Tate, P., & Havelock, P. (1984). *The consultant: An approach to learning and teaching.* Oxford: Oxford University Press.

Pepicello, J. A., & Murphy, E. C. (1996). Integrating medical and operational management. *Physician Executive, 22,* 4–9.

Perry, B. (2002, November). Growth and satisfaction: "I became a nurse because I wanted to help others." *Canadian Business and Current Affairs, 98*(10), np.

Perse, E. M., Nathanson, A. I., & McLeod, D. M. (1996). Effects of spokesperson sex, public announcement appeal, and involvement in safe-sex PSA's. *Health Communication, 8,* 171–189.

Pesky, S., & Blascovich, J. (2007). Immersive virtual environments versus traditional platforms:

Effects of violent and nonviolent video game play. *Media Psychology, 10*(1), 135–156.

Peter, J. (2003, June 16). Pilot launched to increase diversity in medical field. Associated Press. Retrieved August 8, 2003, through LexisNexis.

Peter, J., & Valkenburg, P. M. (2006). Adolescents' exposure to sexually explicit online material and recreational attitudes toward sex. *Journal of Communication, 56*, 639–660.

Peters, E., Lipkus, I., & Diefenbach, M. A. (2006). The functions of affect in health communications and in the construction of health preferences. *Journal of Communication, 56*, S140–S162.

Peterson, E. D., Shah, B. R., Parsons, L., Pollack, C.V., Jr., French, W. J., Canto, J. G., Gibson, C. M., & Rogers, W. J. (2008). Trends in quality of care for patients with acute myocardial infarction in the National Registry of Myocardial Infarction from 1990 to 2006. *American Heart Journal, 156*(6), 1045–1055.

Petraglia, J. (2007). Narrative intervention in behavior and public health. *Journal of Health Communication, 12*(5), 493–505.

Petty, R. E., & Cacioppo, J. T. (1981). *Attitudes and persuasion: Classic and contemporary approaches.* Dubuque, IA: Wm. C. Brown.

Petty, R. E., & Cacioppo, J. T. (1986). *Communication and persuasion: Central and peripheral routes to attitude change.* New York: Springer.

Pexton, C. (nd). Framing the need to improve health care using Six Sigma methodologies. iSixSigma. Retrieved October 16, 2008, from http://healthcare.isixsigma.com/library/content/c030513a.asp

Philpott, A., Knerr, W., & Maher, D. (2006). Promoting protection and pleasure: Amplifying the effectiveness of barriers against sexually transmitted infections and pregnancy. Viewpoint. *The Lancet* (www.thelancet.com), *368*, pp. 1–4. Retrieved September 1, 2008, from http://www.thepleasureproject.org/content/File/Pleasure_Lancet_Dec06.pdf

Physicians and surgeons. (2008). Occupational outlook handbook, 2008–09 edition. Washington, DC: U.S. Department of Labor. Retrieved November 11, 2008, from http://www.bls.gov/oco/ocos074.htm

Physicians are becoming engaged in addressing disparities. (2005, April). Institute for Ethics at the American Medical Association. Retrieved December 3, 2008, from http://www.ama-assn.org/ama/pub/category/14969.html

Physicians divided on impact of CAM on U.S. health care; aromatherapy fares poorly, acupuncture touted. (2005, September 9). *Business Wire*, np. Retrieved October 23, 2008, from http://www.businesswire.com/portal/site/google/index.jsp?ndmViewId=news_view&newsId=20050909005437&newsLang=en

Physicians report growing dissatisfaction with "business" of medicine. (2008). Locum Tenens. Retrieved July 31, 2008, from www.locumtenens.com/physician-careers/Business-of-Medicine.aspx

Physician workforce policy guidelines for the United States, 2000–2020. (2005, January). Rockville, MD: Council on Graduate Medical Education. Retrieved October 20, 2008, from http://www.cogme.gov/report16.htm#sumrec

Pick, S., Givaudan, M., & Poortinga, Y. H. (2003). Sexuality and life skills education: A multistrategy intervention in Mexico. *American Psychologist, 58*(3), 230–234.

Pickering, A. (1995). *The mangle of practice: Time, agency, and science.* Chicago: University of Chicago Press.

Pilling, V. K., & Brannon, L. A. (2007). Assessing college students' attitudes toward responsible drinking messages to identify promising binge drinking intervention strategies. *Health Communication, 22*(3), 265–276.

Pincus, C. R. (1995). Why medicine is driving doctors crazy. *Medical Economics, 72*, 40–44.

Pinkleton, B. E., Austin, E. W., Cohen, M., Miller, A., & Fitzgerald, E. (2007). A statewide evaluation of the effectiveness of media literacy training to prevent tobacco use among adolescents. *Health Communication, 21*(1), 23–34.

Piotrow, P. T., Rimon, J. G., II, Payne Merritt, A., & Saffitz, G. (2003). Advancing health communication: The PCS experience in the field.

Center Publication 103. Baltimore: Johns Hopkins Bloomberg School of Public Health/Center for Communication Programs. Retrieved August 7, 2008, from http://www.jhuccp.org/pubs/cp/103/103.pdf

Piper, I., Shvarts, S., & Lurie, S. (2008). Women's preferences for their gynecologist or obstetrician. *Patient Education and Counseling, 72*(1), 109–114.

Plane passengers sue TB patient. (2007, July 13). CNN.com/health. Retrieved August 26, 2008, from http://www.cnn.com/2007/HEALTH/conditions/07/12/tb.suit/index.html

Platt, F. W. (1992). *Conversational failure: Case studies in doctor–patient communication.* Tacoma, WA: Essential Science.

Platt, F. W. (1995). *Conversation repair: Case studies in doctor–patient communication.* Boston: Little, Brown.

Platt, F. W., & Gordon, G. H. (2004). *Field guide to the difficult patient interview* (2nd ed.). Philadelphia: Lippincott Williams & Wilkins.

Pollar, O. (1998, December). A diverse workforce requires balanced leadership. *Workforce, 77,* S4–S5.

Polonec, L. D., Major, A. M., & Atwood, L. E. (2006). Evaluating the believability and effectiveness of the social norms message "Most students drink 0 to 4 drinks when they party." *Health Communication, 20*(1), 23–34.

Porter-O'Grady, T., Bradley, C., Crow, G., & Hendrich, A. L. (1997, Winter). After a merger: The dilemma of the best leadership approach for nursing. *Nursing Administration Quarterly, 21,* 8–19.

Potter, J. E. (2002). Do ask, do tell. *Annals of Internal Medicine, 137*(5), 341–343.

Potter, W. J. (1998). *Media Literacy.* Thousand Oaks, CA: Sage.

Powell, J. H. (2003, June 17). More minority docs: Representation lacks for races suffering more. *Boston Herald,* p. 28.

Prescription drug trends. (2008, September). Menlo Park, CA: Henry J. Kaiser Family Foundation. Retrieved October 2, 2008, from http://www.kff.org/rxdrugs/upload/3057_07.pdf

Press, I. (2002). *Patient satisfaction: Defining, measuring, and improving the experience of care.* Chicago: Health Administration Press.

Probst, J. C., Greenhouse, D. L., & Selassie, A. W. (1997). Patient and physician satisfaction with an outpatient care visit. *Journal of Family Practice, 45,* 418–426.

Prochaska, J. O., & DiClemente, C. C. (1983). Stages and processes of self-change of smoking: Toward an integrative model of change. *Journal of Consulting and Clinical Psychology, 51,* 390–395.

Prochaska, J. O., DiClemente, C. C., & Norcross, J. C. (1992). In search of how people change applications to the addictive behaviors. *American Psychologist, 47,* 1102–1114.

Prochaska, J. O., Johnson, S., & Lee, P. (1998). The transtheoretical model of behavior change. In S. A. Shumaker, E. B. Schron, J. K. Ockene, & W. L. McBee (Eds.), *The handbook of behavior change* (2nd ed., pp. 59–84). New York: Springer-Verlag.

Purnell, L. D. (2008, February). Traditional Vietnamese health and healing. *Urologic Nursing, 28*(1), 63–67.

Putnam, L., & Poole, M. S. (1987). Conflict and negotiation. In F. Jablin, L. Putnam, K. Roberts, & L. Porter (Eds.), *Handbook of organizational communication* (pp. 549–599). Newbury Park, CA: Sage.

Query, J. L., Jr., & Wright, K. (2003). Assessing communication competence in an online study: Toward informing subsequent interventions among older adults with cancer, their lay caregivers, and peers. *Health Communication, 15*(2), 203–218.

Quesada, A., & Summers, S. L. (1998, January). Literacy in the cyberage: Teaching kids to be media savvy. *Technology & Learning, 18,* 30–36.

Quick, B. L., & Stephenson, M. T. (2007). Authoritative parenting and issue involvement as indicators of ad recall: An empirical investigation of anti-drug ads for parents. *Health Communication, 22*(1), 25–35.

Quittner, J. (1995, April 17). Back to the real world. *Time, 145,* 56–57.

Rabak-Wagener, J., Eickhoff-Shemek, J., & Kelly-Vance, L. (1998, July). The effect of media analysis on attitudes and behaviors regarding body images among college students. *Journal of American College Health, 47*, 29–35.

Raffel, M. W., & Raffel, N. K. (1989). *The U.S. health system: Origins and functions* (3rd ed.). New York: John Wiley & Sons.

Ragan, S. L. (1990). Verbal play and multiple goals in the gynecological exam interaction. *Journal of Language and Social Psychology, 9*, 67–84.

Ragan, S. L., & Goldsmith, J. (2008). End-of-life communication: The drama of pretense in the talk of dying patients and their M.D. In K. B. Wright & S. D. Moore (Eds.), *Applied health communication* (pp. 207–227). Cresskill, NJ: Hampton Press.

Ragan, S. L., Wittenberg, E., & Hall, H. T. (2003). The communication of palliative care for the elderly cancer patient. *Health Communication, 15*(2), 219–226.

Rains, S. A. (2007). Perceptions of traditional information sources and use of the World Wide Web to seek health information: Findings for the Health Information National Trends Survey. *Journal of Health Communication, 12*(7), 667–680.

Rains, S. A. (2008a, January/March). Seeking health information in the information age: The role of Internet self-efficacy. *Western Journal of Communication, 72*(1), 1–18.

Rains, S. A. (2008b, June). Health at high speed: Broadband Internet access, health communication, and the digital divide. *Communication Research, 35*(3), 283–297.

Rains, S. A., & Turner, M. M. (2007). Psychological reactance and persuasive health communication: A test and extension of the intertwined model. *Human Communication Research, 33*(2), 241–269.

Ramanadhan, S., & Viswanath, K. (2006). Health and the information nonseeker: A profile. *Health Communication, 20*(2), 131–139.

Ramirez, A. J., Graham, J., Richards, M. A., Cull, A., & Gregory, W. M. (1996). Mental health of hospital consultants: The effects of stress and satisfaction at work. *The Lancet, 347*, 724–729.

Ramstack, T. (2004, June 22). Court shields HMOs from malpractice; justices limit lawsuits over doctor-ordered care. *Washington Times*, Page One, p. A01.

Ratanawongsa, N., Roter, D., Beach, M. C., Laird, S. L., Larson, S. M., Carson, K. A., & Cooper, L. A. (2008). Physician burnout and patient–physician communication during primary care encounters. *Journal of General Internal Medicine, 23*(10), 1581–1588.

Ratzan, S., & Meltzer, W. (2005). (2005). State of the art in crisis communication: Past lessons and principles of practice. In M. Haider (Ed.), *Global public health communication: Challenges, perspectives, and strategies* (pp. 321–347). Boston: Jones and Bartlett.

Rawlins, W. K. (1989). A dialectical analysis of the tensions, functions, and strategic challenges of communication in young adult friendships. *Communication Yearbook, 12*, 157–189.

Rawlins, W. K. (1992). *Friendship matters: Communication, dialectics, and the life course*. New York: Aldine De Gruyter.

Ray, E. B. (1983). Identifying job stress in a human service organization. *Journal of Applied Communication Research, 11*, 109–119.

Reality check: 2008 survey of health care consumers. (2008). Deloitte. Retrieved November 17, 2008, from http://www.deloitte.com/dtt/article/0,1002,cid=192468,00.html

Reducing health disparities in Asian American and Pacific Islander populations. (2005). Management Sciences of Health. Office of Minority Health and Bureau of Primary Health Care. Retrieved December 23, 2008, from http://erc.msh.org/aapi/ca6.html

Rees, A. M. (1994). Consumer enlightenment or consumer confusion? *Consumer Health Information Source Book, 4*, 10–11.

Reese, S. (2008, April 18). Pick up the mouse, put down the phone: Trading e-mails with patients is easier than playing phone tag, and you may even get paid for it. *Medical Economics, 85*(8), 24–28.

Reflections on health promotion and interactive technology: A discussion with David Gustafson, Jack Wennberg, and Tony Gorry. (1997). In R. L. Street Jr., W. R. Gold, & T. Manning (Eds.), *Health promotion and interactive technology: Theoretical applications and future directions* (pp. 221–236). Mahwah, NJ: Lawrence Erlbaum.

Regan-Smith, M. G., Obenshain, S. S., Woodward, C., Richards, B., Zeitz, H. J., & Parker, A. S., Jr. (1994). Rote learning in medical schools. *Journal of the American Medical Association, 272,* 1380–1381.

Registered nurse population: Findings from the 2004 national sample survey of registered nurses. (2007, March). Washington, DC: U.S. Department of Health and Human Services. Retrieved October 21, 2008, from http://bhpr.hrsa.gov/healthworkforce/rnsurvey04

Reilly, D. R. (2003, Winter). Not just a patient: The dangers of dual relationships. *Canadian Journal of Rural Medicine, 8*(1), np.

Reilly, P. (1987). *To do no harm: A journey through medical school.* Dover, MA: Auburn House.

Reinberg, S. (2008, October 29). U.S. hospitals lag in patient satisfaction. *Health Day* online. Retrieved November 14, 2008, from http://www.healthday.com/Article.asp?AID=620778

Reinhardt, J. P. (Ed.). (2001). *Negative and positive support.* Mahwah, NJ: Lawrence Erlbaum.

Reinhardt, J. P., Boerner, K., & Horowitz, A. (2006). Good to have but not to use: Differential impact of perceived and received support on well-being. *Journal of Social and Personal Relationships, 23*(1), 117–129.

Reis, R. (2008). How Brazilian and North American newspapers frame the stem cell research debate. *Science Communication, 29*(3), 316–334.

Reiser, S. J. (1978). *Medicine and the reign of technology.* Cambridge: Cambridge University Press.

Renganathan, E., Hosein, E., Parks, W., Lloyd, L., Suhaili, M. R., & Odugleh, A. (2005). Communication-for-behavioral-impact (COMB): A review of WHO's experiences with strategic social mobilization and communication in the prevention and control of communicable diseases. In M. Haider (Ed.), *Global public health communication: Challenges, perspectives, and strategies* (pp. 305–320). Boston: Jones and Bartlett.

Residents' decreased duty-hours may have downside. (2007, August 3). *Medical Economics, 85*(15), 12.

Reynolds, B. (2006, August). Response to best practices. *Journal of Applied Communication Research, 34*(4), 249–252.

Rhodes, S. D., Yee, L. J., & Hergenrather, K. C. (2003). Hepatitis A vaccination among young African American men who have sex with men in the deep south: Psychosocial predictors. *Journal of the American Medical Association, 95*(4), 31S–36S.

Rifkin, L. (2008, March 21). Still a privilege to be a doctor: Though not immune to the hassles and hardships of practice, this physician tells why he experiences the joy of medicine. *Medical Economics, 85*(6), 28–29.

Rimal, R. (2000). Closing the knowledge–behavior gap in health promotion: The mediating role of self-efficacy. *Health Communication, 12*(3), 219–238.

Rimal, R. N. (2008, March/April). Modeling the relationship between descriptive norms and behaviors: A test and extension of the theory of normative social behavior (TNSB). *Health Communication, 23*(2), 103–116.

Rimal, R. N., & Adkins, D. A. (2003). Using computers to narrowcast health messages: The role of audience segmentation, targeting, and tailoring in health promotion. In T. L. Thompson, A. M. Dorsey, K. I. Miller, & R. Parrott (Eds.), *Handbook of health communication* (pp. 497–513). Mahwah, NJ: Lawrence Erlbaum.

Rimal, R. N., & Morrison, D. (2006). A uniqueness to personal threat (UPT) hypothesis: How similarity affects perceptions of susceptibility and severity in risk assessment. *Health Communication, 20*(3), 209–219.

Rimal, R. N., Ratzan, S. C., Arnston, P., & Freimuth, V. S. (1997). Reconceptualizing the "patient": Health care promotion as increasing citizens' decision-making competencies. *Health Communication, 9,* 61–74.

Rimal, R. N., & Real, K. (2005, June). How behaviors are influenced by perceived norms: A test of the theory of normative social behavior. *Communication Research, 32,* 389–414.

Rimer, B. K., & Kreuter, M. W. (2006). Advancing tailored health communication: A persuasive and message effects perspective. *Journal of Communication, 56,* S184–S201.

Ritzer, G. (1993). *The McDonaldization of Society.* Thousand Oaks, CA: Pine Forge Press.

Robert Wood Johnson Foundation. (2001). National program project report on urban hospital closing, mergers, and other reconfigurations. Retrieved August 13, 2003, from www.rwjf.org/reports/grr/0208054.htm

Robert Wood Johnson Foundation. (2008, April 29). Cost of insurance far outpaces income. Princeton, NJ: Author. Retrieved August 14, 2008, from www.rwjf.org/programareas/resources/product.jsp?id=28698&pid=1132

Roberto, A. J., Zimmerman, R. S., Carlyle, K. E., Abner, E. L., Cupp, P. K., & Hansen, G. L. (2007). The effects of computer-based pregnancy, STD, and HIV prevention intervention: A nine-school trial. *Health Communication, 21*(2), 115–124.

Roberts, L., & Bucksey, S. J. (2007). Communicating with patients: What happens in practice? *Physical Therapy, 87*(5), 587–594.

Robertson, T. (1999, March 26). Michigan jury gets Kevorkian case: Defendant cites civil rights leaders. *Boston Globe,* p. A3.

Robinson, J. D. (2003). An interactional structure of medical activities during acute visits and its implications for patients' participation. *Health Communication, 15*(1), 27–58.

Robinson, T., Callister, M., Magoffin, D., & Moore, J. (2006). The portrayal of older characters in Disney animated films. *Journal of Aging Studies, 21,* 203–213.

Rodriguez, H. P., Anastario, M. P., Frankel, R. M., Odigie, E. G., Rogers, W. H., von Glahn, T., & Safran, D. G. (2008). Can teaching agenda-setting skills to physicians improve clinical interaction quality? A controlled intervention. *BMC Medical Education, 8,* 3–7.

Rodwin, M. A. (1995). Strains in the fiduciary metaphor: Divided physician loyalties and obligations in a changing health care system. *American Journal of Law & Medicine, 21,* 241–257.

Rogers, E. M. (1973). *Communication strategies for family planning.* New York: Free Press.

Rogers, E. M. (1983). *Diffusion of innovations* (3rd ed.). New York: The Free Press.

Rogers, E. M., & Dearing, J. W. (1988). Agenda-setting research: Where has it been, where is it going? In J. A. Anderson (Ed.), *Communication yearbook* (11th ed., pp. 555–593). Newbury Park, CA: Sage.

Rogers, M. E. (1986). Science of unitary human beings. In V. M. Malinski (Ed.), *Explorations of Martha Rogers' science of unitary human beings* (pp. 3–14). Norwalk, CT: Appleton-Century-Crofts.

Roizen, M. F., & Oz, M. C. (2006). *YOU: The smart patient.* Washington, DC: Free Press.

Rollnick, S., & Miller, W. (1995). What is motivational interviewing? *Behavioural and Cognitive Psychotherapy, 23,* 325–334. Reprinted online. Retrieved October 30, 2008, from http://www.motivationalinterview.org/clinical/whatismi.html

Romer, D., Jamieson, K. H., & Aday, S. (2003, March). Television news and the fear of crime. *Journal of Communication, 53*(1), NA.

Rook, K. S. (1995). Support, companionship, and control in older adults' social networks: Implications for well-being. In J. F. Nussbaum & J. Coupland (Eds.), *Handbook of communication and aging* (pp. 437–463). Mahwah, NJ: Lawrence Erlbaum.

Rooney, J. J., & Vanden Heuvel, L. N. (2004, July). Root cause analysis for beginners. *Quality Progress, 37*(7), 45.

Rose, M., Manser, T., & Ware, J. C. (2008). Effects of call on sleep and mood in internal medicine residents. *Behavioral Sleep Medicine, 6*(2), 75–88.

Rosen, I. M., Gimotty, P. A., Shea, J. A., & Bellini, L. M. (2006). Evolution of sleep quantity, sleep deprivation, mood disturbances, empathy, and burnout among interns. *Academic Medicine, 81*(1), 82–85.

Rosenberg, J. (1996). When patients die. *American Medical News, 39,* 14–18.

Rosenstein, A. H., & O'Daniel, M. (2008). Managing disruptive physician behavior: Impact on staff relationships and patient care. *Neurology, 70*(17), 1564–1570.

Rosenstock, I. M. (1960). What research in motivation suggests for public health. *American Journal of Public Health, 50,* 295–301.

Rosenthal, S. L., Lewis, L. M., Succop, P. A., Burklow, K. A., Nelson, P. R., Shedd, K. D., Heyman, R. B., & Biro, F. M. (1999). Adolescents' views regarding sexual history taking. *Clinical Pediatrics, 38*(4), 227–233.

Rossiter, C. M., Jr. (1975). Defining "therapeutic communication." *Journal of Communication, 25*(3), 127–130.

Roter, D., & Hall, J. A. (1992). Improving talk through interventions. *Doctors talking with patients/patients talking with doctors: Improving communication in medical visits.* Westport, CT: Auburn House.

Roter, D. L., Larson, S., Sands, D. Z., Ford, D. E., & Houston, T. (2008). Can e-mail messages between patients and physicians be patient-centered? *Health Communication, 23*(1), 80–86.

Roter, D. L., Stewart, M., Putnam, S. M., Lipkin, J., Jr., Stiles, W., & Iniu, T. S. (1997). Communication patterns of primary care physicians. *Journal of the American Medical Association, 277,* 350–357.

Rothman, A. J., Bartels, R. D., Wlaschin, J., & Salovey, P. (2006). The strategic use of gain- and loss-framed messages. *Journal of Communication, 56,* S202–S220.

Rothman, A. J., & Salovey, P. (1997). Shaping perceptions to motivate healthy behavior: The role of message framing. *Psychological Bulletin, 121,* 3–19.

Rouner, D., & Lindsey, R. (2006). Female adolescent communication about sexually transmitted diseases. *Health Communication, 19*(1), 29–38.

Rowe, S., & Toner, C. (2003). Dietary supplement use in women: The Role of the media. *Journal of Nutrition, 133*(6), 2008S–2009S.

Rubenstein, D. (2008, March 10). Guidelines to achieving diversity: ACHE points the way to hospitals seeking to broad their workforce. *Modern Healthcare, 38*(10), 48.

Rucinski, D. (2004, August). Community boundedness, personal relevance, and the knowledge gap. *Communication Research, 31*(4), 472–495.

Rudolph, J. (2008, March 7). Bonding with patients when time is scarce: Even the busiest physician can find time to convey caring and concern. *Medical Economics, 85*(5), 50–51.

Ruppert, R. A. (1996, March). Caring for the lay caregiver. *American Journal of Nursing, 96,* 40–46.

Russo, A., Jiang, J., & Barrett, J. (2007, August). Trends in potentially preventable hospitalizations among adults and children, 1997–2004. Rockville, MD: Healthcare Cost and Utilization Project. Retrieved December 1, 2008, from http://www.hcup-us.ahrq.gov/reports/statbriefs/sb36.pdf

Rutledge, M. S., & McLaughlin, C. G. (2008, October). Hispanics and health insurance coverage. Robert Wood Johnson Foundation. Retrieved December 21, 2008, from http://www.rwjf.org/pr/product.jsp?id=35728

Ryan, E. B., Anas, A. P., & Vuckovich, M. (2007). The effects of age, hearing loss, and communication difficulty on first impressions. *Communication Research Reports, 24*(1), 13–19.

Ryan, E. B., & Butler, R. N. (1996). Communication, aging, and health: Toward understanding health provider relationships with older clients. *Health Communication, 8,* 191–197.

Ryff, C. D., & Singer, B. H. (Eds.) (2001). *Emotion, social relationships, and health.* New York: Oxford University Press.

Saha, S., Guiton, G., Wimmers, P. F., & Wilkerson, L. (2008). Student body racial and ethnic composition and diversity-related outcomes in U.S. medical schools. *Journal of the American Medical Association, 300*(10), 1135–1145.

Salamon, J. (2008, May 26). My year inside Maimonides: A hospital with a polyglot patient body learns the importance of communication. *Modern Healthcare, 38*(21), 24.

Salander, P. (2002). Bad news from the patient's perspective: An analysis of the written narratives of newly diagnosed cancer patients. *Social Science & Medicine, 55,* 721–732.

Salmon, C. T., & Atkin, C. (2003). Using media campaigns for health promotion. In T. L. Thompson, A. M. Dorsey, K. I. Miller, & R. Parrott (Eds.), *Handbook of health communication* (pp. 449–472). Mahwah, NJ: Lawrence Erlbaum.

Sandberg, H. (2007). A matter of looks: The framing of obesity in four Swedish daily newspapers. *European Journal of Communication Research, 32*(4), 447–472.

Sanders, L. (2003). The ethics imperative. *Modern Healthcare, 33*(11), 46.

Sandman, P. M. (2006a). Telling 9/11 emergency responders to wear their masks. In Comments and questions (and some answers). The Peter Sandman Risk Communication Website. Retrieved September 1, 2008, from http://www.psandman.com/gst2006.htm

Sandman, P. M. (2006b, August). Crisis communication best practices: Some quibbles and additions. *Journal of Applied Communication Research, 34*(3), 257–262.

Sanghavi, D. (2008, March 9). When science meets the soul. Maria and Jose Azevedo had to choose: Allow their baby to die a preventable death or save him while acting against their religion. The doctor who helped guide them shares their story. *Boston Globe,* p. 28.

Scheide, R. V. (2006, January 25). Viagra and the culture of manhood. *Creating Loafing,* online. Retrieved December 24, 2008, from http://charlotte.creativeloafing.com/gyrobase/Content?oid=oid%3A7280

Schein, E. H. (1986). *Organizational culture and leadership.* San Francisco: Jossey-Bass.

Schmid Mast, M., Hall, J. A., & Roter, D. (2007). Disentangling physician sex and physician communication style: Their effects on patient satisfaction in a virtual medical visit. *Patient Education and Counseling, 68,* 16–22.

Schmid Mast, M., Hall, J. A., & Roter, D. (2008). Caring and dominance affect participants' perceptions and behaviors during a virtual medical visit. *Journal of General Internal Medicine, 23*(5), 523–527.

Schneider, M-J. (2006). *Introduction to public health* (2nd ed.). Boston: Jones and Bartlett.

Schoen, C., Davis, K., & Collins, S. R. (2008, May/June). Building blocks for reform: Achieving universal coverage with private and public health insurance. *Health Affairs, 27*(3), 646–657.

Schoen, C., Osborn, R., Doty, M. M., Bishop, M., Peugh, J., & Murukutla, N. (2007). Toward higher-performance health systems: Adults' health care experiences in seven countries, 2007. Web exclusives. *Health Affairs, 26*(6), w717–w734. Retrieved August 19, 2008, from content.healthaffairs.org/cgi/search?andorexactfulltext=and&resourcetype=1&disp_type=&author1=schoen&fulltext=&pubdate_year=&volume=&firstpage=

Scholl, J. C. (2007). The use of humor to promote patient-centered care. *Journal of Applied Communication Research, 35*(2), 156–176.

Schooler, C., Chaffee, S. H., Flora, J. A., & Roser, C. (1998). Health campaign channels: Tradeoffs among reach, specificity, and impact. *Health Communication Research, 24,* 410–432.

Schopler, J. H., & Galinsky, M. J. (1993). Support groups as open systems: A model for practice and research. *Health and Social Work, 18,* 195–207.

Schreiber, L. (2005). The importance of precision in language: Communication research and (so-called) alternative medicine. *Health Communication, 17*(2), 173–190.

Schulman, K. A., Berlin, J. A., Harless, W., Kerner, J. F., Sistrunk, S., Gersh, B. J., Dubé, R., Taleghani, C. K., Burke, J. E., William, S., Eisenberg, J. M., & Escarce, J. J. (1999). The effect of face and sex on physicians' recommendations for cardiac catheterization. *New England Journal of Medicine, 340,* 618–626.

Schwade, S. (1994, December). Hospitals with the human touch. *Prevention, 46,* 96–99.

Scott, M. K. (2008, September 11). Not-quite-so-thin is in for models at Fashion Week. *Associated Press.* Retrieved October 6, 2008, from http://ap.google.

com/article/ALeqM5iN3K5rOZKX2Oe-XcYhoqPZN5VimAD934LH9G0

Seeger, M. W. (2006, August). Best practices in crisis communication: An expert panel process. *Journal of Applied Communication Research, 34*(3), 232–244.

Senge, P. M. (2006). *The fifth discipline: The art and practice of the learning organization.* New York: Doubleday/Currency.

Sexual health of adolescents and young adults in the United States. (2008, September). Menlo Park: CA: Henry J. Kaiser Family Foundation. Retrieved October 1, 2008, from http://www.kff.org/womenshealth/upload/3040_04.pdf

Shannon, C. K. (2006, November/December). A gender-based study of attitudes and practice characteristics of rural physicians in West Virginia. *West Virginia Medical Journal, 102*(6), 22–25.

Shapiro, R. S., Tym, K. A., Eastwood, D., Derse, A. R., & Klein, J. P. (2003). Managed care, doctors, and patients: Focusing on relationships, not rights. *Cambridge Quarterly of Healthcare Ethics, 12*(3), 300–307.

Sharf, B. F. (1984). *The physician's guide to better communication.* Glenview, IL: Scott, Foresman.

Sharf, B. F., Haidet, P., & Kroll, T. L. (2005). "I want you to put me in the grave with all my limbs": The meaning of active health participation. In E. B. Ray (Ed.), *Health communication in practice: A case study approach* (pp. 39–51). Mahwah, NJ: Lawrence Erlbaum.

Shea, S., Basch, C. E., Wechsler, H., & Lantigua, R. (1996). The Washington Heights–Inwood Healthy Heart Program. A 6-year report from a disadvantaged urban setting. *American Journal of Public Health, 86,* 166–171.

Sheehan, K. H., Sheehan, D. V., White, K., Leibowitz, A., & Baldwin, D. C. (1990). A pilot study of medical student "abuse." *Journal of the American Medical Association, 263,* 533–537.

Shortell, S. M., Gillies, R. R., & Devers, K. J. (1995). Reinventing the American hospital. *Millbank Quarterly, 73,* 131–160.

Shurn, L. J. (Ed.). (2004). *The psychology of entertainment media: Blurring the lines between entertainment and persuasion.* Mahwah, NJ: Lawrence Erlbaum.

Signorielli, N. (1993). *Mass media images and impact on health.* Westport, CT: Greenwood Press.

Signorielli, N., & Staples, J. (1997). Television and children's conceptions of nutrition. *Health Communication, 9,* 289–302.

Silk, K. J., Bigbsy, E., Volkman, J., Kingsley, C., Atkin, C., Ferrara, M., & Goins, L.-A. (2006). Formative research on adolescent and adult perceptions of risk factors for breast cancer. *Social Science & Medicine, 63,* 3124–3136.

Silvester, J., Patterson, F., Koczwara, A., & Ferguson, E. (2007). "Trust me…": Psychological and behavioral predictors or perceived physician empathy. *Journal of Applied Psychology, 92*(2), 519–527.

Simon-Arndt, C. M., Hurtado, S. L., & Patriarca-Troyk, L. A. (2006). Acceptance of Web-based personalized feedback: User ratings of an alcohol misuse prevention program targeting U.S. Marines. *Health Communication, 21*(1), 13–22.

Singer, D. G., & Singer, J. L. (1998). Developing critical viewing skills and media literacy in children. *Annals of the American Academy of Political and Social Science, 557,* 164–179.

Singh, S. N., & Wachter, R. M. (2008). Perspectives on medical outsourcing and telemedicine—rough edges in a flat world? *New England Journal of Medicine, 358*(15), 1622.

Sismondo, S. (2008). How pharmaceutical industry funding affects trial outcomes: Causal structures and responses. *Social Science & Medicine, 66*(9), 1909–1914.

Sixth futures forum on crisis communication. (2004, May). Reykjavik, Iceland. World Health Organization. Retrieved September 25, 2008, from http://www.euro.who.int/document/E85056.pdf

Skluth, M. (2007, September 7). Get patients involved. *Medical Economics, 84*(17), 16.

Skolnick, A. (1990). Christian scientists claim healing efficacy equal if not superior to that of medicine. *Journal of the American Medical Association, 264,* 1379–1381.

Slack, P. (1991). Responses to plague in early modern Europe: The implications of public health.

In A. Mack (Ed.), *In time of plague: The history and social consequences of lethal epidemic disease* (pp. 111–132). New York: New York University Press.

Slater, M. D. (1995). Choosing audience segmentation strategies and methods for health communication In E. Maibach & R. L. Parrot (Eds.), *Designing health messages: Approaches from communication theory and public health practice* (pp. 186–198). Thousand Oaks, CA: Sage.

Slater, M. D. (2006). Specification and misspecification of theoretical foundations and logic models for health communication campaigns. *Health Communication, 20*(2), 149–158.

Slater, M. D., Rouner, D., Domenech-Rodriguez, M., Beauvais, F., Murphy, K., & Van Leuven, J. K. (1997). Adolescent responses to TV beer ads and sports content/context: Gender and ethnic differences. *Journalism & Mass Communication Quarterly, 74*, 108–122.

Slusarz, M. (1996). From fried rice to sushi: To market an integrated delivery system throw out the old menu. *Journal of Health Care Marketing, 16*, 12–15.

Smedley, B. D., Stith, A. Y., & Nelson, A. R. (2003). Unequal treatment: Confronting racial and ethnic disparities in health care. Board on Health Sciences Policy. Institute of Medicine. Retrieved December 3, 2008, from http://books.nap.edu/openbook.php?isbn=030908265X

Smith, D. H., & Pettegrew, L. S. (1986). Mutual persuasion as a model for doctor–patient communication. *Theoretical Medicine, 7*, 127–146.

Smith, K. C., & Wakefield, M. (2006). Newspaper coverage of youth and tobacco: Implications for public health. *Health Communication, 19*(1), 19–28.

Smith, M., Droppleman, P., & Thomas, S. P. (1996, January–March). Under assault: The experience of work-related anger in female registered nurses. *Nursing Forum, 31*, 22–33.

Smith, R. (2007, April/May). Media depictions of health topics: Challenge and stigma formats. *Journal of Health Communication, 12*(3), 233–249.

Smith, R. A., Downs, E., & Witte, K. (2007, June). Drama theory and entertainment education: Exploring the effects of a radio drama on behavioral intentions to limit HIV transmission in Ethiopia. *Communication Monographs, 74*(2), 133–153.

Smith, R. C., & Hoppe, R. B. (1991). The patient's story: Integrating the patient- and physician-centered approaches to interviewing. *Annals of Internal Medicine, 115*, 460–477.

Smith, S. L., Nathanson, A. I., & Wilson, B. J. (2002). Prime-time television: Assessing violence during the most popular viewing hours. *Journal of Communication, 52*(1), 84–111.

Smith, S. W., Kopfman, J. E., Lindsey, L. L. M., Yoo, J., & Morrison, K. (2004). Encouraging family discussion on the decision to donate organs: The role of the willingness to communicate scale. *Health Communication, 16*(3), 333–346.

Smith-du Pré, A., & Beck, C. S. (1996). Enabling patients and physicians to pursue multiple goals in health care encounters: A case study. *Health Communication, 8*, 73–90.

Snyder, L. B., & Rouse, R. A. (1995). The media can have more than an impersonal impact: The case of AIDS risk perceptions and behavior. *Health Communication, 7*, 125–145.

Somma, A. M. (2008, October 10). Organ donor worker arranges gift of life. *Hartford Courant*, online. Retrieved December 15, 2008, from http://www.courant.com/news/health/hc-transplant1210.artdec10,0,539459.story?page=1

Sood, S., Shefner-Rogers, C. L., & Sengupta, M. (2006). The impact of a mass media campaign on HIV/AIDS knowledge and behavior change in North India: Results from a longitudinal study. *Asian Journal of Communication, 16*(3), 231–250.

Sopory, P. (2005). Metaphor in formative evaluation and message design: An application to relationship and alcohol use. *Health Communication, 17*(2), 149–172.

Soule, K. P., & Roloff, M. E. (2000). Help between persons with and without disabilities from a resource theory perspective. In D. O. Braithwaite & T. L. Thompson (Eds.), *Handbook of communication and people with disabilities: Research and applications* (pp. 67–83). Mahwah, NJ: Lawrence Erlbaum.

South, D. (1997). All I really need to know about medicine I learned from my patients. *Patient Care, 31*, 238–240.

Sparks, L., O'Hair, H. D., & Kreps, G. L. (Eds.) (2008). *Cancer communication and aging.* Cresskill, NJ: Hampton Press.

Sparks, L., Villagran, M. M., Parker-Raley, J., & Cunningham, C. B. (2007). A patient-centered approach to breaking bad news: Communication guidelines for health care providers. *Journal of Applied Communication, 35*(2), 177–196.

Spear, S. (2003, April). Where there's hope, there's change. *Journal of Environmental Health, 65*(8), 26–28.

Spector, R. E. (1979). *Cultural diversity in health and illness.* New York: Appleton-Century-Crofts.

Spector, R., & McCarthy, P. (2005). *The Nordstrom way to costumer service excellence: A handbook for implementing great service in your organization.* Hoboken, NJ: John Wiley & Sons.

Stacy, A. W., Zogg, J. B., Unger, J. B., & Dent, C. W. (2004). Exposure to televised alcohol ads and subsequent alcohol use. *American Journal of Health Behavior, 28*(6), 498–509.

Stanos, S., & Houle, T. T. (2006). Multidisciplinary and interdisciplinary management of chronic pain. *Physical Medicine and Rehabilitation Clinics of North America, 17*(2), 435–450.

State scorecard data tables. (2007, June). Supplement to *Aiming Higher*: Results from a state scorecard on health system performance. New York: Commonwealth Fund. Retrieved August 12, 2008, from /www.commonwealthfund.org/usr_doc/State_data_tables.pdf?section=4039

States, R. A., Susman, W. M., Riquelme, L. F., Godwin, E. M., & Greer, E. (2006). Community health education: Reaching ethnically diverse elders. *Journal of Allied Health. 35*(4), 215–222.

Stephens, M. (2004, August 16). E(erectile) D(ysfunction) TV. *PopMatters*, online. Retrieved December 25, 2008, from http://www.alternet.org/mediaculture/19551/

Stephenson, M. T., Morgan, S. E., Roberts-Perez, S. D., Harrison, T., Afifi, W., & Long, S. D. (2008). The role of religiosity, religious norms, subjective norms, and bodily integrity in signing an organ donor card. *Health Communication, 23*(5), 436–447.

Stephenson, M. T., Quick, B. L., Atkinson, J., & Tschida, D. A. (2005). Authoritative parenting and drug-prevention practices: Implications for antidrug ads for parents. *Health Communication, 17*(3), 301–321.

Stevens, L. M., Lynm, C., & Glass, R. M. (2008). Organ donation. *Journal of the American Medical Association, 299*(2), 244.

Stewart, L. P., Lederman, L. C., Golubow, M., Cattafesta, J. L., Godhart, F. W., Powell, R. L., & Laitman, L. (2002, Winter). Applying communication theories to prevent dangerous drinking among college students: The RU SURE campaign. *Communication Studies, 53*(4), 381–399.

Stivers, T. (2002). Presenting the problem in pediatric encounters: "symptoms only" versus "candidate diagnosis" presentations. *Health Communication, 14*(3), 299–338.

Stratton, T. D., Saunders, J. A., & Elam, C. L. (2008). Changes in medical students' emotional intelligence: an exploratory study. *Teaching and Learning in Medicine, 20*(3), 279–284.

Street, R. L., Jr. (1990). Dentist–patient communication: A review and commentary. In D. O'Hair & G. L. Kreps (Eds.), *Applied communication theory and research* (pp. 331–351). Hillsdale, NJ: Lawrence Erlbaum.

Street, R. L., Jr. (1997). Health promotion and technology. (1997). In R. L. Street Jr., W. R. Gold, & T. Manning (Eds.), *Health promotion and interactive technology: Theoretical applications and future directions* (pp. 1–18). Mahwah, NJ: Lawrence Erlbaum.

Street, R. L., Jr., Gold. W. R., & Manning, T. (Eds.) (1997). *Health promotion and interactive technology: Theoretical applications and future directions* (pp. 221–236). Mahwah, NJ: Lawrence Erlbaum.

Street, R. L., Jr., Gordon, H. S., Ward, M. M., Krupat, E., & Kravitz, R. L. (2005). Patient participation in medical consultations: Why some patients are more involved than others. *Medical Care, 43*(10), 960–969.

Street, R. L., Jr., & Manning, T. (1997). Information environments in breast cancer education. In R. L. Street Jr., W. R. Gold, & T. Manning (Eds.), *Health promotion and interactive technology: Theoretical applications and future directions* (pp. 121–139). Mahwah, NJ: Lawrence Erlbaum.

Street, R. L., Jr., & Millay, B. (2001). Analyzing patient participation in medical encounters. *Health Communication, 13*(1), 61–73.

Street, R. L., Jr., & Rimal, R. N. (1997). Health promotion and interactive technology: A conceptual foundation. In R. L. Street Jr., W. R. Gold, & T. Manning (Eds.), *Health promotion and interactive technology: Theoretical applications and future directions* (pp. 1–18). Mahwah, NJ: Lawrence Erlbaum.

Stretcher, V. J., & Rosenstock, I. M. (1997). The health belief model. In K. Glanz, F. M. Lewis, & B. K. Rimer (Eds.), *Health behavior and health education* (pp. 41–59). San Francisco: Jossey-Bass.

Stroebe, M. S. (Ed.). (2001). *Handbook of bereavement research: Consequences, coping, and care.* Washington, DC: American Psychological Association.

Struggling in silence: Physician depression and suicide. (nd). Website. Retrieved November 8, 2008, from www.doctorswithdepression.org/

Studer, Q. (2002, September). Back to the basics: Making service excellence a priority. *AHA [American Hospital Association] Trustee Magazine, 55*(8), 7–10. Retrieved August 13, 2003, from www.hospitalconnect.com/DesktopServlet

Studer, Q. (2003). *Hardwiring excellence: Purpose, worthwhile work, making a difference.* Gulf Breeze, FL: Fire Starter.

Study finds television stations donate an average of 17 seconds an hour to public service advertising. (2008, January). Henry J. Kaiser Family Foundation. Retrieved October 1, 2008, from http://www.kff.org/entmedia/entmedia012408pkg.cfm

Substance Abuse & Mental Health Services Administration (SAMSHA). (2005, July/August). SAMSHA honors film, TV, radio portrayals of mental illness. Washington, DC: Author. Retrieved October 1, 2008, from http://www.samhsa.gov/SAMHSA_NEWS/VolumeXIII_4/article8.htm

Suchman, A. L., Markakis, K., Beckman, H. B., & Frankel, R. (1997). A model of empathic communication in the medical interview. *Journal of the American Medical Association, 277*, 678–683.

Sugai, W. J. (2008, June 20). Taking a hard line with compliant patients. Talk back. Letter to the editor. *Medical Economics, 85*(12), 14.

Sullivan, G. H., & Wolfe, S. (1996). When communication breaks down. *RN, 59*, 61–64.

Swain, K. A. (2007, Summer). Outrage factors and explanations in news coverage of the anthrax attacks. *Journalism and Mass Communication Quarterly, 84*(2), 335–352.

Swedish, J. (April 28, 2008). Our carpe diem moment; execs, clinicians must help policymakers find the way to universal coverage (Opinions Commentary). *Modern Healthcare, 38*(17), 22.

Swiderski, R. M. (1976). The idiom of diagnosis. *Communication Quarterly, 24*, 3–11.

Tai, Z., & Sun, T. (2007, December). Media dependencies in a changing media environment: The case of the 2003 SARS epidemic in China. *New Media & Society, 9*(6), 987–1009.

Tan, G., Jensen, M. P., Thornby, J. I., & Anderson, K. O. (2006). Are patient ratings of chronic pain services related to treatment outcome? *Journal of Rehabilitation Research and Development, 43*(4), 451–460.

Tanner, A. H. (2004a). Agenda building, source selection, and health news at local television stations. *Science Communication, 25*(4), 350–363.

Tanner, A. H. (2004b). Communicating health information and making the news: Health reporters reveal the PR tactics that work. *Public Relations Quarterly, 49*(1), 24–27.

Tardy, C. H. (1994). Counteracting task-induced stress: Studies of instrumental and emotional support in problem-solving contexts. In B. R. Burleson, T. L. Albrecht, & I. G. Sarason (Eds.), *Communication of social support: Messages,* interactions, relationships, and community (pp. 71–87). Thousand Oaks, CA: Sage.

Tarrant, C., Windridge, K., Boulton, J., Baker, R., & Freeman, G. (2003, June 14). How important is personal care in general practice? *British Medical Journal (Clinical Research Edition)*, *326*, 1310.

Taubes, G. (1998). Telling time by the second hand. *Technology Review*, *101*, 76–78.

Taylor, D. (1999). *The writer's guide to everyday life in Colonial America: From 1607 to 1783*. Cincinnati, OH: Writer's Digest Books.

Taylor, S. E., Falke, R. L., Mazel, R. M., & Hilsberg, B. L. (1988). Sources of satisfaction and dissatisfaction among members of cancer support groups. In B. H. Gottlieb (Ed.), *Marshaling social support: Formats, processes, and effects* (pp. 187–208). Newbury Park, CA: Sage.

Television, alcohol ads, and youth, 2001 to 2005. (2006). The Center of Alcohol Marketing and Youth. Retrieved October 6, 2008, from http://camy.org/factsheets/index.php?FactsheetID=23

Teno, J. M., Clarridge, B. R., Casey, V., Welch, L. C., Wetle, T., Shield, R., & Mor, V. (2004). Family perspectives on end-of-life care at the last place of care. *Journal of the American Medical Association*, *291*(1), 88–93.

Terrell, G. E. (2007, September/October). "Can't get no (physician) satisfaction?" *Physician Executive*, pp. 12–15.

Terry, K. (2007, August 3). Doctors are now getting more tech savvy: While EHRs remain uncommon, physicians are taking advantage of many new devices and media, our survey shows. *Medical Economics*, *84*(15), 52–55.

Thomas, E. J., Sexton, J. B., & Helmreich, R. L. (2003). Discrepant attitudes about teamwork among critical care nurses and physicians. *Critical Care Medicine*, *31*(3), 956–959.

Thomas, S. B., Quinn, S. C., Billingsley, A., & Caldwell, C. (1994). *American Journal of Public Health*, *84*, 575–579.

Thompson, C. B. (1996, October). Research to support holistic nursing taxonomies. *Holistic Nursing Practice*, *11*, 31–38.

Thompson, T. L. (1984). The invisible helping hand: The role of communication in the health and social service professions. *Communication Quarterly*, *32*, 148–161.

Thompson, T. L. (1990). Patient health care: Issues in interpersonal communication in the health and social service professions. In E. B. Ray & L. Donohew (Eds.), *Communication and health: Systems and applications* (pp. 27–50). Hillsdale, NJ: Lawrence Erlbaum.

Thompson, T. L. (2006). Seventy-five (count 'em—75) issues of *Health Communication*: An analysis of emerging themes. *Health Communication*, *20*(2), 117–122.

Thompson, T. L., Dorsey, A. M., Miller, K. I., & Parrott, R. (Eds.) (2003). *The handbook of health communication*. Mahwah, NJ: Lawrence Erlbaum.

Thompson, T. L., & Gillotti, C. (2005). Staying out of the line of fire: A medical student learns about bad news delivery. In E. B. Ray (Ed.), *Health communication in practice: A case study approach* (pp. 11–25). Mahwah, NJ: Lawrence Erlbaum.

Thompson, T. L., Robinson, J. D., Anderson, D. J., & Federowicz, M. (2008). Health communication: Where have we been and where can we go? (2008). In K. B. Wright & S. D. Moore (Eds.), *Applied health communication* (pp. 3–33). Cresskill, NJ: Hampton Press.

Thoreau, E. (2006). Ouch!: An examination of the self-representation of disabled people on the Internet. *Journal of Computer-Mediated Communication*, *11*, 442–468.

Thorpe, K., & Loo, P. (2003). Balancing professional and personal satisfaction of nurse managers: Current and future perspectives in a changing health care system. *Journal of Nurse Management*, *11*(5), 321–330.

Thorwald, J. (1962). *Science and secrets of early medicine* (translated by R. Winston & C. Winston). New York: Harcourt, Brace & World.

Threat of bioterrorism: A frustrating and persistent security risk. (2008, August 7). *Government Security*, Online Exclusive, np. Retrieved August 29, 2008, from General OneFile via Gale.

Tichenor, P. J., Donohue, G. A., & Olien, C. N. (1970). Mass media flow and differential growth in knowledge. *Public Opinion Quarterly, 34,* 159–170.

Tieman, J. (2002, January 14). Exec pay gap grows between the sexes. *Modern Healthcare, 32,* 12.

Todd, A. D. (1984). The prescription of contraception: Negotiations between doctors and patients. *Discourse Processes, 7,* 171–200.

Todd, A. D. (1989). *Intimate adversaries: Cultural conflict between doctors and women patients.* Philadelphia: University of Philadelphia Press.

Tourangeau, A. E., & Cranley, L. A. (2005). Nurse intention to remain employed: Understanding and strengthening determinants. *Journal of Advanced Nursing, 55*(4), 497–509.

Tovey, P., & Broom, A. (2007). Oncologists' and specialist cancer nurses' approaches to complementary and alternative medicine and their impact on patient action. *Social Science & Medicine, 64,* 2550–2564.

Transue, E. R. (2004). *On call: A doctor's days and nights in residency.* New York: St. Martin's Griffin.

Trick or treat? Tobacco industry prevention ads don't help curb youth smoking and should be taken off the air, says the American Legacy Foundation®; New study proves tobacco ads claiming prevention may actually have opposite effect. (2006, October 31). *PR Newswire US,* online. Retrieved December 9, 2008, through LexisNexis Academic.

Troth, A., & Peterson, C. C. (2000). Factors predicting safe-sex talk and condom use in early sexual relationships. *Health Communication, 12*(2), 195–218.

Tse, H. (1999). Test your Asian IQ. *Asian-Nation: The landscape of Asian America.* Retrieved December 23, 2008, from http://www.asian-nation.org/asian-iq-quiz.shtml

Tu, H. T. (2005, June). Medicare seniors much less willing to limit physician-hospital choice for lower costs. Center for Studying Health System Change, Issue Brief No. 96, np. Retrieved July 23, 2008, from www.hschange.org/CONTENT/744

Tucker, C. M., Herman, K. C., Pedersen, T. R., Higley, B., Montrichard, M., & Ivery, P. (2003). Cultural sensitivity in physician–patient relationships: Perspectives of an ethnically diverse sample of low-income primary care patients. *Medical Care, 41*(7), 859–870.

Tuffrey-Wijne, I., Hollins, S., & Curfs, L. (2005). Supporting patients who have intellectual disabilities: A survey investigating staff training needs. *International Journal of Palliative Nursing, 11*(4), 182–188.

TV program description. (2004). *The most dangerous woman in America* [video documentary], Nancy Porter (Writer/Director). NOVA in association with WGBH/Boston. Retrieved August 27, 2008, from http://www.pbs.org/wgbh/nova/typhoid/about.html

Twaddle, A. C., & Hessler, R. M. (1987). *A sociology of health* (2nd ed.). New York: Macmillan.

Uba, L. (1992). Cultural barriers to health care for Southeast Asian refugees. *Public Health Reports, 107,* 544–548.

Ulmer, R. R., Seeger, M. W., & Sellnow, T. L. (2007, June). Post-crisis communication and renewal: Expanding the parameters of post-crisis discourse. *Public Relations Review, 33*(2), 130–134.

Ulrich, C. M., Soeken, K. L., & Miller, N. (2003). Ethical conflict associated with managed care: Views of nurse practitioners. *Nursing Research, 52*(3), 168–175.

The ultimate family tree. (2005, May). *National Geographic, 207*(5), np.

UNAIDS: Joint United Nations Programme on HIV/AIDS. (2008, August). Global facts and figures. Retrieved September 1, 2008, from http://data.unaids.org:80/pub/GlobalReport/2008/20080715_fs_global_en.pdf

UNESCO (United Nations Educational, Scientific, and Cultural Organization) Institute for Statistics. (2008). According to the most recent UIS data, there are an estimated 774 million illiterate adults in the world, about 64% of whom are women. Montreal: Author. Retrieved December 6, 2008, from http://www.uis.unesco.org/ev.php?URL_ID=6401&URL_DO=DO_TOPIC&URL_SECTION=201

U.S. Bureau of Labor Statistics. (2003). BLS career information: Nurse. Retrieved August 11, 2003, from www.bls.gov/k12/sci_004t.htm#Jobs

U.S. Bureau of Labor Statistics. (2007a, December 18). Occupational outlook handbook, 2008–2009 edition. Chiropractors. Washington, DC: Author. Retrieved October 23, 2008, from http://www.bls.gov/oco/ocos071.htm

U.S. Bureau of Labor Statistics. (2007b, December 18). Occupational outlook handbook, 2008–2009 edition. Registered nurses. Washington, DC: Author. Retrieved October 23, 2008, from http://www.bls.gov/oco/ocos083.htm

U.S. Bureau of Labor Statistics. (2008, March 12). Career guide to industries. Health care. Retrieved December 29, 2008, from http://www.bls.gov/oco/cg/cgs035.htm

U.S. Census Bureau. (2004). Social assistance: 2002. Washington DC: Author. Retrieved December 14, 2008, from http://www.census.gov/prod/ec02/ec0262i04.pdf

U.S. Census Bureau. (2007). Income, poverty, and health insurance coverage in the United States: 2006. Retrieved July 18, 2008, from www.census.gov/prod/2007pubs/p60-233.pdf

U.S. Census Bureau News. (2008, August 14). An older and more diverse nation by midcentury. Washington, DC: Author. Retrieved October 23, 2008, from http://www.census.gov/Press-Release/www/releases/archives/population/012496.html

U.S. Department of Health and Human Services (DHHS). (2002). Projected supply, demand, and shortages of registered nurses. Health Resources and Services Administration, Bureau of Health Profession, National Center for Health Workforce Analysis.

U.S. Department of Health and Human Services (DHHS). (2005). Overview of the uninsured in the United States: An analysis of the 2005 current population. The uninsured by age. Retrieved July 31, 2008, from http://aspe.hhs.gov/health/reports/05/uninsured-cps/index.htm

U.S. Department of Health and Human Services, Health Resources and Services Administration. (2006). The registered nurse population: Findings from the 2004 national sample survey of registered nurses. Washington, DC: Author. Retrieved October 23, 2008, from http://bhpr.hrsa.gov/healthworkforce/rnsurvey04/2.htm

U.S. Department of Health and Human Services, Office of the Surgeon General. (2007). The surgeon general's call to action to prevent and reduce underage drinking. Washington, DC: U.S. Department of Health and Human Services. Retrieved October 3, 2008, from http://www.surgeongeneral.gov/topics/underagedrinking/calltoaction.pdf

U.S. Department of Labor. (2007, December 18). Occupational outlook handbook, 2008–09 edition. Medical and health services managers. Washington, DC: Author. Retrieved October 16, 2008, from http://www.bls.gov/oco/ocos014.htm#nature

U.S. Food and Drug Administration (FDA). (2001, March 8). Summary of reports of death in Viagra users received form marketing (late March) through mid-November 1998. Washington, DC: Author. Retrieved December 22, 2008, from http://www.fda.gov/cder/consumerinfo/viagra/safety3.htm

U.S. Food and Drug Administration. (2007, October 18). Questions and answers about Viagra, Levitra, Cialis, and Revatio: Possible sudden hearing loss. Washington, DC: Author. Retrieved December 22, 2008, from http://www.fda.gov/cder/drug/infopage/ed_drugs/QA.htm

Unsworth, C. (1996). Team decision-making in rehabilitation. *American Journal of Physical Medicine & Rehabilitation, 75,* 483–486.

Urba, S. (1998). Sometimes the best thing I do is listen. *Medical Economics, 75*(9), 167–170.

Valente, T. W., Paredes, P., & Poppe, P. R. (1998). Matching the message to the process: The relative ordering of knowledge, attitudes, and practices in behavior change research. *Human Communication Research, 24,* 366–385.

Vanden Heuvel, L., & Robinson, C. (2005, Summer). How many causes should you pursue? *Journal for Quality and Participation, 28*(2), 22–23.

Vanderford, M. L., Jenks, E. B., & Sharf, B. F. (1997). Exploring patients' experiences as a primary source of meaning. *Health Communication, 9,* 13–26.

van der Pal-de Bruin, K. M., de Walle, H. E., de Rover, C. M., Jenninga, W., Cornel, M. C., de Jong-van den Berg, L. T., Buitendijk, S. E., & Paulussen, T. G. (2003). Influence of educational level on determinants of folic acid use. *Pediatric and Perinatal Epidemiology, 17*(3), 256–263.

van Zanten, M., Boulet, J. R., & McKinley, D. (2007). Using standardized patients to assess the interpersonal skills of physicians: Six years' experience with a high-stakes certification examination. *Health Communication, 22(3)*, 195–205.

Vardeman, J. E., & Aldoory, L. (2008). A qualitative study of how women make meaning of contradictory media messages about the risks of eating fish. *Health Communication, 23*(3), 282–291.

Veatch, R. M. (1983). The physician as stranger: The ethics of the anonymous patient–physician relationship. In E. E Shelp (Ed.), *The clinical encounter: The moral fabric of the patient–physician relationship* (pp. 187–207). Dordrecht, The Netherlands: D. Reidel.

Veatch, R. M. (1991). *The patient–physician relation: The patient as partner, Part 2.* Bloomington, IN: Indiana University Press.

Vernon, J. A., Trujillo, A., Rosenbaum, S., & DeBuono, B. (2007). Low health literacy: Implications of national health policy. Retrieved December 6, 2008, from http://www.gwumc.edu/sphhs/departments/healthpolicy/chsrp/downloads/LowHealthLiteracyReport10_4_07.pdf

Vesely, R. (2008, June 16). Say what?: Looming mandate in California puts the onus on health insurers to provide their members with language-assistance services. *Modern Healthcare*, 48.

Vest, J. (1997, July 21). Joe Camel walks his last mile. *U.S. News & World Report, 123*, 56.

Vestal, K. W., Fralicx, R. D., & Spreier, S. W. (1997). Organizational culture: The critical link between strategy and results. *Hospital & Health Services Administration, 42*, 339–365.

Viswanath, K., Kahn, E., Finnegan, J. R., Hertog, J., & Potter, J. D. (1993). Motivation and the knowledge gap: Effects of a campaign to reduce diet-related cancer risk. *Communication Research, 20*, 546–563.

Viva Viagra. (2008). TV spots. Pfizer. Retrieved December 24, 2008, from http://www.viagra.com/content/viva-viagra-music.jsp?setShowOn=../content/viva-viagra.jsp&setShowHighlightOn=../content/viva-viagra-music.jsp

Volpintesta, E. J., & Kanterman, L. H. (2008, March 21). Hospitalists: Pro and con. Letter to the editor. *Medical Economics, 85*(6), 10.

Waalen, J. (1997). Women in medicine: Bringing gender issues to the fore. *Journal of the American Medical Association, 277*, 1404–1405.

Wahl, O. F., & Lefkowits, J. Y. (1989). Impact of a television film on attitude toward mental illness. *American Journal of Community Psychology, 17*, 521–528.

Waitzkin, H. (1991). *The politics of medical encounters: How patients and doctors deal with social problems.* New Haven, CT: Yale University Press.

Wakefield, M., Terry-McElrath, Y., Emery, S., Saffer, H., Chaloupka, F. J., Szczypka, G., Flay, B., O'Malley, P. M., & Johnston, L. D. (2006). Effect of televised, tobacco-company-funded smoking prevention advertising on youth smoking-related beliefs, intentions, and behavior. *American Journal of Public Health, 96*(2), 2154–2160.

Walker, K. L., Arnold, C. L., Miller-Day, M., & Webb, L. M. (2002). Investigating the physician–patient relationship: Examining emerging themes. *Health Communication, 14*(1), 45–68.

Waller, L. A., Carlin, B. P., Xia, H., & Gelfand, A. E. (1997, June). Hierarchical spatio-temporal mapping of disease rates. *Journal of the American Statistical Association, 92*(438), 607–617.

Walsh-Burke, K., & Marcusen, C. (1999). Self-advocacy training for cancer survivors. The Cancer Survival Toolbox. *Cancer Practice, 7*(6), 297–301.

Walt, D. (1997, March 17). Standing up for ethics. *American Medical News, 40*, 12–15.

Walters, T. N., Walters, L. M. Kern-Foxworth, M., & Priest, S. H. (1997). The picture of health? Message standardization and recall of televised AIDS public service announcements. *Public Relations Review, 23*, 143–159.

Wang, X., & Arpan, L. M. (2008, January/March). Effects of race and ethnic identity on audience evaluation of HIV public service announcements. *Howard Journal of Communications*, 19(1), 44–63.

Wanzer, M. B., Booth-Butterfield, M., & Gruber, K. (2004). Perceptions of health care providers' communication: Relationships between patient-centered communication and satisfaction. *Health Communication*, 16(3), 363–384.

Warner, K. E. (1987). Television and health education: Stay tuned. *American Journal of Public Health*, 77, 140–142.

Wartella, E. A. (1996). The context of television violence. Paper presented at the annual meeting of the Speech Communication Association in San Antonio.

Wartik, N. (1996). Learning to mourn. *American Health*, 15, 76–81.

Waseem, M., & Ryan, M. (2005). "Doctor" or "doctora": Do patients really care? *Pediatric Emergency Care*, 21(8), 515–517.

Watzlawick, P., Beavin, J. H., & Jackson, D. D. (1967). *Pragmatics of human communication*. New York: W. W. Norton.

Waymer, D., & Heath, R. L. (2007, February). Emergent agents: The forgotten publics in crisis communication and issues management research. *Journal of Applied Communication Research*, 35(1), 88–108.

Weaver, R. R. (2003). Informatics tools and medical communication: Patient perspectives of "knowledge coupling" in primary care. *Health Communication*, 15(1), 59–78.

Webb, T., Jenkins, L., Browne, N., Abdelmonen, A. A., & Kraus, J. (2007). Violent entertainment pitched to adolescents: An analysis of PG-13 films. *Pediatrics*, 119(6), e1219–e1229.

Weber, M. (1946). *From Max Weber: Essays in sociology*. New York: Oxford University Press.

Wechsler, H., Nelson, T. F., Lee, J. E., Seibring, M., Lewis, C., & Keeling, R. P. (2003, July). Perception and reality: A national evaluation of social norms marketing interventions to reduce college students' heavy alcohol use. *Journal of Studies on Alcohol*, 64(4), 484–494.

Wechsler, H., & Wernick, S. M. (1992). A social marketing campaign to promote low-fat milk consumption in an inner-city Latino community. *Public Health Reports*, 107, 202–207.

Weech-Maldonado, R., Morales, L. S., Elliott, M., Spritzer, K., Marshall, G., & Hays, R. D. (2003). Race/ethnicity, language, and patients' assessments of care in Medicaid managed care. *Health Services Research*, 38(3), 789–808.

Weinrich, S., Vijayakumar, S., Powell, I. J., Priest, J., Hamner, C. A., McCloud, L., & Pettaway, C. (2007). Knowledge of hereditary prostate cancer among high-risk African American men. *Oncology Nursing Forum*, 34(4), 854–60.

Weiss, G. G. (2008, June 20). The new doctor–patient paradigm: How the shift from the "physician as wise parent" model to one of more shared responsibility is playing out in the exam room. *Medical Economics*, 85(12), 48–52.

Welch, G., Rose, G., & Ernst, D. (2006). Motivational interviewing and diabetes: What is used, and does it work? *Diabetes Spectrum*, 19(1), 5–11.

Weston, W. W., & Lipkin, M., Jr. (1989). Doctors learning communication skills: Developmental issues. In M. Stewart & D. Roter (Eds.), *Communicating with medical patients. Vol. 9. Interpersonal communication* (pp. 43–57). Newbury Park, CA: Sage.

Whaley, B. B. (1999). Explaining illness to children: Advancing theory and research by determining message content. *Health Communication*, 11, 185–193.

Whaley, B. B. (2000). Explaining illness to children: Theory, strategies, and future inquiry. In B. B. Whaley (Ed.), *Explaining Illness* (pp. 195–207). Mahwah, NJ: Lawrence Erlbaum.

Whaley, B. B., & Edgar, T. (2008). Explaining illness to children. In K. B. Wright & S. D. Moore (Eds.), *Applied health communication* (pp. 145–158). Cresskill, NJ: Hampton Press.

What her friends did when she was dying. (1997, March). *Redbook*, 188, 73–78.

*What's right in health care: 365 stories of purpose, worthwhile work, and making a difference.* (2007). Compiled by Studer Group. Gulf Breeze, FL: Fire Starter.

White, A. D. (1925). *A history of the warfare of science with theology in Christendom* (vol. 2). New York: D. Appleton. (originally published in 1896)

Whitla, D. K. Orfield, G., Silen, W., Teperow, C., Howard, C., & Reede, J. (2003). Educational benefits of diversity in medical school: A survey of students. *Academic Medicine, 78*(5), 460–466.

Whitt, N., Harvey, R., McLeod, G., & Child, S. (2007). How many health professionals does a patient see during an average hospital stay? *New Zealand Medical Journal, 120*(1253), U2517.

Whitten, P., Sypher, B. D., & Patterson, J. D., III. (2000). Transcending the technology of telemedicine: An analysis of telemedicine in North Carolina. *Health Communication, 12*(2), 109–135.

Wicks, R. J. (2008). *The resilient clinician.* Oxford: Oxford University Press.

Wikler, D. (1987). Who should be blamed for being sick? *Health Education Quarterly, 14,* 11–25.

Wilkinson, S., Perry, R., Blanchard, K., & Linsell, L. (2008). Effectiveness of a three-day communication skills course in changing nurses' communication skills with cancer/palliative care patients: A randomized controlled trial. *Palliative Medicine, 22*(4), 365–375.

Willems, S. J., Swinnen, W., & De Maeseneer, J. M. (2005). The GP's perception of poverty: A qualitative study. *Family Practice, 22*(2), 177–183.

Williams, A., & Nussbaum, J. F. (2001). *Intergenerational communication across the life span.* Mahwah, NJ: Lawrence Erlbaum.

Williams, C. (2003, June 30). Retailers find profits in catering to teens. *Post and Courier,* p. 16E.

Williams, J. E., & Flora, J. A. (1995). Health behavior segmentation and campaign planning to reduce cardiovascular disease risk among Hispanics. *Health Education Quarterly, 22,* 33–48.

Williams, M. V., Parker, R. M., Baker, D. W., Parikh, N. S., Pitkin, K., Coates, W. C., & Nurss, J. R. (1995). Inadequate functional health literacy among patients at two public hospitals. *Journal of the American Medical Association, 274,* 1677–1672.

Willies-Jacobo, L. (2007, August). Susto: Acknowledging patient's beliefs about illness. *Virtual Mentor, 9*(8), 532–536.

Willing, R. (1999, April 14). Kevorkian sentenced to 10–25 years. *USA Today,* p. 1A.

Wills, T. A. (1985). Supportive functions of interpersonal relationships. In S. Cohen & S. L. Syme (Eds.), *Social support and health* (pp. 61–82). Orlando, FL: Academic Press.

Willwerth, J. (1993, February 15). It hurts like crazy. *Time, 141,* 53.

Wilson, K. (2003). Therapeutic landscapes and the First Nations people: An exploration of culture, health and place. *Health & Place, 9*(2), 83–93.

Wiltshire, J., Cronin, K., Sarto, G. E., & Brown, R. (2006). Self-advocacy during the medical encounter: Use of health information and racial/ethnic differences. *Medical Care, 44*(2), 100–109.

Wimmer, R. D., & Dominick, J. R. (1997). *Mass communication research* (5th ed.). Belmont, CA: Wadsworth.

Winslow, C.-E. A. (1923). *The evolution and significance of the modern public health campaign.* New Haven, CT: Yale University Press.

Witte, K. (1997). Preventing teen pregnancy through persuasive communications: Realities, myths, and hard-fact truths. *Journal of Community Health, 22,* 137–154.

Witte, K. (2008). Putting the fear back into fear appeals: The extended parallel process model. In L. C. Lederman (Ed.), *Beyond these walls: Readings in health communication* (pp. 273–291). New York: Oxford University Press.

Wolf, M. S., Williams, M. V., Parker, R. M., Parikh, N. S., Nowlan, A. W., & Baker, D. W. (2007). Patients' shame and attitudes toward discussing the results of literacy screening. *Journal of Health Communication, 12*(8), 721–732.

Women most active online audience for health information. (2003). *Datamonitor, M2Presswire.* Retrieved August 1, 2003, through LexisNexis.

Wood, J. (1999). *Gendered lives* (3rd ed.). Belmont, CA: Wadsworth.

Woodbury, B. (2007, August 29). Health savings accounts and high-deductible health plans. The Bell Policy Center, Denver. Retrieved July 28, 2008, from www.thebell.org/PUBS/IssBrf/2007/08-HSAs.php

World-class health care, step by step: Extracts from Health Minister Khaw Boon Wan's replies to MPs on a range of issues, including elderly care and longevity. (2008, March 4). *Straits Times* (Singapore), np. Retrieved July 21, 2008 through LexisNexis Academic Universe.

World Health Organization (WHO). (1948). Preamble to the Constitution of the World Health Organization. Official records of the World Health Organization, no. 2, p. 100. Retrieved September 7, 2003, from www.who.int/about/definition/en

World Health Organization (WHO). (2003). Update 83—one hundred days into the outbreak. Retrieved July 19, 2003, from www.whoi.int/csr/don/2003_16_18/en

World Health Organization. (2003, March 16). Epidemic and pandemic alert and response (EPR). Severe acute respiratory syndrome (SARS). Multi-country Outbreak. Update. Geneva, Switzerland: Author. Retrieved September 1, 2008, from http://www.who.int/csr/don/2003_03_16/en/index.html

World Health Organization. (2003, June 18). Epidemic and pandemic alert and response (EPR). Update 83. One hundred days into the outbreak. Geneva, Switzerland: Author. Retrieved September 1, 2008, from http://www.who.int/csr/don/2003_06_18/en/index.html

World Health Organization. (2007a). Fact sheet. The top ten causes of death. Geneva, Switzerland: Author. Retrieved September 16, 2008, from http://www.who.int/mediacentre/factsheets/fs310.pdf

World Health Organization. (2007b). Why is smoking an issue for non-smokers? Geneva, Switzerland: Author. Retrieved September 12, 2008, from http://www.who.int/features/qa/60/en/index.html

World Health Organization. (2007c). World No Tobacco Day, 2007. Geneva, Switzerland: Author. Retrieved September 12, 2008, from http://www.who.int/tobacco/communications/events/wntd/2007/en/index.html

World Health Organization. (2007d, October). Interim protocol: Rapid operations to contain the initial emergence of pandemic influenza. Geneva, Switzerland: Author. Retrieved September 2, 2008, from http://www.who.int/csr/disease/avian_influenza/guidelines/RapidContProtOct15.pdf

World Health Organization. (2007e, October). Options for the use of human H5N1 influenza vaccines and the WHO H5N1 vaccine stockpile. Geneva, Switzerland: Author. Retrieved September 2, 2008, from http://www.who.int/csr/resources/publications/WHO_HSE_EPR_GIP_2008_1d.pdf

World Health Organization. (2008a). WHO report on the global tobacco epidemic. The global tobacco crisis. Tobacco: Global agent of death. Geneva, Switzerland: Author. Retrieved September 16, 2008, from http://www.who.int/tobacco/mpower/mpower_report_tobacco_crisis_2008.pdf

World Health Organization (WHO). (2008b). World health statistics. Part 2. Global health indicators. Global health indicators. Geneva, Switzerland: Author. Retrieved August 16, 2008, from www.who.int/whosis/whostat/EN_WHS08_Table4_HSR.pdf

World Health Organization Statistical Information System (WHOSIS). (2008). Life expectancy. Geneva, Switzerland: Author. Retrieved December 23, 2008, from http://www.who.int/whosis/data/Search.jsp?countries=[Location].Members

World Health Organization (WHO) wants total ban on tobacco advertising. (2008, May 30). Geneva, Switzerland: Author. Retrieved September 26, 2008, from http://www.who.int/mediacentre/news/releases/2008/pr17/en/index.html

World Health Report, 2000. Health systems: improving performance (2000). Geneva, Switzerland: World Health Organization. Retrieved August 19, 2008, from http://www.who.int/whr/2000/en/

World Health Report, 2007. (2007). A safer future: Global public health security in the 21st century. Geneva, Switzerland: World Health Organization. Retrieved August 23, 2008, from http://www.who.int/whr/2007/en/index.html

World Organisation for Animal Health (OIE). (2008, September 1). Annual incidence rate of bovine spongiform encephalopathy (BSE) in OIE member countries that have reported cases, excluding the United Kingdom. Paris, France: Author. Retrieved September 1, 2008, from http://www.oie.int/eng/info/en_esbincidence.htm

Wright, A. L., Schwindt, L. A., Bassford, T. L., Reyna, V. F., Shisslak, M. M., St. Germain, P. A., & Reed, K. L. (2003). Gender differences in academic advancement: Patterns, causes, and potential solutions in one U.S. College of Medicine. *Academic Medicine, 78*(5), 500–508.

Wright, K. (2002). Social support within an on-line cancer community: An assessment of emotional support, perceptions of advantages and disadvantages, and motives for using the community from a communication perspective. *Journal of Applied Communication Research, 31*(3), 195–209.

Wright, K. B. (2008). New technologies and health communication. In K. B. Wright & S. D. Moore (Eds.), *Applied health communication* (pp. 63–84). Cresskill, NJ: Hampton Press.

Wright, K. B., Frey, L., & Sopory, P. (2007, March). Willingness to communicate about health as an underlying trait of patient self-advocacy: The development of the willingness to communicate about health (WTCH) measure. *Communication Studies, 58*(1), 35–49.

www.thepleasureproject.org. (2004). Oxford: Pleasure Project.

Wyatt, J. C. (1995). Hospital information management: The need for clinical leadership. *British Medical Journal, 311*, 175–178.

Wynia, M. K., VanGeest, J. B., Cummins, D. S., & Wilson, I. B. (2003). Do physicians not offer useful services because of coverage restrictions? *Health Affairs, 22*(4), 190–197.

Yamada, T. (2008, March 27). In search of new ideas for global health. *New England Journal of Medicine, 358*(13), 1324–1325.

Yamba, C. B. (1997). Cosmologists in turmoil: Witchfinding and AIDS in Chiawa, Zambia. *Africa, 22*(4), 190–197.

Yanovitzky, I. (2006, April/May). Sensation seeking and alcohol use by college students: Examining multiple pathways of effects. *Journal of Health Communication, 11*(3), 269–280.

Yanovitzky, I., Stewart, L. P., & Lederman, L. C. (2006). Social distance, perceived drinking by peers, and alcohol use by college students. *Health Communication, 19*(1), 1–10.

Yanovitzky, I., & Stryker, J. (2001, April 2). Mass media, social norms, and health promotion efforts: A longitudinal study of media effects on youth binge drinking. *Communication Research, 28*(2), 208–239.

Yee, A. M., Puntillo, K., Miaskowski, C., & Neighbor, M. L. (2006). What patients with abdominal pain expect about pain relief in the emergency department. *Journal of Emergency Nursing, 32*(4), 281–287.

Young, A. (2004). *What patients taught me: A medical student's journey.* Seattle: Sasquatch Books.

Young, A., & Flower, L. (2002). Patients as partners, patients as problem-solvers. *Health Communication, 14*(1), 69–97.

Young, A. J., & Rodriguez, K. L. (2006). The role of narrative in discussing end-of-life care: Eliciting values and goals from text, context, and subtext. *Health Communication, 19*(1), 49–59.

Youth exposure to alcohol advertising on television, 2001–2007. Executive summary. (2008, June 23). The Center of Alcohol Marketing and Youth. Retrieved October 3, 2008, from http://camy.org/research/tv0608/

Zakrzewski, P. A., Ho, A. L., & Braga-Mele, R. (2008). Should ophthalmologists receive communication skills training in breaking bad news?

*Canadian Journal of Ophthalmology, 43*(4), 419–424.

Zillmann, D., & Vorderer, P. (Eds.) (2000). *Media entertainment: The psychology of its appeal.* Mahwah, NJ: Lawrence Erlbaum.

Zimmerman, F. J. (2008, June). Children's media use and sleep problems: Issues and unanswered questions. Prepaid for the Henry J. Kaiser Family Foundation. Retrieved October 1, 2008, from http://www.kff.org/entmedia/upload/7674.pdf

Zimmermann, S. (1994). Social cognition and evaluations of health care team communication effectiveness. *Western Journal of Communication, 58,* 116–141.

Zimmermann, S., & Applegate, J. L. (1994). Communicating social support in organizations: A message-centered approach. In B. R. Burleson, T. L. Albrecht, & I. G. Sarason (Eds.), *Communication of social support: Messages, interactions, relationships, and community* (pp. 50–70). Thousand Oaks, CA: Sage.

Zipperer, R. (1997, February). Bias and beauty tips? *Consumers' Research Magazine, 80,* 35.

Zook, E. (1993). Diagnosis HIV/AIDS: Caregiver communication in the crisis of terminal illness. In E. B. Ray (Ed.), *Case studies in health communication* (pp. 113–128). Hillsdale, NJ: Lawrence Erlbaum.

Zook, R. (1997, April). Handling in appropriate sexual behavior with confidence: Here are nine tips for keeping the boundaries clear. *Nursing, 27,* 65.

Zorn, T. E., & Gregory, K. W. (2005). Learning the ropes together: Assimilation and friendship development among first-year male medical students. *Health Communication, 17*(3), 211–231.

Zoucha, R., & Broome, B. (2008, April). The significance of culture in nursing: Examples from the Mexican-American culture and knowing the unknown. *Urologic Nursing, 28*(2), 140–142.

Zuckerman, M. (1994). *Behavioral expressions and biosocial bases of sensation seeking.* Cambridge: Cambridge University Press.

# AUTHOR INDEX